Pharmacy Technician

Practice and Procedures

Gail Orum-Alexander, Pharm. D.

Charles Drew University of Medicine and Science
Dean, College of Science and Health
Los Angeles, California

James J. Mizner, Jr., BS, MBA, RPh

ACT College
Pharmacy Technician Program Director
Arlington, VA

Mc Graw Hill
Connect
Learn
Succeed™

The McGraw·Hill Companies

Connect Learn Succeed™

PHARMACY TECHNICIAN: PRACTICE AND PROCEDURES

Some ancillaries, including electronic and print components, may not be available to customers outside the United States.

This book is printed on acid-free paper.

1 2 3 4 5 6 7 8 9 0 WDQ/WDQ 1 0 9 8 7 6 5 4 3 2 1 0

ISBN 978-0-07-352072-8
MHID 0-07-352072-1

Vice president/Editor in chief: *Elizabeth Haefele*
Vice president/Director of marketing: *John E. Biernat*
Publisher: *Kenneth S. Kasee Jr.*
Senior sponsoring editor: *Debbie Fitzgerald*
Senior Developmental Editor, Allied Health: *Patricia Hesse*
Editorial coordinator: *Parissa DJangi*
Marketing manager: *Mary B. Haran*
Lead digital product manager: *Damian Moshak*
Media development editor: *Marc Mattson*
Director, Editing/Design/Production: *Jess Ann Kosic*
Project manager: *Jean R. Starr*
Manager, Media production: *Janean A. Utley*
Senior designer: *Marianna Kinigakis*
Senior photo research coordinator: *John C. Leland*
Photo researcher: *Danny Meldung, Photo Affairs, Inc.*
Cover and interior design: *Ellen Pettengell*
Typeface: *10.5/13 New Aster*
Compositor: *Laserwords Private Limited*
Printer: *Worldcolor Press Inc.*
Cover credit: *©Moodboard*
Credits: The credits section for this book begins on page 545 and is considered an extension of the copyright page.

Library of Congress Cataloging-in-Publication Data

Orum-Alexander, Gail.
Pharmacy technician : practice and procedures / Gail Orum-Alexander, James J. Mizner Jr.
p. ; cm.
Includes bibliographical references and index.
ISBN-13: 978-0-07-352072-8 (alk. paper)
ISBN-10: 0-07-352072-1 (alk. paper)
1. Pharmacy technicians. I. Mizner, James J. II. Title.
[DNLM: 1. Pharmacists' Aides—Problems and Exercises. 2. Technology, Pharmaceutical—methods—Problems and Exercises. QV 18.2 O78p 2011]
RS122.95.O78 2011
615'.1076—dc22
2009049800

WARNING NOTICE: The clinical procedures, medicines, dosages, and other matters described in this publication are based upon research of current literature and consultation with knowledgeable persons in the field. The procedures and matters described in this text reflect currently accepted clinical practice. However, this information cannot and should not be relied upon as necessarily applicable to a given individual's case. Accordingly, each person must be separately diagnosed to discern the patient's unique circumstances. Likewise, the manufacturer's package insert for current drug product information should be consulted before administering any drug. Publisher disclaims all liability for any inaccuracies, omissions, misuse, or misunderstanding of the information contained in this publication. Publisher cautions that this publication is not intended as a substitute for the professional judgment of trained medical personnel.

The Internet addresses listed in the text were accurate at the time of publication. The inclusion of a Web site does not indicate an endorsement by the authors or McGraw-Hill, and McGraw-Hill does not guarantee the accuracy of the information presented at these sites.

www.mhhe.com

Brief Contents

About the Authors viii
Preface ix
What Every Student Needs to Know xvi

Unit 1 The Pharmacy Technician 3

Chapter 1 Overview, Practice Settings, and Organizations 4
Chapter 2 Basic Safety and Standards 28
Chapter 3 Communication and Customer Service 54
Chapter 4 Ethics, Law, and Regulatory Agencies 79

Unit 2 Pharmacology and Medications 125

Chapter 5 Measurements and Calculations 126
Chapter 6 Introduction to Pharmacology 169
Chapter 7 Drug Classifications 195
Chapter 8 Over-the-Counter Agents 225
Chapter 9 Complementary and Alternative Modalities 250

Unit 3 Medication Management and Preparation 267

Chapter 10 Dosage Forms and Routes of Administration 268
Chapter 11 Extemporaneous and Sterile Compounding (IV Admixtures) 295
Chapter 12 Medication Errors 313
Chapter 13 Referencing 346

Unit 4 Practice Settings 371

Chapter 14 Retail Setting 372
Chapter 15 Hospital/Inpatient Setting 397
Chapter 16 Other Environments 412
Chapter 17 Inventory Management 438

Unit 5 Transition from Student to Technician 467

Chapter 18 Preparing for Your Career as a Pharmacy Technician 468
Chapter 19 Career Development 485

Appendix A The 50 Most Common Drugs by Prescriptions Dispensed (2007) 497
Appendix B Common Look-Alike and Sound-Alike Drugs 499
Appendix C Selected Drug Categories 510
Appendix D Measurements, Abbreviations, and Formulas 514
Appendix E PTCB Correlation 516
Glossary 539
Credits 545
Index 548
Flashcards

Contents

About the Authors viii

Preface ix

What Every Student Needs to Know xvi

Unit 1 The Pharmacy Technician 3

Chapter 1 Overview, Practice Settings, and Organizations 4

Introduction 5

The Development of Modern-Day Pharmacy Practice 5

The Practice of Pharmacy and the Pharmacy Technician 8

Pharmacy Technician Training, Education, and Credentialing 16

Pharmacy Practice Settings and Pharmacy Technician Responsibilities 19

Chapter 2 Basic Safety and Standards 28

Introduction 29

Common Infectious Diseases 30

Bloodborne Diseases 31

Airborne Diseases 33

Nosocomial Infections 34

Prevention of Spreading Infectious Diseases 34

Incidents 38

Incident Report 39

Procedures for HIV Prophylaxis 41

Documentation and Reporting Outside Your Organization 42

First Aid and CPR Requirements 42

Hazardous Materials 45

NIOSH Recommendations for Health Care Workers 49

Chapter 3 Communication and Customer Service 54

Introduction 55

Communication 56

Types of Communication 58

Customer Service 63

Stress in the Pharmacy 73

Chapter 4 Ethics, Law, and Regulatory Agencies 79

Introduction 81

Ethics 81

Law 83

Federal Pharmacy Laws 1906–1962 85

Federal Pharmacy Laws 1970 89

Federal Pharmacy Laws 1970–1979 102

Federal Pharmacy Laws 1980–1999 105

Federal Pharmacy Laws 2000–Present 110

Regulatory Agencies 113

Unit 2 Pharmacology and Medications 125

Chapter 5 Measurements and Calculations 126

Introduction 127

Numbering Systems 129

Mathematical Concepts 130

Pharmacy Units of Measurement 135

Other Units of Measurement 142

Dosage Calculations 144

Physician's Orders and Prescriptions 149
Drug Labels 154
Compounding 155
Intravenous Applications 160

Chapter 6 Introduction to Pharmacology 169
Introduction 170
Terms Associated with Pharmacology 171
Pharmacokinetics 176
Absorption 178
Distribution 181
Metabolism 184
Elimination 185
Dosing Considerations 186
Side Effects 189
Pregnancy 190

Chapter 7 Drug Classifications 195
Introduction 196
Drug Classifications 197
Central Nervous System Medications 198
Cardiovascular System Medications 203
Renal/Vascular System Medications 204
Respiratory System Medications 207
Gastrointestinal System Medications 208
Endocrine System Medications 210
Anti-Infective Medications 214
Antineoplastic Medications 218
Immune System Medications 219
Dermatologic, Ophthalmic, and Otic Medications 220

Chapter 8 Over-the-Counter (OTC) Agents 225
Introduction 226
Legal Requirements for OTC Agents 227
Types of OTC Agents 230

Chapter 9 Complementary and Alternative Modalities 250
Introduction 251
Significance of Complementary and Alternative Modalities 253
Dietary Supplements 254

Unit 3 Medication Management and Preparation 267

Chapter 10 Dosage Forms and Routes of Administration 268
Introduction 269
Routes of Administration 270
Dosage Forms 275
Dosage Form Abbreviations 290

Chapter 11 Extemporaneous and Sterile Compounding (IV Admixtures) 295
Introduction 296
Exemporaneous Compounding 297
Sterile Compounding 301
Techniques Used in Sterile Compounding 304

Chapter 12 Medication Errors 313
Introduction 314
Medication Errors 314
Types of Errors 317
Causes of Errors 320
Consequences of Errors 321
Methods to Reduce Prescription Errors 323
Prevention of Prescribing Errors 329
Regulatory Oversight 334

Chapter 13 Referencing 346
Introduction 347
Types of Reference Sources 347
Commonly Used Pharmacy Reference Books 350
Internet References 360
Personal Digital Assistants (PDAs) and Pharmacy Software 364

Unit 4 Practice Settings 371

Chapter 14 Retail Setting 372
Introduction 374
Retail Pharmacy 375
Flow of Service 377
Computer Usage in Retail Pharmacy 389
Customer Service 391
OTC (Over-the-Counter) Medications 392

Chapter 15 Hospital/Inpatient Setting 397
Introduction 398
Inpatient Facility Classifications 398
Policies and Procedures 400
Medication Orders 401
Pharmacy Technician–Inpatient Setting 404
Other Responsibilities of the Pharmacy Technician 407

Chapter 16 Other Environments 412
Introduction 413
Long-Term Care Pharmacy 414
Home Infusion Pharmacy 418
Managed-Care Pharmacy 423
Mail-Order Pharmacy 428
Federal Pharmacy 432
Pharmaceutical Industry 433

Chapter 17 Inventory Management 438
Introduction 439
Overview of Inventory Management 440
Retail Inventory Management 444
Hospital Inventory Management 449
Controlled Substances 452
Investigational Drugs 457
Drug Recalls 460

Unit 5 Transition from Student to Technician 467

Chapter 18 Preparing for Your Career as a Pharmacy Technician 468
Introduction 469
Pharmacy Technician Training Programs 469
Finding a Position 473
Your Resume 473
The Application Process 476
Pre-Employment Requirements 478

Chapter 19 Career Development 485
Introduction 486
On the Job 486
Continuing Education 490
Professional Organizations 492

Appendix A The 50 Most Common Drugs by Prescriptions Dispensed (2007) 497
Appendix B Common Look-Alike and Sound-Alike Drugs 499
Appendix C Selected Drug Categories 510
Appendix D Measurements, Abbreviations, and Formulas 514
Appendix E PTCB Correlation 516
Glossary 539
Credits 545
Index 548
Flashcards

About the Authors

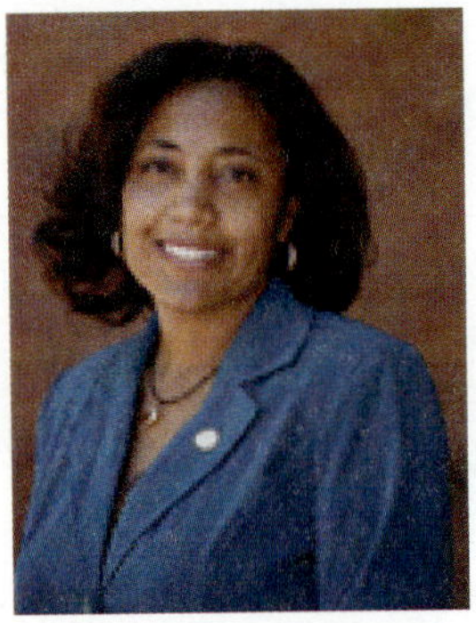

Gail Orum-Alexander

Gail Orum-Alexander has a Doctor of Pharmacy degree from the University of Southern California, School of Pharmacy and is a registered pharmacist in the state of California. She is the Dean of the College of Science and Health at Charles R. Drew University of Medicine and Science. She also serves as director of the Pharmacy Technology Program. She has published and reviewed articles on the pharmacologic management of obesity and obesity in children and adolescents.

Dr. Orum-Alexander is actively involved in local and national organizations, as well as community programs that focus on minority health issues. She is a member of the American Society of Health-System Pharmacists and has served as a site visitor for pharmacy technician program accreditation. She is a member of the Pharmacy Technician Educators Council and has served as an item writer for the Pharmacy Technician Certification Examination. Her honors include Most Outstanding Faculty Award, Charles R. Drew University, College of Science and Health (1997 and 1998), Recognition Awards from Physician Assistant Students (2002 and 2003), and the Outstanding Faculty Service Award, Charles R. Drew University (2004).

Dr. Orum-Alexander resides in Alhambra, California, and enjoys reading, needle arts, and walking.

James Mizner

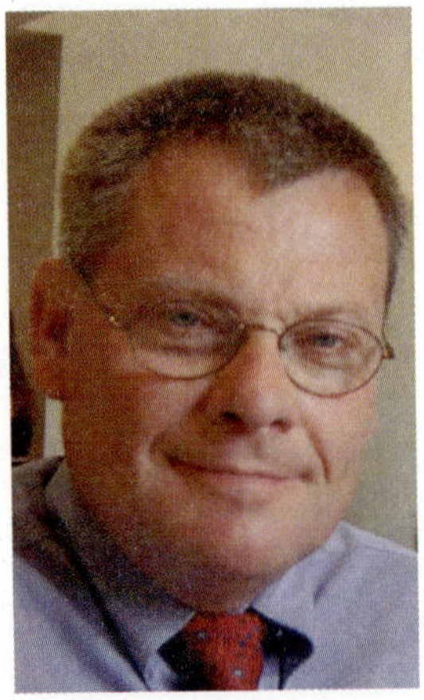

Jim Mizner received a BS in Pharmacy from Duquesne University and an MBA from Keller Graduate School of Business. He is a licensed pharmacist in the state of Virginia with experience in both retail and hospital pharmacy. He is the director for the Pharmacy Technician and the Allied Health Technology Programs at ACT College located in Rosslyn, Virginia. He is also an online adjunct pharmacy technician professor for National University.

In addition to teaching, Mizner is a pharmacy technician program specialist for both the Accrediting Bureau of Health Education Schools (ABHES) and the Ohio Board of Regents. In his spare time, he studies Tae Kwon Do with his son. He resides in Reston, Virginia, with his wife and son.

Preface

When you visit your local pharmacy to refill a prescription, whom do you meet first? In most situations, you will meet a very valuable member of the pharmacy team, the pharmacy technician.

According to the U.S. Department of Labor Statistics Occupational Outlook, 2008–2009, employment for pharmacy technicians is expected to increase much faster than the average through 2016, and job opportunities are expected to be good.

Due to this rapid growth and increased need for pharmacy technicians, the *Pharmacy Technician: Practice and Procedures* text has evolved. This rapid growth and increased need for pharmacy technicians is based upon two primary factors:

- Increased use of medications
- Shortage of registered pharmacists

The aging population and the advancement and augmented use of prescription medications have consequently increased the need for dispensing of medications whether it is in long-term care, acute care, or outpatient pharmacy practice. Although automation and centralization of services was predicted to decrease the need for registered pharmacists, the amplified use of medications by the population has outweighed these factors.

Pharmacists are in high demand and the shortage of pharmacists is expected to increase over the next decade. Pharmacists require well-trained pharmacy technicians to assist them with basic tasks, so they can be available to perform counseling and other higher-level functions. In order for pharmacy technicians to be well trained, they need exceptional educational materials—thus the magnified need for McGraw-Hill's *Pharmacy Technician: Practice and Procedures 1e*.

> “*The real-life scenarios involving pharmacy technicians are well done and thought-provoking.*
>
> **Mary Ann Stuhan**
> **Cuyahoga Community College**

> “*The tables that have actual product names are helpful, as these are the names that the technician hears on a daily basis. The author does a great job of delivering the material to make it interesting. It is easy to read and follow. The information is understandable and not too detailed for pharmacy technicians.*
>
> **Sandi Tschritter**
> **Spokane Community College**

Student-Based Learning

With McGraw-Hill's *Pharmacy Technician: Practice and Procedures* text, pharmacy technician training is brought to a new level. The easy-to-understand language and format was created to make this challenging content interesting as well as comprehensive. Students in the pharmacy technician program need to be stimulated and motivated to learn the necessary information to enter the field.

Gone are the typical read the chapter, listen to the lecture, and memorize for the test *teaching* strategies. The focus is on *learning* strategies and McGraw-Hill has infused these new learning strategies as well as technology throughout the product. These educational methods help the learning process become student based as well as meet the needs of students with all types of learning styles.

> *I feel the text is complete and contains valuable information. The material is up-to-date and accurate, making it an asset for the pharmacy professional.*
>
> **Nancy L. Needham**
> **American Career College**

Organization

The textbook and educational materials written for *Pharmacy Technician: Practice and Procedures* are intended for entry-level students as well as seasoned learners who want to prepare themselves for the pharmacy technician profession. In addition to **learning outcomes** and a **correlation to the knowledge statements for the Pharmacy Technician Certification Board** exam, each chapter starts with a **Case Study** to apply the content within the chapter and begin the process of critical thinking and problem solving. Case study questions are listed and act as an anticipatory set for the chapter. (Student must answer these questions in the chapter review.)

Following the theme of encouraging student-based learning as well as interaction with the content, the textbook includes many other essential features.

- **At Your Service** features focus on customer service as well as communication within pharmacy practice.
- **Tech Check** questions are presented after every major topic to help the student grasp small portions of content.
- **Caution boxes** point out critical information relative to the practice of pharmacy.
- **Marginal key terms** provide the learner with important terms and definitions as they are learning the content. They do not have to look in the back of the book or try to find the definition in the paragraph where the term is introduced.
- **Bulleted chapter summaries** highlight the key points of the chapters and provide a quick review of the learning outcomes of the chapter.
- **Multiple choice** questions help the student master the content as well as prepare for the certification examination.
- **Acronyms, abbreviations, and matching activities** reinforce key chapter concepts.
- **Critical thinking** questions reinforce the application of chapter content.
- **HIPAA scenarios** challenge the student to think about and respond to real-life situations where patient privacy issues are at stake.
- **Internet activities** keep the student up-to-date with the pharmacy practice as well as the new and updated medications and health care trends.
- **Application activities on the student CD-ROM** make the content come alive and reinforce the content presented in an interesting and interactive way.
- **320 end-of-book flashcards** provide quick and easy review of key content.

> *A strength of the chapter on medication errors is getting the point across that medication errors are way too prevalent in this field, and how important the technician's part is in cutting down on errors. I think the examples of medication errors are interesting for the students to read (real life examples).*
>
> **Mindy Koppel**
> **Pennsylvania Institute of Technology**

Teaching and Learning Supplements

You will find many useful teaching and learning supplements with McGraw-Hill's *Pharmacy Technician: Practice and Procedures*. These supplements create a complete package for today's learner whether they are learning on the job, on their own, through distance education, or in the typical classroom setting.

- **Laboratory Manual to Accompany *Pharmacy Technician: Practice and Procedures*** provides students with the opportunity to test their recall of text concepts and applications. The Laboratory Manual features include:
    - Learning Outcomes
    - Test Your Knowledge
        - Multiple choice questions
        - True/false questions
        - Matching
        - Fill in the blank
    - Apply Your Knowledge
        - Research information on the Web
        - Answer questions that require critical thinking
    - Practice Your Knowledge
        - Complete a research task using specific pharmacy reference books
        - Complete a laboratory procedure
    - Calculation Corner
        - Work out solutions to common pharmacy calculation problems

> *This book includes some topics that others omit. Also, it is the most up-to-date with the newest information. The features like case studies and "at your service" make it seem more personal.*
>
> **Coelle Harper**
> **Career Centers of Texas—Fort Worth**

- **McGraw-Hill *Connect Plus*** is a Web-based assignment and assessment platform that gives students the means to better connect with their coursework, with their instructors, and with the important concepts that they will need to know for success now and in the future. With *Connect Plus* instructors can deliver assignments, quizzes, and tests easily online. Students can practice important skills at their own pace and on their own schedule. With *Connect Plus*, students also get 24/7 online access to an eBook—an online edition of the text—to aid them in successfully completing their work, wherever and whenever they choose.
- **McGraw-Hill LearnSmart: Pharmacology** is a diagnostic learning system that determines the level of student knowledge, then feeds the student appropriate content. Students learn faster and study more efficiently.

  As a student works within the system, LearnSmart develops a personal learning path adapted to what the student has learned and retained. LearnSmart is also able to recommend additional study resources to help the student master topics.

  In addition to being an innovative, outstanding study tool, LearnSmart has features for instructors. There is a Course Gauge where the instructor can see exactly what students have accomplished as well as a built-in assessment tool for graded assignments.

  Students and instructors will be able to access LearnSmart anywhere via a web browser. And for students on the go, it will also be available through any iPhone or iPod Touch.
- **Online Learning Center (OLC)**, www.mhhe.com/pharmacytech, contains the following instructor resources:
    - Instructor's Manual
    - McGraw-Hill's EZTest Test Generator
    - PowerPoint presentations
    - Image bank featuring selected textbook images

Student and Instructor CD-ROMs

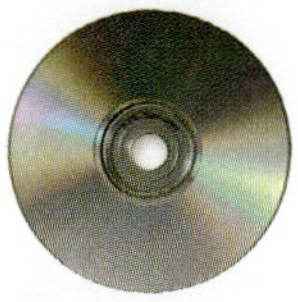

- **Student Applications CD-ROM** accompanies the main text. This CD assists the student in learning the content presented in the textbook as well as preparing for their certification test. This easy to use CD promotes critical thinking, learning of skills and provides drill and practice activities all in one.

  Over *75 Topic Specific Activities* are correlated to the textbook learning objectives as well as the ASHP Modules and PTCB Knowledge Statements. These activities include videos, photos, matching, drag and drop, and completion exercises. Each activity is graded and student scores are tracked on any writable media. Results can be emailed to the instructor and/or printed to be included in the student's portfolio.

  Interactive Games require knowledge of the chapter content, a good memory and an interest in having fun while learning. Games can be used for enrichment, reinforcement, and/or review and support the current edutainment trend of today's high tech learner.

Chapter	CD Activity Name	Learning Outcome(s)	PCTB Statement(s)	ASHP Module(s)
1	Do You Know Your Duties?	1.1, 1.2	III-7, III-9	1
	Where Do I Practice	1.7	III-7, III-9	1
2	Incident Report	2.10	II-35	28
	Hand washing and Hand Hygiene	2.6, 2.7	III-18	28
3	Listening and Angry Customer	3.4, 3.5, 3.6, 3.9	I-71, I-72, II-24, III-2, III-5	24, 30, 37
	Understanding Non Verbal Communication	3.1, 3.2, 3.3	I-71, I-72, II-24, III-2, III-5	30, 34, 35, 36, 37
4	Do not use Abbreviations	4.8	I-1, I-2	18
	Verifying a DEA number	4.2	I-23	18
	Pharmacy Legislations	4.3	I-1, I-2	1,15,18
5	Parts of a prescription	5.9, 5.26	I-36	18
	Drug Labels	5.11	I-36, II-18	18
	Roman Numerals	5.1	I-50, I-51	20
	Multiplying Fractions	5.2	I-50, I-51	20
	Dividing Fractions	5.2	I-50, I-51	20
	Converting Fraction to Decimals	5.3	I-50, I-51	20
	Convert Decimal to Percent	5.4	I-50, I-51	20
	Convert Fraction to Percent	5.4	I-50, I-51	20
	Convert to Ratio to Percent	5.4	I-50, I-51	20
	Metric Abbreviations	5.5	I-50, I-51	20
	Converting Between Metric Measurements	5.6	I-50, I-51	20
	Converting Between Temperature Systems	5.7	I-50, I-51	20
	Using the 24-hour clock	5.8	I-50, I-51	20
	Calculating Estimated Days Supply	5.10	I-50, I-51	20
	Converting by the Fraction Proportion Method	5.13	I-50, I-51	20
	Converting by the Ratio Proportion Method	5.13	I-50, I-51	20
	Converting by the Dimensional Analysis Method	5.13, 5.24	I-50, I-51	20
	Amount to Dispense by Fraction Proportion Method	5.14	I-50, I-51	20
	Amount to Dispense by the Ratio Proportion	5.14	I-50, I-51	20
	Amount to Dispense by Dimensional Analysis	5.14, 5.24	I-50, I-51	20
	Amount to Dispense by Formula Method	5.14	I-50,I-51	20
	Calculating Dosage Based on Weight	5.15	I-50, I-51	20
	Pediatric Specific Dosage Calculations	5.15	I-50, I-51	20
	Calculating Dose Based on BSA	5.15	I-50, I-51	20
	Preparing Dilutions from a Concentration	5.17	I-50, I-51	20
	Alligations	5.18	I-50, I-51	20
	Formula Method for Concentrations	5.17	I-50, I-51	20
	Calculating Flow Rates mL/hour	5.19	I-50, I-51	21
	Calculating Flow Rates gtt/min	5.21	I-50, I-51	20
6	Pharmacokinetics	6.3, 6.4, 6.5, 6.6, 6.7	I-16, II-8	2, 3, 4, 5, 6, 7, 8, 9, 10, 11, 12, 13, 14
	Medications in Pregnancy	6.20	I-17	2, 3, 4, 5, 6, 7, 8, 9, 10, 11, 12, 13, 14
	Altered Affects of Medications	6.10	I-16, I-17	2, 3, 4, 5, 6, 7, 8, 9, 10, 11, 12, 13, 14
7	Reading Generic and Trade Names	7.5	I-5	2, 3, 4, 5, 6, 7,
	Controlled Substances	7.6, 7.7	I-44	8, 9, 10, 11, 12, 13, 14, 18
	Classify of Common Drugs	7.5	I-18, I-44	2, 3, 4, 5, 6, 7, 8, 9, 10, 11, 12, 13, 14
8	Classify OTC Agents	8.5, 8.6	I-28	2, 3, 4, 5, 6, 7, 8, 9, 10, 11, 12, 13, 14
	Can They Take this Medication?	8.6	I-28	2, 3, 4, 5, 6, 7, 8, 9, 10, 11, 12, 13, 14
9	Labeling Requirements for Dietary Supplements	9.1	I-19	2
	CAM Treatments	9.3	I-19	2

Chapter	CD Activity Name	Learning Outcome(s)	PCTB Statement(s)	ASHP Module(s)
10	Dosage Forms How Do We Abbreviate? Routes of Administration	10. 2 10.6 10.1	I-13, II-4 I-4 I-13, I-39, I-4	2, 3, 4, 5, 6, 7, 8, 9, 10, 11, 12, 13, 14 2, 3, 4, 5, 6, 7, 8, 9, 10, 11, 12, 13, 14 2, 3, 4, 5, 6, 7, 8, 9, 10, 11, 12, 13, 14
11	How the Hood Works? Equipment	11.1 11.6	I-55, I-57, I-58 I-55, I-57, I-58	21 17
12	Prescription Errors Look or Sound Alike Drugs	12.2, 12.3, 12.4 12.2, 12.3, 12.4	I-20, I-24 I-20, I-24	1, 25 1, 25
13	Which Reference Would You Use? The Monograph	13.3 13.4	I-15, III-8 I-15, III-8	1, 16 1,16
14	Calculating Days Supply Prescription Translation	14.4 14.5	I-20, I-36 I-20, I-36	18, 23, 19, 37 18, 23, 19, 37
15	Medication Orders Inpatient Duties	15.7 15.1, 15.7	I-20, I-36, I-70 I-43, III-22	18, 23, 34 18, 34
16	Understanding Other Environments Managed Care Pharmacy	16.1, 16.2, 16.3 16.5, 16.6	I-1, I-20 I-1, I-20, I-36 I-70	34, 35, 36, 37 34, 35, 36, 37
17	Calculating Inventory Drug Recall Terms Drug Recall Steps	17.1, 17.2, 17.10 17.1, 17.2, 17.3 17.1, 17.2, 17.3	II-11, II-25 II-11, II-25 II-11, II-25	17 17 17
18	Interviewing Techniques Parts of a Resume	18.7 18.5	III-7 III-7	30 30
19	Stress Management Understanding Pharmacy Organizations	19.1 19.6	III-3 III-6	30 32

- **Spin the Wheel Game** A learning game that infuses a bit of chance; this game can be used for classroom or student review. Users can select one or multiple chapters. Play the game with one, two, three, or four players or teams. Questions are created from the chapter objectives. This game can be used for classroom or individual review. It will allow the user to choose the chapter and/or chapters they would like to review and split the students into teams for classroom or small group activity. (The Instructor Productivity CD allows the instructor to change, add or delete questions for this game.)

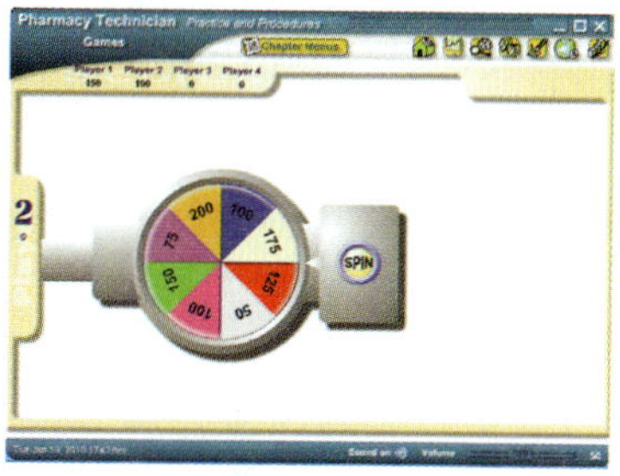

- **Brand Generic Concentration Game** An interactive matching game that helps the student learn common Brand and Generic drug names as well as drug categories. The user matches drugs to uncover a picture. With each match, part of the picture is revealed and you must answer a question related to the picture for extra points. The computer monitors the number of matches. All matches must be completed before the picture is revealed and the student can play again. Each time the puzzle is created the medications are randomized from a master list so no two games are alike. The game is designed for two players or teams.

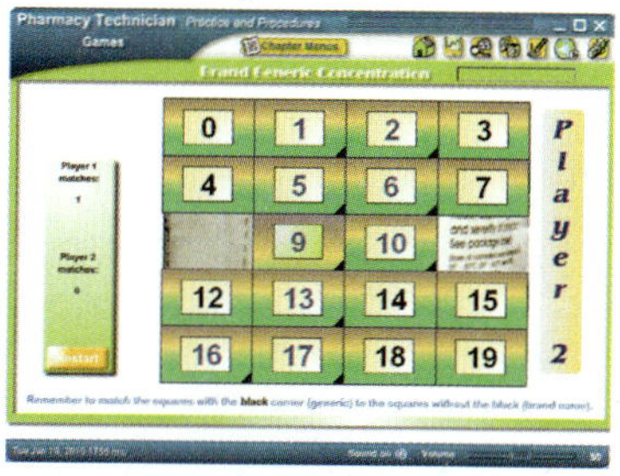

- **Pharm Tech Challenge** A jeopardy-like game that provides lots of fun for up to three players.

  An *audio glossary, brand-generic flash cards, presentation reviews, key terms quizzes,* and *chapter tests* round out the educational content and provide additional multiple review and learning activities for the user.

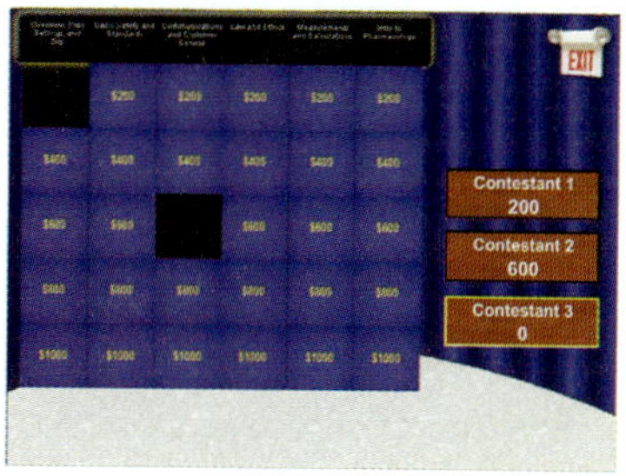

- **Instructor Resource CD-ROM** includes easy-to-use resources for class preparation. The CD includes the following:
  - PowerPoint® presentations with *Apply Your Knowledge* questions and Instructor notes.
  - McGraw-Hill's EZTest Test Generator with over 500 questions and answer rationales and correlations to PTCB and ASHP competencies. The flexible electronic testing program allows instructors to create tests from book-specific items. It accommodates a wide range of

question types, and instructors may add their own questions. Multiple versions of the test can be created and any test can be exported for use with course management systems such as WebCT, BlackBoard, or PageOut. EZTest Online gives instructors a chance to easily administer EZTest-created exams and quizzes online. EZTest Online is available for Windows and Macintosh environments.

- Electronic resources including answers to the textbook questions, lesson plans, and correlation charts to PTCB and ASHP
- Image Bank with selected figures from the textbook that can be utilized in classroom presentations, handouts, or questions.

Acknowledgments

For insightful reviews, helpful suggestions, and information, we would like to acknowledge the following:

Robert W. Aanonsen, CPhT
Platt College

Lori Andrews
Ivy Tech Community College

Trisha Autry, CPhT
Clover Park Technical College

Sybil Barnes
Long Technical College

Nora Chan, PharmD
City College of San Francisco

Chris P. Crigger, CPhT
San Antonio College

Charleen A. Daniel
Sixth Avenue Medical Pharmacy
Pharmacy Technician/Trainer
Washington State Pharmacy Association

Karen Davis, CPhT
Consultant

Cathy L. Dease, BS, MS, MBA
Pharmacy Branch
Army Medical Department Center and School

Lynn Egler, RMA, AHI, CPhT,
Medical Coordinator/ Externship Coordinator
Dorsey Schools

Donna Fresnilla, BA
Community College of Rhode Island

Jill M. Frost, BS, CPhT
Tennessee Technology Center

Coelle Lynette Harper Deaton, BSE
Career Centers of Texas–Fort Worth

Linda Hart, CPhT, AS/Pt
High-Tech Institute

Gary W. Haworth, MEd, RPh
Linn-Benton Community College

Michael M. Hayter, Pharm D., MBA
Virginia Highlands Community College

A. G. Hirst, AA, BA
North Georgia Technical College

Eddy van Hunnik, PhD
Gibbs College of Boston

Jennifer L. Jiminey, MA
Choice House Calls

Linda C. Kelley, CPhT
MedVance Institute

Mindy Koppel, CPhT
CHI Institute Southampton

Barbara Lacher, BS
North Dakota State College of Science

Danny D. Lame, MA, BA, AA
Platt College

James P. Lear, AA
National Institute of Technology

Tonya Lewis, CPhT
Georgia Medical Institute

Barbara A. Lipp, CPhT
Bryman College

Jemey Martin
Georgia Medical Institute

Michelle C. McCranie, CPhT
Ogeechee Technical College

Janet McGregor Liles, BS
Arkansas State University–Beebe

"*This retail chapter was absolutely beautiful! Great detail, and explanations.*

Chris P. Crigger
San Antonio College

Earl R. McKinstry, RPh, MS
Western Dakota Technical Institute

Tara G. McManaway, MDiv, LPC ALPS (WV), LMT (WV) CMT (MD)
College of Southern Maryland

Michael Meir, MD
Director HIT
TCI College

Salvatore J. Monopoli, DPM
The Cittone Institute

Nancy L. Needham, MEd, CPhT
American Career College

Hieu T. Nguyen, BS
Western Career College

Joshua Owens, BA
Bridgerland Applied Technology College

Christina Rauberts Conklin, AA, RMA
Florida Metropolitan University

David R. Reiter, AS
Pueblo Community College

Phil Rushing, BSPharm
Community Care College

Patricia A. Schommer, MA, CPhT
National American University

Douglas Scribner, BA, CPhT
TVI Community College

Susan M. Shorey, BA, MA
Valley Career College

Karen A. Smith, CPhT
Bryman College

Jason P. Sparks, BA, CPhT
Austin Community College

Cynthia J. Steffen, RPh
Milwaukee Area Technical College

Cardiece Sylvan, CPhT
Pharmacy Technician Program Director
MedVance Institute

Lisa R. Thompson, CPhT
MedVance Institute

Joseph A. Tinervia, CPhT, MBA
Tulsa Job Corps Pharmacy Technician

Sandi Tschritter, BA, CPhT
Spokane Community College

Cindy Turner, CPhT
Western Career College

Pedro A. Valentin, CPhT, BBA
Columbus Technical College

Ray Vellenga, RPh, MS
Century College

Janice Vermiglio-Smith, RN, MS, PhD
Central Arizona College

Marvin L. Walker, AAS
Austin Community College

Judy S. Weisbard, MPA, CPhT
Chaffey College

Denise A. Wilfong, MHS, NREMT-P
Western Carolina University

Marsha L. Wilson, MA, BS, MEd
Clarian Health

Richard L. Witt, BS
Allegany College of Maryland

Hwa H. Yeon, AA
Everest College

Dr. Betty Yarhi, PharmD, BS
ACT College

“

Chapter 4 covers law with terms and a writing style that are easy to read. I believe it would be difficult for someone reading this chapter to misinterpret the facts because clarity is present.

Jill Frost
Tennessee Technology Center

“

The author covers most of the topics that presently aren't covered in most technician textbooks.

The end of the chapter exercises are very helpful.

Joseph Tinervia
Tulsa Job Corps Center

“

I think the author has great ideas. This textbook would be an excellent addition to any pharmacy technology program.

The writing is very clear. It is easy to read and understand. The reading flows and the instructions provided are very clear.

Michelle C. McCranie
Ogeechee Technical College

What Every Student Needs to Know

Many tools to help you learn have been integrated into your text.

Chapter Features

Learning Outcomes

Upon completion of this chapter, you will be able to:

11.1 Define *extemporaneous compounding.*
11.2 Define *sterile compounding.*
11.3 Identify types of products produced by sterile compounding.
11.4 Identify pharmacy settings where nonsterile compounding occurs.
11.5 Identify common pharmacy equipment or supplies used in extemporaneous compounding.
11.6 Articulate which types of preparations must be prepared using aseptic technique and which do not require aseptic technique.
11.7 Identify pharmacy settings where sterile compounding occurs.
11.8 Define *aseptic technique.*
11.9 Describe how aseptic technique relates to infection control.
11.10 Explain and describe cleaning and use of the laminar flow hood.
11.11 Describe the use of personal protective equipment in sterile compounding.
11.12 Identify the regulations associated with sterile compounding.

Key Terms

alligation
aseptic technique
extemporaneous compounding
infection control
IV
IV piggyback
laminar flow hood
levigation
reconstitution
sepsis
sterile compounding
TPN
triturate
USP<797>

PTCB

In preparation for the certification examination, you should understand and perform activities associated with the following PTCB Knowledge Statements:

PTCB Knowledge Statement — *Domain I. Assisting the Pharmacist in Serving Patients*

Knowledge of practice site policies and procedures regarding prescriptions or medication orders (20)
Knowledge of procedures to prepare IV admixtures (55)
Knowledge of procedures to prepare total parenteral nutrition (57)
Knowledge of procedures to prepare reconstituted injectable medications (58)
Knowledge of aseptic technique (65)
Knowledge of infection control procedures (66)

Marginal Key Terms

highlight important terminology that will assist you in understanding the content.

Learning Outcomes

present a list of the key points you should focus on in the chapter.

PTCB Knowledge Statements

correlate to the chapter content.

Case Studies

begin the process of critical thinking and problem solving.

Case Study

Marcos, CPhT, has been the senior pharmacy technician at ABC for the past 5 years. ABC Infusion Services provides intravenous TPNs for patients who receive the medications at home. Nurses home with medication administration. As the senior technician, four other pharmacy technicians and works closely with the ph ers. Marcos is responsible for checking the laminar flow hoods a biologic studies in the sterile compounding area, as well as IV a during a busy period, Marcos noticed that the newest technicia labels to be adhered to the IV bags in the hood to speed proces to keep a pen in the hood so he can easily initial his work.

While reading this chapter, keep the following questions in min

1. Is Jack using proper aseptic technique?(LO 11.2, 11.8)
2. What are the potential risks that can occur?(LO 11.9, 11.10)
3. What is Marcos's responsibility as the senior technician?(LO 11

At Your Service

Pat is a pharmacy technician at Community Medical Center. She often prepares intravenous admixture products, including total parenteral nutrition (TPN) and chemotherapy. Pat recently received a written order from the nurses' station for IV hydration fluids for a patient. It does not take Pat much time to prepare the IV. A nurse comes from the nurses' station asking if the IV is ready for the patient. The nurse says the patient needs it right away and does not understand why Pat will not hand her the prepared IV until after the pharmacist checks it. After all, Pat is a very experienced technician. The nurse says she will check the IV before she gives it to the patient anyway.

While reading this chapter, keep the following questions in mind.

1. Is the nurse right or wrong? Explain.(LO 11.3)
2. How should Pat respond to the nurse?(LO 11.12)
3. What should Pat do?(LO 11.12)

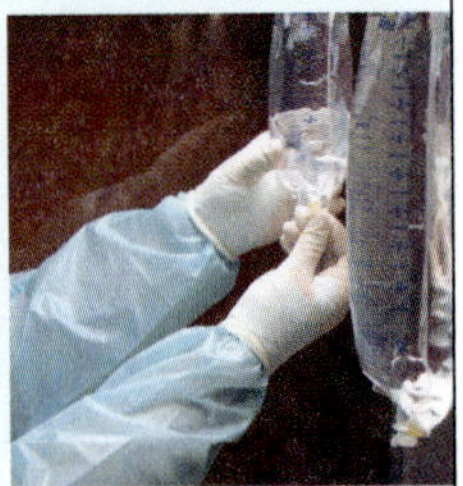

Tech Check

1. List three pieces of equipment that may be used in compounding.(LO 11.5)
2. List three types of supplies that may be used in compounding.(LO 11.5)
3. Which item is always used while compounding, regardless of the product?(LO 11.11)

At Your Service

focuses on customer service as well as communication within pharmacy practice.

Tech Check questions

are presented after every major topic to help you grasp small portions of content.

Tables

summarize data and help organize concepts.

Table 11-1 Common Equipment and Supplies Used for Extemporaneous Compounding

Equipment	Supplies
Class A balance	Suppository molds
Pipette	Filters
Mortar and pestle	Parchment paper
Spatula	Gelatin capsules
Graduated cylinders	Containers
Beakers	Labels
Bunsen burner	Syringes
Compounding slab	Weighing papers
Thermometers	Flasks

Caution boxes

point out critical information relative to the practice of pharmacy.

Caution

The pharmacy technician should always wear gloves while compounding a medication to limit the risk of contamination of the product prior to dispensing.

Bulleted chapter summaries

highlight the key points of the chapters and provide a quick review of the learning outcomes of the chapter.

Chapter Summary

Understanding the uses and procedures of sterile and nonsterile compounding is vital to the pharmacy technician. Important points to remember are:

- Compounding is the manufacture of pharmaceutical preparations and may involve both sterile and nonsterile methods.
- Dosage forms produced by nonsterile compounding are those used in situations where the risk of infection is low, and include agents for topical or ...ments or creams.
- ...rile compounding ...ophthalmic preparations, ...n to the patient is high. ...sterile compounding
- Aseptic technique is utilized by health professio... to minimize the transfer of pathogens to the pa...
- As proper cleaning of the laminar flow hood i... critical element of infection control, its cleani... and maintenance must be documented and k... on file as part of the pharmacy's records.
- The proper use of personal protective equipm... in sterile compounding is important to limit transfer of pathogens from the pharmacy tec... cian into the product being compounded.
- USP <797> is a set of enforceable regulations

Multiple Choice

1. Topical creams requiring compounding usually do *not* require ______ (LO 11.6)
   a. laminar flow hood.
   b. accurate calculations.
   c. wearing gloves.
   d. cleaning equipment after use.
2. Levigation refers to ______ (LO 11.5)
   a. increasing solid particle size.
   b. decreasing solid particle size.
   c. filtering solids from a liquid mixture.
   d. incorporating a solid into a diluent.
3. The pharmacy technician should always wear ______ while doing any type of

Critical Thinking Questions

1. If you observed someone using inappropriate aseptic technique, what would you do or say? (LO 11.8) What risks are presented if you do or say nothing? (L...
2. Why is it impo...
3. Would you be afra... peutic agents? (LO 11...

End-of-chapter review

includes a variety of question formats, critical thinking, and research and Internet activities.

Internet Activities

1. Access **www.ashp.org.** Locate information on USP<797>. Choose one article on the Web site. Read the article and identify how the issues discussed impact the practice of pharmacy technicians. Be prepared to discuss your article and comments in class. (LO 11.12)
2. Access **www.usp.org.** ... link. Write a brief par... *United States Pharma...* services it provides. (LO...

HIPAA Scenario

After a patient, Larry Newsome, picked up his compounded nicotine lollipops for smoking cessation, the pharmacist realized that the caution label "Keep out of the reach of children" was not included

Discussion Q...

1. In what ... law for P...

HIPAA scenarios

challenge you to think about and respond to real-life situations where patient privacy issues are at stake.

Appendices

offer additional information that is pertinent to the pharmacy technician.

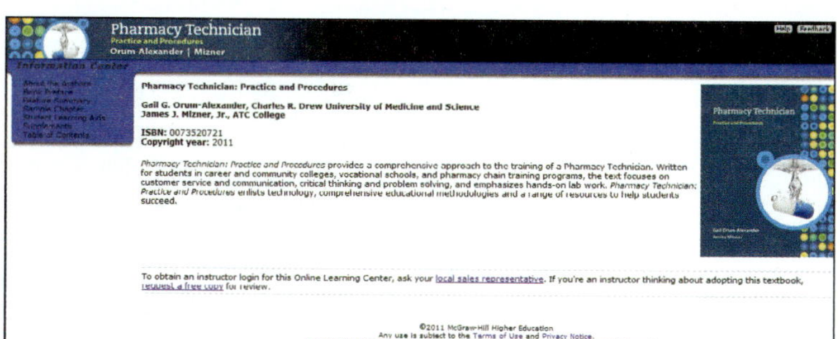

Online Learning Center (www.mhhe.com/pharmacytech)

offers additional teaching tools.

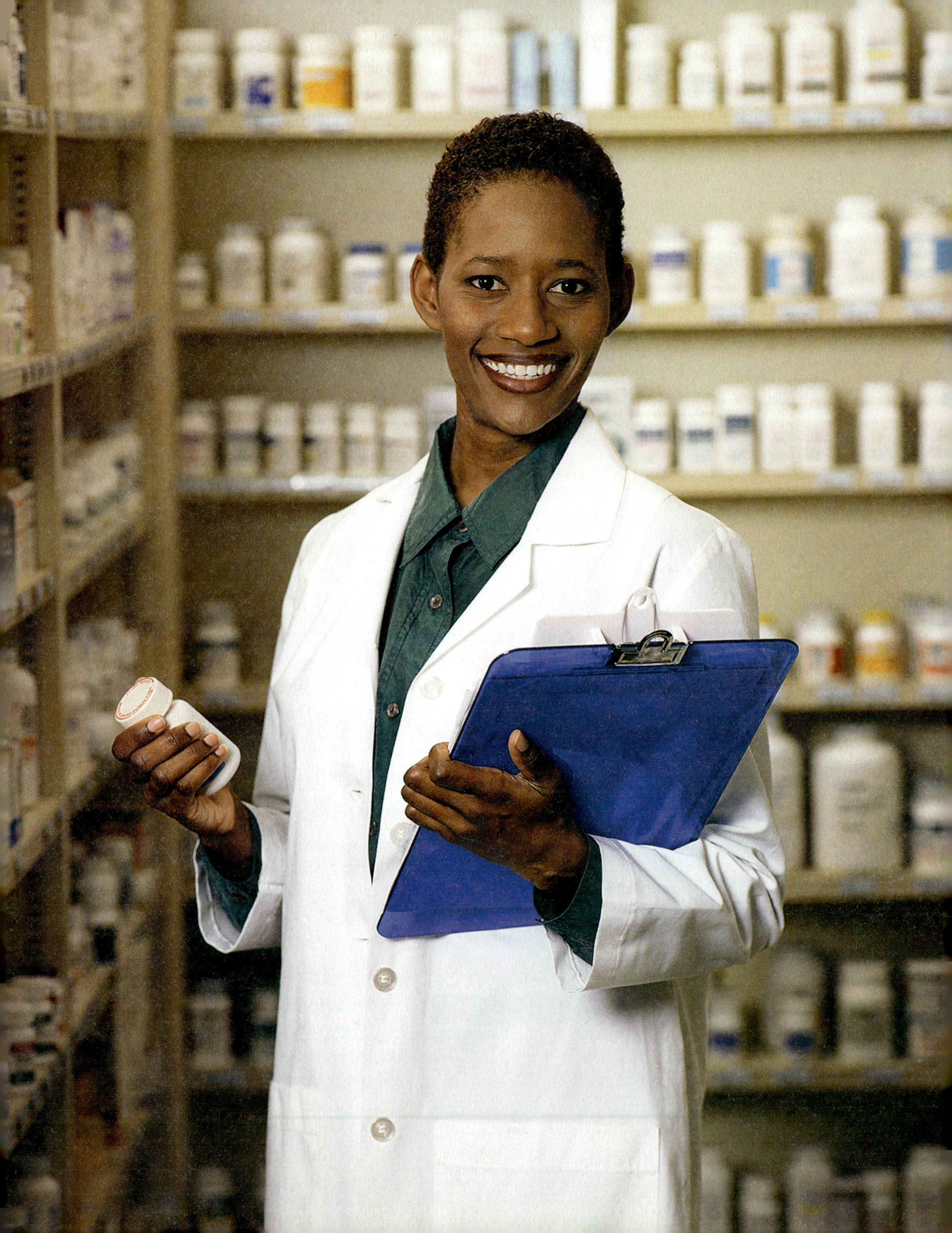

Unit 1

The Pharmacy Technician

Chapter 1 Overview, Practice Settings, and Organizations

Chapter 2 Basic Safety and Standards

Chapter 3 Communication and Customer Service

Chapter 4 Law and Ethics

1

Overview, Practice Settings, and Organizations

Key Terms

accreditation
certification
chain pharmacy
continuing education
credentialing
externship
franchise pharmacy
independent pharmacy
internship
licensure
on-the-job training
prescription
registering

Learning Outcomes

Upon completion of this chapter, you will be able to:

1.1 Explain and demonstrate characteristics associated with a pharmacy technician.

1.2 Explain the role of the pharmacy technician as it exists today in the practice of pharmacy.

1.3 Differentiate between the duties of a pharmacy technician and a pharmacist.

1.4 Demonstrate an appreciation of the evolvement of the practice of pharmacy from the beginning of humanity to its present-day form.

1.5 Differentiate between certification, licensure, and registration with a state board of pharmacy.

1.6 Describe the various types of training pharmacy technicians may experience in the preparation of their career.

1.7 Differentiate between the various pharmacy settings where a pharmacy technician may practice and the responsibilities found in each setting.

PTCB

In preparation for the certification examination, you should understand and perform activities associated with the following PTCB Knowledge Statements:

PTCB Knowledge Statement

Domain I. Assisting the Pharmacist in Serving Patients

Knowledge of pharmaceutical, medical, and legal developments that impact on the practice of pharmacy (2)

PTCB Knowledge Statement

Domain III. Participation in the Administration and Management of Pharmacy Practice

Knowledge of required operational licenses and certificates (6)

Knowledge of roles and responsibilities of pharmacists, pharmacy technicians, and other pharmacy employees (7)

Knowledge of professional standards for personnel, facilities equipment, and supplies (9)

Case Study

A young man met with his career counselor at his local high school to discuss what he would like to do upon graduation. The career counselor asked the young man to describe himself. He provided her with the following list: strong people skills, a desire to assist people, detail oriented, a solid math background, willingness to learn. During their meeting, the young man stated that his uncle owned a small pharmacy and had offered him a job as a pharmacy technician, but he was uncertain whether he would take the job. The career counselor then asked him about his hesitancy, and the young man stated that he did not know what a pharmacy technician's responsibilities were, and if he would need additional education.

While reading this chapter, keep the following questions in mind:

1. Where could he find information about pharmacy technicians?(LO 1.2)
2. What type of career opportunities exist for pharmacy technicians?(LO 1.7)
3. What personal characteristics are required for pharmacy technicians?(LO 1.1)
4. What are some of the tasks a pharmacy technician performs?(LO 1.3)

Introduction to Pharmacy(LO 1.4)

Pharmacy is the art and science of preparing and dispensing medications and providing drug-related information to the public. It involves:

- Interpreting of prescriptions and medication orders
- Compounding, labeling, and dispensing of drugs and devices
- Drug product selection and drug utilization review
- Patient monitoring and intervention
- Provision of cognitive services related to use of medications and devices

According to the American Pharmacists Association (APhA), formerly the American Pharmaceutical Association, the mission of pharmacy is to serve society as "the profession responsible for the appropriate use of medications, devices and services to achieve optimal therapeutic outcomes."

The Development of Modern-Day Pharmacy Practice(LO 1.4)

The practice of pharmacy originated thousands of years ago, but educational requirements and roles of both pharmacists and pharmacy technicians continue to change today. Table 1-1 highlights a chronological history of pharmacy and its milestones.

The practice of pharmacy originated very early in civilization, but the recognition and usage of pharmacy technicians has existed only in the last 50 years. Table 1-2 reviews the milestones for pharmacy technicians and their role in the practice of pharmacy. This role will continue to evolve in the years to come.

Table 1-1 Historical Perspectives of the Practice of Pharmacy

2600 B.C.–Babylonia 	Medical texts on clay tablets include symptoms of illness, prescriptions, and directions for compounding.
2000 B.C.–China	Shen Nung investigates the medicinal value of herbs and writes *Pen T-Sao,* a recording of 365 drugs.
1500 B.C.–Egypt	*Ebers Papyrus*, a collection of 800 prescription, is written in hieroglyphics mentioning over 700 remedies.
300 B.C.–Greece 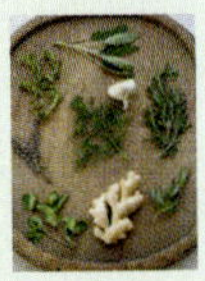	Theophrastus' (father of botany) writings deal with the medicinal qualities of herbs.
100 B.C.–Asia Minor	Mithridates develops an antidote for various poisons.
First century A.D.	Dioscorides writes about the collection of drugs, their storage, and use.
130–200 A.D.	Galen teaches and practices both medicine and pharmacy.
Eighth century A.D.	First apothecary shops appear in Baghdad.
1240 A.D.	Frederick II of Hohenstaufen issues edict of prescribing regulations for pharmacists.
1617–England 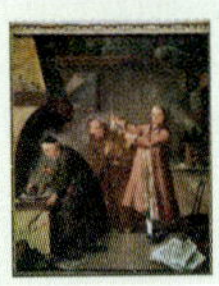	*Masters, Wardens, and Society of the Art and Mystery of the Apothecaries of the City of London* is the first organization of pharmacists in the Anglo-Saxon world.
1729	The Marshall Apothecary shop, a forerunner of retail pharmacy and training school for pharmacists, is established in Philadelphia.
1752	The first American hospital pharmacy is established in Philadelphia.
1777	Andrew Craigie is First Apothecary General.
1816	Friedrich Wilhelm Adam Serturner develops morphine and discovers alkaloids.
1820 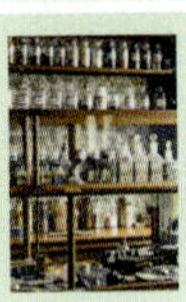	Caventou and Pelletier discover methods of separating quinine from cinchona bark.
1821	America's first pharmacy educational institution is established in Philadelphia.
1852	American Pharmaceutical Association is formed; renamed American Pharmacists Association in 2003.
1868	Pharmacy course at the University of Michigan is established, but the program does not require a pre-graduation apprenticeship.
1904	National Association of Boards of Pharmacy is established.

Table 1-2 Milestones for Pharmacy Technicians

January 1967	American Society of Health-System Pharmacists (ASHP) and the American Association of Colleges of Pharmacy (AACP) Joint Committees recommend that national pharmacy organizations "explore and study the need for, the use of, and the educational and training requirements of sub-professional pharmacy personnel." Members of the American Pharmaceutical Association (APhA), the National Association of Retail Druggists (NARD), the ASHP, and the AACP recommend that that the APhA "initiate a crash program to study the role technicians should have in the profession of pharmacy."
March 1970	ASHP releases the *ASHP Statement on Supportive Personnel in Hospital Pharmacy.*
April 1971	ASHP establishes a mechanism to accredit pharmacy technician training programs in its hospitals.
November 1975	ASHP releases *Training Guidelines for Hospital Pharmacy Supportive Personnel.*
June 1977	ASHP publishes *Manual for Hospital Pharmacy Technicians: A Programmed Course in Basic Skills.*
November 1980	ASHP creates *Minimum Competencies for Institutional Pharmacy Technicians with Training Guidelines.*
May 1981	ASHP recommends that an **accreditation** standard be established for pharmacy technician training programs.
September 1983	ASHP accredits the first technician-training program at Thomas Jefferson University Hospital in Philadelphia.
June 1983	ASHP approves a resolution that endorses **certification** and registration of pharmacy technicians, but opposes state licensure.
1995	ASHP, in conjunction with APhA, the Illinois Council of Health-System Pharmacists (ICHP), and the Michigan Pharmacists Association (MPA), creates the Pharmacy Technician Certification Board (PTCB).
March 1996	ASHP and APhA release the *White Paper on Pharmacy Technicians.*
December 2001	NABP becomes a partner with the PTCB.
January 2003	*The White Paper on Pharmacy Technicians 2002: Needed Changes Can No Longer Wait* is released.
February 2007	The PTCB examination is converted from a paper-based examination to that of a computer-based examination.

accreditation The process by which a private association, organization or government agency, after initial and periodic evaluations, grants recognition to an organization that has met certain established criteria.

certification The process by which a nongovernmental agency or association grants recognition to an individual who has met certain predetermined qualifications specified by that agency or association.

Tech Check

1. When did pharmacy organizations in the United States begin examining the need for sub-professional pharmacy personnel?(LO 1.4)
2. When was the PTCB formed?(LO 1.4)
3. When did the ASHP and APhA release the *White Paper on Pharmacy Technicians?*(LO 1.4)

At Your Service

You are working as a new pharmacy technician for an independent retail pharmacy that processes approximately 400 prescriptions a day. One day you observe one of the other pharmacy technicians answering a customer's question about the medication he or she is taking. Some of these questions include:

- What is the name of the medication I am taking? (LO 1.3)
- When should I take this drug? (LO 1.3)
- Will it interact with another medication that I am taking? (LO 1.3)
- What should I do if I forget to take my medication? (LO 1.3)

While reading this chapter, keep the following question in mind:

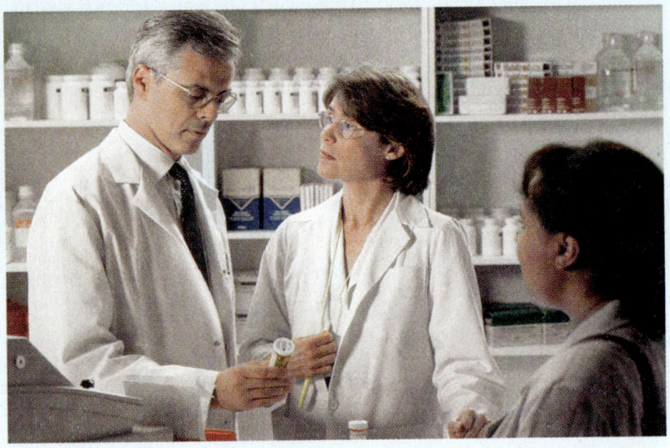

1. Was the pharmacy technician correct in answering the customer's question, or should he have informed the pharmacist of these questions? Why?

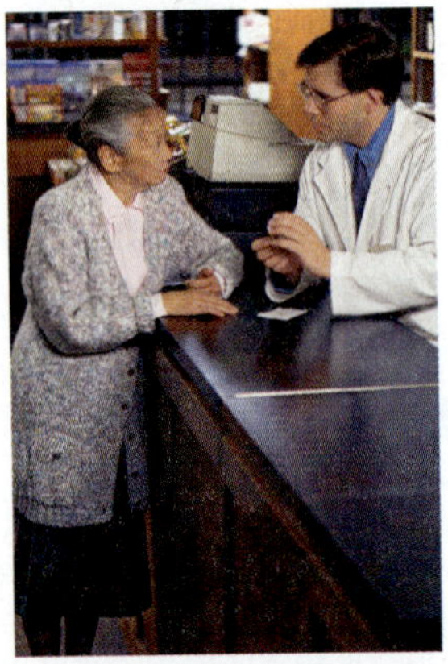

Figure 1-1 Pharmacist advising customer.

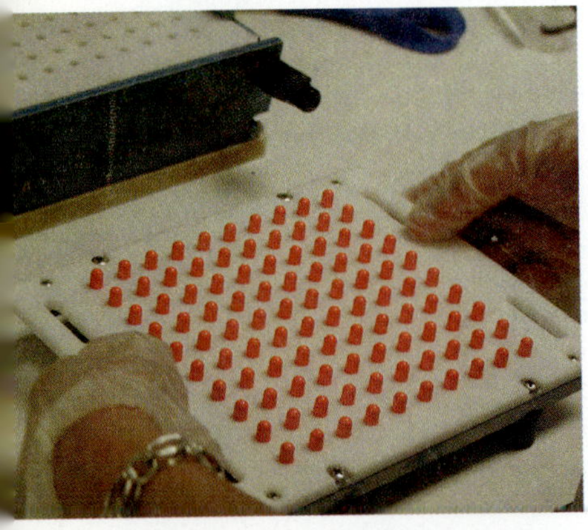

Figure 1-2 Pharmacist creating capsules.

The Practice of Pharmacy and the Pharmacy Technician (LO 1.1, 1.2, 1.3)

The Pharmacist

The primary role of the pharmacy technicians is to assist the pharmacist in the practice of pharmacy. However, what does a pharmacist do? What is the practice of pharmacy?

Pharmacists distribute drugs prescribed by physicians and other health practitioners (e.g., physician assistants and nurse practitioners) and provide information to patients about medications and their use. They advise physicians and other health practitioners on the selection, dosages, interactions, and side effects of medications (Figure 1-1). Pharmacists also monitor the health and progress of patients in response to drug therapy to ensure the safe and effective use of medication.

Pharmacists must understand the use, clinical effects, and composition of drugs, including their chemical, biological, and physical properties. Compounding, the actual mixing of ingredients to form powders, tablets, capsules, ointments, and solutions, is a small part of a pharmacist's practice. Most medicines are now produced by pharmaceutical companies in standard dosages and drug delivery forms (Figure 1-2). Most pharmacists work in a community setting, such as a retail drugstore, or in a health care facility, such as a hospital, nursing home, mental health institution, or neighborhood health clinic.

Pharmacists must be high school graduates or have obtained their GED. They must attend an approved pharmacy school in the United States. The curriculum is a minimum of six years (usually 2 years pharmacy prerequisite courses and 4 years of pharmacy school). Upon graduation they are awarded a PharmD degree. Pharmacists graduating prior to 1996 received a BS degree in pharmacy that took 5 years to obtain. Both degrees allow a pharmacist to perform the same tasks. While pharmacy students are in school they may perform an **internship** in a pharmacy to obtain pharmacy experience. Upon graduating from pharmacy school all pharmacists must complete a pharmacy **externship** to gain practical experience prior to taking their pharmacy boards to become licensed as a pharmacist. After pharmacists pass their pharmacy boards, they are licensed to practice pharmacy in that state only. If a pharmacist wishes to practice in another state, he or she may reciprocate the license to that state if the state pharmacy regulations permit or the pharmacist may need to retake the state pharmacy board examination for that particular state. Prior to renewing the license, a pharmacist must complete the required **continuing education** requirements of that state.

The majority of pharmacists work in retail (community) pharmacies (Figure 1-3). They counsel patients and answer questions about **prescription** drugs, including questions regarding possible side effects or interactions among various drugs. They provide information about over-the-counter (OTC) drugs and make recommendations after talking with the patient. They also may provide advice about the patient's diet, exercise, or stress management or about durable medical equipment and home health care supplies. In addition, they may be required to complete paperwork associated with the practice of pharmacy. Those who own or manage community pharmacies may sell non-health-related merchandise, hire and supervise personnel, and oversee the general operation of the pharmacy. Some community pharmacists provide specialized services to help patients manage conditions such as diabetes, asthma, smoking cessation, or high blood pressure. Some community pharmacists also are trained to administer vaccinations. Retail pharmacy is discussed in more detail in Chapter 14.

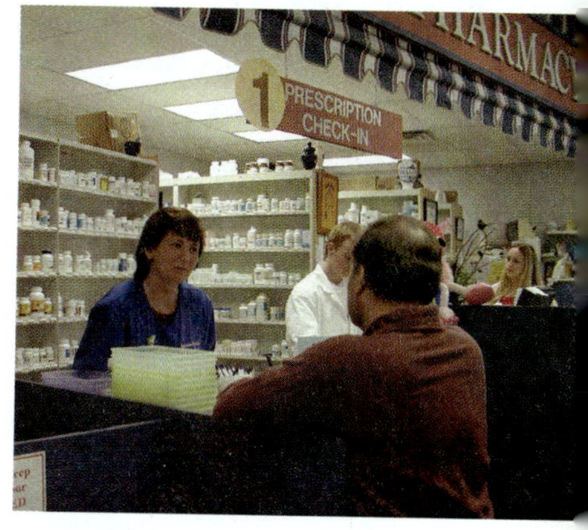

Figure 1-3 The retail pharmacy.

Some pharmacists work in health care facilities (such as hospitals) and dispense medications and advise the medical staff on the proper selection, usage, and effects of drugs. They may make sterile solutions to be administered intravenously. They assess, plan, and monitor drug programs or regimens. Pharmacists counsel hospitalized patients on the proper usage of medications upon being discharged from the hospital. Pharmacists evaluate the prescribing patterns by physicians in hospitals and their outcomes. Hospital pharmacy is discussed in more detail in Chapter 15.

Pharmacists working in a home health care environment monitor drug therapies and prepare infusions (solutions that are administered intravenously into patients) and other medications for use in the home. Some pharmacists specialize in specific drug therapy areas, such as intravenous nutrition support, oncology (cancer), nuclear pharmacy (used for chemotherapy), geriatric pharmacy, and psycho-pharmacotherapy (the treatment of mental disorders by means of drugs). Other pharmacy environments are discussed in more detail in Chapter 16.

Pharmacists are required to maintain confidential computerized records of patients' drug therapies to prevent harmful drug interactions. They are responsible for the accuracy of every prescription filled, but they often rely upon pharmacy technicians to assist them in the dispensing process. The pharmacist may delegate prescription filling and administrative tasks and supervise their completion.

internship Practical experience obtained while an individual is obtaining education or training.

externship Practical experience obtained after an individual has completed education or classroom training.

continuing education Ongoing, required education after one receives a degree, certification, or licensure in a particular discipline.

prescription A written directive by a licensed medical doctor for the preparation and administration of a remedy in the home setting. In some states, physician assistants and nurse practitioners may have the authority to prescribe medications.

The Pharmacy Technician

Pharmacists are responsible for many different tasks, and they cannot do everything by themselves. Pharmacy technicians play an integral role in the practice of pharmacy. The role of the pharmacy technician is to assist the pharmacist. Without the assistance of pharmacy technicians, the pharmacist would not be able to perform his or her duties as expected.

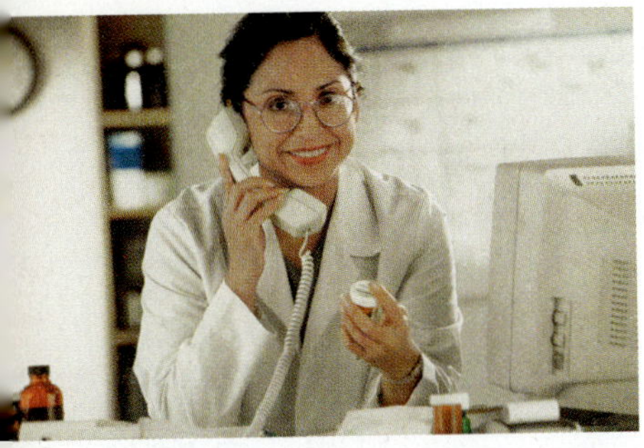

Figure 1-4 The pharmacy technician assisting patients.

Pharmacy technicians greet patients at the counter when they drop off or pick up a prescription. They relay important information to the pharmacist and may answer telephone calls from patients (Figure 1-4).

Pharmacy technicians perform technical duties in a pharmacy regardless of the setting. In contrast, the pharmacist performs both technical and judgmental tasks. The major differences between a pharmacist and a pharmacy technician are the judgmental tasks. Judgmental tasks involve the pharmacist making a decision on the pharmaceutical care of the patient. It is the pharmacist who makes the decision when a warning appears during a drug utilization evaluation of a patient's profile. It is the pharmacist who makes an OTC recommendation to a patient after collecting information from the patient and determining if the OTC therapy is appropriate. It is the duty of the pharmacist to counsel a patient regarding his or her medication because of the Omnibus Budget Reconciliation Act of 1990 (OBRA-90).

Duties of the Pharmacy Technician

Each state board of pharmacy will determine the duties a pharmacy technician may perform in the various pharmacy settings in the state. This information is presented in Tables 1-3 and 1-4. The pharmacist and the pharmacy technician must work as a team to provide optimum pharmaceutical care to patients.

Table 1-3 Duties of Pharmacy Technicians in Community Pharmacies by State

State	Accept Called-In Prescription from Physician's Office	Enter Prescription into Computer	Check the Work of Other Pharmacy Technicians	Call Physician for Refill Authorization	Compound Medications for Dispensing	Transfer Prescription Orders
Alabama	No	Yes	No	Yes	Yes	No
Alaska	No	Yes	No	Yes	Yes	No
Arizona	No	Yes	No	Yes	Yes	No
Arkansas	No	Yes	No	Yes	Yes	No
California	No	Yes	No	Yes	Yes	No
Colorado	No	Yes	Yes	Yes	Yes	No
Connecticut	No	Yes	No	Yes	Yes	No
Delaware	No	Yes	No	No	Yes	No
District of Columbia	Yes	Yes	No	Yes	Yes	No
Florida	No	Yes	No	Yes	Yes	No
Georgia	No	Yes	No	No	No	No
Hawaii	No	Yes	No	No	Yes	No

(Continued)

Table 1-3 Duties of Pharmacy Technicians in Community Pharmacies by State *(Continued)*

State	Accept Called-In Prescription from Physician's Office	Enter Prescription into Computer	Check the Work of Other Pharmacy Technicians	Call Physician for Refill Authorization	Compound Medications for Dispensing	Transfer Prescription Orders
Idaho	No	Yes	No	Yes	Yes	No
Illinois	*	Yes	No	Yes	Yes	No
Indiana	No	Yes	No	Yes	Yes	No
Iowa	Yes	Yes	No	Yes	Yes	No
Kansas	No	Yes	No	Yes	Yes	No
Kentucky	No	Yes	No	Yes	Yes	No
Louisiana	Yes	Yes	No	Yes	Yes	Yes
Maine	No	Yes	No	Yes	Yes	No
Maryland	No	Yes	*	Yes	Yes	No
Massachusetts	Yes	Yes	No	Yes	Yes	Yes
Michigan	Yes	Yes	Yes	No	Yes	No
Minnesota	No	Yes	No	Yes	No	Yes
Mississippi	No	Yes	No	Yes	Yes	No
Missouri	Yes	Yes	No	Yes	Yes	Yes
Montana	*	Yes	No	Yes	Yes	No
Nebraska	No	Yes	No	Yes	Yes	No
Nevada	No	Yes	No	Yes	Yes	No
New Hampshire	No	Yes	No	No	Yes	No
New Jersey	No	Yes	No	Yes	Yes	No
New Mexico	No	Yes	No	Yes	Yes	No
New York	No	Yes	No	No	No	No
North Carolina	Yes	Yes	No	Yes	Yes	Yes
North Dakota	Yes	Yes	Yes	Yes	Yes	Yes
Ohio	No	Yes	No	No	Yes	No
Oklahoma	No	Yes	No	Yes	Yes	No
Oregon	No	Yes	No	Yes	Yes	No
Pennsylvania	No	Yes	No	No	Yes	No
Puerto Rico	May key in but not enter	May key in but not enter	*	May key in but not enter	May key in but not enter	*
Rhode Island	*	Yes	No	Yes	Yes	No
South Carolina	Yes	Yes	Yes	Yes	Yes	Yes
South Dakota	No	No	No	No	Yes	No

(Continued)

Table 1-3 Duties of Pharmacy Technicians in Community Pharmacies by State *(Continued)*

State	Accept Called-In Prescription from Physician's Office	Enter Prescription into Computer	Check the Work of Other Pharmacy Technicians	Call Physician for Refill Authorization	Compound Medications for Dispensing	Transfer Prescription Orders
Tennessee	Yes	Yes	No	Yes	Yes	Yes
Texas	No	Yes	No	Yes	Yes	No
Utah	No	Yes	No	Yes	Yes	Yes
Vermont	No	Yes	No	Yes	Yes	No
Virginia	No	Yes	No	Yes	Yes	No
Washington	No	Yes	No	Yes	Yes	No
West Virginia	No	Yes	No	Yes	No	No
Wisconsin	*	Yes	No	Yes	Yes	No
Wyoming	No	Yes	N/A	Yes	Yes	No

* Check with the state board of pharmacy for specific details.

Source: **www.ptcb.org.**

Table 1-4 Duties of a Pharmacy Technician in a Hospital/Institutional Setting

State	Accept Called-In Prescription from Physician's Office	Enter Prescription into Computer	Check the Work of Other Pharmacy Technicians	Call Physician for Refill Authorization	Compound Medications for Dispensing	Transfer Prescription Orders
Alabama	No	Yes	No	Yes	Yes	No
Alaska	No	Yes	No	Yes	Yes	No
Arizona	No	Yes	No	Yes	Yes	No
Arkansas	No	Yes	No	Yes	Yes	No
California	No	Yes	No	Yes	Yes	No
Colorado	No	Yes	Yes	Yes	Yes	No
Connecticut	No	Yes	No	Yes	Yes	No
Delaware	No	Yes	No	No	Yes	No
District of Columbia	Yes	Yes	No	Yes	Yes	No
Florida	No	Yes	No	Yes	Yes	No
Georgia	No	Yes	No	No	No	No
Hawaii	No	Yes	No	No	Yes	No
Idaho	No	Yes	No	Yes	Yes	No
Illinois	*	Yes	No	Yes	Yes	No
Indiana	No	Yes	No	Yes	Yes	No
Iowa	Yes	Yes	No	Yes	Yes	No

(Continued)

Table 1-4 Duties of a Pharmacy Technician in a Hospital/Institutional Setting *(Continued)*

State	Accept Called-In Prescription from Physician's Office	Enter Prescription into Computer	Check the Work of Other Pharmacy Technicians	Call Physician for Refill Authorization	Compound Medications for Dispensing	Transfer Prescription Orders
Kansas	No	Yes	*	Yes	Yes	No
Kentucky	No	Yes	Yes	Yes	Yes	No
Louisiana	Yes	Yes	No	Yes	Yes	Yes
Maine	No	Yes	No	Yes	Yes	No
Maryland	No	Yes	No	Yes	Yes	No
Massachusetts	Yes	Yes	No	Yes	Yes	No
Michigan	Yes	Yes	Yes	No	Yes	Yes
Minnesota	No	Yes	Yes	Yes	No	No
Mississippi	No	Yes	No	Yes	Yes	No
Missouri	Yes	Yes	No	Yes	Yes	Yes
Montana	*	Yes	No	Yes	Yes	No
Nebraska	No	Yes	No	Yes	Yes	No
Nevada	No	Yes	No	Yes	Yes	No
New Hampshire	No	Yes	No	No	Yes	No
New Jersey	No	Yes	No	Yes	Yes	No
New Mexico	No	Yes	No	Yes	Yes	No
New York	No	Yes	No	No	No	No
North Carolina	Yes	Yes	No	Yes	Yes	Yes
North Dakota	Yes	Yes	Yes	Yes	Yes	Yes
Ohio	No	Yes	No	No	Yes	No
Oklahoma	No	Yes	No	Yes	Yes	No
Oregon	No	Yes	No	Yes	Yes	No
Pennsylvania	No	Yes	No	Yes	Yes	No
Puerto Rico	*	*	No	*	*	*
Rhode Island	No	Yes	No	Yes	Yes	No
South Carolina	Yes	Yes	Yes	Yes	Yes	Yes
South Dakota	No	No	No	No	Yes	No
Tennessee	Yes	Yes	No	Yes	Yes	Yes
Texas	No	Yes	No	Yes	Yes	No
Utah	No	Yes	No	Yes	Yes	Yes
Vermont	No	Yes	No	No	Yes	No
Virginia	No	Yes	No	Yes	Yes	No

(Continued)

Table 1-4 Duties of a Pharmacy Technician in a Hospital/Institutional Setting *(Continued)*

State	Accept Called-In Prescription from Physician's Office	Enter Prescription into Computer	Check the Work of Other Pharmacy Technicians	Call Physician for Refill Authorization	Compound Medications for Dispensing	Transfer Prescription Orders
Washington	No	Yes	Yes	Yes	Yes	No
West Virginia	No	Yes	No	Yes	Yes	No
Wisconsin	*	Yes	No	*	Yes	No
Wyoming	No	Yes	*	Yes	Yes	No

* Check with the state board of pharmacy for specific details.
Source: **www.ptcb.org.**

Occupational Outlook for Pharmacy Technicians

According to the Bureau of Labor Statistics, good job opportunities are expected for full-time and part-time work, especially for technicians with formal training or previous experience. These job openings for pharmacy technicians will result from the expansion of retail pharmacies and other employment settings and from the need to replace workers who transfer to other occupations or leave the labor force.

Employment of pharmacy technicians is expected to grow much faster than the average for all occupations through 2016 because as the population grows and ages, demand for pharmaceuticals will increase dramatically. The increased number of middle-aged and elderly people—who use more prescription drugs than younger people—will spur demand for technicians in all practice settings. With advances in science, more medications are becoming available to treat a greater number of conditions.

In addition, cost-conscious insurers, pharmacies, and health systems will continue to expand the role of technicians. As a result, pharmacy technicians will assume responsibility for some of the more routine tasks previously performed by pharmacists. Pharmacy technicians also will need to learn and master new pharmacy technology as it emerges. For example, robotic machines are being increasingly used to dispense medicine into containers. Technicians must oversee the machines, stock the bins, and label the containers. Although automation is increasingly incorporated into the job, it will not necessarily reduce the need for technicians.

Characteristics of a Pharmacy Technician

The practice of pharmacy is a conservative profession. Pharmacy technicians are required to maintain high ethical standards and are expected to present a neat, clean, and wholesome appearance (Figure 1-5).

Appearance

- Clothing is kept clean and wrinkle-free.
- White lab jacket may be worn.
- Hair is properly groomed.
- Hair color is not extreme in nature.
- Fingernails are kept short.
- Acrylic nails are not permitted due to OSHA (Occupational Safety and Health) regulations.

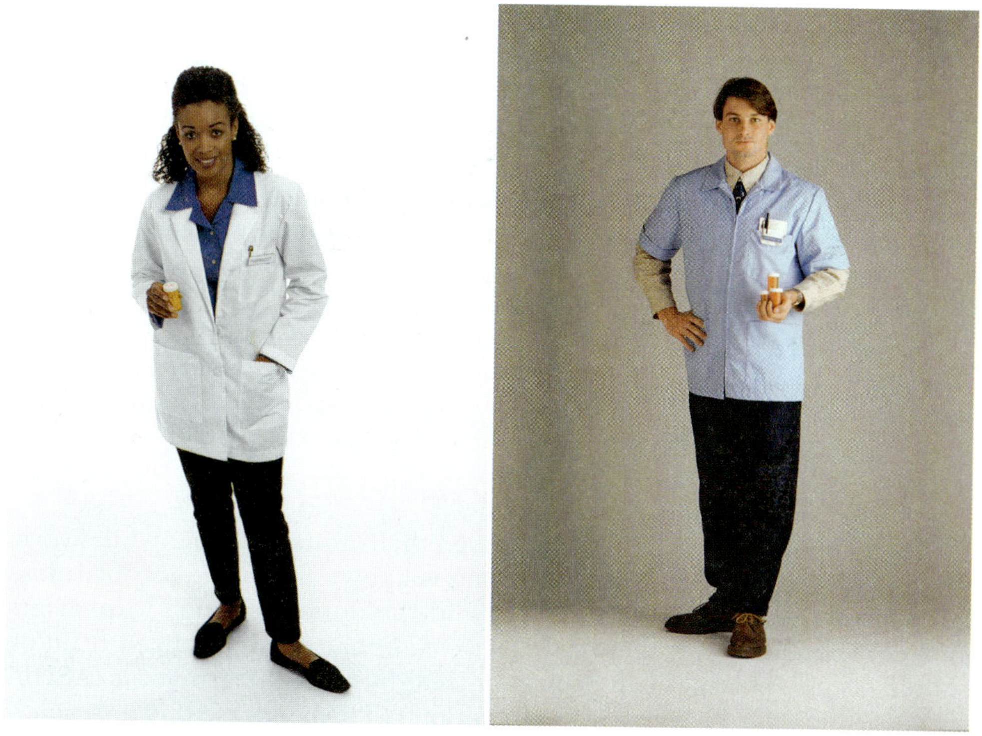

Figure 1-5 Pharmacy technician's appearance.

- Jewelry is kept to a minimum, especially in hospital settings.
- Body piercing and tattoos are hidden from the view of the patient.

Pharmacy technicians possess strong communication skills, which includes both speaking and listening. They maintain a courteous attitude at all times to patients and other health care practitioners. Pharmacy customers and patients possess some type of medical problem, and they are seeking a solution for that problem. Therefore, pharmacy technicians must be able to assist patients with their needs.

Approximately 30% of a pharmacy technician's time is spent performing tasks that require mathematical calculations. Much of the pharmacy math performed can be solved using proportions. Examples of math applications in pharmacy include:

- Calculating the proper quantity of a medication to be dispensed
- Calculating the amount of ingredients during compounding
- Performing calculations in preparing intravenous mixtures
- Proper billing of prescriptions to third-party payers.

Pharmacy calculations are discussed in greater detail in Chapter 5.

The practice of pharmacy requires that individuals are dependable and accountable for their actions. They are detail-oriented and are very conscientious in their work. Pharmacy technicians possess the ability to respect confidential patient data. Maintaining confidentiality is one of the most important aspects of the federal legislation related to health care called HIPAA. HIPAA will be discussed in detail in chapter 4. They must be able to adjust to their work pace if large influxes of prescriptions are suddenly received. Pharmacy technicians show a desire to learn about new drug therapies and their impact on disease. As part of the health care team, pharmacy technicians must be able to work as a member of that team and also be able to work independently in specific situations.

Tech Check

4. What pharmacy technician duties are legally permitted by the state board of pharmacy in your state if you are working in a retail pharmacy?(LO 1.3)
5. What pharmacy technician duties are legally permitted by the state board of pharmacy in your state if you are working in a hospital setting?(LO 1.3)
6. List three adjectives that describe a pharmacy technician.(LO 1.1)

Pharmacy Technician Training, Education, and Credentialing(LO 1.5, 1.6)

The early pharmacy technicians received their initial training while working in a pharmacy. This type of training is known as **on-the-job training.** As the practice of pharmacy evolves and the duties assigned to pharmacy technicians expand, there is a consensus that a standardized training should occur. The American Society of Health-System Pharmacists (ASHP) and the American Pharmacists Association (APhA) endorse this position.

In 2002, approximately 247 schools and training institutions offered a wide range of credentials for pharmacy technicians, ranging from diplomas or certificates to associate degrees. The Armed Forces provides formal training for all of their pharmacy technicians. Formal pharmacy technician training programs range in length from 540 to 2145 contact hours. The ASHP is one of several organizations that accredits pharmacy technician training programs and requires a minimum of 600 contact hours and a minimum of 15 weeks in length. The Pharmacy Technicians Educators Council (PTEC) endorses the ASHP minimum requirements.

In recent years, there has been a strong movement toward the standardization of training for pharmacy technicians. The ASHP, APhA, PTEC, the American Association of Colleges of Pharmacy (AACP), and the National Association of Chain Drug Stores (NACDS) have worked on developing the *Model Curriculum for Pharmacy Technician Training.* All groups believe that both pharmacy technician education and training should be standards-based.

Diploma and Certificate Programs

Formal pharmacy technician education programs require classroom and laboratory work in a variety of areas including:

- Medical and pharmaceutical terminology
- Pharmaceutical calculations
- Pharmacy record keeping
- Pharmaceutical techniques
- Pharmacy law and ethics

Technicians also are required to learn medication names, actions, uses, and doses. Many training programs include internships, where students gain hands-on experience in actual pharmacies while they are taking courses, or externships, which provide hands-on experience after a student has completed his or her classroom education. Students receive a diploma, a certificate, or an

on-the-job training The training obtained from working in a specific job. This form of training is informal in nature and may lack structure.

associate degree, depending on the program. Recently, some pharmacy technician programs have been approved to be taught online.

Associate Degree Programs

Many pharmacy technician educational programs are awarding an associate degree for pharmacy technicians. These programs are normally 2 years in length. The program requirements may vary from institution to institution. They possess two distinct phases:

- Pharmacy technician courses
- Core of general education courses include requirements in English composition, psychology, sociology, biology, chemistry, or business

On-the-Job Training (Externship)

After a pharmacy technician has completed an approved pharmacy technician program, he or she may be required to perform an externship. Unlike an internship, where the pharmacy technician obtains work experience while still taking classes, the externship occurs after the student has completed all assigned classroom and lab work.

Both an internship and externship allow students to apply the knowledge they have learned from their studies. In both situations, the pharmacy technician is exposed to real-life situations in the practice of pharmacy. Pharmacy technicians will assist the pharmacist in the performance of their duties (Figure 1-6). They will:

- Enter patient information into a computer system.
- Interpret prescriptions and medication orders.
- Pour, count, and package medications.
- Prepare extemporaneous compounds and intravenous admixtures.
- Bill insurance providers.

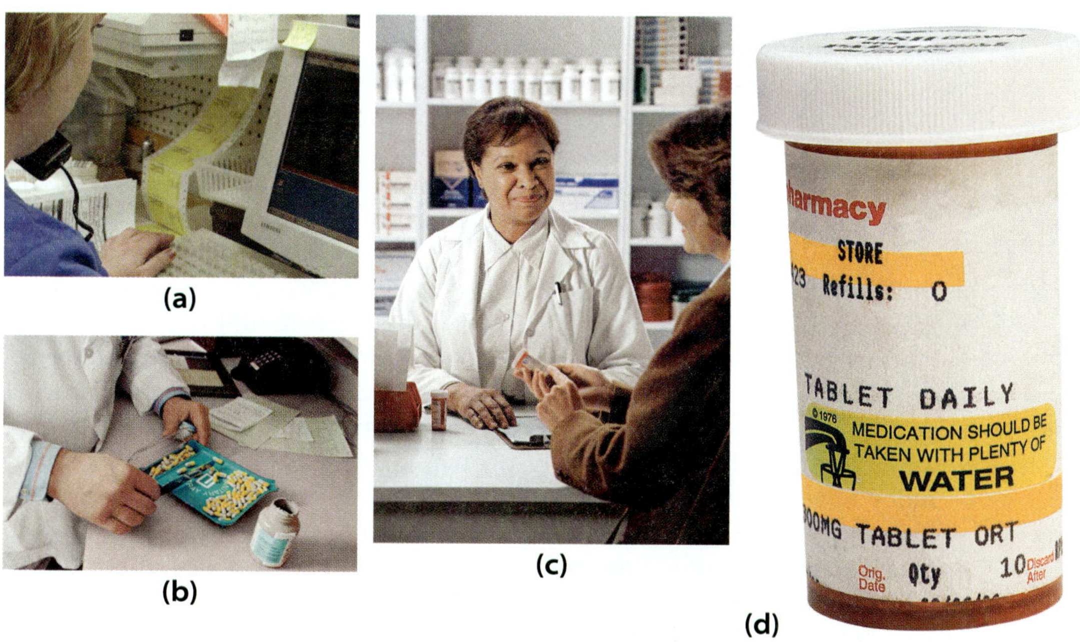

Figure 1-6 (*a*) Entering patient information into a computer. (*b*) Counting medication. (*c*) Assisting the patient. (*d*) Interpreting medication orders.

- Reorder medications.
- Stock the pharmacy with medications and pharmacy supplies.
- Assist the patient.

At all times, the pharmacy technician must be supervised by the pharmacist.

Credentialing

The National Association of Boards of Pharmacy (NABP) establishes task forces to examine issues in the practice of pharmacy in the United States. The NABP has issued statements to formally recognize pharmacy technicians, requested a national technician certification examination, and has been active in changing the language in state's statutes regarding pharmacy technicians. The NABP believes that pharmacy technicians should be registered.

The American Society of Health-System Pharmacists Task Force on Technical Personnel in Pharmacy has established the following definitions:

- **Credentialing** is the process of formally recognizing professional or technical competence. After a pharmacy technician has satisfactorily passed the Pharmacy Technician Certification Board's (PTCB) Pharmacy Technician Certification Examination (PTCE), he or she is awarded the CPhT credential. Pharmacists receive the credential of RPh upon being licensed by the state board of pharmacy.
- Accreditation is the process of granting recognition or vouching for conformance with a standard (usually refers to recognition of an institution). In some states, the board of pharmacy recognizes pharmacy technician programs if specific standards are met. Accrediting Bureau of Health Education Schools (ABHES) is an accrediting body for career schools with allied health programs to include pharmacy technician programs. All hospitals and long-term care facilities must be accredited by The Joint Commission (TJC), formerly the Joint Commission on Accreditation of Healthcare Organizations (JCAHO). Without this accreditation, their existence would cease to exist because they would not be able to participate under the Centers for Medicare and Medicaid Services.
- Certification is the process by which a government agency grants recognition to an individual who has met predetermined qualifications specified by the agency or association. Pharmacy technicians can become certified by the PTCB based upon their knowledge of core pharmacy competencies.
- **Licensure** is the process by which a nongovernmental agency or association grants permission to an individual to engage in a particular occupation based upon finding that the individual has attained a minimal degree of competency necessary to ensure that the public health, safety, and welfare will be reasonably protected. A few state boards of pharmacy have begun to license pharmacy technicians. The state boards of pharmacy issue both pharmacy and pharmacist licenses.
- **Registering** is defined as the process of making a list or being included on a list. Pharmacy technicians must submit an application, which indicates their PTCB or other agency's certification number with its expiration date, if they took a state pharmacy technician examination or if they completed a pharmacy board–approved training program. The

credentialing The general process of formally recognizing professional or technical competence.

licensure The process by which a government agency grants permission to an individual to engage in a given occupation based upon the finding that the applicant has attained the minimal degree of competency necessary to ensure that the public health, safety, and welfare will be reasonably protected.

registering The process of making a list or being included on an existing list. In many states, a pharmacy technician may be required to register with the state board of pharmacy.

registration process may vary among the states. In an occupational setting, such as pharmacy, it may or may not be illegal to carry out a particular function without being registered.

These topics are discussed in more detail in Chapter 19.

Tech Check

7. What is the meaning of ASHP?(LO 1.5, 1.6)

8. What is the meaning of APhA?(LO 1.5, 1.6)

9. What is the meaning of PTEC?(LO 1.5, 1.6)

Pharmacy Practice Settings and Pharmacy Technician Responsibilities(LO 1.7)

Community (Retail) Setting

Community pharmacies are found in a variety of locations to include urban, suburban, and rural areas. A community pharmacy maintains a physician-pharmacist-patient relationship. A community pharmacy may take the form of an independent pharmacy, **chain pharmacy,** or franchise pharmacy. An **independent pharmacy** is privately owned and functions, in varying degrees, to serve society's need for both drug products and pharmaceutical services. Independent pharmacies were once known as the neighborhood drug store.

The U.S. Department of Commerce defines a chain pharmacy as those units with prescription departments that are centrally owned by individuals or organizations who own 11 or more units. Chain pharmacies offer a wider range of goods than an independent pharmacy. Grocery stores, mass merchandisers, and discounters have included a pharmacy as one of their store's departments. Examples of chain pharmacies include CVS, Walgreens, and Rite Aid (Figure 1-7).

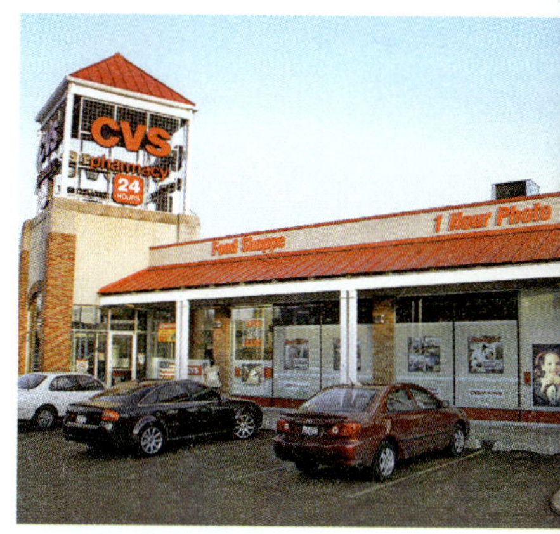

Figure 1-7 CVS Pharmacy.

A **franchise pharmacy** is one where the franchisor (or licensor) licenses another party (franchisee or licensee) to use the franchisor's trade name, trademarks, commercial symbols, patents, copyrights, and other property in the distribution and selling goods and services. An example of a franchise pharmacy is *Medicine Shoppe*. According to the Bureau of Labor Statistics, 7 out of 10 (70%) pharmacy positions are found in retail pharmacies.

According to the PTCB, a pharmacy technician practicing in a retail setting may have the following responsibilities:

- Help patients who are dropping off or picking up prescription orders.
- Enter prescription orders into the computer.
- Create and update patient's health and insurance information in the computer.
- Assist the pharmacist, under direct supervision, in the practice of pharmacy, in accordance with local, state, federal, and company regulations.
- Communicate with insurance carriers to obtain payment for prescription claims.
- At point of sale, verify that customer receives correct prescription(s).

chain pharmacy A retail unit containing prescription departments that are centrally owned by individuals or organizations with 11 or more units.

independent pharmacy A privately owned pharmacy, whose function is to serve society's need for both drug products and pharmaceutical services.

franchise pharmacy A pharmacy where the owner of a trademark, a patent, or a product licenses another party to sell products or services under the franchisor.

- Complete weekly distribution center medication orders, place orders on shelves, and verify all associated paperwork.
- Assist the pharmacist with filling and labeling prescriptions.
- Prepare the pharmacy inventory.
- Screen telephone calls for the pharmacist.
- Communicate with prescribers and their agents to obtain refill authorization.
- Compound oral solutions, ointments, and creams.
- Prepackage bulk medications.
- Maintain an awareness of developments in the community and pharmaceutical fields that relate to job responsibilities and integrate them into practice.
- Assist in training new employees.
- Assist other pharmacy technicians.
- Assist pharmacist in scheduling and maintaining workflow.
- Maintain knowledge of loss prevention technique.

Retail pharmacy is discussed in more detail in Chapter 14.

Hospital/Institutional Setting

A hospital is an institution for treatment of persons who are sick. A hospital's organizational structure generally has a formalized pattern of authority, responsibility, and coordination that affects all departments of the hospital, including the pharmacy. A board of directors oversees the operation of the hospital, and a chief executive officer (CEO) oversees and runs the hospital. Hospitals provide many different types of services to patients. All hospitals have a variety of departments to which specialized functions are performed, such as the emergency department, the radiology department, respiratory therapy, physical therapy, medical services, pharmacy services, nursing services, and a nutritional staff, to name a few (Figure 1-8).

A hospital is open 24 hours a day, 7 days a week, and 365 days a year. A hospital may be either for-profit or nonprofit. Hospitals may treat patients with a specific condition such as a burn; psychiatric hospitals treat persons with mental illnesses; other hospitals may treat active and retired military personnel, such as the Veterans Administration (VA) hospital; others may treat a specific demographic such as a children's or women's hospital. One commonality among all hospitals, however, is the treatment of patients with some form of illness. A hospital has physician-pharmacist-nurse-patient relationships. These relationships illustrate the interdependency of various health care practitioners and the importance of teamwork in our health care system.

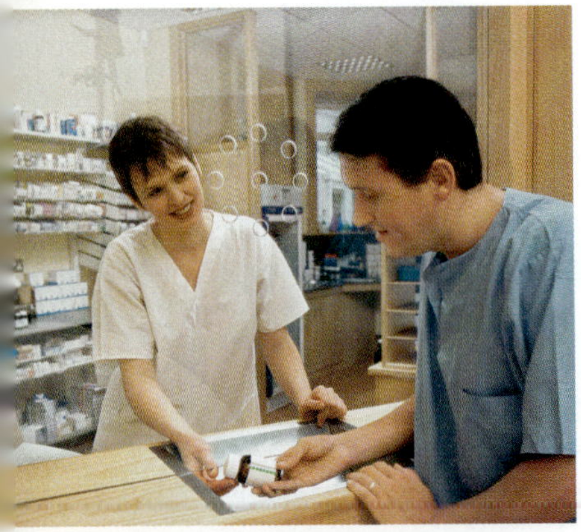

Figure 1-8 Hospital pharmacy.

The director of pharmacy reports to the hospital administrator. In many situations, the pharmacy director will oversee professional and clinical services, educational and technical services, and research and support services. Educational and technical services may oversee the hiring and training of pharmacy technicians. Under the direction of a pharmacist, the pharmacy technician performs pharmacy-related functions, in compliance with department policies and procedures that provide optimal pharmaceutical care.

Responsibilities of hospital pharmacy technicians may include:

- Rotate through all work areas of the pharmacy.
- Transport medications, drug delivery devices, and other pharmacy equipment from the pharmacy to nursing units and clinics.
- Pick up copies of physician orders, automated medication administra-

tion records, and unused medications from the nursing units and return them to the pharmacy.
- Fill patient medication cassettes.
- Prepare medications and supplies for dispensing, including:
    - Prepacking bulk medications.
    - Compounding ointments, creams, oral solutions, and other medications.
    - Preparing chemotherapeutic agents.
    - Compounding total parenteral nutrition solutions.
    - Compounding large-volume intravenous mixtures.
    - Packaging and preparing drugs being used in clinical investigations.
    - Preparing prescriptions for outpatients.
    - Checking continuous unit-dose medications.
    - Controlling and auditing narcotics, and stocking substance.
- Assist pharmacists in entering medication orders into the computer system.
- Prepare inventories, order drugs and supplies from the storeroom; receive drugs and stock shelves in various pharmacy locations.
- Screen telephone calls.
- Perform monthly nursing unit inspections, maintain workload records, and collect quality assurance data.
- Assist in training new employees.
- Assist other pharmacy technicians.
- Coordinate insurance billing including third-party prescriptions.
- Delivering and placing unit dose medications in automated dispensing equipment (machines).
- Handle triage telephone/window inquiries.

Hospital pharmacy is discussed in more detail in Chapter 15.

Long-Term Care Pharmacy

Long-term care is defined as a range of health and health-related services provided to individuals who, because of their physical and mental conditions, require medical, nursing, or supportive care for a prolonged period of 30 or more days (Figure 1-9). Long-term care will continue to expand in the United States as we see individuals living longer.

Within the past several decades there has been an increase in chronic disease conditions with associated social and emotional conditions. Presently there are more beds in long-term care facilities than there are in acute-care facilities.

Long-term care facilities encompass a wide range of facilities. These include:

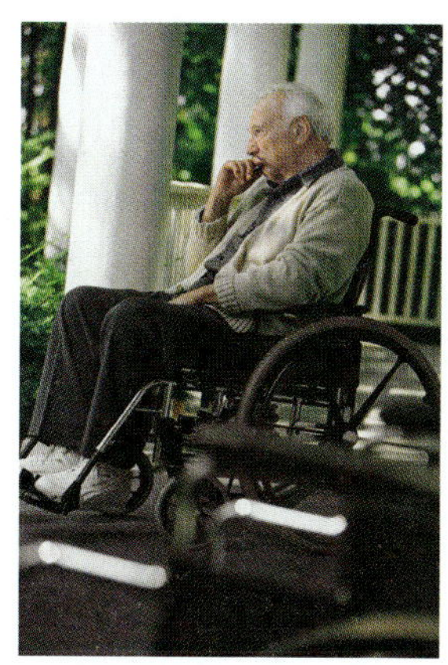

Figure 1-9 Long-term care.

- Long-term care facility (LTCF) formerly known as "nursing home." A LTCF provides nursing, personal, and residential care for the residents.
- Extended-care facility (ECF) is a nursing home that qualifies for participation in Medicare.
- Skilled nursing facility (SNF) is a nursing home that meets the qualifications for both Medicaid and Medicare.
- Intermediate-care facility (ICF) is defined according to the *Congressional Discursive Dictionary of Healthcare* as "an institution recognized under the Medicaid program which is licensed state laws to provide, on a regu-

lar basis, health related care and services to individuals who do not require the degree of care and treatment which a hospital or skilled nursing facility is designed to provide, but who, because of their mental or physical condition require services (above the level of room and board) which can be made available to them in only institutional facilities."

Long-term care pharmacy is the pharmacy services provided to long-term care facilities. The American Society of Consultant Pharmacists has recognized the importance of utilizing pharmacy technicians effectively in the long-term care pharmacy setting. Consultant pharmacists are now able to focus on medication-related issues of their patients. Many of the tasks that were previously performed by pharmacists have been delegated to qualified pharmacy technicians. Consultant pharmacists have identified five key areas where pharmacy technicians can greatly assist the pharmacist in their duties. These areas include:

Data collection and reporting

- Conduct customer satisfaction assessments.
- Assist in collection of data for patient assessment tools.
- Compile continuous quality improvement data.
- Perform drug utilization evaluation (DUE).
- Maintain computerized information between dispensing and consultant pharmacists.
- Prepare pharmacy reports.
- Prepare billing statements.

Surveys and inspections

- Conduct medication room inspections.
- Conduct narcotic audits.
- Check emergency boxes and replace outdated medications.
- Check orders for completeness.
- Assist with medication pass evaluation.

Education

- Assist in facility meetings (such as quality assurance committees).
- Help organize and maintain medical library.
- Provide in-services to facility personnel.

Maintenance

- Assist in maintenance of devices (fax machines, automated dispensing systems, medication carts, etc.).

Dispensing/inventory

- Order medication stock.
- Package medications.
- Mix intravenous solutions.
- Fill and label prescriptions.
- Call for refills.

Mail-Order Pharmacy

Pharmacy technicians who work in mail-order pharmacies have varying responsibilities depending on state regulations. Technicians receive written prescriptions or requests for prescription refills from patients

(Figure 1-10). They also may receive prescriptions sent electronically from the doctor's office. They must verify that the information on the prescription is complete and accurate. To prepare the prescription, technicians must retrieve, count, pour, weigh, measure, and sometimes mix the medication. Then, they prepare the prescription labels, select the type of prescription container, and affix the prescription and auxiliary labels to the container. Once the prescription is filled, technicians price and file the prescription, which must be checked by a pharmacist before it is mailed to the patient. Technicians may establish and maintain patient profiles, prepare insurance claim forms, and stock and take inventory of prescription and OTC medications.

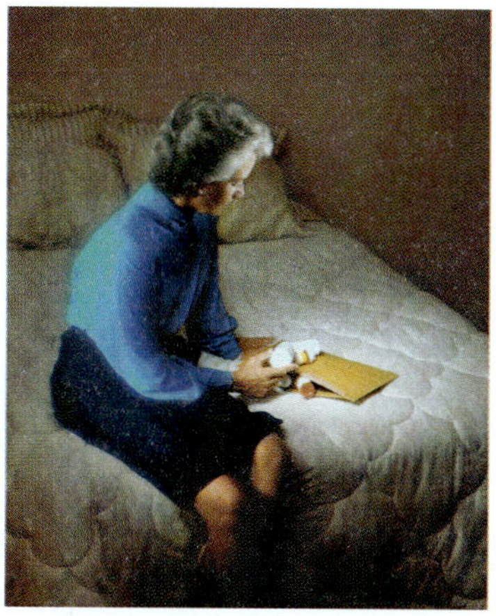

Figure 1-10 Mail-order prescriptions.

Managed-Care Pharmacy

Managed-care pharmacy is the practice of pharmacy that involves both clinical and administrative activities performed in a managed-care pharmacy. Under the supervision of a pharmacist, the pharmacy technician:

- Handles daily the ongoing pharmacy benefit telephone calls from members, pharmacy providers, and physicians.
- Troubleshoots third-party prescription claim questions with an understanding of online rejections and plan parameters.
- Develops and maintains an electronic service log on all telephone calls with complete follow-up history.
- Develops a trending report on the service calls and identifies possible trends in pharmacy service.
- Provides as needed telephone and administrative support for the department.

Home Infusion Pharmacy

Home infusion therapy involves the administration of medications, nutrients, or other solutions in the home. Infusion therapy always originates with a prescription from a qualified physician, who is overseeing the care of the patient. Infusion therapy is designed to achieve positive therapeutic results. A provider of infusion therapy must be a licensed health care professional such as a nurse, physician, or pharmacist. Home nursing services are also provided to ensure proper patient education and training and to monitor the care of the patient in the home. These may be provided directly by infusion pharmacy nursing staff or by a qualified home health agency (Figure 1-11).

Home infusion therapies include anti-infectives for the treatment of infections such as pneumonia, pain management for cancer-related pain, and blood transfusions for the treatment of hemophilia. Pharmacy technicians working in home infusion pharmacies order the supplies needed to compound intravenous admixtures and prepare the intravenous admixtures in addition to other tasks that a pharmacy technician might be responsible for doing in a retail pharmacy setting. Home infusion pharmacies will continue to grow as more physicians continue to approve of this type of therapy, and third-party providers acknowledge the savings of having the patient receive these services at home.

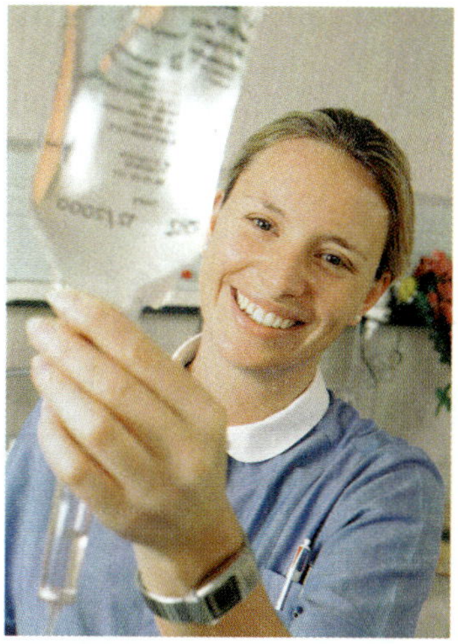

Figure 1-11 Nurse with an IV drip.

Department of Defense

All of the branches of the Department of Defense utilize civilian pharmacy technicians in addition to those members of the military that are pharmacy technicians. Civilian pharmacy technicians may work in military base medical clinic hospital pharmacies. These pharmacies process medication orders in pharmacies and prescriptions for current members of the military, retired members of the military, and family members of the military members.

Pharmaceutical Companies

Pharmacy technicians may work for the drug manufacturers in the marketing department, or as a pharmaceutical salesperson, where they visit health care provider's office offices to inform the physician of their company's line of products. They may also call on pharmacies to provide information and to collect information on the sales of their products.

Tech Check

10. Which practice setting employs 70% of the U.S. pharmacy positions?(LO 1.7)

11. What are some of the responsibilities of a hospital pharmacy technician?(LO 1.7)

12. What are some of the responsibilities of a pharmacy technician who works in a mail-order pharmacy?(LO 1.7)

Chapter Summary

Understanding the participation in the administration and management of pharmacy practice is vital to the pharmacy technician. Important points to know are the following:

- The profession of pharmacy has its roots at the beginning of civilization.
- The role of the pharmacist has evolved resulting in an increase for the need for pharmacy technicians.
- The primary task of pharmacy technicians is to assist the pharmacist.
- Pharmacy technicians are responsible for technical tasks in the pharmacy.
- Certification is being required by many employers and by the various state boards of pharmacy.
- There are many different career options for pharmacy technicians. Many of these career options may require special education or training for the pharmacy technicians.

Chapter Review

Case Study Questions

1. Where could he find information about pharmacy technicians?(LO 1.2)
2. What type of career opportunities exist for pharmacy technicians?(LO 1.7)
3. What personal characteristics are required for pharmacy technicians?(LO 1.1)
4. What are some of the tasks a pharmacy technician performs?(LO 1.3)

At Your Service Question

1. Was the pharmacy technician correct in answering the customer's question, or should he have informed the pharmacist of these questions? Why?(LO 1.3)

Multiple Choice

Select the best answer.

1. Which of the following best defines the practice of pharmacy?(LO 1.4)
   a. Art and science of preparing and dispensing medications
   b. Art and science of preparing and dispensing medications and providing drug-related information to the public
   c. Providing medical care to the public
   d. Providing pharmaceutical information to the public
2. What is the primary task for pharmacy technicians?(LO 1.2)
   a. Assist the pharmacist
   b. Counsel patients
   c. Manage inventory
   d. Process prescriptions
3. What type of duties does a pharmacy technician perform regardless of the pharmacy setting?(LO 1.3)
   a. Consultative
   b. Judgmental
   c. Technical
   d. All of the above
4. What is the purpose of certification?(LO 1.5)
   a. Certification is the process of registering with a nongovernmental agency or association.
   b. Certification is the process of providing information to a nongovernmental agency or association that one has specific talents.
   c. Certification is the process by which a nongovernmental agency or association grants recognition to an individual who has met specific qualifications of that association.
   d. Certification is the process of submitting of information to a regulatory agency that one possesses specific skills for a particular profession.
5. If a pharmacy technician were working in a CVS Pharmacy, in what type of pharmacy setting would he or she be working?(LO 1.7)
   a. Community pharmacy
   b. Institutional pharmacy
   c. Long-term care pharmacy
   d. Managed-care pharmacy
6. Which of the following would be an example of a franchise pharmacy?(LO 1.7)
   a. CVS Pharmacy
   b. Medicine Shoppe
   c. Omnicare Pharmacy
   d. Rodman's Pharmacy
7. If a pharmacy technician were preparing IVs to be administered in the patient's home, what type of setting would it be?(LO 1.7)
   a. Home infusion pharmacy
   b. Institutional pharmacy
   c. Long-term care pharmacy
   d. Mail-order pharmacy
8. If a pharmacy technician were working for Pfizer pharmaceuticals as a pharmacy salesperson, what type of practice would it be?(LO 1.7)
   a. Community pharmacy
   b. Drug manufacturer
   c. Institutional pharmacy
   d. Long-term care pharmacy
9. What is the minimum number of days that a person must be hospitalized to be considered for a long-term care facility?(LO 1.7)
   a. 7 days
   b. 14 days
   c. 21 days
   d. 30 days
10. In what type of pharmacy setting would a pharmacy technician be working in a US Army base hospital pharmacy?(LO 1.7)
    a. Chain pharmacy
    b. Military pharmacy
    c. Mail-order pharmacy
    d. Managed-care pharmacy
11. Which of the following would least likely be a pharmacy technician task associated with a mail-order pharmacy?(LO 1.7)
    a. Data entry
    b. IV preparation
    c. Prescription billing
    d. Prescription processing

12. Which of the following tasks would a pharmacy technician perform in a community pharmacy?(LO 1.7)
    a. Bill prescriptions to a third-party provider
    b. Contact a physician's office for a new prescription for a patient
    c. Prepare prescriptions for mailing
    d. Intravenous preparation

13. Which of the following tasks would a pharmacy technician least likely perform in a community pharmacy?(LO 1.7)
    a. Count medication
    b. Pour medication
    c. Measure medication
    d. Prepare IVs

14. Which of the following routes could be used for home infusion products?(LO 1.7)
    a. Enterally
    b. Intravenously
    c. Subcutaneously
    d. All of the above

15. Which of following tasks might a pharmacy technician perform in a managed-care setting?(LO 1.7)
    a. Handles pharmacy benefit telephone calls from members, pharmacy providers, and physicians
    b. Troubleshoot third-party prescription claim questions with an understanding of online rejections and plan parameters
    c. Develop and maintain an electronic service log on all telephone calls with complete follow-up history
    d. All of the above

16. Which of the following types of tasks might a pharmacy technician perform in a long-term care pharmacy?(LO 1.7)
    a. Collect data
    b. Conduct surveys
    c. Perform surveys
    d. All of the above

17. Which of the following tasks might a pharmacy technician perform in a hospital?(LO 1.7)
    a. Fill patient medication cassettes
    b. Prepare medications and supplies for dispensing
    c. Prepackage bulk medications
    d. All of the above

18. Which of the following terms refers to obtaining practical experience upon completion of a formalized pharmacy technician education?(LO 1.6)
    a. Externship
    b. Internship
    c. On-the-job training
    d. Work study

19. Which type of pharmacy setting would a pharmacy technician transport medications, drug-delivery devices, and other pharmacy equipment from the pharmacy to nursing units and clinics?(LO 1.7)
    a. Community pharmacy
    b. Hospital pharmacy
    c. Home infusion pharmacy
    d. Managed-care pharmacy

20. Which of the following is least likely a task a pharmacy technician would perform?(LO 1.3)
    a. Counsel a patient
    b. Enter patient information into a computer system
    c. Interpret prescriptions and medication orders
    d. Pour and count medications

Definitions

Print the meaning of the following acronyms.

APhA ______________________

ASHP ______________________

DUE ______________________

ECF ______________________

ICF ______________________

LTCF ______________________

PTCB ______________________

PTEC ______________________

SNF ______________________

TPN ______________________

Critical Thinking Questions

1. Go to a local pharmacy and ask the pharmacist what he or she looks for when interviewing pharmacy technicians.(LO 1.1)
2. What three characteristics of pharmacy technicians do you feel are the most important and why?(LO 1.1)
3. Why is certification important to the pharmacy technician?(LO 1.5)
4. Does it make a difference to the patient if a pharmacy technician is certified?(LO 1.5)
5. Which pharmacy setting do you find exciting as a pharmacy technician? Why?(LO 1.7)

HIPAA Scenario

Susan Taylor is the mother of a 16-year-old girl. She suspects that her daughter Pamela has begun to take birth control pills without her permission and goes to the local pharmacy her family uses and asks if her daughter has filled a prescription recently. The new pharmacy technician looks up Pamela's profile and informs Susan that Pamela filled a prescription for a birth control patch 3 weeks ago. Susan confronts an enraged Pamela, who calls the pharmacy supervisor and demands that the pharmacy technician be fired for giving her mother information about her prescription history without her permission.

Discussion Questions(PTCB II. 73)

1. Should the pharmacy technician have given Susan Taylor information about the drugs her daughter was taking?
2. What actions should the technician have taken?
3. How should the technician be disciplined?

Internet Activities

1. Go to **www.caremark.com** and identify the type of services provided by Caremark.
2. Compare the required knowledge skills for pharmacy technicians by the PTCB and ASHP, which are found on their Web sites: **www.ptcb.org, www.ashp.org.**(LO 1.5)
3. Select a pharmacy continuing education article of your interest from one of the many pharmacy Web sites mentioned in this chapter. Report to your classmates what you learned from the article.(LO 1.5)

2

Basic Safety and Standards

Key Terms

antiretroviral
antiseptic agent
aseptic technique
bloodborne
bloodstream infection
cardiopulmonary resuscitation (CPR)
Centers for Disease Control and Prevention (CDC)
hand hygiene
incident report
multidrug-resistant pathogens
nosocomial
Occupational Safety and Health Administration (OSHA)
pathogen
postexposure prophylaxis (PEP)

Learning Outcomes

Upon completion of this chapter, you will be able to:

2.1 Describe the role of regulatory agencies (CDC, OSHA) as they pertain to safety and standards in health care settings.

2.2 Define *infectious disease*, *nosocomial infections*, and *airborne* and *bloodborne diseases*.

2.3 List the four major types of nosocomial infections.

2.4 Describe methods to prevent airborne and bloodborne disease transmission.

2.5 Discuss the role of prevention in the spread of disease.

2.6 Discuss the role of hand hygiene in the prevention of disease.

2.7 Describe the proper technique for hand washing.

2.8 List and identify the proper use of personal protective equipment (PPE).

2.9 Define and explain the significance of policies and procedures as they pertain to documentation, reporting, and the prevention of disease transmission in health care organizations.

2.10 Describe the activities related to the incident report.

2.11 Describe HIV prophylaxis.

2.12 Discuss the importance of emergency preparedness (for example, first aid and CPR training).

2.13 Describe the proper handling, storage, and disposal of hazardous materials.

PTCB

In preparation for the certification examination, you should understand and perform activities associated with the following PTCB Knowledge Statements:

PTCB Knowledge Statement

Domain I. Assisting the Pharmacist in Serving Patients

Knowledge of federal, state, and/or practice site regulations, codes of ethics, and standards related to the practice of pharmacy (1)

PTCB Knowledge Statement	***Domain II. Maintaining Medication and Inventory Control Systems*** Knowledge of risk management opportunities (13) Knowledge of policies, procedures, and practices regarding storage and handling of hazardous materials and wastes (22)
PTCB Knowledge Statement	***Domain III. Participating in the Administration and Management of Pharmacy Practice*** Knowledge of storage and handling requirements for hazardous substances (13) Knowledge of hazardous waste disposal requirements (14) Knowledge of infection control policies and procedures (18)

Case Study

Bob a senior pharmacy technician at a small local community hospital, is responsible for calibrating blood glucose monitors for nursing staff use for the patients. As Bob has been a pharmacy technician at this facility for 9 years, he is very familiar with the nursing staff. Bob does not wear gloves during the calibrations. Sometimes he performs the calibrations in the pharmacy. As he performs the calibrations first thing in the morning, he often enjoys a doughnut at the same time. Occasionally, Bob performs the calibrations in a patient's room.

While reading this chapter, keep the following questions in mind:

1. What modes of infectious disease transmission could Bob be exposed to?(LO 2.2)
2. How can Bob reduce his risk?(LO 2.5, 2.8)
3. What is Bob's responsibility as a senior technician to reduce the risk of spread of infectious disease?(LO 2.5)

Introduction to Basic Safety and Standards(LO 2.1, 2.5)

Pharmacy technicians have a critical role in the promotion and maintenance of safety in the clinical setting. The technician must not only know the criteria for a safe environment, but must also be able to take action in the event of an emergency. These actions must comply with federal and state laws, in addition to the policies and procedures of the institution where the technician is employed. Pharmacy policies and procedures must be in effect to govern infection surveillance, prevention, and control in the pharmacy. The Joint Commission (TJC) standards regarding infection control policy and procedures represent minimum standards to be met in any institution. Pharmacy technicians who function effectively in any health care facility must be mindful of all of the regulations, standards, and policies in order to implement the appropriate procedure (action) for a particular situation.

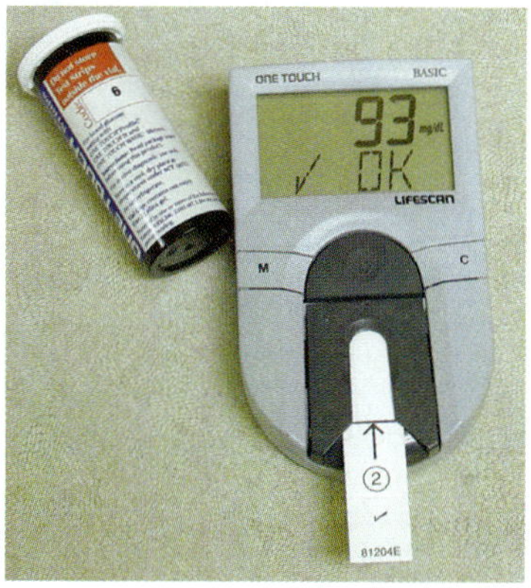

A pharmacy technician may be responsible for calibrating a blood glucose monitor such as the one pictured here.

The **Centers for Disease Control and Prevention (CDC)** is the primary organization concerned with controlling and preventing all types of disease. The CDC is recognized as the leading federal agency for protecting and promoting health and safety, providing credible information to enhance health

At Your Service

Elizabeth K., pharmacy technician at a large medical center, frequently goes to the wards to collect medication orders for the pharmacy. Recently, while Elizabeth was performing her duties on the ward, she observed a nurse who had just administered medication to a patient by injection intentionally break the needle on the syringe and toss the broken syringe and needle into a wastepaper basket. When Elizabeth questioned the actions of the nurse, the nurse replied that no one could use the syringe, now that she had broken the needle.

While reading this chapter, keep the following questions in mind.

1. What should the nurse have done?(LO 2.5)
2. What is Elizabeth's responsibility as the pharmacy technician?(LO 2.2, 2.5)

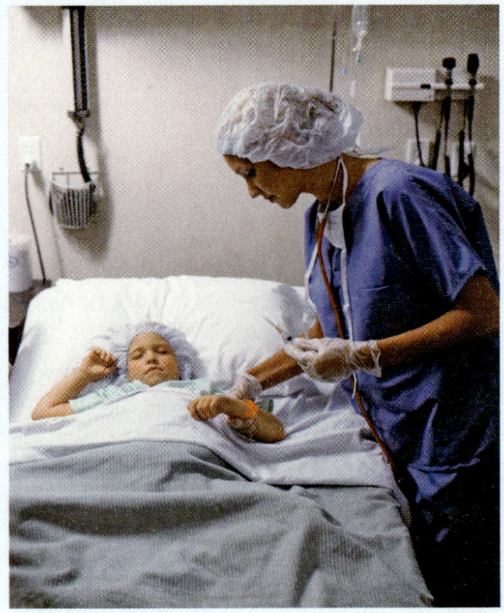

decisions, and promoting health through strong partnerships. The CDC provides a national focus for developing and applying disease prevention and control, environmental health, and health promotion and education activities designed to improve the health of the people of the United States. The CDC's particular areas of interest involve limiting the spread of infectious disease and decreasing pathogen resistance to antimicrobial drug therapy. In particular, the CDC provides updates on infectious disease trends for the education of health care professionals. Pharmacy personnel need to be aware of the methods by which infection spread can be reduced.

The **Occupational Safety and Health Administration (OSHA)** is an organization responsible for developing standards for safety in the workplace. OSHA's mission is to ensure the safety and health of America's workers by setting and enforcing standards; providing training, outreach, and education; establishing partnerships; and encouraging continual improvement in workplace safety and health. OSHA also develops guidelines to enable organizations to provide safer work environments.

Common Infectious Diseases(LO 2.2, 2.3, 2.5)

In every health care facility, care must be taken to control the spread of infectious disease. The CDC provides information or precautions to health care providers to restrict the uncontrolled spread of disease. In this chapter, three types of infectious disease will be discussed: bloodborne diseases, airborne diseases, and **nosocomial** infections. Pharmacy technicians who are employed in the inpatient setting, for example, are at greater risk for contracting diseases as a result of being in close proximity with patients.

Centers for Disease Control and Prevention (CDC) The Centers for Disease Control and Prevention is the primary organization concerned with controlling disease transmission to prevent its spread and impact on society.

pathogen Microbial agent causing disease.

Occupational Safety and Health Administration (OSHA) Organization responsible for developing standards for safety in the workplace.

nosocomial Originating or taking place in a hospital or other health care setting.

As pharmacy technicians work in various settings, they need to be aware of the modes of disease transmission.

Bloodborne Diseases(LO 2.1, 2.4, 2.5)

Bloodborne diseases are transmitted through exchange of blood or blood containing body fluids. Pathogens contained in these fluids cause disease. Examples of viral pathogens causing bloodborne disease are human immunodeficiency virus (HIV) (Figure 2-1), hepatitis B virus (HBV), and hepatitis C virus (HCV). Exposures placing individuals at risk for infection with HIV, HBV, and HCV include percutaneous injury (needlestick or cut) or contact of mucous membrane or nonintact skin with blood, tissue, or other body fluids. In the event of health care worker exposure to these pathogens, an **incident report** should be completed immediately (Figure 2-2, p. 32). Specific components of the incident report will be itemized later in this chapter. Appropriate management of the exposure is critical to the health of the exposed individual. **Postexposure prophylaxis** (PEP) may be warranted.

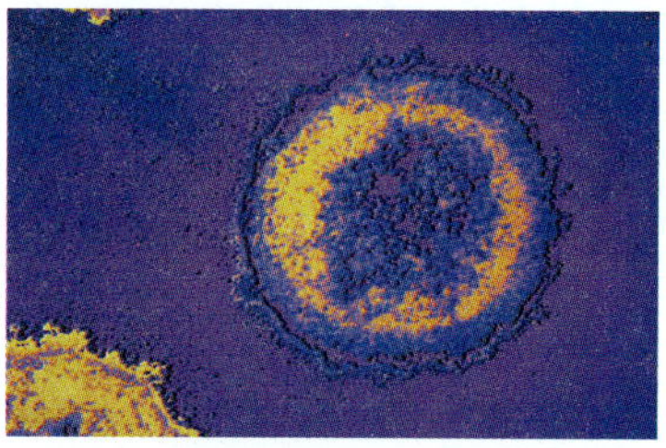

Figure 2-1 HIV micrograph.

Standard Precautions

Standard precautions are designed to reduce the risk of transmission of bloodborne pathogens and reduce the risk of transmission of microorganisms from moist body surfaces. Standard precautions apply to all patients, regardless of their infectious disease status. These precautions apply to blood, all body fluids, secretions, and excretions except sweat, nonintact skin, and mucous membranes. The goal of standard precautions is to decrease the risk of pathogen transmission from all sources in health care facilities. Compliance to standard precautions is necessary to reduce the risk of spread of bloodborne pathogens.

Potentially infectious body fluids

- Amniotic fluid
- Blood
- Cerebrospinal fluid
- Pericardial fluid
- Peritoneal fluid
- Pleural fluid
- Semen
- Synovial fluid
- Vaginal secretions

Not considered infectious unless containing blood

- Feces
- Nasal secretions
- Saliva
- Sputum
- Sweat
- Tears
- Urine
- Vomitus

bloodborne Pathogens or disease carried in blood and other body fluids.

incident report Document used for internal reporting of injury or accident.

postexposure prophylaxis (PEP) Using preventative measures, such as medications, to prevent a disease or infection after a person has had an accidental exposure to the disease or infection.

Figure 2-2 **Incident report. In the event of an accident or exposure incident, OSHA regulations require completion of an incident report form.**

Millstone Industries

Central State Division
Incident Report

Name of Injured Employee ______________________

Department ______________ Job Title ______________

Supervisor ______________________

Date of Accident ______________ Time ______________

Nature of Injury ______________________

Was injured acting in a regular line of duty? ______________

Was first aid given? ________ By whom? ______________

Was designated emergency contact notified? ______________

Did injured receive medical treatment? ______________

Was injured tested for infection? ________ If no, why not? ________

Did injured go to ER? ________ Other? ________

Did injured leave work? ________ Date ________ Hour ________ A.M. P.M.

Did injured return to work? ________ Date ________ Hour ________ A.M. P.M.

Other Parties Involved ______________________

Names of Witnesses ______________________

Describe where and how accident occurred. ______________________

What, in your opinion, caused the accident? ______________________

Has anything been done to prevent a similar accident? ______________________

Has the hazard causing the injury been reported by telephone or in writing? ______________

Date ______________ Employee's Signature ______________

Date ______________ Supervisor's Signature ______________

IF TREATMENT IS NEEDED, TAKE THE ORIGINAL AND DUPLICATE OF THIS FORM TO THE EMERGENCY ROOM.

This part for Employee Health Office use only

Was incident investigated? ______________________

Has injured had follow-up medical care? ______________________

Comments ______________________

Original copy to Employee Health Office *Duplicate copy to supervisor*

Caution

Avoid needlestick injuries. Do not recap or break needles!

Tech Check

1. What is the mission of OSHA?(LO 2.1)
2. For which patients are standard precautions taken?(LO 2.5)
3. List three diseases transmitted via the bloodborne route.(LO 2.4)
4. For which bloodborne pathogens is postexposure prophylaxis recommended?(LO 2.4)
5. In the event of an accident or exposure incident OSHA requires the completion of what document?(LO 2.1)

Airborne Diseases(LO 2.2, 2.4, 2.5)

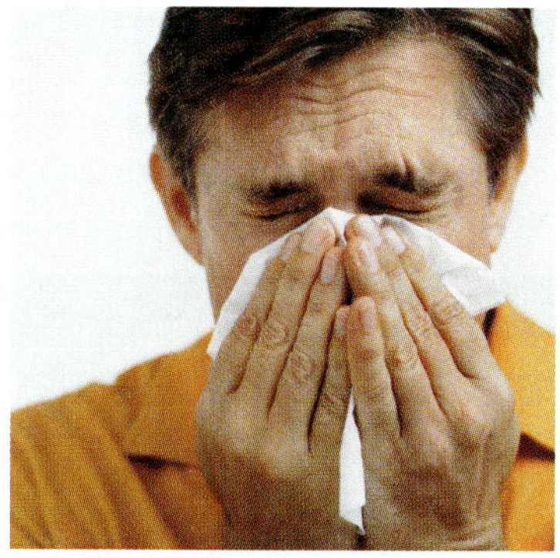

Airborne diseases, such as pneumonia and tuberculosis, are spread by infectious microbes contained in air that is inhaled. This type of transmission may occur either by dissemination of small droplet particles (less than 5 micrometers) or dust particles containing pathogens. Dispersion of these particles may be enhanced by air currents and may be deposited on or inhaled by an individual in the same room as the patient, or someone in the retail pharmacy with a bad cough or sneeze.

Airborne Precautions

Airborne precautions are applied to patients suspected or known to have diseases that are spread via the airborne route, such as influenza, tuberculosis, and pneumonia. Aspects of airborne precautions include:

- Close monitoring of airflow in a private room for the patient. The door should be kept closed and the patient should remain in the room as much as possible.
- Appropriate respiratory protection (N95 respirator) should be worn by any individual entering the room of a patient with known or suspected infectious pulmonary tuberculosis.
- Patient transport from the room should be limited. If the patient must be moved, a surgical mask should be placed on the patient to minimize the spread of pathogens.

Droplet Precautions

Droplet precautions are designed to minimize the risk of droplet transmission of infectious agents. Droplet transmission should be differentiated from airborne transmission. In airborne transmission, the droplet particles are small in size (less than 5 micrometers). Droplet transmission involves contact with mucous membranes of the mouth and nose with large (greater than 5 micrometers) particles. These large particles contain pathogens and are generated from an individual with disease through coughing, sneezing, and talking. The particles may also be dispersed through various procedures like suctioning and bronchoscopy. These particles do not remain suspended in the air, and therefore transmission of microorganisms via this route requires close (less than 3 feet) contact between individuals. Individuals coming within 5 feet of a patient with disease transmitted via the droplet route should wear masks. Influenza is transmitted via droplet transmission. Special air handling and ventilation are not required for droplet precautions as the particles do not remain suspended long enough to warrant these interventions. Although it is highly unlikely that pharmacy technicians would be at risk for droplet transmission, technicians should be aware that the risk for droplet transmission increases with closer proximity to infected individuals.

Tech Check

6. Why is monitoring of airflow critical to reduce the spread of pathogens via the airborne route?(LO 2.4)

7. List diseases that may be spread via the airborne route.(LO 2.2)

8. Which procedures may cause a potential risk in droplet transmission of microorganisms?(LO 2.4)

Figure 2-3 Scanning electron micrograph (SEM) of a number of *Pseudomonas aeruginosa* bacteria.

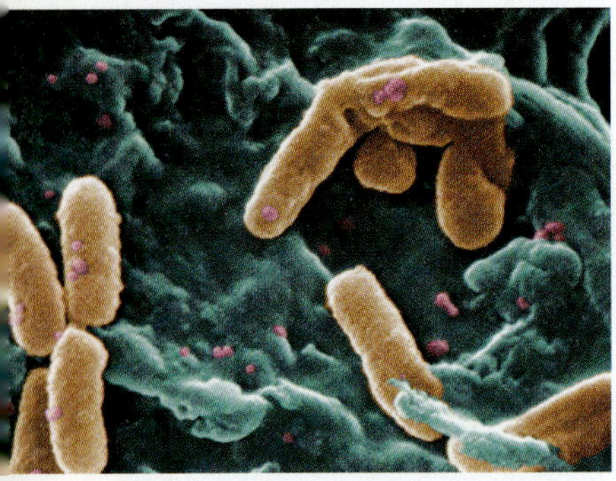

CDC/Janice Haney Carr

Nosocomial Infections(LO 2.3)

A nosocomial infection is one that originates in a health care facility. The patient is exposed to the infecting organism while in the facility and as a result develops an infection. Nosocomial infections result in increased morbidity and mortality in patients, longer hospitals stays, and increased risk of transmission of these pathogens to other patients and hospital staff. Lack of control of nosocomial infections may lead to **multidrug-resistant pathogens,** particularly with infections caused by *Pseudomonas aeruginosa* (Figure 2-3). Prevention and control of nosocomial infections is a critical issue in any health care facility. Through use of proper precautions and **aseptic technique,** the transmission of pathogens is reduced along with the potential for nosocomial infections.

There are four major types of nosocomial infections:

- Surgical wound infections
- Lower respiratory tract infections
- Urinary tract infections
- **Bloodstream infections**

Pathogens often associated with nosocomial infections are *Pseudomonas aeruginosa*, Methicillin-resistant *Staphylococcus aureus* (MRSA) (Figure 2-4), *Escherichia coli*, *Klebsiella*, and *Candida* species. MRSA is a pathogen that was primarily associated with nosocomial infections, as its spread was limited to inpatients. Lack of control of this pathogen has lead to community-associated MRSA infections, meaning that community members now have risk of contracting infections from a pathogen that was previously confined to institutional settings. Effective infection control policies and procedures reduce the incidence of nosocomial infections, and therefore provide for a safer environment for health care.

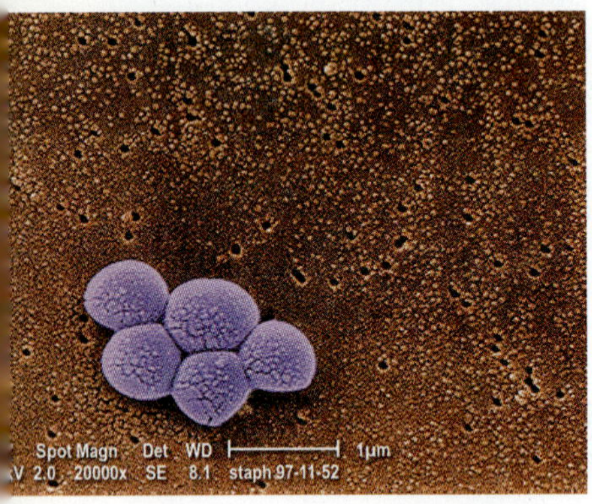

Figure 2-4 Methicillin-resistant *Staphylococcus aureus* (MRSA) bacteria.

Tech Check

9. What is a nosocomial infection?(LO 2.2)
10. List the four major types of nosocomial infections.(LO 2.3)
11. List three pathogens associated with nosocomial infections.(LO 2.3)
12. Name a pathogen associated with multiple-drug resistance.(LO 2.3)
13. Name a pathogen that demonstrates expansion from primarily nosocomial to the community.(LO 2.3)

Prevention of Spreading Infectious Diseases(LO 2.5, 2.6, 2.7, 2.8)

In the 1840s, Ignaz Semmelweis demonstrated that infections in the hospital could be reduced through hand washing between patients. Hand washing is the primary means to control the transmission of pathogens in hospitals and in the community, now part of a proper **hand hygiene** regimen for medical professionals. Hands should be washed between patients and between multiple procedures on the same patient to avoid cross-contamination. Hands should be washed even if gloves are worn, to reduce the risk of pathogen transmission in the event that a small

multidrug-resistant pathogens Bacteria impervious to multiple antibacterial agents.

aseptic technique Processes to maintain sterility of product.

bloodstream infection Bacteria from infected site in the body invade bloodstream.

hand hygiene Hand washing, antiseptic hand rub, and antiseptic hand wash.

tear or hole has occurred in the glove. To prevent the spread of infection, frequent hand washing should be performed throughout the shift while working as a pharmacy technician.

Hand Washing and Disease Containment

There are three routes by which hand washing reduces the spread of infection between people:

1. Fecal-oral transmission occurs when an individual neglects to wash hands after having a bowel movement and touches food, beverages, and other inanimate objects. Pathogens are transferred to individuals who touch the same items at a later time. Microbes transmitted via this route include giardia, hepatitis A, shigella, and salmonella.
2. Indirect contact with respiratory secretions. An infected individual coughs or sneezes into his or her hands, depositing microbes that can then be spread to others through touching or shaking hands. Illnesses that are transmitted via this route include the common cold, influenza, and respiratory syncytial virus (RSV).
3. Contact with body fluids. Urine, saliva, and other body fluids may contain microbes that can be transmitted directly from person to person, or indirectly through touching objects contaminated through touch by an infected individual. Microbes spread in this manner include cytomegalovirus, staphylococcal species, and Epstein-Barr virus (EBV).

When Should Hands Be Washed?

Hands should be washed:

- When they are visibly soiled or dirty
- Before and after contact with a patient
- Prior to donning gloves for working in the laminar flow hood
- Prior to eating
- After using the restroom

Other Aspects of Hand Hygiene

- The use of gloves does not eliminate the need for hand washing.
- Liquid soap is preferred, as a bar of soap in a dish tends to colonize bacteria.
- Alcohol preparations (hand rubs) are effective if hands are not visibly dirty, and soap and water are not available.
- Alcohol-based antiseptics should be applied to all surfaces of hands and fingers, which should then be allowed to dry.
- Health care workers should not wear artificial nails, and natural nails should be kept less than ¼-inch long. Nail polish should not be chipped.

Hand Washing Technique

What Constitutes Proper Hand Washing Technique? (Figures 2-5a and 2-5b)

1. Wet hands with warm running water.
2. Apply soap and thoroughly distribute over hands.
3. Vigorously rub hands together for 10 to 15 seconds, generating friction on all surfaces of the hands and fingers, including the backs of the hands, backs of fingers, and under the fingernails.

Figure 2-5 (*a*) **When you wash your hands, be sure to clean all surfaces, including the palms, between the fingers, and under the fingernails. (*b*) The nails and cuticles require additional attention to ensure that all dirt is removed.**

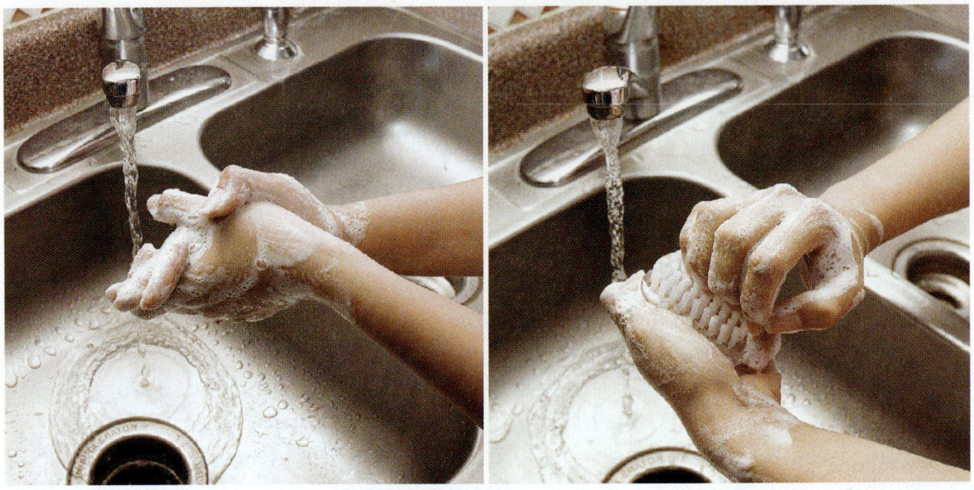

(a) (b)

4. Rinse hands completely to remove all traces of soap, especially under rings and between fingers.
5. Dry hands using clean and dry paper towels.
6. Use a paper towel to turn off the faucet in the event that there are no foot controls or automatic shutoff.

Hand Hygiene Antiseptic Agents

An **antiseptic agent** is an antimicrobial substance that, when applied to the skin, causes a reduction in the number of microbial flora. As microbes may be capable of surviving for some time on hands and inanimate objects, antiseptic agents play a role in the reduction of pathogens transmitted through touch. Antiseptic agents include:

- Alcohols
- Chlorhexidine
- Chlorine
- Hexachlorophene
- Iodophors
- Chloroxylenol
- Quaternary ammonium compounds
- Triclosan

When hands are visibly dirty, soap and water should be used to wash the hands. Antiseptic agents will not be as effective on visibly dirty as on clean appearing hands; however, they may still demonstrate antibacterial effect.

Antiseptic Drug Products

The Food and Drug Administration (FDA) has categorized antiseptic drug products into three categories:

1. *Patient preoperative skin preparation*—fast-acting, broad-spectrum, and persistent antiseptic substance that substantially reduces the number of microorganisms on intact skin.
2. *Antiseptic hand wash*—an antiseptic-containing preparation designed for frequent use to reduce the number of microorganisms on intact

antiseptic agent Antimicrobial substance applied to skin to reduce microbial flora.

Table 2-1 Characteristics and Antimicrobial Spectrum of Hand Hygiene Antiseptic Agents.

Group	Gram-Positive Bacteria	Gram-Negative Bacteria	Mycobacteria	Fungi	Viruses	Speed of Action
Alcohols	+ + +	+ + +	+ + +	+ + +	+ + +	fast
Chlorhexidine	+ + +	+ +	+	+	+ + +	intermediate
Iodine Compounds	+ + +	+ + +	+ + +	+ +	+ + +	intermediate
Iodophors	+ + +	+ + +	+	+ +	+ +	intermediate
Phenols	+ + +	+	+	+	+	intermediate
Triclosan	+ + +	+ +	+	–	+ + +	intermediate
Quaternary ammonium compounds	+	+ +	–	–	+	slow

Note: + + + = excellent; + + = good; + = weak; – = no activity.

skin to an initial baseline level after adequate washing, rinsing, and drying. It is broad spectrum, fast acting, and may be persistent.

3. *Surgical hand scrub*—an antiseptic containing preparation that substantially reduces the number of microorganisms on intact skin. It is broad spectrum, fast acting, and persistent. Table 2-1 outlines the characteristics and antimicrobial spectrum of hand hygiene antiseptic agents.

Protective Wear

Protective wear, commonly referred to as personal protective equipment (PPE), generally consists of items that create a barrier between the contamination source and the health care worker. The PPE worn by pharmacy technicians varies depending upon the pharmacy setting in which the technician is employed. Retail pharmacy technicians typically wear lab coats or gowns. However, pharmacy technicians who perform sterile compounding must wear gloves, hair covers, gowns, and shoe covers. Proper technique must be used in the donning of certain types of protective wear in order to preserve their effectiveness; for example, gloves. Disposable PPE such as masks and gloves, should never be reused or reworn. Other items serve as a barrier to minimize the spread or contact with the contamination source but must be removed as soon as possible if soiled: for example, gown or lab coat.

Personal protective equipment (PPE) includes the following (Figure 2-6):

- Face shields
- Full face respirators
- Gloves
- Gowns or lab coats
- Masks
- Protective glasses or goggles
- Shoe covers
- Hair covers

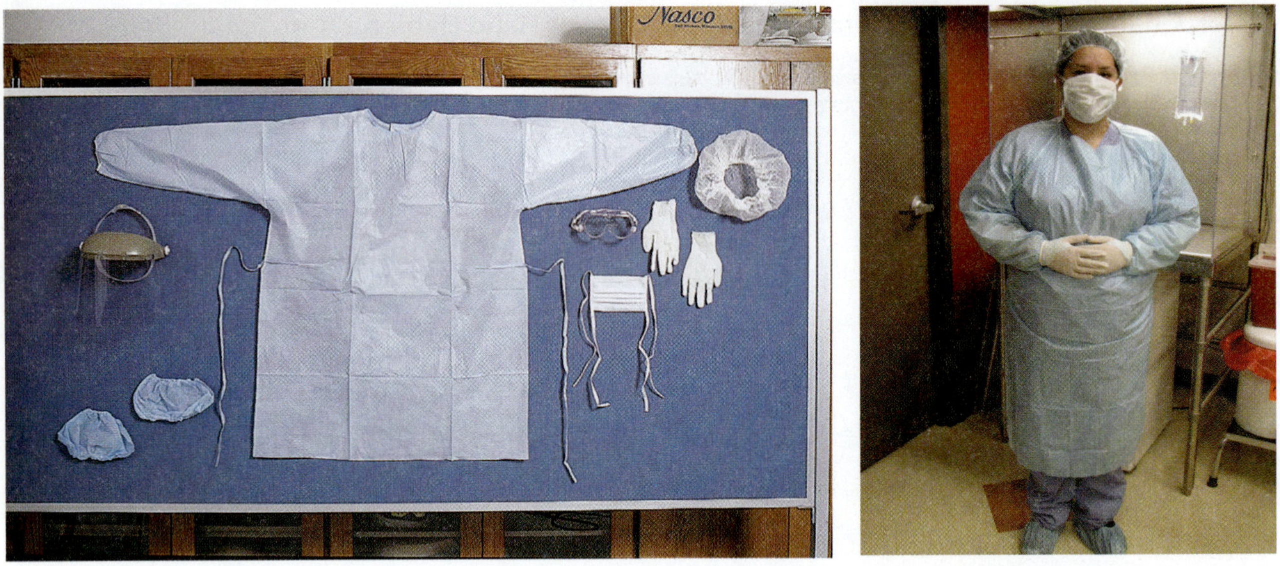

Figure 2-6 Pharmacy technicians may need to use various types of personal protective equipment including gloves, masks and protective face shields, gowns, and other protective clothing.

Tech Check

14. How long should hands be rubbed together creating friction during hand washing?(LO 2.7)

15. What are the three routes of pathogen transmission that are affected by hand washing?(LO 2.6)

16. Should hands be washed prior to donning gloves?(LO 2.7)

17. Define *antiseptic agent.* (LO 2.6)

18. List five items of PPE. (LO 2.8)

19. List the three FDA categories of antiseptic drug products. (LO 2.6)

Incidents(LO 2.9, 2.10)

Documentation and Reporting Within Your Organization

Policy and procedure manuals exist in every health care organization. Pharmacy policies and procedures regarding infectious disease control and surveillance are critical to the control of infectious disease in a given facility. The policy indicates the goals and objectives of the health care organization. Procedures are the implementation or how the policy is carried out. Both policies and procedures must be in compliance with federal and state regulations. TJC standards for infection control in the pharmacy represent the minimum standards to be met by institutions. TJC is discussed in more detail in Chapter 4.

The pharmacy technician is responsible for assisting the pharmacist in controlling pathogen transmission and preventing infection in the pharmacy. The pharmacy technician may perform these functions by ensuring that medicinal agents are properly stored, adhering to proper aseptic technique, and controlling pathogen transmission and preventing infection through complying with pharmacy policies and procedures as they relate to infection control.

According to TJC recommendations, Pharmacy Infection Control Policies and Procedures must at least address the following:

- Infection surveillance, prevention, and control for the pharmacy.
- Shelf-life of all sterile items in storage.
- Hand washing technique and personal hygiene requirements.
- Use of single-dose and multiple-dose containers.
- Sterile product preparation (including aseptic technique).
- Requirement for assessing sterile technique of personnel and frequency assessed.
- Irrigation solution preparation.
- Preparation of parenteral nutrition products.
- Storage of sterile medication products.
- Traffic control of sterile medication preparation areas.
- Proper use of laminar flow hoods (including cleaning and checking for operational efficiency).
- Microbiological monitoring of laminar flow hoods, if required.
- Testing for microbial contamination of hospital-prepared sterile products, if required.
- Routine cleaning of pharmacy facilities (e.g., cleaning responsibilities, procedures, schedules, and agents approved by the infection control committee).
- Reporting of unsanitary conditions and practices.
- Containment and disposal of waste.

Source: From CP Coe, JP Uselton: *Preparing the Pharmacy for a Joint Commission Survey*, 5th ed. Bethesda, MD: ASHP, 2003, p. 106.

Tech Check

20. List five TJC recommendations for Pharmacy Infection Control Policies and Procedures that pertain to pharmacy technicians. (LO 2.9)

Incident Report (LO 2.10)

What Is an Incident Report?

Accidents or events involving employees, students, visitor injury, property damage, and/or occupational illness are reported to the pharmacy supervisor by the technician. An incident report is completed, then reviewed by an oversight committee (e.g., Hospital Safety Committee) in order to determine what factors that might have lead to the incident and how it might have been prevented. If an accident- or work-related injury occurs in a retail pharmacy, an incident report is filed with the immediate supervisor, who is typically the pharmacist-in-charge. Typically, incident reports are general forms that contain three main areas (Figure 2-7):

1. Information about the person involved in the incident (name, contact information, whether or not the person is an employee, student, or visitor, and identification information).
2. Information about the incident (date, time, whether or not police were notified, location of incident, description of what occurred, type of

Patient's ID number:	
Date:	Location:
Description of incident:	
Plan of action followed:	
Additional comments:	
Pharmacist's name and initials, and name of pharmacy:	

Figure 2-7 **Pharmacy incident report form.**

injury, whether or not treatment was provided, if work will be missed, if there were any witnesses).

3. Reporter/supervisor information (printed name with signature of supervisor or individual taking the report, title, date).

Pharmacy Incident Report Form

Additionally, the CDC has published recommendations for the contents of an occupational exposure report to microbial pathogens. The following items should be included in addition to those in a general incident report:

- Date and time of exposure.
- Details of procedure being performed, including where and how exposure occurred; if related to a sharp device, the type and brand of device and how and when in the course of handling the device the exposure occurred.
- Details of the exposure, including the type and amount of fluid or material and the severity of the exposure.
- Details about the exposure source (e.g., HBV, HIV, **antiretroviral** resistance information).
- Details about exposed person (e.g., hepatitis B vaccination).
- Details about counseling, postexposure management, and follow-up.

Tech Check

21. List the three primary components of an incident report. (LO 2.10)

22. For which types of situations are incident reports submitted? (LO 2.10)

antiretroviral Agents used in the management of HIV.

Procedures for HIV Prophylaxis(LO 2.11)

Postexposure Prophylaxis

The CDC recommends that HIV postexposure prophylaxis (PEP) consist of treatment with at least two antiretroviral agents over a period of 4 weeks. It is also recommended that the prophylactic regimen begin within hours of exposure.

Possible combinations include:

Lamivudine or Emtricitabine

PLUS

Zidovudine, Stavudine, or Tenofovir.

Three drug regimens are recommended when the risk of transmission is high or when antiretroviral agent resistance is suspected.

Monitoring the Patient

Monitoring of the patient must include parameters pertaining to HIV status (e.g., viral load, CD4 cell counts) as well as numerous adverse drug reactions and drug interactions of the antiretroviral agents. The recommendations for prophylaxis are based upon the use of the nucleoside reverse transcriptase inhibitors (NRTIs). In HIV-positive patients and for those patients with AIDS, other categories (nonnucleoside reverse transcriptase inhibitors [NNRTIs], protease inhibitors [PIs], and integrase inhibitors) of antiretroviral medications are necessary to manage their conditions. These medicines are used in combination with each other to suppress the viral load while minimizing the risk of viral resistance to antiretroviral agents. For more on antiretroviral drug classification, see Chapter 7.

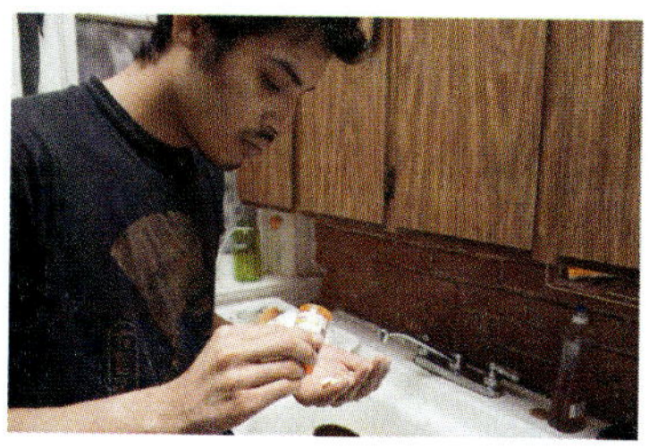

Table 2-2 outlines the common adverse drug reactions of antiretroviral agents for HIV PEP.

Although PEP for occupational exposure to HIV is an attempt to safeguard against infection, there are situations that warrant expert consultation for HIV PEP. They are:

- Delayed exposure report
- Unknown source

Table 2-2 Common Adverse Drug Reactions of Antiretroviral Agents for HIV PEP

Drug	Reaction
Zidovudine (Retrovir®)	Anemia, neutropenia, nausea, headache, insomnia, muscle pain, weakness
Lamivudine (Epivir®)	Abdominal pain, nausea, diarrhea, rash, pancreatitis
Stavudine (Zerit®)	Peripheral neuropathy, headache, diarrhea, nausea, insomnia, anorexia, pancreatitis, increased liver function tests, anemia, neutropenia
Didanosine (Videx®)	Pancreatitis, lactic acidosis, neuropathy, diarrhea, abdominal pain, nausea

- Known or suspected pregnancy in the exposed person
- Resistance of the source virus to antiretroviral agents
- Toxicity of the initial PEP regimen

Tech Check

23. What is PEP?(LO 2.11)

24. Components of HIV PEP for occupational exposure are from where? (LO 2.11)

25. Describe the adverse drug reaction profile of lamivudine. (LO 2.11)

26. Are the NRTIs the only type of antiretroviral therapy available?(LO 2.11)

27. Discuss situations warranting expert consultation for HIV PEP. (LO 2.11)

Documentation and Reporting Outside Your Organization(LO 2.9)

FBI and CDC

An incident report is the internal reporting mechanism for a hospital or health care organization. Certain incidents warrant outside reporting to health departments, the Federal Bureau of Investigation (FBI), and/or the CDC. Requirements for reporting of individual instances of infectious disease vary by state (Figure 2-8). Individual cases of occupationally acquired HIV infections and HIV PEP failures are reportable to the CDC. In the event of outbreaks of infectious disease, the local health departments, local police and fire departments, and the CDC would be notified. The CDC recommends that local health departments are the first to be notified in the event of an epidemic or outbreak. In the event of suspected bioterrorism, the FBI would be notified in addition to those bodies notified in the event of an outbreak or epidemic. Every pharmacy should have a "chain of contacts" to be notified in the event of the above incidences. Every member of the pharmacy staff, particularly the pharmacy technician, should be aware of the location of the contact information and be prepared to work along with other health care professionals in the event of a crisis.

Tech Check

28. Describe a situation in which the hospital pharmacy would contact the FBI. (LO 2.9)

29. Describe two situations warranting the notification of the CDC. (LO 2.9)

First Aid and CPR Requirements(LO 2.12)

cardiopulmonary resuscitation (CPR) To provide ventilations (breaths) and chest compressions (blood circulation) for a person who shows no signs of breathing or having a heartbeat.

Pharmacy technicians, as health care paraprofessionals, should have basic first aid training and **cardiopulmonary resuscitation (CPR)** certification. Both the American Heart Association (AHA) and the American Red Cross offer training for CPR, as well as provide for recertification. The CPR certification must be kept current and is renewable. Pharmacy technicians are strongly encouraged to have both CPR and first aid training. This type of

ARIZONA DEPARTMENT OF HEALTH SERVICES
COMMUNICABLE DISEASE REPORT
Important Instructions on Reverse Side
PLEASE PRINT OR TYPE

County/IHS ID Number/Chapter | State ID Number

PATIENT'S NAME (Last) (First) | DATE OF BIRTH | SEX ☐ Male ☐ Female | ETHNICITY ☐ Hispanic ☐ Non-Hispanic

STREET ADDRESS | CENSUS TRACT | CITY | RACE ☐ White ☐ Am. Indian ☐ Asian ☐ Black ☐ Other ☐ Unknown

COUNTY | STATE | ZIP CODE | PHONE NO.

DIAGNOSIS OR SUSPECT REPORTABLE CONDITION

DATE ONSET | DATE OF DIAGNOSIS | LAB RESULTS

COUNTY USE ONLY:
LAB CONFIRMATION DATE:________
☐ Negative
☐ Positive
☐ Not Done
☐ Unknown

PATIENT OCCUPATION OR SCHOOL

PHYSICIAN OR OTHER REPORTING SOURCE | PHONE NUMBER

STREET ADDRESS | CITY | STATE | ZIP CODE

COUNTY USE ONLY:
☐ Confirmed case
☐ Probable case
☐ Outbreak Associated
☐ Ruled Out

Original and 1st copy to County Health Department ☐ CHECK IF ADDITIONAL FORMS ARE NEEDED (Quantity)________

REPORTABLE DISEASES

Arizona Revised Statutes and Arizona Administrative Code require the following diseases to be reported to the County Health Department or Indian Health Services within 5 business days of diagnosis or treatment.

AIDS[3]
Amebiasis[1]
Anthrax
Aseptic meningitis
Botulism*
Brucellosis
Campylobacteriosis[1]
Chancroid[3]
Chlamydial infections (genital)[3]
Cholera*
Coccidioidomycosis
Colorado tick fever
Conjunctivitis, acute[2]
Cryptosporidiosis
Dengue
Diphtheria*
Ehrlichiosis
Encephalitis, viral
Foodborne illness/ Waterborne illness*
Giardiasis[1]
Gonorrhea[3]
Haemophilus influenzae*
Hemolytic Uremic Syndrome[1]
Hepatitis A[1]
Hepatitis B, Delta Hepatitis
Hepatitis Non-A, Non-B
Herpes Genitalis[3]
HIV[3]
Lead Poisoning[3]
Legionellosis
Leprosy
Listeriosis
Lyme Disease
Malaria
Measles*
Meningococcal disease*
Mumps
Pediculosis[2]
Pertussis*
Pesticide poisoning[3]
Plague*
Poliomyelitis*
Psittacosis
Q Fever
Rabies in humans*
Relapsing fever
Reye's Syndrome
Rocky Mt. spotted fever
Rubella*
Congenital rubella syn.
Salmonellosis[1]
Scabies[2]
Shigellosis[1]
Staphylococcal disease[1,2]
Streptococcal diseases[1,2]
Syphilis[3]
Tetanus
Toxic Shock Syndrome
Trichinosis
Tuberculosis[3]
Tuberculosis infection in children <6 yrs of age
Tularemia
Typhoid Fever[1]
Typhus fever
Varicella
Yellow Fever*

*Telephone report required to the County Health Department or Indian Health Services within 24 hours.

[1] Report within 24 hours of diagnosis if in food handler.

[2] Outbreak reports only

[3] These conditions are reported on other forms, call 1-800-334-1540 for a supply

ADHS/DPS/OIDS/IDES-1 (Rev. 11-94)

Figure 2-8 Each state has its own communicable disease report.

training prepares individuals to recognize emergencies and respond appropriately to provide care to those in need (Figure 2-9).

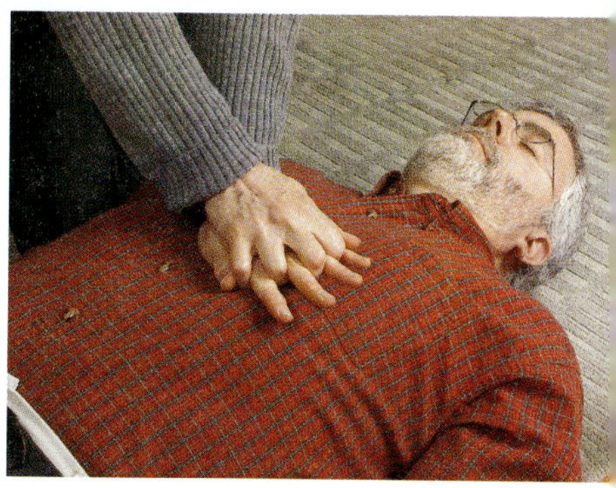

Figure 2-9 CPR.

Bioterrorism Considerations

Health care workers, such as pharmacists and pharmacy technicians, need to be aware of what to do in the event of bioterrorist attacks not only for their own protection, but also for the protection of coworkers and patients. Pharmacy technicians need to be aware of pharmacy policies and procedures with respect to managing such emergencies as well as other unexpected events that may occur (e.g., fire, evacuation, natural disasters). Pharmacy personnel may be called upon in emergencies to help provide medications, information, and assistance to patients and other health care professionals.

Biological agents associated with bioterrorism include:

- Anthrax (Figure 2-10)
- Avian flu

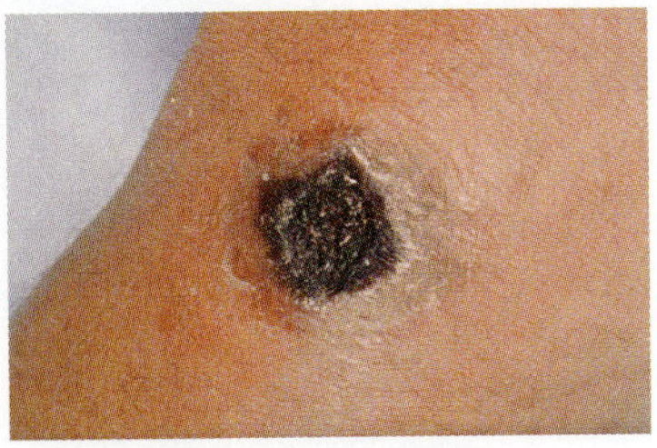

Figure 2-10 **Anthrax lesion on the skin of the forearm caused by the bacterium *Bacillus anthracis*.**

- Bloodborne pathogens
    - Hepatitis B
    - Hepatitis C
    - HIV
- Foodborne pathogens
    - Salmonella
    - Botulism
    - Shigella
- Hantavirus
- Legionnaires' disease
- Molds and fungi
- Plague
- Ricin
- Severe acute respiratory syndrome (SARS) (Figure 2-11)
- Smallpox
- Tularemia
- Viral hemorrhagic fever (VHF)

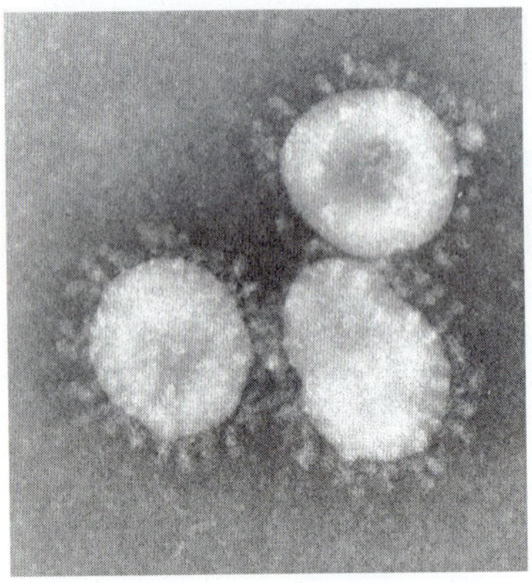

Figure 2-11 **SARS virus.**

Emergency Action Plan

Emergency events may or may not involve biological agents. In any event, according to OSHA standards, employers must have an Emergency Action Plan (EAP) and a Fire Prevention Plan (FPP). The purpose of an EAP is to facilitate and organize employer and employee actions during workplace emergencies. An EAP is a written document that is required by the OSHA standard.

The elements of the plan shall include but are not limited to:

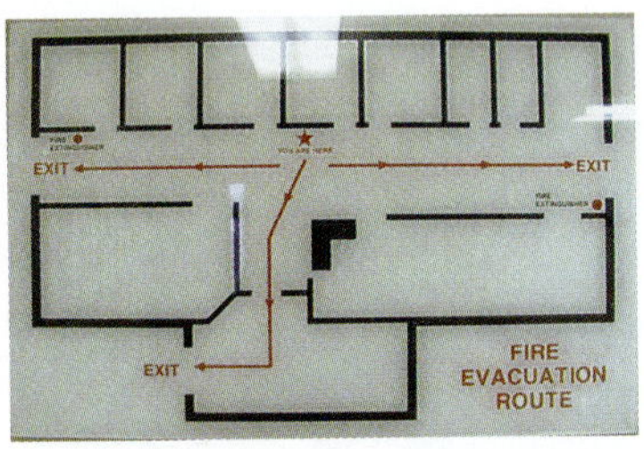

Figure 2-12 **While working as a pharmacy technician, you should be aware of the fire and emergency escape routes.**

1. Escape procedures and emergency escape route assignments (Figure 2-12).
2. Procedures to be followed by employees who remain to operate critical plant operations before they evacuate.
3. Procedures to account for all employees after emergency evacuation has been completed.
4. Rescue and medical duties for those employees who are to perform them.
5. Means of reporting fires and other emergencies.
6. Names or job titles of persons who can be contacted for further information or explanation of duties under the plan.

Fire Prevention Plan

Portable fire extinguishers and sprinkler systems are employed in the event of a fire. These items must be checked periodically to ensure proper functioning in case of an emergency.

An FPP is a hazard prevention plan that ensures advanced planning for evacuations in fire and other emergencies. An FPP is a written document required by the OSHA standard.

The elements of the plan include, but are not limited to:

1. A list of major workplace fire hazards and their proper handling and storage procedures, potential ignition sources, their control procedures, and the type of fire protection equipment or systems that can control a fire.

2. Names or job titles of those persons responsible for maintenance of equipment and systems installed to prevent or control ignition of fires.
3. Names or job titles of those persons responsible for control of fuel source hazards.

Tech Check

30. List five biological agents that have been associated with bioterrorism. (LO 2.12)

31. What type of plan does OSHA require to facilitate and organize workers in the event of any emergency? (LO 2.12)

Hazardous Materials (LO 2.13)

Hazardous Drugs

The American Society of Health-System Pharmacists (ASHP) defines hazardous drugs as those that exhibit one or more of the following effects in humans or animals:

- Carcinogenicity
- Teratogenicity or developmental toxicity
- Reproductive toxicity
- Organ toxicity at low doses
- Genotoxicity
- Structure and toxicity profiles of new drugs mimicking existing drugs determined hazardous by the above criteria

Storage

The proper procedures are critical to limit the risk of exposure to hazardous drugs where drugs are stored. The *OSHA Technical Manual* recommends limiting access to areas where hazardous drugs are stored to authorized personnel only. Signs should be posted indicating that entry to these areas is restricted (Figure 2-13).

Bins or shelves where hazardous drugs are stored should be designed to prevent breakage and limit contamination in the event of leakage. Bins should have barrier fronts to reduce the chance of containers falling to the floor. Bins with solid, as opposed to slotted, bottoms may help limit spills or waste due to leakage. Warning labels should be applied to all hazardous drug containers, shelves, and bins, where the containers are stored.

ASHP recommends hazardous drugs requiring refrigeration be stored separately from nonhazardous drugs in individual bins designed to prevent breakage and contain leakage. At no time should food or beverages be stored in refrigerators designated for drug storage, whether or not the drugs are defined as hazardous.

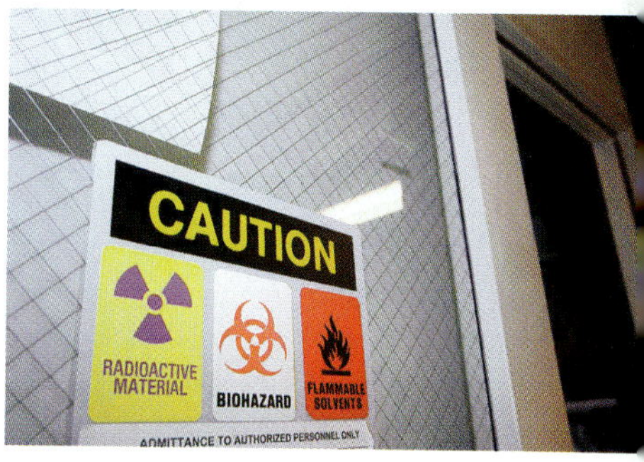

Figure 2-13 Caution. Authorized personnel only.

Tech Check

32. What are the recommendations of the *OSHA* with respect to access to areas where hazardous drugs are stored? (LO 2.13)

33. What are some desirable characteristics of shelving and bins used in the storage of hazardous drugs? (LO 2.13)

Handling

Pharmacy technicians must be aware that exposure to hazardous drugs during preparation may be due to ineffective work practice controls and failure to properly don personal protective equipment (PPE). Exposure can occur from

- Not using recommended biological safety cabinets
- Not using appropriate PPE
- Hazardous handling practices
- Improper practices in drug preparation areas

Approved biological safety cabinets (BSCs) must be used when preparing hazardous drugs. Class II, type B, or class III BSCs that vent to the outside are recommended by OSHA for use when preparing hazardous drugs. OSHA does not recommend horizontal BSCs for the preparation of hazardous drugs as they increase the risk of drug exposure. The BSC should contain covered needle containers for disposal, and a covered waste container for excess fluids disposal. It is also critical that the pharmacy technician follow the proper policies and procedures when using BSCs, as noncompliance increases risk for exposure. The policies and procedures established by individual sites are designed to ensure compliance with OSHA regulations. Types of noncompliance include poor cleaning technique of the BSC, unnecessary items or clutter in the BSC, and blocking of the BSC vent. The pharmacy technician should consult the BSC user's manual, as well as the pharmacy policy and procedure manual to ensure compliance in this area (Figure 2-14).

OSHA Requirements

OSHA requires employers to assess potential hazards, to select and use appropriate PPE, and to protect employees from hazardous drugs and chemicals. Examples of PPE include lab coats, gloves, masks, and goggles. Other requirements include:

- Latex gloves without powder should be doubled and worn at all times while handling hazardous drugs.
- The employer must ensure that hypoallergenic (nonlatex) gloves and liners are available to employees who are allergic to latex.
- The proper technique with double gloving requires that the inner glove is placed under the sleeve of the lab coat, and the outer glove is to be placed over the sleeve of the lab coat.

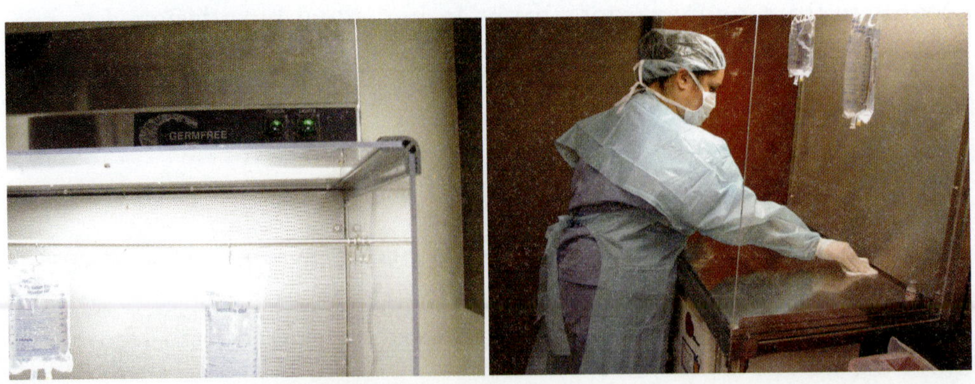

Figure 2-14 **To protect technicians from hazardous material contamination, work is carried out beneath a ventilated filtration hood.**

- Gloves should be changed hourly, or immediately following contamination.
- Removal of gloves should be performed in such a way as to avoid direct skin contact with the outside of the glove.
- Hands should be washed before donning and after removal of gloves. (Please refer to the section in this chapter on proper hand washing technique.)
- Lab coats should cover the clothing of the technician, be disposable with tight-fitting cuffs, and have a solid front.
- OSHA also requires the use of face and eye protection whenever splashes, sprays, or aerosols of hazardous drugs could result in eye, nose, or mouth contamination.

Hazardous handling practices and improper activities while preparing hazardous drugs increase risk of exposure to the agent. OSHA and the ASHP require that the area where hazardous drugs are prepared have restricted access, and that signs are displayed indicating the restriction of access to authorized personnel. In addition, smoking, drinking, eating, mouth pipetting, manipulating contact lenses, and applying cosmetics or lip balm is prohibited where hazardous drugs are prepared, stored, or used to reduce risk of exposure (Figure 2-15).

Hazardous drugs should be prepared in the pharmacy by pharmacists and/or pharmacy technicians who use the proper BSCs and PPE. The risk of exposure to hazardous drugs through inhalation or direct skin contact may occur when transferring hazardous drugs from one container to the other in reconstitution or manipulation, withdrawal of needles from drug vials, and expulsion of air from a drug-filled syringe. All syringes and needles used in the course of preparation should be placed in "sharps" containers for disposal without being crushed, clipped, or capped. The *OSHA Technical Manual* recommends that drug administration sets be attached and primed within the BSC prior to addition of the drug. Priming should be performed with a non-drug-containing solution or using the back-flow closed system. After preparation, syringes and intravenous bags containing hazardous drugs should be labeled with a distinctive warning label.

Resources employers may use to evaluate the hazard potential of a drug include material safety data sheets (MSDS), package inserts provided by the FDA, health warnings for manufacturers, reports, and/or case studies published in medical journals, and evidence-based recommendations from other facilities.

HAZARDOUS DRUGS PRESENT!!!

- **NO** EATING.
- **NO** DRINKING.
- **NO** SMOKING.
- **NO** MOUTH PIPETTING.
- DO **NOT** APPLY COSMETICS OR LIP BALM.
- DO **NOT** MANIPULATE CONTACT LENSES.

Figure 2-15 The warning sign alerts personnel to the presence of potentially hazardous substances and advises them about safety guidelines.

Table 2-3 Partial List of Drugs to Be Handled as Hazardous

Drug	Therapeutic Classification
Asparaginase	Antineoplastic
Azathioprine	Immunosuppressant
Bicalutamide	Antineoplastic
Bleomycin	Antineoplastic
Carmustine	Antineoplastic
Chloramphenicol	Antibiotic
Dacarbazine	Antineoplastic
Estradiol	Estrogen
Fluoxymesterone	Androgen
Lomustine	Antineoplastic
Mifepristone	Oxytocic
Mitomycin	Antineoplastic
Nafarelin	Gonadotropin
Oxytocin	Oxytocic
Progesterone	Progestin
Raloxifene	Estrogen agonist
Ribavirin	Antiviral
Tacrolimus	Immunosuppressant
Thioguanine	Antineoplastic
Tretinoin	Anti-acne
Vidarabine	Antiviral
Vincristine	Antineoplastic
Zidovudine	Antiretroviral

Tech Check

34. Define *hazardous drugs.* (LO 2.13)

35. What type of horizontal BSC is *not* recommended by OSHA for the preparation of hazardous drugs? Why? (LO 2.13)

36. What type of container should be used for the disposal of needles and syringes? (LO 2.13)

An extensive list of hazardous drugs may be found on the National Institute for Occupational Safety and Health (NIOSH) Web site at **www.cdc.gov/niosh/docs/2004-165/2004-165d.html**.

Table 2-3 represents a partial listing of hazardous agents.

NIOSH Recommendations for Health Care Workers(LO 2.13)

Protection

The National Institute for Occupational Safety and Health (NIOSH) recommends that health care workers take the following steps to protect themselves from hazardous drugs. Read all information and MSDS your employer provides to you for the hazardous drugs you handle.

- Participate in any training your employer provides on the hazards of the drugs you handle and the equipment and procedures you should use to prevent exposure.
- Be familiar with and able to recognize sources of exposure to hazardous drugs. Sources of exposure include
  - all procedures involving hazardous drugs (including preparation, administration, and cleaning), and
  - all materials that come into contact with hazardous drugs (including work surfaces, equipment, protective wear, intravenous bags and tubing, patient waste, and soiled linens).
- Prepare hazardous drugs in an area that is devoted to that purpose alone and is restricted to authorized personnel.
- Prepare hazardous drugs inside a ventilated cabinet designed to protect workers and others from exposure and to protect all drugs that require sterile handling.
- Use two pairs of powder-free, disposable chemotherapy gloves, with the outer one covering the gown cuff whenever there is risk of exposure to hazardous drugs.
- Avoid skin contact by using a disposable gown made of polyethylene-coated polypropylene material (which is nonlinting and nonabsorbent). Make sure the gown has a closed front, long sleeves, and elastic or knit closed cuffs. Do not reuse gowns.
- Wear a face shield when splashes to the eyes, nose, or mouth may occur and when adequate engineering controls (such as the sash or window on a ventilated cabinet) are not available.
- Wash hands with soap and water immediately before using personal protective clothing (such as disposable gloves and gowns) and after removing it.
- Use syringes and intravenous sets with Luer-Lok™ fittings for preparing and administering hazardous drugs.
- Place drug-contaminated syringes and needles in chemotherapy sharps containers for disposal.
- When supplemental protection is needed, use closed-system drug-transfer devices, glove bags, and needleless systems inside the ventilated cabinet.
- Handle hazardous wastes and contaminated materials separately from other trash.
- Clean and decontaminate work areas before and after each activity involving hazardous drugs and at the end of each shift.
- Clean up small spills of hazardous drugs immediately, using proper safety precautions and PPE.
- Clean up large spills of hazardous drugs with the help of an environmental services specialist.

Source: **www.cdc.gov/niosh/docs/2004-165/2004-165d.html.**

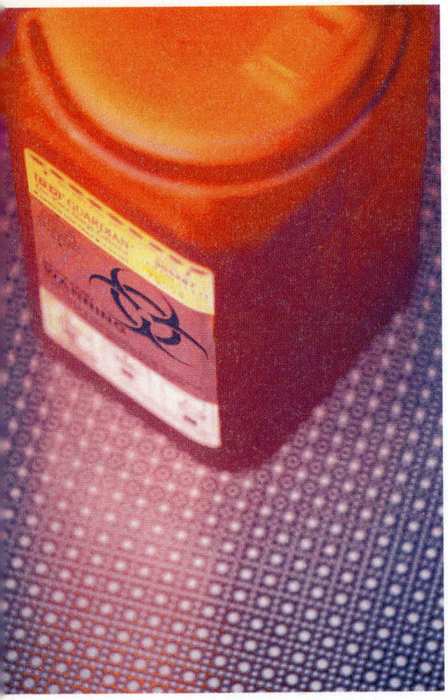

Figure 2-16 **Hazardous waste container.**

Disposal of Hazardous Drugs

Proper disposal of hazardous drugs is critical to maintaining safety in the workplace. Exposure to hazardous drugs may occur during disposal while bagging and labeling products and through improper waste disposal and use of containers.

OSHA requires that bags containing materials contaminated with hazardous drugs be labeled "Hazardous Drug Waste."

- The bags must be thick, leak-proof, and colored differently than other hospital trash bags.
- The bags should be used for routine collection of discarded gloves, gowns, and other disposable material.
- The hazardous waste bag should be kept inside a covered waste container clearly labeled "Hazardous Drug Waste."
- At least one receptacle should be located in every area where such agents are prepared or administered.
- The bag should be sealed when filled and the covered waste container should be securely taped.

Containers for the disposal of needles and breakable items containing hazardous waste should be labeled "Hazardous Drug Waste Only." Personnel should be trained in the use of properly labeled, sealed, and covered disposal containers to meet the requirements of the bloodborne pathogens standard, if items are contaminated with blood. The technician must be aware of the safety and standards in order to apply them in the workplace (Figure 2-16).

Hazardous drug-related wastes should be disposed of according to the Environmental Protection Agency (EPA) regulations for hazardous waste. While awaiting transfer to the appropriate site for final disposal, hazardous waste should remain in a secure area in covered, labeled drums with plastic liners.

Caution

Only hazardous waste should be placed in containers labeled for their disposal!

Tech Check

37. Describe methods of possible exposure to hazardous drugs while disposing of those agents. (LO 2.13)

38. Describe the characteristics of the hazardous waste disposal bags. (LO 2.13)

The pharmacy technician plays a critical role in the prevention of workplace accidents and infection control. The methods the technician employs to perform this role will vary by pharmacy setting. In the retail setting, for instance, a technician will simply wear a lab coat and will clean up spills with clean paper towels. In an inpatient setting, technicians will wear lab coats with gloves most of the time, and will also use caution when cleaning up spills that may contain contaminants, pathogens, or toxic chemicals. In any pharmacy setting, the technician has the responsibility to assist the pharmacist in achieving and maintaining a safe pharmacy environment for both pharmacy staff and patients.

Chapter Summary

Understanding the management of infectious disease in the workplace is vital to the pharmacy technician. Since the pharmacy technician works closely with other health care professionals and patients, it is important for the pharmacy technician to understand the impact of the following on pharmacy practice:

- Regulatory agencies (The Joint Commission, OSHA, CDC) play a critical role to ensure infection control and workplace safety.
- Use of standard precautions limits the spread of infectious disease, including bloodborne and airborne disease transmission.
- The four major types of nosocomial infections are surgical wound infections, lower respiratory tract infections, urinary tract infections, and bloodstream infections.
- Hand hygiene, including hand washing, wearing gloves, and using antiseptics, helps limit the spread of pathogens that cause infectious disease.
- Personal protective equipment, when used appropriately, protect both patients and pharmacy technicians by decreasing transport of microbes and risk of contamination with hazardous materials.
- Proper documentation and reporting, as described in the institution's policies and procedures, are a part of the pharmacy technician's job duties.
- Human Immunodeficiency Virus (HIV) Postexposure Prophylaxis (PEP) is most successful when antiretroviral agents are initiated within hours of occupational exposure.
- Emergency preparedness includes first aid, CPR, bioterrorism training, Emergency Action Plan and the Fire Prevention Plan.
- Proper handling, storage and disposal of hazardous materials is vital to maintaining a safe healthcare workplace.

Chapter Review

Case Study Questions

1. What modes of infectious disease transmission could Bob be exposed to?(LO 2.2)
2. How can Bob reduce his risk?(LO 2.5, 2.8)
3. What is Bob's responsibility as a senior technician to reduce the risk of spread of infectious disease?(LO 2.5)

At Your Service Questions

1. What should the nurse have done?(LO 2.5)
2. What is the pharmacy technician's responsibility?(LO 2.2, 2.5)

Multiple Choice

Select the best answer.

1. Which of the following pathogens is *not* transferred via the bloodborne route?(LO 2.4)
   a. HBV
   b. HIV
   c. TB
   d. HCV
2. Which of the following agents is *not* a component of PEP for HIV?(LO 2.11)
   a. Zidovudine
   b. Triclosan
   c. Lamivudine
   d. Stavudine

3. In the proper technique for hand washing, how long should the hands be rubbed together with a soap causing friction?(LO 2.7)
   a. 1–5 seconds
   b. 5–10 seconds
   c. 10–15 seconds
   d. 20–30 seconds
4. Which is *not* a biological agent associated with bioterrorism?(LO 2.12)
   a. SARS
   b. Ricin
   c. Anthrax
   d. Chicken pox
5. Which of the following agencies is primarily focused on the prevention of disease transmission?(LO 2.1)
   a. NIOSH
   b. CDC
   c. ASHP
   d. OSHA
6. Used needles and syringes should be placed in a.(LO 2.4)
   a. regular trash bag.
   b. hazardous waste bag.
   c. "sharps" container.
   d. storage bin.
7. Which of the following agents is *not* recommended for hand hygiene in a health care facility?(LO 2.6)
   a. Alcohol-based hand rubs
   b. Antibacterial soap
   c. Water
   d. Scented soap
8. Which of the following is generally *not* included in an incident report?(LO 2.10)
   a. The name and identifying information of the injured party
   b. The description of the injury, event, or exposure
   c. The name of a witness
   d. The name of the person at fault
9. Which is true regarding outside reporting of infectious disease outbreaks?(LO 2.9)
   a. The first agency to be notified is the FBI.
   b. Reportable infectious diseases vary by state.
   c. State health departments should not be notified in the event of an outbreak.
   d. The CDC should be notified before the local health department.
10. Which of the following conditions warrants reporting to the CDC?(LO 2.9)
    a. Antiretroviral drug resistance
    b. PEP for HIV failure
    c. PEP for HIV adverse drug reactions
    d. A and B
11. Which is true of both the EAP and FPP?(LO 2.12)
    a. They are used only in the case of fire.
    b. They must be written.
    c. They must be available via e-mail.
    d. None of the above.
12. Which of the following is *not* a recommendation of NIOSH for health care workers handling hazardous materials?(LO 2.13)
    a. Two pairs of gloves should be worn.
    b. A horizontal BSC should always be used.
    c. Any spills should be cleaned up immediately.
    d. Hazardous waste should be handled separately from other trash.
13. Which of the following is *not* a foodborne pathogen?(LO 2.12)
    a. Shigella
    b. Salmonella
    c. Botulism
    d. Hantavirus
14. Which of the following is false?(LO 2.6)
    a. Pharmacy technicians should wash their hands before and after handling dangerous drugs, even if gloves are worn.
    b. Pharmacy technicians should not wear artificial nails if they are engaged in the handling of dangerous drugs and/or sterile compounding.
    c. Nail polish, if worn, should not be chipped.
    d. Needles and syringes contaminated with hazardous materials may be disposed of in the nonchemo sharps container.
15. Which of the following is *not* an airborne disease?(LO 2.2)
    a. Influenza
    b. Tuberculosis
    c. Hepatitis
    d. Pneumonia

Critical Thinking Questions

1. What is your understanding of the role of OSHA and how the standards relate to workplace safety?(LO 2.1)
2. After learning about the various precautions discussed in this chapter, will this impact your typical hand hygiene behavior?(LO 2.6)

3. Have you ever known someone who was admitted to a hospital and contracted an infection while in the hospital? If so, do you know how the infection was managed? What was the patient told?(LO 2.3)

4. What is your understanding of an epidemic or outbreak of infectious disease? Why is it so dangerous?(LO 2.12)

5. Have you ever been in an emergency situation? Were you able to take appropriate action? Were certain departments contacted (fire, police, etc.)? How do you feel about the response of these departments?(LO 2.9, 2.12)

HIPAA Scenario

Carl Henning is an inpatient at Burles Medical Center. His physician called the hospital where Fran works in the pharmacy and asked if he could get a copy of the medication profile that had been created for Carl at Fran's hospital. His intention is to compare Carl's two drug profiles to ensure that he is aware of all the medications Carl has been taking. Fran politely declines the physician's request, saying that the Health Insurance Portability and Accountability Act (HIPAA) prevents her from disseminating that information to anyone outside of her facility.

Discussion Questions (PTCB II. 73)

1. Are physicians legally entitled to access the medical records of their patients that were compiled at another health care entity?

2. Did Fran take the correct action in refusing to give the doctor the information he requested?

Internet Activities

1. Go to the Centers for Disease Control and Prevention Web site (**www.cdc.gov**) and click on the Emergency Preparedness and Response link. In this link find the contact protocol flowchart and print it out. Summarize your findings in other areas at this link. (LO 2.1)

2. Go to the Centers for Disease Control and Prevention Web site at **www.cdc.gov/ncphi/disss/nndss/nndsshis.htm** to search for nationally notifiable diseases by state. List the reportable infectious diseases in your state that are reportable by the health care provider only. Discuss your findings in class. (LO 2.2)

3. Access the Centers for Disease Control and Prevention Web site at **www.cdc.gov/niosh/docs/2004-165/#sum**. Scroll down to case studies. Select a case study and list the possible ways the exposure could have been avoided. Also discuss what actions you might have taken if you were exposed to the agent or if you witnessed exposure to an agent. (LO 2.1, 2.2, 2.11, 2.13)

3

Communication and Customer Service

Key Terms

compassion
customer service
empathy
encoding
kinesics
oculesics
proxemics
receiver
sender

Learning Outcomes

Upon completion of this chapter, you will be able to:

3.1 Identify and explain the components of the communication process.

3.2 Differentiate between the various types of communication used in pharmacy.

3.3 Identify various forms of nonverbal communication.

3.4 Explain the importance of effective communication in the practice of pharmacy.

3.5 Explain the results that may occur due to poor communication in the practice of pharmacy.

3.6 Identify various solutions to communication problems in a pharmacy.

3.7 Explain the meaning of customer service in the practice of pharmacy.

3.8 Define and identify the customer in the practice of pharmacy.

3.9 Identify tools used to provide outstanding customer service.

3.10 Explain the need for patient privacy and confidentiality in the practice of pharmacy.

PTCB

In preparation for the certification examination, you should understand and perform activities associated with the following PTCB Knowledge Statements:

PTCB Knowledge Statement

Domain I. Assisting the Pharmacist in Serving Patients

Knowledge of customer service principles (71)

Knowledge of communication techniques (72)

Knowledge of confidentiality requirements (73)

PTCB Knowledge Statement

Domain II. Maintaining Medication and Inventory Control Systems

Knowledge of the written, oral, and electronic communication channels necessary to ensure appropriate follow-up and problem resolution (24)

PTCB Knowledge Statement

Domain III. Participation in the Administration and Management of Pharmacy Practice

Knowledge of lines of communication throughout the organization (2)

Knowledge of written, oral, and electronic communications (5)

Case Study

Robert is a 50-year-old white male who suffers from cardiovascular disease (hypertension and cardiac arrhythmias). He is a certified public accountant, owns a small investment company, and is a workaholic. He has two children in college. In the past, you have noted that he does not take his medication properly. You notice Robert walking toward the pharmacy and he is looking at the ground. His skin color is extremely pale, he is clutching his chest, and his words sound slurred. He approaches the pharmacy counter and asks if his physician has called in his refills. After checking the filled prescriptions and realizing the physician has not called yet, you ask him what medication needs to be refilled. He informs you that it is something for his heart. You check his profile and notice that he is taking 10 cardiovascular medications.

While reading this chapter, keep the following questions in mind:

1. What forms of communication were used during this incident?(LO 3.2, 3.3, 3.6)
2. What did his nonverbal actions demonstrate?(LO 3.3)

Introduction to Communication and Customer Service(LO 3.1)

The ability to recognize human behaviors and the ability to communicate effectively are vital to a pharmacy technician and the pursuit for success. In the practice of pharmacy, the pharmacy technician works with patients. In some cases, these patients are also customers. In this chapter about communication and customer service, the terms *patient* and *customer* are used interchangeably. Patients will often have their first interaction with the pharmacy technician in the pharmacy or other health care facility. It is important that patients develop a good rapport and feel confident in the care they are receiving. The pharmacy technician sets the tone for the communication cycle and must be aware of all the obstacles that can affect human communication. As a pharmacy technician, you are often exposed to all kinds of patients. You will see patients from different cultures, socioeconomic backgrounds, educational levels, ages, and lifestyles. You must be able to communicate with each patient with professionalism and diplomacy.

At Your Service

It is Monday morning and Brandon, the pharmacy technician, has started his shift. Brandon knows that customer service is the foundation for success in the practice of pharmacy. As a pharmacy technician, he plans to provide excellent customer service to all of his patients. The telephone rings, and Brandon answers the telephone.

"Good morning, Your Neighborhood Pharmacy, Brandon speaking. How may I help you?"

"This is Mary Sanders, and I am calling to see if my physician has called in a new prescription for me."

"Let me check the records in our computer, Ms. Sanders. I will be back with you in a moment."

Less than a minute later, Brandon returns to the telephone.

"Ms. Sanders, your physician did call in your prescription for you this morning. Unfortunately, we are temporarily out of the medication, but we have ordered it from our wholesaler. It will be ready for you to pick up this afternoon after 4 P.M. I can call you when your medication arrives. Is that alright with you, Ms. Sanders?"

"That will be fine; the number I can be reached at is 703-555-5555, ext. 555. I will be at that number until 5 P.M. My cell phone number is 703-111-1111," replied Ms. Sanders.

Later that day at 3:45 P.M., the wholesaler order arrives at the pharmacy. Brandon checks the order and begins to process the prescriptions that are awaiting medications from the order.

He fills Ms. Sanders's prescription, calls her at her office, and leaves a message on her telephone. Brandon then calls Ms. Sanders on her cell phone, reaches her, and informs her that the prescription is ready. Ms. Sanders is extremely appreciative of everything Brandon has done for her regarding her prescription.

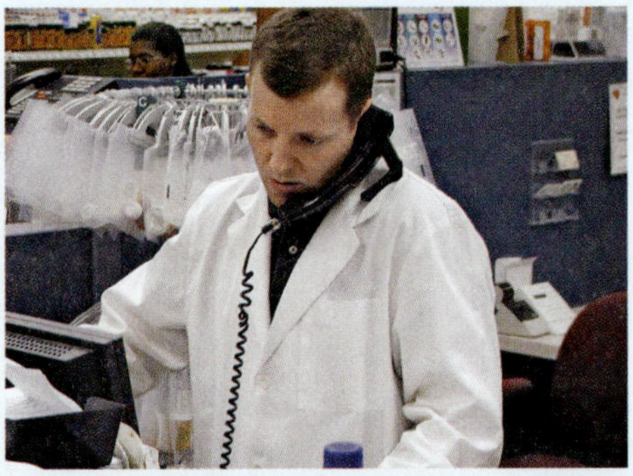

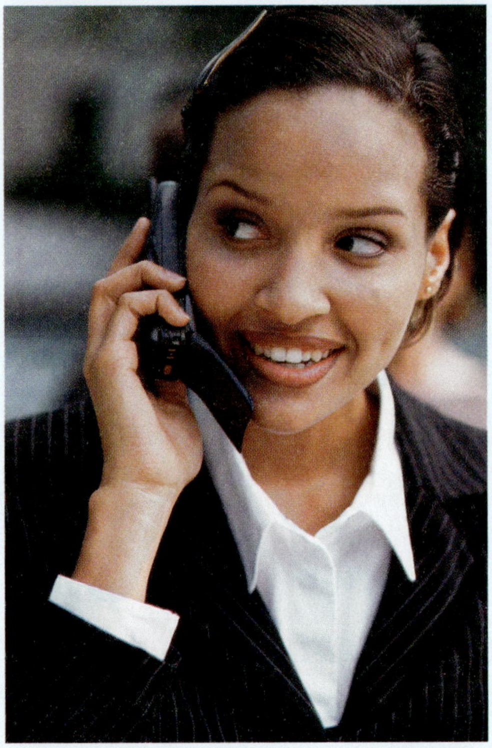

While reading this chapter, keep the following question in mind.

1. What are examples of good **customer service** exemplified by Brandon?(LO 3.9)

Communication(LO 3.1, 3.4, 3.5)

customer service Meeting the specific needs of the patient, who in this situation is considered the customer (one who pays for goods or services).

Communication is the process by which information is exchanged between individuals through a common system of symbols, signs, or behavior. Communication consists of both verbal and nonverbal forms of expression. Nonverbal communication involves facial expressions, body movements, eye contact, and other physical gestures.

One-on-one communication is the most common form of communication in the practice of pharmacy. Examples of pharmacy communication include:

- A patient presenting a written prescription to the pharmacy technician or pharmacist.
- A patient calling in a refill to the pharmacy.
- A physician's office calling or faxing in a prescription to the pharmacy.
- A pharmacy technician asking a patient if she may help him or her.

The communication cycle consists of a source, a message, a **receiver,** feedback, and barriers (Figure 3-1). Messages can be planned or spontaneous. The source initiates the process by formulating or **encoding** a message before it is sent. A message may be a thought, an idea, an emotion, or information that can be conveyed verbally or nonverbally.

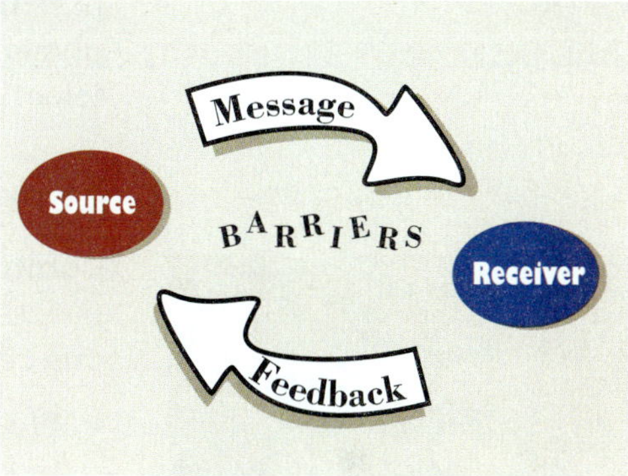

Figure 3-1 The process of communication involves an exchange of messages through verbal and nonverbal means.

The receiver receives the message, decodes it, and interprets its meaning. It is extremely important that the receiver listen closely to what the **sender** is saying. There may be times when the interpretation of the message may be entirely different from what the sender intended. We cannot make assumptions of what is being said by an individual. False assumption may pose consequences to the customer.

Feedback is the process by which the receiver communicates back to the sender his or her understanding of the sender's message. Feedback can be either verbal or nonverbal. It is in this situation that the roles of the sender and receiver are reversed. Meanings are assigned to both verbal and nonverbal communication based upon our experiences.

Feedback plays an important part of the communication process because it demonstrates whether the initial message was received properly.

Communication can flow vertically (upward or downward) or laterally. Downward communication flows from one level of the organization to a lower level. Downward communication may include the usage of written memos, electronic memos via e-mail, or even a letter. Examples of downward communication in a pharmacy may include the pharmacist

- Instructing the pharmacy technician to do a specific task or the steps taken to perform a specific duty.
- Informing the pharmacy staff on specific goals of the pharmacy.
- Giving instructions on handling a specific situation.

Upward communication occurs from a lower level to a higher level within an organization. Upward communication may be used to solicit feedback from the employees or provide employees with a vehicle to recommend solutions to a problem. Methods used to obtain upward communication include employee surveys, "brown bag lunches" with the employees, or even a suggestion box. Examples of upward communication in a pharmacy include the pharmacy technician

- Informing the pharmacist whether a patient is waiting or will return later.
- Telling the pharmacist that a physician or patient is waiting on the telephone for them.
- Informing the pharmacist that a patient has a question.

Lateral communication occurs among members of the same work group such as pharmacy technicians. Lateral communication is necessary to save

receiver The individual who responds to the sender's communication.

encoding The process of converting information from one system of communication into another system.

sender The individual who initiates the communication.

time and facilitate coordination of the prescription-filling process. Examples of lateral communication include the pharmacy technician

- Informing a coworker about waiting prescriptions.
- Telling a fellow technician of medications that need to be ordered.
- Notifying a coworker of changes in prescribing habits of a doctor.

All pharmacy communication must take place at the proper time. Information must be accurately and promptly provided to the pharmacist, patient, or fellow pharmacy technician. You should never interrupt the pharmacist with questions when he or she is talking to a physician on the telephone or counseling a patient.

Communication Barriers

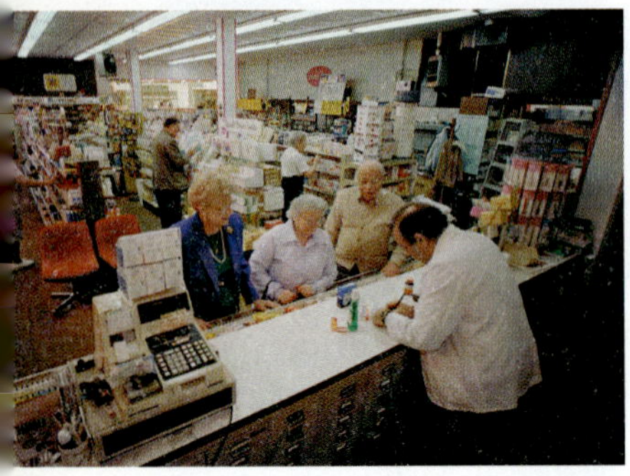

Figure 3-2 The pharmacy counter can be a communication barrier.

Communication barriers are things that may prevent the communication process from being interpreted correctly by an individual. There are various types of communication barriers which include the following:

- Physical distractions, such as the telephone ringing, customers talking in front of the pharmacy counter, or music being played throughout the pharmacy (Figure 3-2).
- Language problems, such as a non-English speaking patient in a pharmacy where the primary language spoken is English and using the wrong choice of words (medical or pharmaceutical terms) to the patient.
- Mixed messages, where the customer's verbal communication does not coincide with their nonverbal communication.
- Cultural differences, especially when the customers come from different heritages.
- Absence or lack of feedback from the patient. It is the responsibility of the pharmacy staff to make sure the patient and/or customer understands how to take the prescription or nonprescription medication they have received or purchased.
- Patient's mental or physical disabilities. It may be necessary move from behind the counter to speak to the physically handicapped patient. The pharmacy staff may need to provide the directions to a care giver in the case of a mentally disabled patient.

Tech Check

1. Visit your local pharmacy and observe the actions of the pharmacy staff. What barriers are present at the pharmacy?(LO 3.1, 3.4)
2. What are your recommendations to eliminate these barriers?(LO 3.1, 3.5)

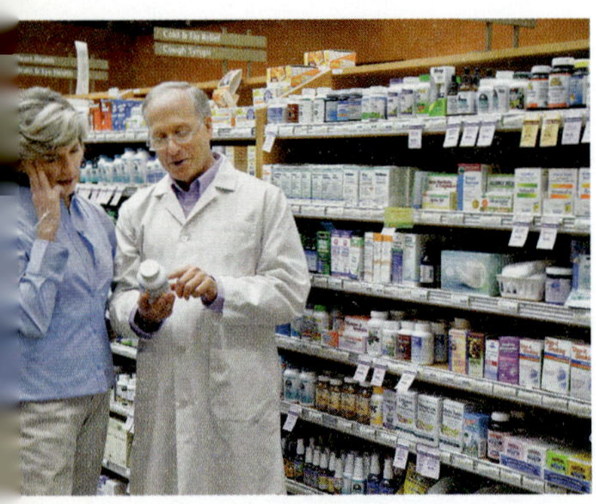

Figure 3-3 Store pharmacist assisting patient.

Types of Communication(LO 3.2, 3.3, 3.6)

Verbal Communication

Every day we communicate with others using words. We assign specific meanings to words based upon our understanding. The meaning of a word may vary from individual to individual; our background, values, or experiences can affect our understanding of a word (Figure 3-2). Individual differences in meaning and understanding can cause a misunderstanding. To prevent misunderstanding is to predict how an individual will translate the message. Pharmacy technicians can obtain feedback by asking customers questions to see if they truly understand what is being said. For example, they may ask customers how they take their medication to verify if they understand.

Verbal Communication Tools

Active Listening

When a patient/customer is talking to us, we are hearing him or her but that does not mean that we are listening. Hearing is a passive process while listening is an active process. Often, individuals hear what is being said but they may not be listening to an individual. Active listening requires concentrating on what the patient/customer is saying. The following tips will help the pharmacy technician actively listen to patients and/or customers.

- Listen for content.
- Listen and respond to the customer's feelings.
- Note all cues by the customer.
- Reflect back on what the customer said.
- Make eye contact with the customer.
- Use positive head nods and appropriate facial expressions.
- Avoid distracting gestures to the customer.
- Ask the customer questions.
- Paraphrase what the customer is saying.
- Avoid interrupting the customer.

Speak Clearly

When we respond to customers' statements, it is extremely important that we speak clearly. Have you ever failed to understand what someone was saying? Was it because the person was speaking too fast? Did it appear that the individual's words were mumbled? Did he or she speak in a monotone voice? Was the individual using terms with which you were not familiar? Did the person have an accent? These situations focus on the problem of trying to understand the patient. Is it possible that the customer is saying the same things about you? It is important that we use terms that are specific and precise, but the customer must be able to understand them.

Display Empathy

Empathy is being able to communicate to an individual that you are able to understand his or her feelings in a caring manner. Empathy expresses understanding in a compassionate, patient, and nonjudgmental manner. This relationship develops rapport between you and the customer. The trust, which is demonstrated, must be authentic and sincere. If the customer is unable to perceive your sincerity, trust may not be established. If one's verbal and nonverbal communication is not in balance, the patient will perceive that empathy does not exist.

A second condition necessary in establishing empathy is the demonstration of respect toward the customer as being a worthwhile individual. Pharmacy technicians who demonstrate a positive feeling toward customers will find that customers are more open with them. In contrast, if customers believe they are being judged by you, they will be less likely to confide in you.

empathy The action of understanding, being aware of, and being sensitive to the feelings, thoughts, and experience of another.

Once empathy is conveyed to customers:

- They will trust you as an individual who cares about them.
- They will better understand their own feelings.
- They will be better able to solve their own problems.

It is the customers' perception that determines if the practitioner is exhibiting empathy.

Nonverbal Communication

Body Language

It has been estimated that 60% to 95% of all communication is nonverbal. Nonverbal communication consists of a complete mix of behaviors, psychological responses, and environmental interactions through which a person relates to another individual. Nonverbal communications are those in which words are neither spoken nor written by an individual. Nonverbal communication allows one to express both thoughts and feelings. During nonverbal communication, the customer is able to perceive and interpret messages in a personal manner. These interpretations are based upon various social, psychological, and cultural factors. In many situations, these interpretations are universal. Examples of nonverbal communication are found in Table 3-1.

Nonverbal communication has many different parts. These parts include kinesics, proxemics, oculesics, the environment, and various distracting factors.

Table 3-1 Nonverbal Communication (Body Language)

Nonverbal Behavior	Interpretation
Brisk, erect walk	Confidence 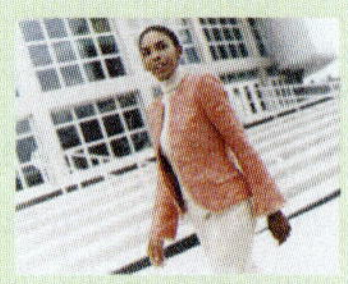
Hand to cheek	Evaluation, thinking
Sitting with hands clasped behind head, legs crossed	Confidence, superiority 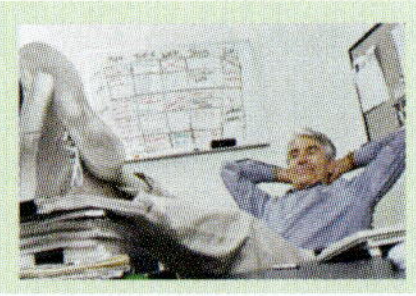
Sitting legs apart	Open, relaxed
Open palm	Sincerity, openness, innocence
Steeping fingers	Authoritative
Tilted head	Interest 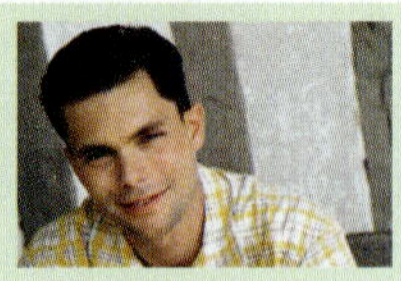
Standing with hands on hips	Readiness, aggression
Sitting with legs crossed, foot kicking slightly	Boredom
Arms crossed on chest	Defensiveness 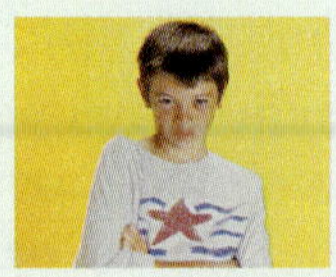

(Continued)

Table 3-1 **Nonverbal Communication (Body Language) *(Continued)***

Nonverbal Behavior	Interpretation
Walking with hands in pockets, shoulders hunched	Dejection
Rubbing the eye	Doubt, disbelief
Hands resting in hand, eyes downcast	Boredom 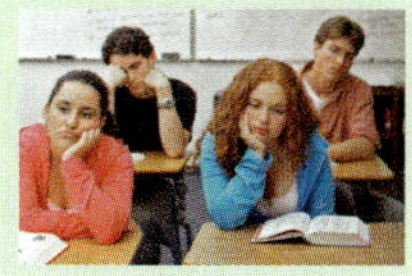
Rubbing hands	Anticipation
Looking down, face turned away	Disbelief
Pulling or tugging at ear	Indecision
Stroking chin	Trying to make a decision 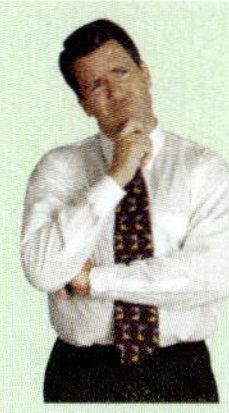
Tapping or drumming fingers	Impatience
Biting nails	Insecurity, nervousness

Kinesics

Kinesics is the study of communication through body movement and facial expression (Figure 3-4). Primary areas examined include eye contact, posture, and gestures. As a health care practitioner, pharmacy technicians must be able to demonstrate empathy and commitment to helping those individuals who are not healthy. Maintaining an open stance demonstrates empathy, sincerity, and respect toward a customer.

There are many things individuals can do to create a warm and friendly environment for a customer. They include:

- Vary eye contact.
- Maintain a relaxed posture.
- Use appropriate gestures when explaining things to a customer.
- Lean slightly toward the customer, instead of away from them.
- Stand straight, head looking toward the customer, and keep arms uncrossed.

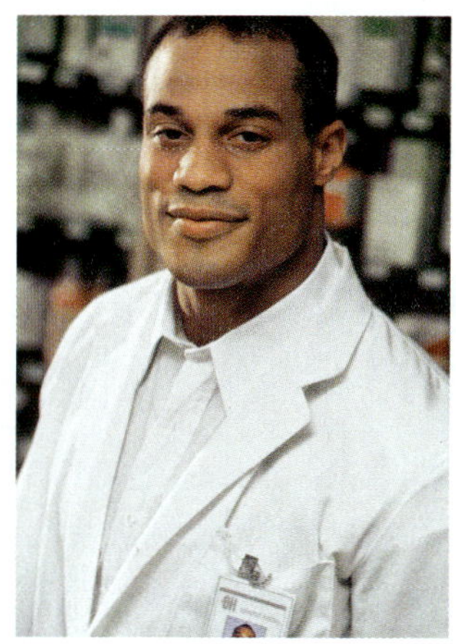

Figure 3-4 Positive communication through facial expression.

kinesics A systematic study of the relationship between nonlinguistic body motions (as blushes, shrugs, or eye movement) and communication.

proxemics The study of the nature, degree, and effect of the spatial separation individuals naturally maintain (as in various social and interpersonal situations).

Proxemics

Proxemics is the way individuals use physical space to convey messages. In the United States there are four different distances used in communicating face-to-face situations: intimate, personal, social, and public distance. Intimate distance is the distance between people that is used for confidential communications. Personal distances are used for talking with family and close friends. Social distance is used in handling business communications, and public distance is used in communicating with individuals across the room.

The pharmacy layout is an example of proxemics. Many pharmacy interactions occur within 4 to 12 feet. The patient consultation area allows the

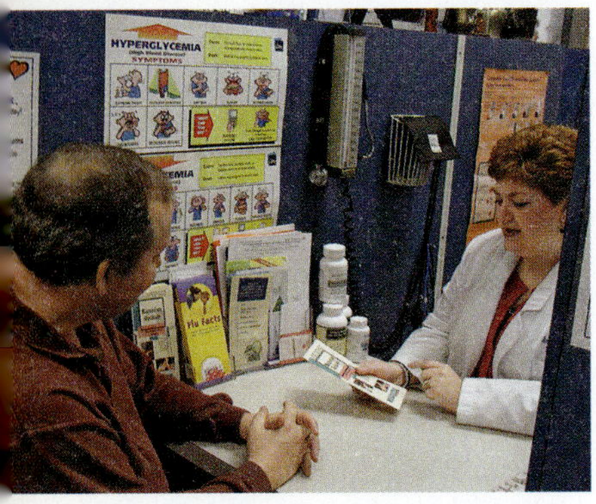

Figure 3-5 The patient consultation area is one example of proxemics.

pharmacist to stand close enough to the customer to allow for confidentiality yet allows the individual to feel comfortable. The patient counseling area, the prescription intake, and pickup areas are specifically designed using both intimate and personal distances (Figure 3-5). The pharmacy should be designed to allow both the pharmacy staff and customer to feel comfortable during their conversations.

Oculesics

Oculesics is a form of communication that involves conveying messages with eye contact. It is good practice for a pharmacy technician to maintain eye contact with the customer at all times. Failing to maintain proper eye contact may signal to the customer that you may not truly care what he or she is saying. Second, failing to maintain proper eye contact prevents you from observing the patient's nonverbal communication (Figure 3-6).

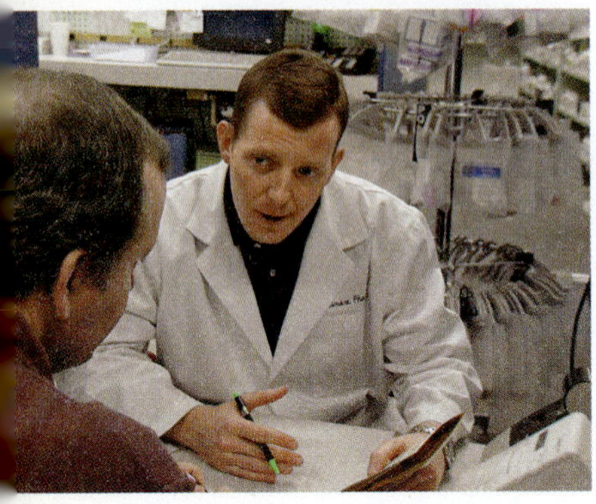

Figure 3-6 The pharmacy technician should maintain good eye contact with the patient.

Environment

The physical appearance of a pharmacy is an important form of nonverbal communication (Figure 3-7). Lighting and the effective usage of space are nonverbal forms of communication. The general appearance of the pharmacy's condition is another nonverbal form of communication. Is the counter dusty, cluttered, or clean? Is the pharmacy appropriately lit or are there burnt-out bulbs? Is there trash on the floor near the pharmacy? Is the area behind the pickup window neat or cluttered with boxes? Are the shelves stocked neatly or are they in disarray? Is music playing? If so, is it overwhelming?

Written Communication

From time to time, a pharmacy technician may be required to provide a written communication either to other allied health personnel or to patient and/or customers. Examples of written communications include faxes, electronic mail, letters, and memos (Figure 3-8). Written communications are both tangible and verifiable. A written communication can be stored for an unspecified period, and often both the sender and receiver have a record of it. A written communication can be retrieved and verified of its content if questions arise. In most situations, an individual will think more carefully, about what is said in a written communication than in an oral communication. A written communication may be revised several times before it is sent.

Some shortcomings to written communications include the time required to write one, which exceeds the amount time for oral communications. Written communications lack instantaneous feedback, compared to oral communications and may not be interpreted in the same manner as oral communications. Finally, written communications do not contain nonverbal communications.

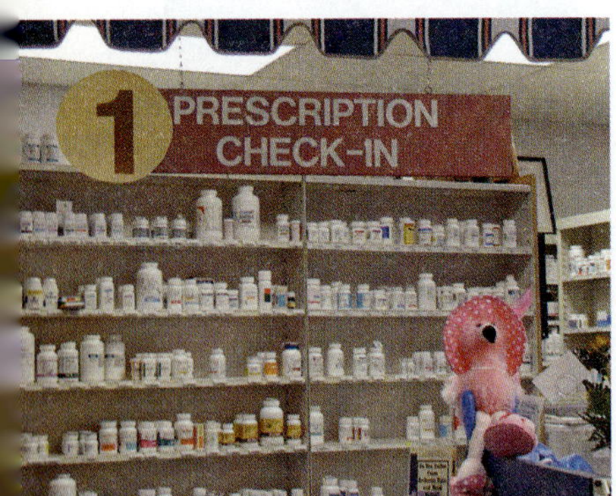

Figure 3-7 The pharmacy appearance.

Communication Obstacles

Environmental Barriers

One of the most noticeable barriers in pharmacy is the pharmacy counter itself. In a retail setting, the pharmacy counter is located in the back of the store; it is generally above ground level and the distance between the patient and pharmacist or pharmacy technician is noticeable (Figure 3-9). The noise level of the area surrounding the pharmacy counter may limit one-on-one communication between the pharmacy staff and the patient and/or customer. Often, individuals are hesitant with ask questions regarding their medication if they are unable to speak at ease with the pharmacist.

oculesics The use of the eyes in a communication setting. In most Western cultures, the use of direct eye contact symbolizes listening and attention.

Personal Barriers

Personal barriers can hinder communication in the practice of pharmacy. If an individual lacks confidence in his or her ability to communicate effectively, the person will demonstrate this to the customer. Individuals are able to learn and improve their communication skills. Shyness is a personal barrier affecting many pharmacy technicians and may precipitate an individual's anxiety level when communicating with customers. However, shyness can be overcome with time and effort.

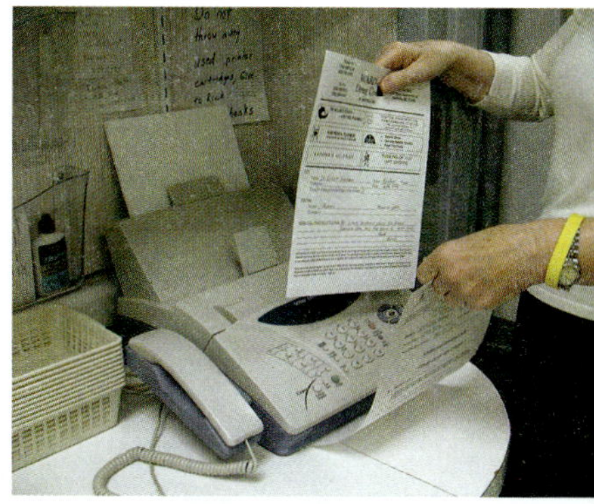

Figure 3-8 **Written communication via fax.**

Customer Barriers

Customer barriers are based upon the experiences of the patients and their perceptions. First, if customers believe the pharmacy staff is not knowledgeable about a specific condition and appropriate therapy, they may be hesitant to ask questions. The pharmacy staff must convey to the customers that they are knowledgeable. Second, if customers perceive the staff is unwilling to communicate with them, they may not ask questions regarding their therapy. Everything we do in the practice of pharmacy must demonstrate to customers that we are there to assist them. A customer's question should not be interpreted as an interruption but rather as an opportunity for the staff to demonstrate their knowledge and desire to assist them. Third, managed health care has caused many individuals to believe that health care has become extremely impersonal. Many patients believe that practitioners do not view them as individuals, but rather as a number. They may sense the pharmacy staff lacks empathy toward them because they are always in a hurry to process them.

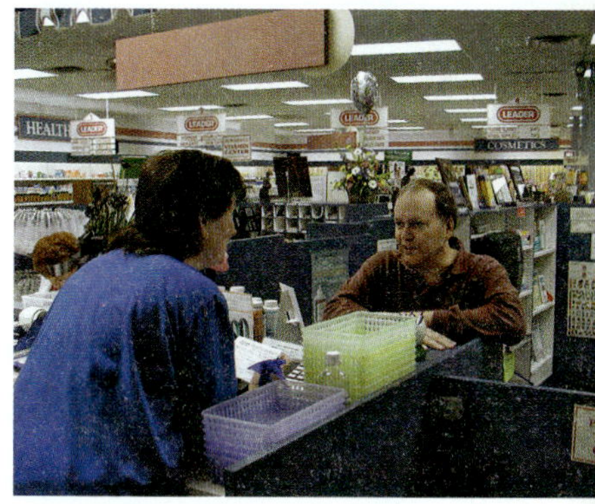

Figure 3-9 **The pharmacy counter is an environmental barrier.**

Finally, customers may be embarrassed to talk about specific conditions. Some customers have trouble discussing sexual dysfunctions, depression, or cancer. This may be attributed to their culture or personal experiences. It is extremely important that the pharmacy staff be observant of patients' verbal and nonverbal communications to overcome the customer barriers.

Tech Check

3. What are three examples of nonverbal communication?(LO 3.3)
4. What are three obstacles to communication?(LO 3.6)
5. What is one thing an individual can do to improve his or her verbal communication skills?(LO 3.6)

Customer Service(LO 3.6, 3.7, 3.8, 3.9, 3.10)

Customer service is the foundation for the success of a pharmacy organization. A pharmacy cannot and will not survive without customers. It is the customers who determine whether a pharmacy becomes profitable or not. Pharmacy customers have many options as to where they have their prescriptions processed: at independent, franchise, or chain drugstores; or at pharmacies located in grocery stores, mass merchandisers, discounters, and membership clubs. Pharmacy customers also may have their prescriptions filled by mail-order pharmacies. It is the organization that provides the best customer service in the eyes of the customer that will survive.

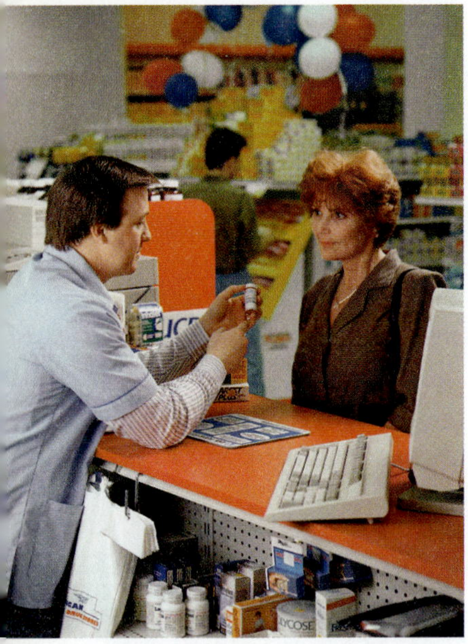

Figure 3-10 Explaining prescription to customer.

Customer service can be defined as meeting the needs of the patient, who is considered a customer (Figure 3-10). Everything one does in the practice of pharmacy is geared toward meeting the needs of the customer. Customer service is more than smiling and saying hello and thank you to the patient. Every customer who walks up to the pharmacy counter has a specific need. This includes filling a prescription or obtaining information about his or her medication.

Every pharmacy customer is entitled to a few basic rights, which include:

- Receiving the correct medication prescribed
- Receiving the correct medication dose
- Receiving the correct dosage form
- Being instructed on the proper route of administration
- Being instructed on taking the drug at the correct time

Every time you encounter a customer, think how you would like to be treated if you were the customer (Table 3-2).

The following are examples of customer service at a pharmacy:

- Acknowledging the customers as they approach the pharmacy counter
- Answering the telephone promptly
- Collecting and entering the patients' information correctly
- Contacting a patient's physician for refills promptly
- Filing a patient's filled prescription properly
- Informing patients as soon as possible of any problems regarding the filling of a prescription

Table 3-2 Customer Service Facts

• It costs anywhere from 6 to 30 times more to get a new customer than it does to keep the ones you currently have.
• For every compliant received, the average company has 26 customers with problems, 6 of which are serious in nature.
• Customers who have complained to an organization and had their complaints satisfactorily resolved tell an average of 5 people about the treatment they receive.
• Reducing customer defections can boost profits by 25% to 85%. In 73% of the cases, the organization made no attempt to persuade dissatisfied customers to stay even though 35% said that a simple apology would have prevented them from moving to the competition.
• A customer whose problem is solved on the spot is very likely (95%) to continue to do business with you again.
• For every customer who complains about an issue, 26 more customers with the same problem have not complained.
• Of customers who register a complaint, between 54% and 70% will do business again with the organization if their complaint is resolved. The figure goes up to 95% if the customer feels that the complaint was resolved quickly.
• An unhappy customer tells more than twice as many people about the experience than if he or she were happy about it.
• Customer service is the key to profitability—creating consistently positive experiences repeatedly.

Source: Adapted from MA Aun: *Thirteen Customer Service Facts,* © 2006.

- Maintaining proper on-hand quantities of medications
- Notifying the pharmacist as soon as possible of any patient questions
- Processing prescriptions promptly
- Reporting to work on time
- Smiling at the customers
- Thanking the patients for having their prescriptions filled at your pharmacy

Types of Customers

There are two basic types of customers: external and internal. External customers are individuals who do business with a particular organization. Internal customers are the people you work with in providing good customer service to your external customers.

External Customers

Physician The physician is a customer of the pharmacy. Everything in our health care system is initiated by the actions of physicians. The physician diagnoses a patient's condition and prescribes the appropriate treatment for the patient. A pharmacy needs to be familiar with the prescribing habits of physicians in the area so it may stock the appropriate medication. If a pharmacy does not stock a particular medication, the physician may advise patients to take their prescriptions to another pharmacy.

Patient The second customer a pharmacy serves is the patient. It is the patient who makes the decision to bring the prescription to us to fill. Without the prescription customer the operations of the pharmacy would cease to exist. Another pharmacy customer is the individual who is attempting to purchase an over-the-counter (OTC) product or is seeking information about a product (Figure 3-11). Other retail establishments may sell OTC products but not everyone contains a pharmacy where the customer may seek advice from a qualified individual.

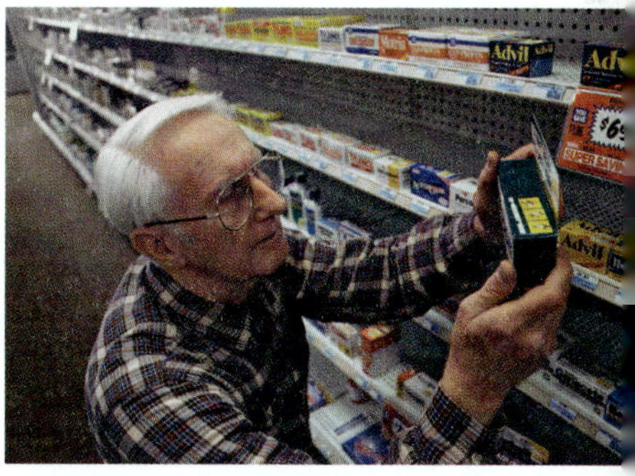

Figure 3-11 **Elderly man reads drug box labels.**

Nurse A nurse is an agent of the physician and therefore is our customer. It is the nurse who may call in a new prescription or authorize a refill for a patient. It is the nurse who checks a patient's chart when we are seeking clarification on a prescription. It is the nurse who acts as a contact between the physician, the patient, and the pharmacy. In a hospital, the nursing staff on the floor is our customer; it is the pharmacy's responsibility to provide them with the products and services needed to take care of the patients. The nursing home staff is our customer when they place an order for residents.

Drug Manufacturer Pharmacy has evolved from a product-driven provider to an information provider. Drug manufacturers and their representatives provide not only the products but also valuable information to pharmacy personnel. This information allows the pharmacy staff to be aware of changes in indications, appropriate dosing regiments, and adverse reactions. The information may have a significant impact on the treatment a patient receives and his or her recovery.

Internal Customers

Internal customers are your coworkers who support you in providing customer service to your external customers. Examples of internal customers include information technology (IT) personnel who make sure that your computer system is working properly. Without your computer, it would be difficult to process, price, or bill prescriptions to the appropriate provider. The accounts payable department is responsible for seeing that accounts are paid on a timely basis to prevent an interruption in service to your external customers. A company's legal department ensures that compliance issues are met. Finally, the human resource department is an internal customer. It is the department's responsibility to make sure that you are compensated appropriately and on a timely basis. Your internal customers provide you with the tools to treat your external customers properly.

Quality Customer Service

Professionalism

In 2000, the *White Paper on Pharmacy Student Professionalism* was released by the American Pharmaceutical Association that defined a profession, a professional, and professionalism. A profession is an occupation that shares 10 common characteristics. These characteristics include:

- Prolonged specialized training in a body of abstract knowledge
- A service orientation
- An ideology based on the original faith professed by members
- An ethic that is binding on the practitioners
- A body of knowledge unique to the members
- A set of skills that forms the technique of the profession
- An association of those entitled to practice the profession
- Authority granted by a society in the form of licensure or certification
- A recognized setting where the profession is practiced
- A theory of societal benefits derived from the ideology

A professional is a member of a profession who displays the following 10 traits:

1. Knowledge and skills of a profession
2. Commitment of self-improvement of skills and knowledge
3. Service orientation
4. Pride in profession
5. Covenantal relationship with the client
6. Creativity and innovation
7. Conscience and trustworthiness
8. Accountability for his or her work
9. Ethically sound decision making
10. Leadership

Professionalism is the active demonstration of the traits of a professional.

Knowledge Base and Understanding

Pharmacy technicians possess a vast amount of pharmacy knowledge. The application of their knowledge base is demonstrated in their ability to read and interpret prescriptions/medication orders, perform pharmacy calculations, and be able to identify the correct generic or brand name of a medication and its usage in the treatment of disease. Pharmacy technicians are capable of compounding medications extemporaneously or using aseptic techniques for sterile medications. For a complete listing of a pharmacy technician's knowledge base, refer to **www.ptcb.org.**

All pharmacy technicians are expected to maintain their competency in their practice. This is accomplished through continuing education programs. There are several different providers of continuing education, many of which are free to pharmacy technicians. The American Council of Pharmacy Education (ACPE) recognizes those approved programs of continuing education and awards continuing education units (CEUs) for the satisfactory completion of the program. Each ACPE-approved program has a brief assessment to be taken upon completion of the program, which requires a minimum passing score of 70%. ACPE programs may include attending seminars or reading educational pharmacy articles. These articles are found in pharmacy magazines or on the Internet. Sources of continuing education include:

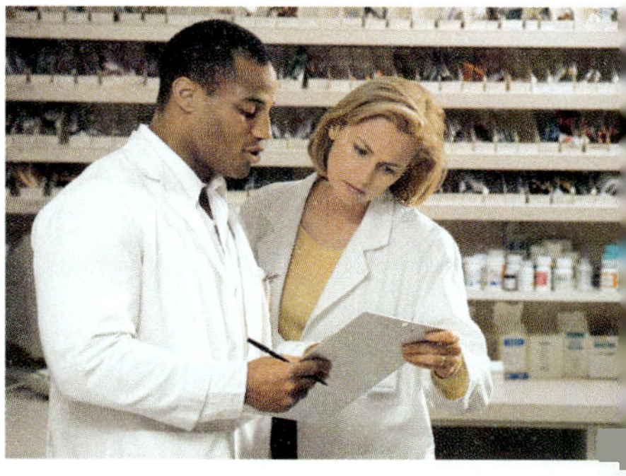

Figure 3-12 Pharmacy technicians have a vast knowledge base.

- **www.ptcb.org**
- **www.powerpak.com**
- **www.pharmacytimes.com**
- **www.uspharmacist.com**

Approximately 30 state boards of pharmacy require that pharmacy technicians be certified to practice in that state. Certification is the process by which a nongovernmental association or agency grants recognition to an individual who has met predetermined qualifications by that association or agency. Certification demonstrates that an individual possesses the necessary knowledge and skills to practice in a particular profession. There is pending legislation that will require all pharmacy technicians to be certified by the PTCB.

Attitude

Pharmacy customer service begins with the attitude of the staff. When the pharmacy team members possess and maintain a positive attitude, they are creating a positive experience for customers as well as for their coworkers and themselves (Figure 3-13). A positive attitude makes changes easier to take. The practice of pharmacy is facing changes every day. If a pharmacy organization fails to keep up with the changes, it will fall behind and lose numerous opportunities—opportunities that do not present themselves again. Enjoy the benefits of maintaining a positive attitude. Individuals with a positive attitude have higher energy levels, stronger immune systems, and they live longer. A positive attitude stimulates the brain, resulting in the development of new ideas. Positive people are able to learn from their mistakes much quicker than those who have negative attitudes. They view problems as challenges, not as obstacles in their life. Other people prefer positive people to grumpy people. Your customers do not want to be around a grumpy individual; neither do your coworkers or even your boss! Positive people attract positive people and obtain positive results in life.

A pharmacy team with a positive attitude attracts customers resulting in customer loyalty, additional prescriptions filled, and an increase in profitability of the organization.

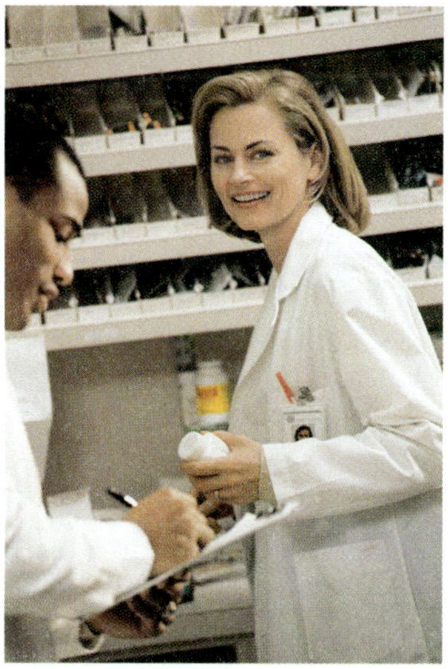

Figure 3-13 Customer service begins with a positive attitude of the staff members.

Remember to do the following:

- Make positive thinking a choice. A pharmacy technician has a choice of maintaining a positive attitude or a negative attitude.
- Make positive thinking a habit. Once an individual has made a choice to become positive, he or she can make that choice a lifelong habit.

Habits and Work Ethics

A habit is a behavior pattern acquired by frequent repetition or physiologic exposure that shows itself in regularity or increased facility of performance. It is an action that has become nearly or completely involuntary. Some of the desired habits of pharmacy technicians include:

- Prioritizing tasks
- Acting proactively
- Being able to develop mutually beneficial solutions for both the customer and your organization
- Being empathetic when dealing with a customer or colleague
- Being able to work on a team
- Possessing effective problem-solving skills

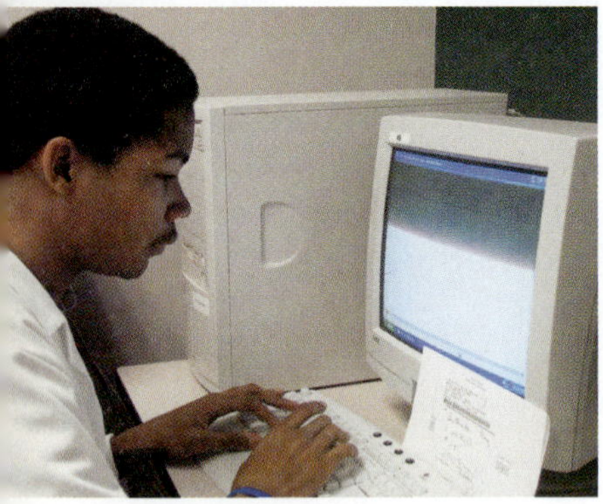

Figure 3-14 Pharmacy Technician with a good work ethic.

A work ethic is a cultural norm that places a positive moral value on doing a good job and that views work itself as having its own built-in value (Figure 3-14). An individual's work ethic is influenced during childhood and adolescence. It is through one's family and friends that a person begins to place a sense of value on work in situations demanding increased responsibility. The praise or criticism of an individual will affect his or her attitude toward work later on in life.

Compassionate Health Care

Terminally Ill

As a pharmacy technician, you must be prepared for the day when a patient is informed that he or she has a terminal illness, such as acquired immune deficiency syndrome (AIDS) or cancer, and come into the pharmacy to have a prescription filled. Some pharmacy staff may have difficulty in communicating with a terminally ill patient and may not know what to say or do for fear of upsetting the patient (Figure 3-15).

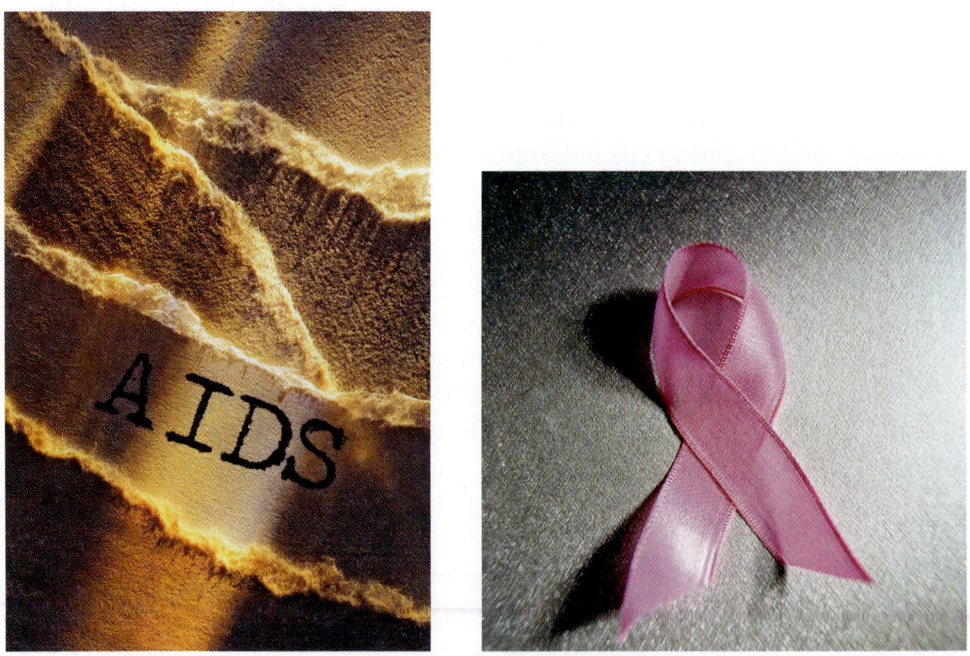

(a) (b)

Figure 3-15 (*a*) AIDS and (*b*) pink ribbon—breast cancer.

The pharmacy staff must have an understanding of the dying process to communicate with the patient. In 1969 Elizabeth Kübler-Ross published the book *On Death and Dying*, in which she describes the five stages of dying. The dying process commences when the patient is informed of a terminal condition. The patient undergoes a transition during these five stages: denial, anger, bargaining, depression, and acceptance.

- Stage 1. Denial is the initial response upon receiving the bad news, "No, not me; It can't be true; Are you sure that a mistake wasn't made; I don't feel sick" are common statements made by the patient.
- Stage 2. Anger is the second stage where one will find the patient asking "Why me!" The patient may display signs of rage, resentment, and anger toward family, friends, and possibly God.
- Stage 3. Bargaining follows anger. The individual begins to ask for an extension of his or her life, whether it is living through the holidays, a birthday, or an anniversary. The patient is seeking divine intervention.
- Stage 4. Depression follows and the patient begins to experience increasing physical weakness, discomfort, and body deterioration. The patient may begin to acknowledge he or she is not recovering from the illness. The patient may begin to feel unworthy and to fear the dying process.
- Stage 5. Acceptance is the final stage in the dying process. It is during this time that the patient lets go.

Patients may or may not fully comprehend what the physician has told them about their condition. Some terminally ill patients may not have the ability to process the information provided to them. The degree of involvement with the terminally ill patient is affected by the pharmacy staff's relationship with the patient. The pharmacy staff should use open-ended questions when talking to the patient. An example of an open-ended question would be "how are you doing today?" or "tell me how you feel" or "how may I help you?" One should try to avoid questions that result in a simple "yes" or "no." Questions that result in a simple "yes" or "no" answer are close-ended questions.

The pharmacy team should focus on both the verbal and nonverbal communication from customers. They must be sensitive to their thoughts and feelings. Terminally ill customers may not behave as they have in the past; at times, they may appear to be argumentative or angry. It is extremely important that the pharmacy team members demonstrate **compassion** to terminally ill patients. Finally, one should not avoid talking to these individuals unless that is their request; failure to interact with them continues to isolate them.

compassion The sympathetic consciousness of others' distress together with a desire to alleviate it.

Prescription Errors

The pharmacy technician is often the first person a customer encounters when approaching the pharmacy counter (Figure 3-16). How would you act if a customer informed you that a mistake was made on his or her prescription? What would you say? How would you say it? Dispensing errors are not acceptable nor are they welcomed, but errors do happen. The trust between the customer and pharmacist has been damaged when an error occurs. It is important that the pharmacy staff work to rebuild the trust with the patient.

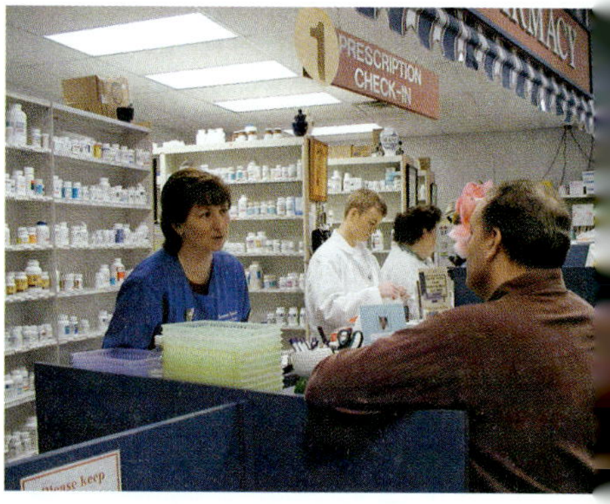

Figure 3-16 Concerned patient at pharmacy counter.

Once a customer has informed you a prescription mishap has occurred, it is EXTREMELY important that the pharmacist be notified IMMEDIATELY.

During your conversation, it is important to maintain good eye contact with the customer and to demonstrate a warm and caring body language. You must also demonstrate to the customer that the pharmacy staff is empathetic and is willing to help resolve the problem. The customer will be more receptive to the pharmacist's explanation if the stage is properly set by the pharmacy technician.

The customer should be directed to a private area where the pharmacist can talk with him or her. The pharmacist should not be disturbed during this time, when he or she is collecting information from the customer about the incident. Overall, how the pharmacy staff members deal with the incident is the key to helping prevent errors in the future.

Patient Confidentiality and Privacy

Whenever customers present a prescription at the pharmacy, they are placing their trust in both the pharmacist and the pharmacy technician. The customer expects that we will maintain all of their personal, identifiable medical information as being confidential. This patient right is guaranteed under the Health Insurance Portability and Accountability Act (HIPAA) of 2003. HIPAA is discussed in more detail in Chapter 4.

All customer conversations should be conducted to ensure the customers' privacy is maintained. When a new customer presents a prescription to be filled, the pharmacy technician will need to collect specific information from the customer. The manner of obtaining this information should not make the customer feel uneasy in disclosing it. When a customer has a specific question for the pharmacist, it is important that the customer be directed to an area where the pharmacist can speak with him or her without interruption or distraction. Some pharmacies have established counseling areas for the customer. Proper customer counseling helps improve a customer's adherence to the drug therapy, eliminate any misunderstanding about taking the medication, and can reduce prescription errors. Privacy is an expectation of all pharmacy customers and is important in providing customer service.

Conflict

Sometimes in the practice of pharmacy, a conflict may develop between two parties (Figure 3-17). A conflict is defined as a process that begins when one party perceives that another party has negatively affected something about which the first party cares. A conflict may arise over differences in the interpretation of facts or disagreements based on behavioral expectations. These conflicts may involve the customer, other medical health care providers, or coworkers.

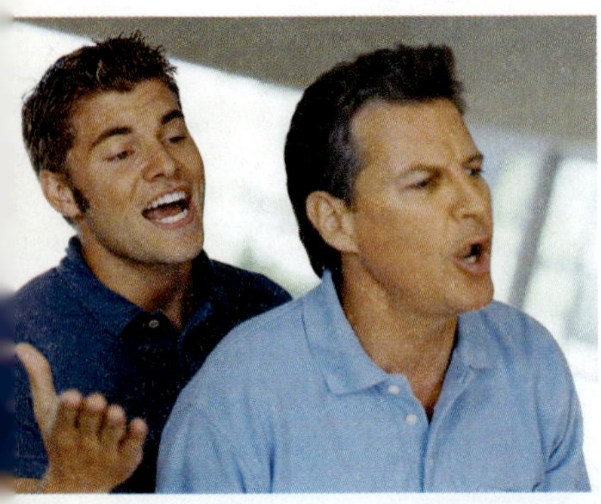

Figure 3-17 Conflict may develop in the practice of pharmacy.

The following are examples of situations that may result in a conflict at a pharmacy:

- A customer does not understand why it will take 15 minutes to fill a prescription.
- A customer is told that there are no refills remaining on the prescription, but it is a medicine that the customer needs to take.
- The pharmacy needs to order a medication for the customer.

- The customer informs you that he or she has a prescription drug card after you have filled the prescription. The customer does not understand why you must bill it to the insurance provider first.
- The customer wishes to refill the prescription early but the insurance provider will not pay for it.

How would you handle the above situations?

All of the situations can be resolved by using the communication skills discussed earlier in this chapter. The pharmacy technician must be open and willing to listen to customers when they are talking about their health and medications. It is extremely important for the pharmacy technician to remain polite and professional to every customer.

Conflict in the pharmacy can be prevented by doing the following:

- Do not pass judgment on a customer. Passing judgment is not a duty of either a pharmacist or a pharmacy technician.
- Do not jump to conclusions as to why a customer is taking a specific medication; many medications have multiple indications.
- All patient information is to remain confidential. The pharmacist and pharmacy technician should never tell anyone about a customer's condition, medications being taken, or the side effects that a patient has experienced.
- Never gossip about a customer, a physician, or even a coworker.
- Be supportive of a customer's decision regarding taking the medication.

Remember that conflicts can be avoided.

Customer Service Solutions

Communication

Communication is essential to good pharmacy service to ensure an ongoing relationship between the customer and the pharmacy staff. The practice of pharmacy is built upon the trust that the customer has given the pharmacist and pharmacy technician. Second, communication between the customer and the pharmacy staff ensures an improvement in the quality of life of the customer.

The practice of pharmacy is customer-centered. In order for the pharmacist and pharmacy technician to provide customer-centered care, they must be able to:

- Understand the customer's illness.
- Recognize each customer as being distinct.
- Develop a relationship with the customer so they may have a better understanding of the customer's health situation and the means to improve his or her quality of life.
- Improve their awareness of communication with the patient and how it may affect the customer.

The pharmacy team should encourage customers to share their experiences with their therapy with the team. They may have many unanswered questions regarding their illness or their treatment and may be hesitant to ask questions of their physician or the pharmacy staff. However, we must encourage them to ask questions to avoid any misunderstandings.

Although the pharmacist and pharmacy technician have undergone specific training regarding illnesses and their treatments, the customers have not. Explain things in terms they can understand. They may have trouble following the prescribed drug therapy, whether it is how often they are to take their medication or how to take it.

The following prescription uses abbreviation that a patient may not understand.

Dr. Andrew J. Shedlock
400 Forest Edge Way
Reston, VA 20194-1215
703-470-3199
FS5555555

Marcus Webb   Date

Address

Ampicillin   500 mg   #40

1 cap po ac qid and hs

Refill   Andrew J. Shedlock

It is our responsibility to make sure that the customer actually understands how to take the medicine. The customer must recognize that the success of the treatment is through the efforts of the physician, pharmacy staff, and himself or herself. All parties need to be actively involved with decisions made regarding the customer's therapy. It is the duty of the pharmacy staff to begin the discussion with the customer.

Telephone Etiquette

The telephone is an important tool used every day in the practice of pharmacy. The telephone is used to receive new prescriptions from a physician's office, to receive refills from a customer, to seek approval for prescription refills, to order medications, resolve adjudication problems with an insurance provider, and to assist in solving a customer's prescription problems (Figure 3-18). Many times an individual's first experience with a pharmacy is through the telephone. It is important this first experience is a positive one.

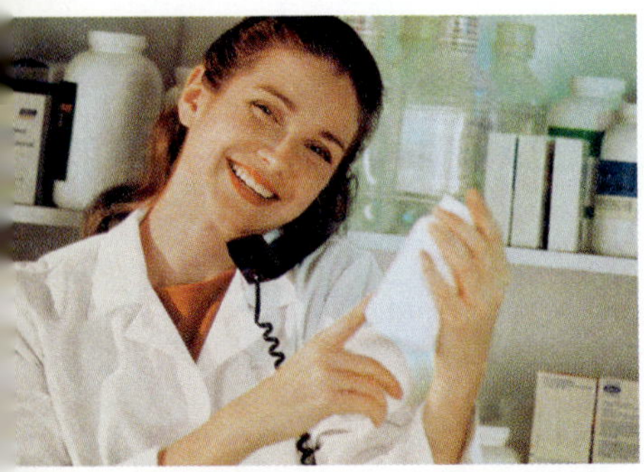

Figure 3-18 **Pharmacist assisting a patient on the phone.**

Good telephone customer service contains many different components. These include:

- Answer the telephone promptly; the telephone should always be answered on the third ring. Failing to answer the telephone promptly may cause customers to become impatient and angry. They may perceive he or she is being ignored.
- Identify the pharmacy and your name. It is important to answer the phone professionally. When answering, state the pharmacy name, its location, and your name. An example would be "Hello, CVS Pharmacy at Plaza America, this is Mathew Krishand; how may I help you?"

- Be friendly. A friendly voice will demonstrate to customers that you wish to help them. If you sound disgruntled, they may perceive that you feel they are interrupting you. Practice pretending to answer the phone in front of the mirror. If you appear to be smiling, your voice will convey friendliness, but if you are frowning, your voice may sound depressed.
- Use the caller's name throughout the telephone call. Using a person's name shows that you are interested in him or her.
- Have your resources available. What equipment do you need to answer the phone? Do you have a pen and paper to write information? Do you have prescription bags to write down prescription numbers?
- Get as much information as possible from customers. Computers allow us to help them in ways we could never do before. For instance, a customer could call in for a refill without the prescription number, but we do need information such as the name and strength of the drug or the physician's name, to fill it. Ask questions to make sure the correct medication is filled.
- Do not interrupt customers. Allow them to provide you with all of the information. When we interrupt patients, it signals to them that we may not be listening to them. Interrupting demonstrates rudeness.
- Give accurate and complete information. Pharmacy technicians provide technical assistance in the pharmacy, not judgmental assistance. If a customer asks if his or her prescription is ready or if the physician called in a prescription, you may answer that question. However, if a customer asks what a medication is being used to treat, inform the pharmacist of the question.
- Indicate your regret if it is appropriate.
- Hang up the phone gently. Allow the customer to hang up first before you place the receiver down. Do not drop the phone.

Tech Check

6. What are three examples of good customer service displayed in a pharmacy?(LO 3.7, 3.8, 3.9, 3.10)
7. What are three things that one should remember when using the telephone?(LO 3.9, 3.10)
8. What do you think is the most important thing a pharmacy technician can do to provide excellent customer service? Why?(LO 3.7, 3.9)

Stress in the Pharmacy(LO 3.6)

Every day we find stress in our lives, whether it is at work, at home, or during other activities. There are two types of stress: positive stress (eustress) and negative stress. Positive stress can motivate an individual to perform better in various activities, such as learning something new, studying for a quiz, or improving one's performance in a sports activity. Positive stress may actually increase productivity in the pharmacy. Negative stress, on the other hand, can have detrimental effects on an individual. The top three stressors in our lives based upon various surveys are death of a spouse, family member, or loved one; a divorce or separation; and the loss of a job. Table 3-3 lists other major potential causes of stress.

Table 3-3 Potential Causes of Stress

Potential Causes of Stress
Hospitalization (yours or a family member's) due to injury or illness
Marriage or reconciliation from a separation
Sexual problems
Having a new baby
Significant change in your financial status (for better or worse)
Job change
Children leaving or returning home
Significant personal success, such as a promotion at work
Moving or remodeling your home
Problems at work, such as your boss's retiring, that may put your job at risk
Substantial debt, such as a mortgage or overspending on credit cards

Continual stress in an individual's life may cause physical, mental, and emotional problems. Continual stress may result in the following:

- Hypertension
- Rapid heart rate
- Shortness of breath
- Unhealthy eating habits that may result in weight gain and possibly develop into type II diabetes
- Development of ulcers and gastrointestinal problems such as constipation and diarrhea
- Headaches and tightness throughout the body
- Increased possibility of affective disorders
- Anxiety attacks that may lead to panic attacks
- Insomnia and other sleep disorders
- Loss of short-term memory

The practice of pharmacy can be stressful. The pharmacy staff is under pressure to fill prescriptions as quickly as possible. Customers are unaware of the steps in filling a prescription and do not realize that other customers are waiting for their prescriptions. Stress may lead to prescription errors, which is discussed in Chapter 12. It is important the pharmacy team members find methods to remove stress in their lives. Table 3-4 lists examples of stress reducers.

Table 3-4 Tips for Reducing Stress

Maintain a healthy balance in your life among work, family, and leisure activities.	Redirect excess energy constructively—clean your closet, work in the garden, do volunteer work, have friends over for dinner, exercise.
Exercise regularly.	Change some of the things you have control over.

(Continued)

Table 3-4 Tips for Reducing Stress *(Continued)*

Eat balanced, nutritious meals and healthful snacks. Avoid foods high in caffeine, salt, sugar, and fat.	Keep yourself focused. Focus your full energy on one thing at a time, and finish one project before starting another.
Get enough sleep.	Identify sources of conflict, and try to resolve them.
Allow time for yourself, and plan time to relax.	Learn and use relaxation techniques, such as deep breathing, meditation, or imagining yourself in a quiet, peaceful place. Choose what works for you.
Rely on the support that family, friends, and coworkers have to offer. Don't be afraid to share your feelings.	Maintain a healthy sense of humor. Laughter can help relieve stress. Joke with friends after work. Go see a funny movie.
Try to be realistic about what you can and cannot do. Do not be afraid to admit that you cannot take on another responsibility.	Try not to overreact. Ask yourself if a situation is really worth getting upset or worried about.
Try to set realistic goals for yourself.	Seek help from social or professional support groups, if necessary.
Be organized. Good planning can help you manage your workload.	Remember that there are always choices, even when there appear to be none.

Source: Adapted from *Medical Assisting Administrative and Clinical Competencies*, 2nd ed., New York, New York, McGraw-Hill Higher Education, page 75, © 2005.

Tech Check

9. What are three things that might contribute to stress?(LO 3.6)
10. What three things can happen to an individual as a result of stress?(LO 3.6)
11. What are three stress reducers?(LO 3.6)

Chapter Summary

The pharmacy customer is the basis of a pharmacy's existence. Using appropriate verbal and nonverbal communication can ensure excellent customer service. It is important to remember that all pharmacy customers are entitled to

- Be treated with quality medications and service
- The full focus and attention of the pharmacy staff
- The freedom to ask questions and receive appropriate feedback
- The right to file a complaint if a member of the pharmacy team has made an error
- Receive respect, fairness, and courtesy

Chapter Review

Case Study Questions

1. What forms of communication were used during this incident?(LO 3.2, 3.3, 3.6)
2. What did his nonverbal actions demonstrate?(LO 3.3)

At Your Service Question

1. What are examples of good customer service exemplified by Brandon?(LO 3.9)

Multiple Choice

Select the best answer.

1. Which of the following is *not* a component of the communication process?(LO 3.1)
   a. A message
   b. A receiver
   c. Feedback
   d. Noise
2. Which of the following is an example of a message?(LO 3.1)
   a. An action
   b. An emotion
   c. A word
   d. All of the above
3. Which of the following functions does a receiver perform?(LO 3.1)
   a. Decodes a message
   b. Interprets a message
   c. Receives a message
   d. All of the above
4. Which of the following is *least likely* an example of upward communication in a pharmacy?(LO 3.2)
   a. Contacting a patient about a recalled prescription medication
   b. Informing the pharmacist that a schedule II medication needs to be reordered
   c. Informing the pharmacist that a patient is waiting for a prescription refill
   d. Making a suggestion to the pharmacist on ways to improve customer service in the pharmacy
5. Which of the following examples of body language may convey to a customer the pharmacy technician is being defensive?(LO 3.3)
   a. Arms crossed on chest
   b. Head tilted
   c. Pulling or tugging at ear
   d. Rubbing hands
6. Which of the following are examples of customer service provided by a pharmacy?(LO 3.9)
   a. Acknowledging the customer
   b. Contacting a patient's physician for a new or refill prescription
   c. Maintaining proper quantities of medication in the pharmacy
   d. All of the above
7. How many different types of customers does a pharmacy serve?(LO 3.8)
   a. One
   b. Two
   c. Depends on the number of prescriptions processed in a given day
   d. The number of different patients contained in the patient base
8. Which of the following is *least likely* an example of an external customer?(LO 3.8)
   a. The insurance provider
   b. The patient
   c. The pharmacy technician
   d. The physician
9. Which of the following is an advantage of having a positive attitude (may select more than one)?(LO 3.6, 3.9)
   a. Increased energy to deal with the problems of the day
   b. General preference toward positive people
   c. Stronger immune system
   d. All of the above
10. Which of the following is a result of hiring individuals with a positive attitude (may select more than one)?(LO 3.6, 3.9)
    a. Improved customer retention
    b. Increased number of prescriptions filled by a pharmacy
    c. Increased profitability for the pharmacy
    d. All of the above
11. Which of the following is *not* a characteristic of a profession?(LO 3.7)
    a. Authority granted by a society in the form of licensure or certification
    b. Creativity and innovation
    c. Prolonged specialized training in a body of abstract knowledge
    d. A set of skills that forms the technique of the profession

12. Which of the following is a trait of a professional (may select more than one)?(LO 3.7)
    a. Commitment of self-improvement
    b. Conscience and trustworthiness
    c. Pride in profession
    d. All of the above

13. Which of the following is *not* appropriate to be worn in a pharmacy (may select more than one)?(LO 3.7, 3.9)
    a. Clothing that is ripped and contains numerous holes or noticeable patches
    b. Matted hair
    c. Pierced eyebrows and lips
    d. All are inappropriate for a pharmacy

14. Which organization recognizes approved continuing education units for pharmacy technicians?(LO 3.9)
    a. ACPE
    b. APhA
    c. ASHP
    d. PTCB

15. Which of the following will influence an individual's work ethic?(LO 3.9)
    a. Childhood experiences
    b. Family life
    c. Praise
    d. All of the above

Critical Thinking Questions

1. A managed-care patient has brought a prescription into the pharmacy to be filled. The pharmacy technician is attempting to adjudicate the claim. The claim is rejected by the third-party provider with the following explanation—INVALID CARDHOLDER. How would you handle the situation?(LO 3.6)

2. A patient drops off a prescription to be filled early in the morning and informs you that he or she will pick it up at the end of the day. When you go to fill the prescription, you realize that you are temporarily out of the medication. You order the medication for the patient and it will be delivered by the wholesaler the next day. The patient returns at the end of the day to find out that the prescription has not been filled and that he or she was not notified of the problem during the day, even though you had a contact telephone number. What would you do?(LO 3.6, 3.9)

3. A new patient brings a prescription to be filled at your pharmacy. While you are collecting information from the patient, you realize that he or she does not speak English. How would you collect information for the patient profile?(LO 3.6, 3.9)

4. A patient returns to the pharmacy in the morning with a filled prescription from the previous evening. The patient informs you that he or she received the wrong medication. How would you handle the situation?(LO 3.9)

5. A patient brings in a new prescription to be filled and you know that you do not carry that particular medication. What options would you give the patient regarding filling the prescription?(LO 3.6, 3.9)

6. It is Monday afternoon and the pharmacy is extremely busy. The pharmacy is giving a wait time of 90-minutes. Patients are impatiently standing around the pharmacy counter. A patient approaches your pharmacy counter with an ice pack to his left jaw and appears to be in pain. He hands you his Percocet prescription and informs you that he has left his dentist's office after having all of his wisdom teeth removed an hour ago. You inform him of the long wait. He asks if it can be done any faster. What do you do?(LO 3.9)

7. A woman who is a very good customer enters the pharmacy to have a prescription filled. She does not appear to be her normal jovial self and you ask if there is something wrong. She replies that her husband died a week ago. How would you handle the situation?

8. A very good patient brings in some prescriptions to be filled. Upon receiving and looking at the prescriptions, you realize that the individual has been diagnosed with human immunodeficiency virus (HIV). What do you say to the patient?(LO 3.4, 3.9, 3.10)

9. Identify stressors in your life and discuss how you reduce this stress.(LO 3.9)

10. Which communication skill is the most important in providing excellent customer service? Why?(LO 3.2, 3.9)

11. Which communication barrier do you find poses the greatest number of problems in providing customer service?(LO 3.6)

12. As a pharmacy technician, what area of communication do you need to work on the most to provide excellent customer service? Why?(LO 3.4)
13. How does maintaining a positive attitude improve customer service?(LO 3.9)
14. A profession is defined as an occupation that shares 10 common characteristics. Explain how each of these characteristics relates to being a pharmacy technician.(LO 3.6, 3.9, 3.10)
15. Evaluate the appearance of a classmate as though you were a customer. Is his or her appearance professional? Why or why not? What would you recommend the person do to make his or her appearance more professional?(LO 3.9)

HIPAA Scenario

Two pharmacy technicians and a pharmacy clerk were overheard discussing a coworker's medical condition in the break room. One of the pharmacy technicians, Michael, filled a prescription for Carol, the coworker, for prenatal vitamins and assumed that Carol was pregnant. He then proceeded to discuss the issue with his friends at work. When Carol, who was not pregnant, entered the break room and realized she was the topic of discussion, she immediately went to find her supervisor. Returning to the break room with the supervisor, she confronted the gossiping trio. The supervisor asked the technicians and the clerk to wait in his office. He then called the hospital's privacy officer to inquire about actions he could take to reprimand his staff.

Discussion Questions (PTCB II. 73)

1. Did the gossiping pharmacy technicians break a law or were they merely guilty of unprofessional behavior?
2. What actions might a supervisor take in such a situation?

Internet Activities

1. Visit the Web site of your state board of pharmacy and review the cases where complaints have been filed against either a pharmacist or pharmacy technician.(LO 3.5)
    a. How many of these cases could have been prevented if better communication skills had been applied?(LO 3.5)
    b. What would you have done to prevent these complaints from being filed?(LO 3.6)

Ethics, Law, and Regulatory Agencies

4

Learning Outcomes

Upon completion of this chapter, you will be able to:

4.1 Explain *ethics*.

4.2 Identify the ethical conduct required of pharmacy technicians.

4.3 Explain the importance of the following pharmacy legislation:

- **a.** Pure Food and Drug Act; Sherley Amendment; Harrison Narcotic Act; Food, Drug and Cosmetic Act
- **b.** Durham-Humphrey Act; Kefauver-Harris Act
- **c.** Controlled Substance Act; Poison Prevention Packaging Act
- **d.** Occupational Safety and Health Act; Drug Listing Act; Medical Device Amendments
- **e.** Orphan Drug Act; Drug Price Competition and Patent Term Restoration Act; Prescription Drug Marketing Act; Omnibus Budget Reconciliation Act of 1987
- **f.** Omnibus Budget Reconciliation Act of 1990; Dietary Supplement Health and Education Act of 1994
- **g.** Health Insurance Portability and Accountability Act of 1996; Comprehensive Methamphetamine Control Act; FDA Modernization Act
- **h.** Medicare Modernization Act; USP <797>; Anabolic Steroid Control Act
- **i.** Isotretinoin Safety and Risk Management Act

4.4 Relate the meaning of *schedule* to the Controlled Substance Act of 1970 and the criteria for placing a medication in a particular schedule.

4.5 Differentiate between an initial inventory, biennial inventory, and perpetual inventory as they relate to pharmacy.

4.6 Describe the methods of filing prescription and pharmacy records.

4.7 Explain the requirements issued by the CMS for Medicaid Tamper Resistant prescription pads.

4.8 Identify the following regulatory agencies and their role in the practice of pharmacy:

- **a.** Food and Drug Administration (FDA); Drug Enforcement Administration (DEA)
- **b.** Occupational Safety and Health Administration (OSHA); Centers for Medicare and Medicaid Services (CMS) and The Joint Commission (TJC) (formerly The Joint Commission Accreditation of Healthcare Organizations, JCAHO)

Key Terms

controlled substance
Drug Enforcement Administration (DEA)
Ethics
Food and Drug Administration (FDA)
Law
legend drugs
malpractice
Medicare
narcotic
National Drug Code (NDC)
negligence
patent
prescription
Protected Health Information (PHI)
respondeat superior

4.9 Identify the role of the state board of pharmacy in each state and the National Association of Boards of Pharmacy.

4.10 Explain *law.*

4.11 Differentiate between federal law, state law, and torts.

4.12 Explain *respondeat superior.*

PTCB

In preparation for the certification examination, you should understand and perform activities associated with the following PTCB Knowledge Statements:

PTCB Knowledge Statement

Domain I. Assisting the Pharmacist in Serving Patients

Knowledge of federal, state, and/or practice site regulations, code of ethics, and standards pertaining to the practice of pharmacy (1)

Knowledge of pharmaceutical, medical, and legal developments that affect the practice of pharmacy (2)

Knowledge of state-specific prescription transfer regulations (3)

Knowledge of information to be obtained from patient/patient's representative (21)

Knowledge of required prescription order refill information (22)

Knowledge of formula to verify the validity of a prescriber's DEA number (23)

Knowledge of techniques for detecting forged or altered prescriptions (24)

Knowledge of National Drug Code (NDC) components (34)

Knowledge of special directions and precautions for patient/patient's representative regarding preparation and use of medications (39)

Knowledge of requirements for mailing a prescription (42)

Knowledge of requirements for dispensing controlled substances (44)

Knowledge of record-keeping requirements for medication dispensing (46)

Knowledge of documentation requirements for controlled substances, investigational drugs, and hazardous waste (68)

Knowledge of confidentiality requirements (73)

PTCB Knowledge Statement

Domain II. Maintaining Medication and Inventory Control Systems

Knowledge of drug product laws and regulations and professional standards related to obtaining medication supplies, durable medical equipment, and products (4)

Knowledge of the use of DEA controlled substance ordering forms (9)

Knowledge of policies, procedures, and practices for inventory systems (11)

Knowledge of legal and regulatory requirements and professional standards for preparing, labeling, dispensing, distributing, and administering medications (18)

Knowledge of medication distribution and control systems requirements for controlled substances, investigational drugs, and hazardous materials and wastes (23)

PTCB Knowledge Statement

Domain III. Participation in the Administration and Management of Pharmacy Practice

Knowledge of state board of pharmacy regulations (11)

Knowledge of the Americans with Disabilities Act requirements (25)

Knowledge of security procedures related to data integrity, security, and confidentiality (26)

Knowledge of legal requirements regarding archiving (30)

Case Study

It is Friday morning at Your Neighborhood Pharmacy, and A.J., the pharmacy technician, is assisting the pharmacist. Mr. Dagit arrives to pick up his prescription. While A.J. is looking for the prescription, he notices a prescription for Mr. Dagit's daughter in the bins. He finds Mr. Dagit's prescription and quietly asks the pharmacist if he should give the daughter's prescription to Mr. Dagit. The pharmacist tells A.J. not to offer the daughter's prescription to the father. A.J. is confused.

While reading this chapter, keep the following questions in mind:

1. Is it good customer service to inform the patient of his daughter's prescription? Why or why not?(LO 4.3g)

Introduction to Ethics, Law, and Regulatory Agencies(LO 4.1)

The practice of pharmacy is regulated by both federal and state laws and pharmacy regulations. Both pharmacists and pharmacy technicians must have a firm knowledge of all the laws and regulations affecting pharmacy practice. This chapter focuses on the ethical behavior expected of both pharmacists and pharmacy technicians and the evolution of pharmacy laws in the United States.

Ethics(LO 4.1, 4.2)

Ethics are a set of moral principles or values that govern the conduct of an individual or group. Factors that affect an individual's ethics include religion, society, and education. Both pharmacists and pharmacy technicians have a code of ethics and must abide by them.

Code of Ethics for Pharmacists

Pharmacists are health professionals who assist individuals in making the best use of medications. This code, prepared and supported by pharmacists, is intended to state publicly the principles that form the fundamental basis of the roles and responsibilities of pharmacists. These principles, based on moral obligations and virtues, are established to guide pharmacists in relationships with patients, health professionals, and society.

Ethics a set of moral principles or values that govern the conduct of an individual or group.

Principles

- A pharmacist respects the covenantal relationships between patient and pharmacist.
- A pharmacist promotes the good of every patient in a caring, compassionate, and confidential manner.
- A pharmacist respects the autonomy and dignity of each patient.
- A pharmacist acts with honesty and integrity in professional relationships.
- A pharmacist maintains professional competence.
- A pharmacist respects the values and abilities of colleagues and other health professionals.
- A pharmacist serves individual, community, and societal needs.
- A pharmacist seeks justice in the distribution of health resources.

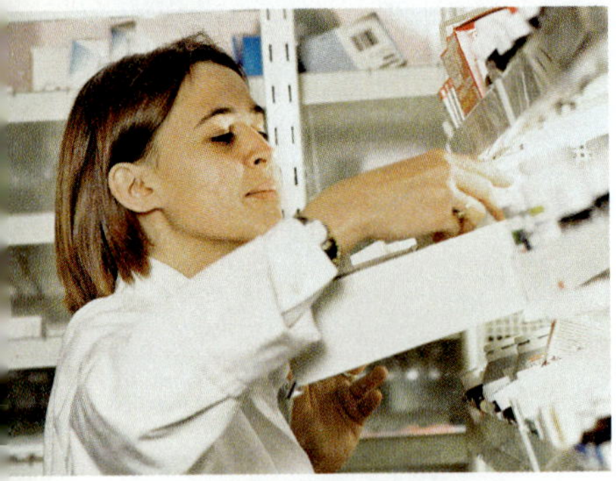

Figure 4-1 Pharmacy technician using ethical practices.

Code of Ethics for Pharmacy Technicians

Pharmacy technicians are health care professionals who assist pharmacists in providing possible care for patients. The principles of this code, which apply to pharmacy technicians working in all settings, are based on the application and support of the moral obligations that guide the pharmacy

At Your Service

John Ebert is a 45-year-old patient who has been a customer of Your Neighborhood Pharmacy for 15 years. He is prescribed Ambien CR 6.25 mg for sleep by Dr. Stone. This is a Schedule IV medication.

John calls in his prescription to be refilled on Saturday at 1:15 P.M. He arrives at the pharmacy at 3:00 P.M. to pick up his prescription, but he is informed by the pharmacy technician that no refills remain on the prescription.

The pharmacy technician informs John that the pharmacy faxed a refill request to his physician at 1:22 P.M. John informs the pharmacy technician that his physician has told him that he may have the prescription filled anytime. He becomes extremely upset that his prescription is not ready, and he demands to see the pharmacist.

The pharmacy technician informs the pharmacist of the situation. Before speaking to the patient, the pharmacist reviews the prescription and notices that the patient received a 30-day supply of medication 10 days ago. The pharmacist speaks to John and attempts to explain to him why they must contact the physician. John demands that the pharmacy return the physician's prescription to him. He becomes irate and informs the pharmacist that he is going to contact the Board of Pharmacy and will have his prescription filled at another pharmacy. While reading this chapter, keep the following questions in mind.

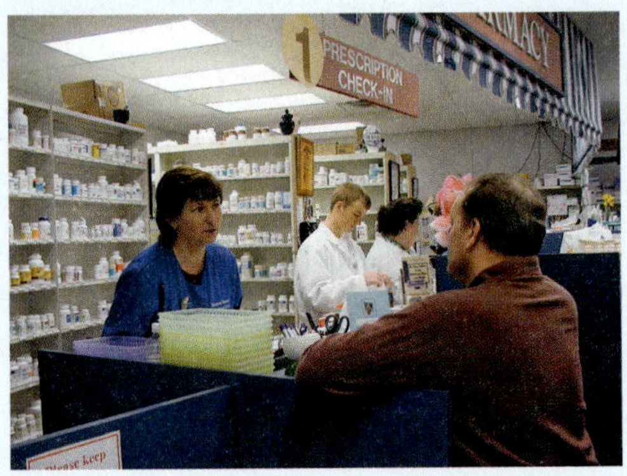

1. Did the pharmacy technician handle the situation correctly? (LO 4.3c)
2. Why is this medication a controlled substance? (LO 4.3c)

profession in relationships with patients, health care professionals, and society (Figure 4-1).

Principles

- A pharmacy technician's first consideration is to ensure the health and safety of the patient and to use knowledge and skills to the best of his or her ability in serving others.
- A pharmacy technician supports and promotes honesty and integrity in the profession, which includes a duty to observe the law, maintain the highest moral and ethical conduct at all times, and uphold the ethical principles of the profession.
- A pharmacy technician assists and supports the pharmacist in the safe, efficacious, and cost-effective distribution of health services and health care resources.
- A pharmacy technician respects and values the abilities of pharmacists, colleagues, and other health care professionals.
- A pharmacy technician maintains competency in his or her practice, and continually enhances his or her professional knowledge and expertise.
- A pharmacy technician respects and supports the confidentiality of a patient's records and discloses pertinent information only with proper authorization.
- A pharmacy technician never assists in the dispensing, promoting, or distribution of medications or medical devices that are not of good quality or do not meet the standards required by law.
- A pharmacy technician does not engage in any activity that will discredit the profession, and will expose, without fear or favor, illegal or unethical conduct in the profession.
- A pharmacy technician associates with and engages in the support of organizations that promote the pharmacy profession through the utilization and enhancement of pharmacy technicians.

Tech Check

1. Which principle of the pharmacy technician code of ethics do you feel is most important? Why? (LO 4.2)
2. Suppose a pharmacy technician goes out on Friday night with his or her friends and consumes multiple alcoholic drinks during the evening. The next morning, the technician is still under the influence of alcohol and goes to work at the pharmacy knowing there is no one to assist the pharmacist. Is this an ethical action? (LO 4.2)

Law (LO 4.10, 4.11, 4.12)

According to *Black's Law Dictionary*, a **law** is a body of rules of action or conduct prescribed by a controlling authority and having binding legal force. A law must be obeyed and followed by citizens subject to sanctions, or legal consequences may occur. Laws protect society. In the practice of pharmacy, laws shape moral standards, promote social justice, facilitate orderly change, and maximize individual freedom. Pharmacy practice is regulated by both federal and state laws.

Law a body of rules of action or conduct prescribed by a controlling authority and having binding legal force.

Federal Law

The U.S. Constitution established the federal government. The federal government is composed of three branches: the executive (president), the legislative (Congress), and the judicial (court system). The president has the authority to enforce the laws that have been enacted by Congress, and the court system has the authority to interpret the validity of these laws. Any power not authorized by the Constitution is reserved to the state governments.

Federal law takes precedence over state laws unless state laws are more stringent than the federal government.

Recently, several states have enacted legislation affecting marijuana and pseudoephedrine that conflicted with federal law. The Supreme Court ruled in favor of the federal law. Examples of federal law affecting pharmacy include:

- Controlled Substance Act
- Poison Prevention Packaging Act
- Health Insurance Portability and Accountability Act (HIPAA)

State Law

The practice of pharmacy is regulated by each individual state, not the federal government. Each state is able to enact laws and Board of Pharmacy regulations as long as they do not conflict with the federal laws. The state laws are consistent with one another regarding the principles, purposes, aims, and objectives of pharmacy practice.

State pharmacy laws provide for:

- The educational qualifications that pharmacists must meet at the examination or registration
- The role of the state board of pharmacy and its ability to administer and enforce pharmacy regulations
- The granting of permits for community pharmacy
- Registration of pharmacists
- The conditions by which a pharmacy permit or license may be suspended or revoked
- Penalties for violations of state pharmacy laws and regulations
    - These may include the imposition of monetary fines, suspension or revocation of a license, or criminal proceedings
- Reciprocation of a pharmacy license from another state
- Registration of pharmacy technicians

Tort Law

Tort law is a category of civil law involving relationships between two individuals. In the practice of pharmacy, the concept of **negligence** may be observed. Negligence is failing to do something that a reasonable individual would do, or doing something that a reasonable and prudent individual would not do. The action of negligence is typically not intentional.

In order to demonstrate negligence, the following four conditions must be met:

- Duty
- Dereliction

negligence The failure to do something that a reasonable person would do, or doing something that a reasonable person would not do.

- Damages
- Direct cause

An example of negligence occurs whenever a prescription error takes place. Another example of a tort law occurs when an individual's privacy is violated. If a pharmacist or pharmacy technician fails to keep a patient's information confidential, tort law may be broken.

Malpractice is an act of the continuing conduct of a professional that does not meet the standard of professional competence and results in provable damages to his or her client or patient. This error or omission may be through negligence, ignorance (when the professional should have known), or intentional wrongdoing. Malpractice does not include the exercise of professional judgment even when the results are detrimental to the client or patient.

Respondeat Superior

Respondeat superior is a Latin phrase meaning "let the master answer." It is the responsibility of the pharmacist to oversee the work of the pharmacy technicians. The pharmacist must check every prescription to ensure that the pharmacy technician correctly enters it into the computer system, counts out the medication, labels the medication container, and performs pharmacy calculations correctly. If a pharmacy technician makes an error during the prescription filling process, the pharmacist will be held liable (Figure 4-2). If the pharmacy technician knowingly does something wrong and the pharmacist is not aware of the incident, the pharmacy technician may be held accountable. Another example of this principle would be if a chain pharmacy knows that a pharmacist is making prescription errors and takes no action to remedy the situation. The chain pharmacy would be held accountable.

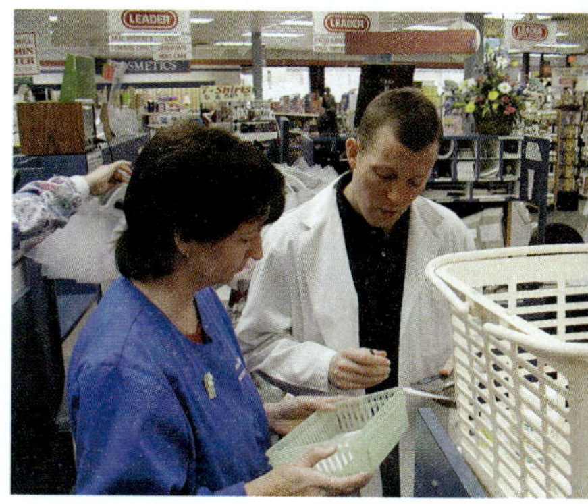

Figure 4-2 The pharmacist is responsible for the pharmacy technician's actions.

Tech Check

3. What four conditions must be present for a suit of malpractice to occur in a civil suit? (LO 4.11)
4. What legal term holds the pharmacist responsible for the action of the pharmacy technicians? (LO 4.12)

Federal Pharmacy Laws 1906–1962 (LO 4.3a, 4.3b)

1906 – Pure Food and Drug Act
1912 – Sherley Amendment
1914 – Harrison Narcotic Act
1938 – Food, Drug and Cosmetic Act (FDCA 1938)
1952 – Durham-Humphrey Amendment
1962 – Kefauver-Harris Amendment

malpractice An act of continuing conduct of a professional that does not meet the standard of professional competence and results in provable damages to his or her client or patient.

respondeat superior A Latin term meaning "let the master answer," a key doctrine in the law of agency that states that a principal (employer) is responsible for the actions of his or her agent (employee) in the "course of employment."

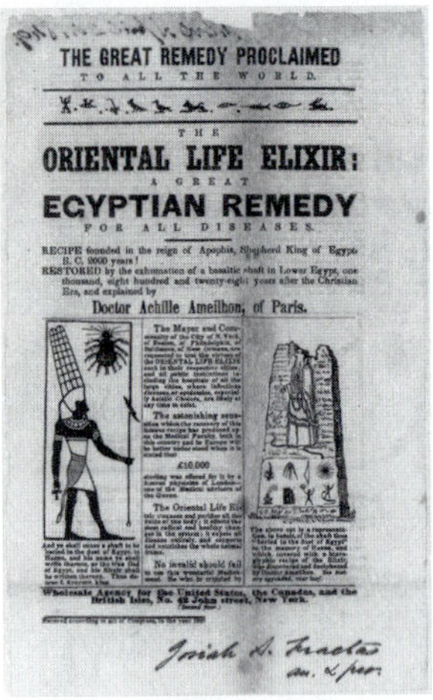

Figure 4-3 The Oriental life elixir: a great Egyptian remedy for all diseases.

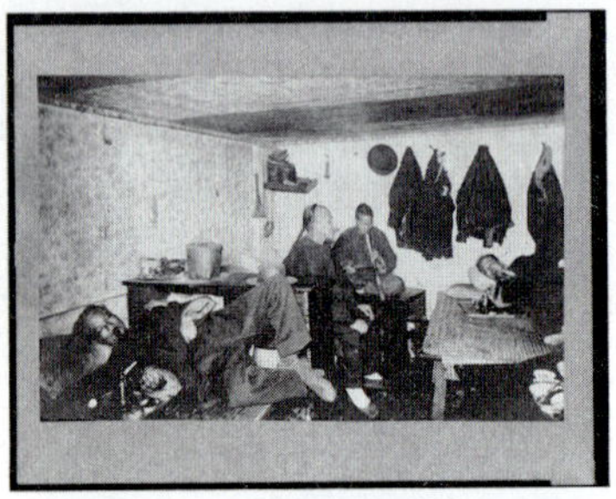

Figure 4-4 Interior of opium den, San Francisco, California.

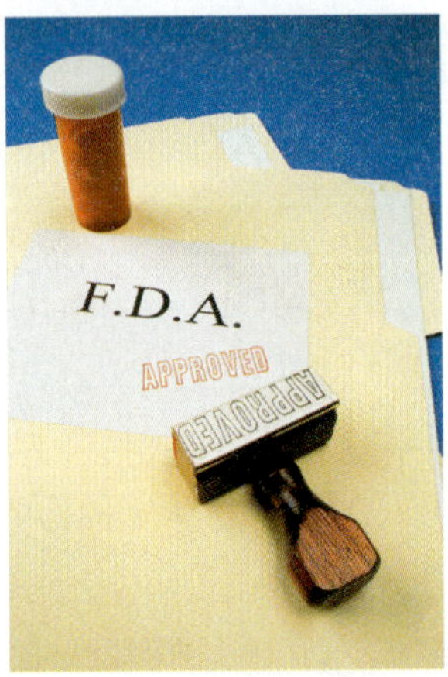

Figure 4-5 The FDA approves all new drug products.

Food and Drug Administration (FDA) The federal administrative agency that administers and enforces the federal Food, Drug and Cosmetic Act and other federal consumer protection laws.

Pure Food and Drug Act of 1906

Prior to 1906, salesmen would travel from community to community selling products to the townspeople. These sales representatives would make promises about their products to the customer without any scientific or medical backing (Figure 4-3). A given product might be used to cure a headache, reduce a fever, kill an infection, settle a stomachache, heal a scar, or make a woman fertile. These products may have been compounded in the back of a home or outdoors. The water may have been secured from a local stream or lake, and the quantities of the ingredients would vary in each batch. Often, the traveling salesmen would cross state lines to sell their products.

The Pure Food and Drug Act was enacted in 1906. It required that drugs marketed in interstate commerce meet their professed minimal standards of strength, purity, and quality.

Sherley Amendment of 1912

The Sherley Amendment was enacted to combat fraudulent, false, or misleading claims of therapeutic effects of a medication, which was known as misbranding.

Harrison Narcotic Act of 1914

The government attempted to limit the amount of opium imported into the United States (Figure 4-4). After this date, an individual required a prescription to purchase opium.

Food, Drug and Cosmetic Act of 1938 (FDCA 1938)

The Pure Food and Drug Act of 1906 required that all drugs be safe before being shipped to other states. As a continuation of the Pure Food and Drug Act of 1906, the Food, Drug and Cosmetic Act of 1938 was enacted. Prior to 1938, the **Food and Drug Administration (FDA)** did not exist, as we know of it today. Because of this act, the FDA was created (Figure 4-5). The FDA initiated a process that all new drug products must follow in order to be approved. This process included the performance of clinical studies, and required that drug manufacturers submit a New Drug Application (NDA) to the FDA before the drug entity would be approved. A discussion on the process of introducing a new drug product in the United States will be discussed in more detail in Chapter 17.

Any product on the market prior to 1938 did not need these requirements unless petitioned by the FDA. Vitamins and nutritional supplements are not required to undergo this process due to the Dietary Supplement Health and Education Act of 1994 that will be discussed later in the chapter.

The Pure Food and Drug Act of 1906 mentioned adulteration and misbranding, but neither of these terms were clearly defined until the Food, Drug and Cosmetic Act of 1938 was enacted act.

Adulteration

According to the Federal Food, Drug and Cosmetic Act, adulteration of any drug or drug product includes:

- Consisting in whole or in part of any filthy, putrid, or decomposed substance
- Prepared, packed, or held under unsanitary conditions

- Prepared in containers composed, in whole or in part, of any poisonous or deleterious substance
- Containing unsafe color additives
- Claiming to be or represented as drugs recognized in an official Compendium but differing in strength, quality, or purity of the drugs

Misbranding

According to the Federal Food, Drug and Cosmetic Act, misbranding of a drug is:

- Labeling that is false or misleading in any way.
- Packaging that does not bear a label containing the name and place of business of the manufacturer, packer, distributor, or an accurate quantity of contents conspicuously and clearly labeled with information by the act (Figure 4-6).
- Failing to state Warning—May be habit forming, if the product is habit forming (Figure 4-7).
- Failing to bear the established name of the drug. In case the drug carries more than two or more active ingredients, the quantities of the ingredients and the amount of alcohol must be included, and also, whether active or not, the established name and quantity of certain other substances described in the act.
- Failing to label adequate directions for use or adequate warnings against use in certain pathological conditions.
- Proving dangerous to health when used in the dosage, manner, or duration prescribed, recommended or suggested in the labeling.

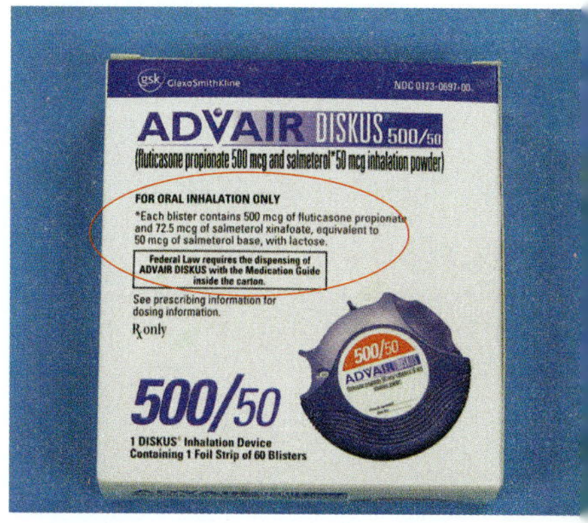

Figure 4-6 Drug package information.

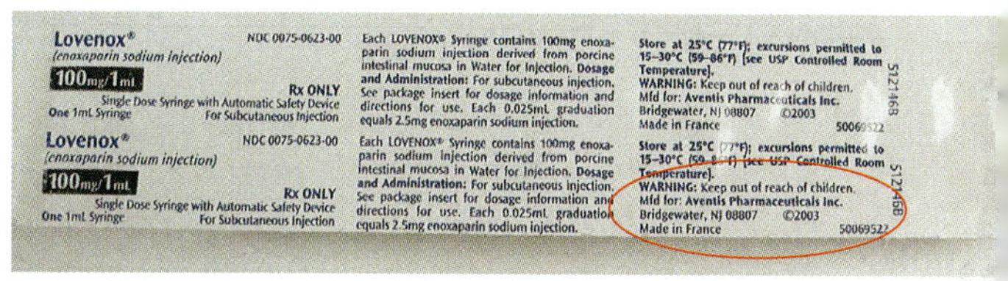

Figure 4-7 Display of warning statement.

Labeling

All medications must be labeled properly. If a drug manufacturer or a pharmacy fails to label a medication properly, they are guilty of misbranding (Figure 4-8). A retail pharmacy dispenses prescriptions and therefore the following information is required on a prescription label:

- Name and address of the pharmacy
- Prescription number or serial number
- Date of prescription filling or refilling
- Name of prescriber
- Name of patient
- Directions for use
- Cautionary statements

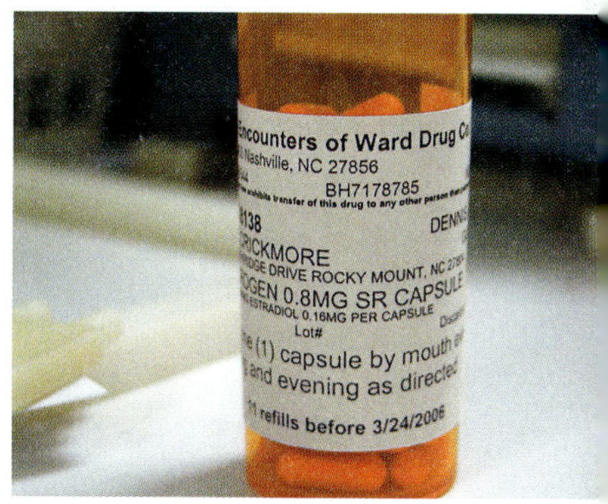

Figure 4-8 Medication label.

Medication orders are dispensed to patients in hospitals and long-term care facilities. The labels for a patient's medication in these settings may require different information to appear on the label. It is extremely important that a pharmacy technician working in either a hospital or long-term care facility be familiar with the label requirements of that institution. These requirements may be found in the institution's policy and procedure manual.

Durham-Humphrey Amendment of 1952

The Durham-Humphrey Act of 1952 was an amendment to the Food, Drug and Cosmetic Act of 1938 (FDCA 1938). The Durham-Humphrey Act separated drugs into two categories, legend and non-legend. A **legend drug**

legend drug A prescription medication bearing the federal legend (federal law prohibits the dispensing of this medication without a prescription).

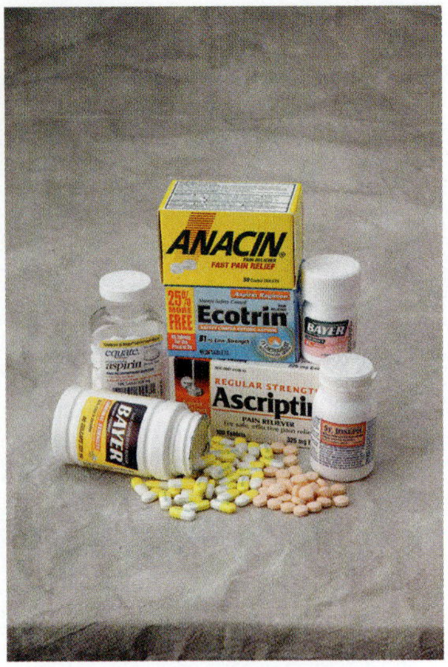

Figure 4-9 Over-the-counter (OTC) drugs.

contains the federal legend and requires that the patient be under a physician's care. A legend drug requires a **prescription**, which is a written directive or order for the preparation and administration of a medication or other remedy.

Non-legend medications, also referred to as over-the-counter (OTC) medications, medications do not require a physician's supervision, and these products can be purchased without a prescription (Figure 4-9). For a medication to be placed as a legend drug, it must show the following:

- The drug is habit forming.
- The drug is not safe for self-medication because of its toxicity or other potentiality for harmful effect, or the method of its use or the collateral measures to its use.
- The drug is a new drug that has not been shown to be safe and is restricted to prescription-only distribution by the FDA when it issues the NDA.

OTC

Examples of OTCs include Tylenol, Benadryl, Robitussin, and Metamucil. The Durham-Humphrey Amendment resulted in the inclusion of the federal legend "Caution: Federal law prohibits dispensing without a prescription" to be included on all prescription medications. At that time, all new medications were classified as prescription medications but could be converted to OTC status later. When this conversion from prescription to OTC status occurred, the medication was formulated at a lower dosage than the prescription medication. Examples of medications being converted from prescription to OTC status included ibuprofen, cimetidine, loperamide, and miconazole and hydrocortisone cream.

An OTC medication's label must include the following:

- The name of the product
- The name and address of the manufacturer, packager, or distributor
- The net contents of the package
- The established name of all active ingredients, and the quantity of certain other ingredients whether active or not, such as alcohol
- The name of any habit-forming drug contained in the preparation
- Cautions and warnings needed for the protection of the user
- Adequate directions for safe and effective use

If, for some reason, a pharmacy wishes to repackage an OTC medication from a stock bottle, the pharmacy would be required to label the medication exactly as the manufacturer had done. If a physician has written a prescription for an OTC medication, a prescription label may be affixed to the OTC package. If a patient were to ask the pharmacy to place a prescription label on an OTC medication without a valid prescription, the pharmacy cannot do this. It would be a violation of the Food, Drug and Cosmetic Act of 1938, because it would be an example of misbranding.

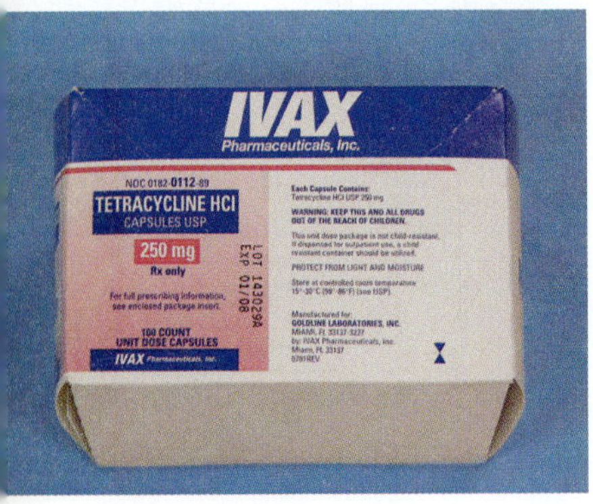

Figure 4-10 Prescription drug package.

prescription A written directive for the preparation and administration of a remedy.

proprietary drug denoting a medicine protected against free competition as to name, composition, or manufacturing process by patent, trademark, copyright, or secrecy. Also known as a brand name or trade drug.

Prescription or Legend Drugs

All prescription or legend drugs must contain the following information when they are sold to a pharmacy (Figure 4-10):

- Generic and brand names (drug names will be discussed more in-depth in chapter 5)
- Ingredient information
- Weight measure of drug (e.g., 25 mg)
- Size of container (e.g., 480 mL, 100 tablets, 30 g)

- Dosage information or a reference to the package insert for dosage information
- Manufacturer, packager, or distributor's name and address
- Expiration date
- Lot number

The Durham-Humphrey Amendment prevented a prescription from being refilled unless it was indicated on the original prescription or authorized from the prescriber. This amendment allowed a prescriber to telephone a prescription into the patient's choice of pharmacy.

Kefauver-Harris Amendment of 1962

The Kefauver-Harris Amendment was enacted because of the marketing of thalidomide in Europe to pregnant women, which resulted in birth defects of their children. These birth defects included disfiguration of the eyes, nose, and ears, and missing limbs. The Kefauver-Harris Amendment requires that all medications (prescription and nonprescription) be pure, safe, and effective. It is the duty of the drug manufacturers to prove that a medication is safe and effective before the FDA will approve it. Any medication marketed between 1938 and 1962 had to show that it was pure, safe, and effective. Medications marketed prior to 1938 were exempted from this act.

Tech Check

5. Define *adulteration* and the conditions associated with it.(LO 4.3a)
6. Define *misbranding* and the conditions associated with it.(LO 4.3a)
7. Explain the conditions for a drug to be considered a prescription medication.(LO 4.3b)
8. What information must be found on the label of an OTC medication? (LO 4.3b)

Federal Pharmacy Laws 1970 (LO 4.3c, 4.4, 4.5, 4.6)

Comprehensive Drug Abuse Prevention and Control Act (Controlled Substance Act of 1970)

The Controlled Substance Act was enacted because of impending drug problems facing the United States and to control addicting drugs. A **controlled substance** is a drug that has been declared illegal for sale or use but may be dispensed by a physician's prescription. **Narcotics**, which are the most common controlled substances, are addictive, dull the senses, reduce pain, alter mood or behavior, and usually induce sleep or stupor. Under the Controlled Substance Act, medications were placed into one of five "schedules" based upon their potential for abuse or addiction.

controlled substance A drug that has been declared illegal for sale or use but may be dispensed by a physician's prescription.

narcotic An addictive drug that dulls the senses, reduces pain, alters mood or behavior, and usually induces sleep or stupor.

Drug Schedules

Schedule I Drugs Schedule I drugs have a high abuse potential and do not possess an accepted medical use in the United States. These medications cannot be prescribed by a physician, dispensed by a pharmacist, or administered by a qualified individual. Schedule I drugs are illegal in the United States.

Unlike Schedule I medications, drugs placed in Schedules II to V do possess a medical use in the United States. These medications are available to be prescribed, dispensed, and administered by qualified providers.

Schedule II Drugs Schedule II medications possess both severe psychological and physical dependence.

Schedule III Drugs Schedule III medications have an abuse potential, which is less than that of Schedule II, but greater than that of Schedule IV drugs. Schedule III medications contain less than 15 mg of hydrocodone per dosage unit and not more than 90 mg of codeine per dosage unit.

Schedule IV Drugs Schedule IV drugs' potential for abuse is less than that of Schedule III but greater than Schedule V.

Schedule V Drugs Schedule V drugs have an abuse potential less than that of Schedule IV and contain small quantities of specific narcotics used in cough and antidiarrheal medications. Schedule V medications are sometimes referred to as "exempt narcotics." Refer to Table 4-1 for a list of controlled substances.

Prescription Requirements for Controlled Substances

A prescription for a controlled substance is one that is dispensed to the ultimate user. Prescriptions for controlled substances can be dispensed only by a physician, dentist, podiatrist, or other mid-level practitioner who is authorized within a specific jurisdiction. A prescription for controlled substance must contain the following information:

- Date
- Patient's full name and address
- Practitioner's name, address, and DEA registration number
- Drug name, strength, dosage form, and quantity prescribed
- Directions for use
- Number of refills
- Signature of the practitioner

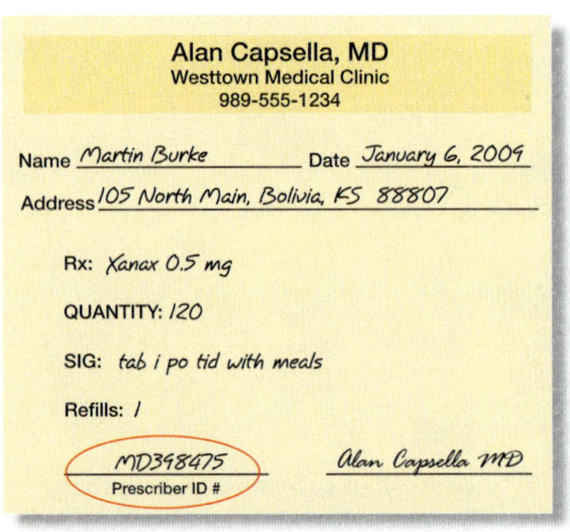

Alan Capsella, MD
Westtown Medical Clinic
989-555-1234

Name Martin Burke Date January 6, 2009
Address 105 North Main, Bolivia, KS 88807

Rx: Xanax 0.5 mg
QUANTITY: 120
SIG: tab i po tid with meals
Refills: 1

MD348475
Prescriber ID #
Alan Capsella MD

Figure 4-11 A prescription for a controlled substance must include a DEA number.

DEA Numbers

A practitioner who is authorized to prescribe controlled substances will be assigned a DEA number upon completion and approval of an application submitted to the DEA (Figure 4-11). A DEA number begins with two letters followed by seven numbers. DEA numbers for physicians, dentists, veterinarians, and other practitioners begin with a letter "A" if they applied prior to October 1985. Practitioners who applied after October 1, 1985, will begin with a "B." Effective October 2006, the letter "F" will be used in issuing new DEA numbers. Mid-level practitioners, DEA numbers begin with an "M." The second letter is the first letter of the practitioner's last name when he or she applied for a DEA number. A mathematical formula is used to verify if a DEA number is valid.

To verify if a DEA number is valid, add the first, third, and fifth digits found in the number. Next add the second, fourth, and sixth digits; multiply this sum by two. Add the sum of the first set and second set of numbers. The number found in the one's column of the sum should be the same as the seventh digit of a valid DEA number.

Table 4-1 Examples of Controlled Substances

Generic Name	Brand Name	Schedule
China White		I
"Crack" Cocaine		I
DMT		I
Ecstasy, MDMA, XTC		I
Hashish		I
Heroin		I
LSD		I
MDA		I
PCE		I
THC		I
amobarbital	Amytal, Tuinal	II
amphetamine	Biphetamine, Dexedrine	II
cocaine		II
codeine		II
fentanyl	Duragesic, Innovar, Sublimaze	II
hydromorphone		II
meperidine	Demerol	II
methamphetamine	Desoxyn, "crank," "speed"	
methylphenidate	Ritalin	II
morphine sulfate	MS Contin, Roxanol, Duramorph, RMS, MSIR	II
oxycodone	OxyContin	II
oxycodone/acetaminophen	Percocet, Roxicet, Tylox	II
pentobarbital	Nembutal	II
phenmetrazine	Preludin	II
secobarbital	Seconal, Tuinal	II
barbituric		III
butabarbital	Butisol, Butibel	III
butalbital	Fiorinal	III
codeine combination products	Empirin, Fiorinal, Tylenol	III
dihydrocodeine	Synalgos-DC	III
hydrocodone	Hycodan	III
hydrocodone combinations	Vicodin, Lortab, Tussionex, Tussend	III
ibuprofen/hydrocodone	Vicoprofen	III
ketamine	Ketaset, Ketalar	III
methyltestosterone	Android, Oreton, Testred, Virilon	III
methyprylon	Noludar	III

(Continued)

Table 4-1 Examples of Controlled Substances *(Continued)*

Generic Name	Brand Name	Schedule
nandrolone	Deca-Durabolin, Durabolin	III
opium containing products	Paregoric	III
oxymetholone	Anadrol	III
phendimetrazine	Plegine, Prelu-2, Bontril, Melfiat, Statobex	III
testosterone	Delatestryl	III
alprazolam	Xanax	IV
butorphanol	Stadol	IV
butalbital/acetaminophen/ codeine	Fioricet	IV
chloral hydrate	Noctec	IV
chlordiazepoxide	Librium	IV
clonazepam	Klonopin	IV
clorazepate	Tranxene	IV
dextropropoxyphene	Darvon, Darvocet	IV
diazepam	Valium	IV
diethylpropion	Tenuate	IV
estazolam	ProSom	IV
flurazepam	Dalmane	IV
lorazepam	Ativan	IV
mazindol	Sanorex, Mazanor	IV
meprobamate	Miltown, Equanil, Equagesic	IV
oxazepam	Serax	IV
pemoline	Cylert	IV
pentazocine	Talwin, Talwin NX	IV
phenobarbital	Luminal	IV
phentermine	Ionamin, Fastin	IV
temazepam	Restoril	IV
triazolam	Halcion	IV
zaleplon	Sonata	IV
zolpidem	Ambien, Ambien CR	IV
codeine preparations: 200 mg/100 mL or g	Robitussin AC, Cheracol	V
difenoxin preparations	Motofen	V
diphenoxylate preparations	Lomotil	V
opium preparations: 100 mg/100 mL or g	Parepectolin, Kapectolin PG, Kaolin Pectin PG	

EXAMPLE

Dr. Andrew James Shedlock has the following DEA number—BS1103972; is it correct? The DEA number begins with a letter "B" signifying that the Doctor Shedlock applied for his DEA number after 1985. The second letter is an "S," which is the first letter of the physician's last name.

Add the first, third, and fifth digits:	$1+0+9=10$
Add the second, fourth, and sixth digits and multiply by 2:	$(1+3+7)(2)=22$
Total	*32*

The number found in the one's column is a two; the DEA number is valid!

Methods of Receiving a Controlled Substance Prescription

All Schedule II medications require a written prescription from a practitioner with a valid DEA number. In the practice of pharmacy, state law over rules federal law. Federal law states that Schedule II medications are valid for 60 days. However, many states laws rule that prescriptions for Schedule II medications are only valid for 7 days from the date it is written. It is necessary for the pharmacy technician to know the state law regarding prescriptions for Schedule II medications. A physician's office may fax a Schedule II prescription to a pharmacy, but the original prescription must be presented at the time of the pickup of the prescription.

In situations where the pharmacy provides Schedule II medications to patients in a long-term care facility and are delivered by the pharmacy, the physician may fax a Schedule II prescription to the pharmacy. In this situation, the faxed prescription will serve as the original prescription and no further prescription will be required.

If a patient is under hospice care, the prescriber may fax a prescription for Schedule II medications, whether or not the patient is in a hospice care, long-term, or other facility. In this situation, it must be noted on the prescription that the patient is a hospice patient.

Prescriptions for Schedules III to V medications may be telephoned in to the pharmacy by the physician or a designated person from the physician's office. Only a pharmacist may accept a telephoned prescription at this time. A prescription for medications in these schedules may be faxed to the pharmacy of the patient's choice. Finally, a physician may write a prescription for a patient with all of the required information. Presently the DEA does not allow prescriptions for controlled substances to be received by way of the Internet.

Partial Dispensing of Controlled Substances

Pharmacists may provide a partial filling of a Schedule II medication if they are unable to fill the entire quantity as prescribed by the physician. The remaining quantity must be provided within 72 hours of receipt of the original prescription or else the remaining quantity becomes void. The patient must be made aware of this situation prior to the filling of the prescription. The pharmacist must note on the hard copy of the prescription the quantity dispensed. If the pharmacist is unable to provide the entire quantity, the physician should be notified of this situation.

A pharmacist may dispense a partial quantity of Schedules III to V medications by notating on the back of the prescription the quantity to be dispensed. The partial dispensing of these medications cannot exceed the total quantity permitted by the original prescription. The remaining refills must be dispensed within 6 months from the date the prescription was written. If a patient requests a partial filling of the prescription, there must be appropriate refills on that prescription.

Emergency Dispensing of Schedule II Medications

In the case of an emergency, a physician may telephone a prescription for a Schedule II medication for a patient. It is the responsibility of the pharmacist to ensure that it is a valid prescription from a legitimate prescriber with a bona fide physician–patient relationship. The quantity of drug prescribed must be limited to the amount needed during this period of emergency. The pharmacist must promptly reduce the emergency prescription to writing and the following notation must appear on the prescription "Authorization for Emergency Dispensing." The physician must provide a written prescription to the pharmacy within 7 days of calling in the prescription to the pharmacy. In the situation that the physician fails to provide a valid prescription to the pharmacy, the DEA is to be notified.

Controlled Substance Prescription Refills

Schedule II medications cannot be refilled, the physician or prescriber must issue a new prescription to the patient. Schedules III to V medications may be refilled up to five times within 6 months of the date of the prescription being written and this must be indicated on the prescription. A patient may obtain multiple refills at a particular filling if such refills exist and a managed-care organization is not paying for the prescription. Refills must be noted on the original prescription; if there are no refills authorized, the pharmacy may contact the physician by either telephone or fax to seek additional refills for schedules III through V medciations.

Transferring a Prescription for Controlled Substances

Prescriptions in Schedules III, IV, and V may be transferred to another pharmacy one time only. The transfer of a prescription must include all of the information contained on a valid prescription. When a prescription is transferred, the prescription at the original pharmacy becomes void and all remaining refills are transferred to the receiving pharmacy. The original pharmacy must note "void" on the original prescription and indicate the date the prescription was transferred, the receiving pharmacy's name, DEA number, telephone number, and individual who accepted the prescription.

The receiving pharmacy must write "Transferred" on the face of the prescription and must include the original date of the prescription, the name, DEA number, and telephone number of the pharmacy of origin, the name of the pharmacist who transferred the prescription, and the number of refills remaining.

Prescription Label for Controlled Substances

All prescription containers for controlled substances must show the pharmacy name and address; the prescription number assigned to the prescription; the date of the initial dispensing; the name of the patient; the name of the prescribing physician; the name, strength, and quantity of the medication; directions for use; and cautionary statements. In addition, the following legend must be included: "Caution: Federal law prohibits the transfer of this drug to any person other than the patient for whom it was prescribed."

Exempt Narcotics

An "exempt narcotic" is a Schedule V medication, which may be dispensed without a prescription by the pharmacist. The following conditions apply to exempt narcotics:

- The pharmacist oversees the transaction.
- The pharmacist ensures that a medical necessity exists that warrants the use of such product.
- Not more than 240 mL or 48 solid dosage units of any substance containing opium or not more than 120 mL or 24 solid dosage units of any controlled substance may be dispensed to the same purchaser within a 48-hour time period.
- Purchaser must be at least 18 years of age.
- Purchaser must provide appropriate identification.
- A Schedule V record book must be completed with the following information: name and address of the purchaser, name and quantity of controlled substance, date of the sale, and initials of the seller.

Ordering of Controlled Substances

An Official Order Form (DEA Form 222) is required in ordering all Schedule II medications. The DEA Form 222 is used to purchase, distribute, or transfer all Schedule II medications. The DEA Form 222 can be ordered by contacting the DEA Headquarters Registration Unit or the nearest DEA Registration Field Office. A book of forms contains seven DEA Form 222s and a maximum of six books can be ordered at one time.

The DEA Form 222 is a three-part form (refer to Figure 4-12) that must be completed by the pharmacist. The pharmacist is required to enter the name of the medication, the number of packages being ordered, and the number of tablets in each package. A maximum of 10 different drugs may be ordered at one time. According to the Code of Federal Regulations, the DEA Form 222 must be "complete, legible and properly prepared, with no signs of alteration, erasure or change of any description."

The DEA Form 222 must be signed by the individual designated with the Power of Attorney to sign an Official Order. Any registrant (e.g., pharmacy) may authorize an individual to obtain and execute an Official Order. In some situations, a pharmacy technician has received the Power of Attorney to sign the Official Order. The power of attorney must be signed by the same person who signed the most recent application for registration or renewal registration, as well as the individual being authorized to obtain and execute Official Order Forms.

Upon receipt of the medication, the receiving pharmacist must date and indicate on each line the number of bottles received. A pharmacist cannot use ditto marks to indicate the date the medication was received.

Figure 4-12 DEA Form 222.

DEA 222 Form Sample

See Reverse of PURCHASER's Copy for Instructions	No order form may be issued for Schedule I and II substances unless completed application form has been received, (21 CFR, 1305.04)	OMD APPROVAL No. 1117-0010

TO: 1) Sun Belt Medical/Energi-Source		STREET ADDRESS 2) 20 Capital Drive
CITY and STATE: 3) Hillon Head Island, SC 29926	DATE 4) Today's Date	TO BE FILLED IN BY SUPPLIERS SUPPLIERS DEA REGISTRATION No.

L I N E No.	TO BE FILLED IN BY PURCHASER					
	No. of Packages	Size of Package	Name of Item	National Drug Code	Package Shipped	Date Shipped
1	5) 1	6) 10 Cpj	7) Morphine Sul 10mg/ml, 1ml LL			
2	1	1	Morphine Sul 10mg/ml, 1ml Stick Guard			
3	1	1	Morphine Sul 10mg/ml, 1ml Luer Jet			
4	1	25x1ml V	Morphine Sul 10mg/ml, 1ml VIAL			
5	1	25x1ml A	Morphine Sul 10mg/ml, 1ml AMPULE			
6	1	10x2ml A	Fentany 10.05mg/ml, AMPULE			
7	1	10 Cpj	Fentany 10.05mg/ml, 2ml LL			
8	1	10 Cpj	Demerol 25mg/ml, 1ml LL			
9	1	25x1ml A	Demerol 50mg/ml, 1ml AMPULE			
10						

8) ◀ LAST LINE COMPLETED	*(MUST BE 10 OR LESS)*	SIGNATURE OF PURCHASER OR ATTORNEY OR AGENT	9)

Date ------	DEA Registration No.	Name and Address of Registrant
Schedules		
Registered as a	No. of the Order Form	

DEA Form -222
(Oct. 1992)

U.S. OFFICIAL ORDER FORMS - SCHEDULES I & II
DRUG ENFORCEMENT ADMINISTRATION
SUPPLIER'S Copy 1

To purchase **Class IV** narcotics, a signed authorization form must be on file as well as a current copy of your Medical Director's or your agency's Federal DEA certificate. When purchasing Class IV narcotics, simply phone, fax or e-mail your order. ***Please be aware that all narcotics will ship to the address on your DEA Certificate.***

With each **Class II** order, a form 222 must be completed and mailed to Sun Belt Medical/Emergi-Source. Forms 222 are issued by your local DEA office. If your Medical Director or authorized purchasing agent does not have any of these forms, call your local DEA office to order the forms.

Please use the following steps when ordering **CLASS II** Narcotics (Morphine, Demerol, Fentanyl):

1) Name of Supplier-Sun Belt Medical/Emergi-Source
2) Street Address- 20 Capital Drive
3) City and State- Hilton Head Island, SC 29926
4) Date-Date the form is completed
*5) Number of Packages-if product is sold in boxes, indicate the number of boxes needed. If product is sold individually, indicate the units needed.
6) Size of package-if sold in boxes, indicate units per box. If sold individually, indicate the packaging size per unit.
7) Description of Product.
8) Last Line Completed-write the number of the last line completed. (Only one line should be completed for each type ordered.)
9) Signature-The Medical Director, agent or person authorized by power of attorney must sign the form.

Helpful Hints:

- Forms 222 are for Class II narcotics only. Class IV narcotics can be phoned or faxed in with other pharmaceuticals
- If an error is made on your form 222, please void the form and begin again with a new form. Any form that has been altered will be returned.
- Sun Belt Medical/Emergi-Source will fill in the Supplier's DEA Registration Number, NDC and shipping information on the forms 222.
- The form 222 is a triplicate form. Retain copy 3 for your records and forward copies 1&2 to Sun Belt Medical/Emergi-Source
- If a purchase order number is needed on the packing slip, please include a note with your form 222 when mailing to Sun Belt Medical/Emergi-Source.
- Narcotics are non-returnable. Please be very specific with description and quantity needed when placing an order.
- All narcotics will ship to the address printed on the forms 222 and Federal DEAlicense.

Destruction of Controlled Substances

A retail pharmacy may seek permission to destroy outdated or damaged controlled substances from the DEA by completing a DEA Form 41 (refer to Figure 4-13) at least 2 weeks prior to the proposed destruction. When seeking authorization the pharmacy must submit a date for the destruction, the method of destruction, and identify the individuals who will witness the destruction. Upon receipt of the request, the DEA will respond in writing to the pharmacy of their decision. Upon completion of the destruction, the pharmacy will forward signed copies of the DEA Form 41 and retain one copy of the form for a minimum of 2 years.

A "blanket authorization" for the destruction of controlled substances may be approved by the DEA for pharmacies in hospitals or clinics for the disposition of needles, syringes, and other injectable objects that may have been exposed to body fluids. The DEA's decision to approve a blanket authorization will be based upon the following:

- Frequency of destruction
- Method of destruction
- Pharmacy's past history of destruction
- Pharmacy security
- Individuals responsible for the destruction

Controlled Substance Inventories

The Controlled Substance Act requires that specific inventories be maintained for all controlled substances. These inventories must be maintained for a minimum of 2 years at the registered pharmacy.

An Initial Inventory is an actual physical count of all controlled substances by a registrant when the registrant takes possession of the pharmacy. If there are no stocks of controlled substances on hand, the registrant must indicate such as zero. Components of this inventory include:

- Inventory date
- The time the inventory was taken (i.e., opening or close of business)
- The drug name
- The drug strength
- The drug form (e.g., tablet, capsule)
- The number of units/volume
- The total quantity
- The name, address, and DEA registration number of the registrant
- The signature of the person or persons responsible for taking the inventory

This record is to be maintained at the pharmacy. Refer to Figure 4-14, which shows an example of a Controlled Substance Inventory page.

A biennial inventory is required to be taken every 2 years after an initial inventory. It contains the same information to be recorded, as the initial inventory requires. This inventory must be taken on any date within 2 years of the previous inventory date. An actual physical count must be taken for all Schedule II medications; an estimated count must be taken for all Schedules III, IV, and V medications. The only exception to the estimated count is when the container holds more than 1000 units and has been opened.

Figure 4-13 DEA Form 41.

OMB Approval No. 1117-0007	U.S. Department of Justice / Drug Enforcement Administration **REGISTRANTS INVENTORY OF DRUGS SURRENDERED**	PACKAGE NO.

The following schedule is an inventory of controlled substances which is hereby surrendered to you for proper disposition.

FROM: *(include Name, Street, City, State and ZIP Code in space provided below.)*

Signature of applicant or authorized agent

Registrant's DEA Number

Registrant's Telephone Number

NOTE: CERTIFIED MAIL (Return Receipt Requested) IS REQUIRED FOR SHIPMENTS OF DRUGS VIA U.S. POSTAL SERVICE. See instructions on reverse (page 2) of form.

NAME OF DRUGS OR PREPARATION Registrants will fill in Columns 1,2,3 and 4 ONLY.	Number of Containers	CONTENTS *(Number of grams, tablets; ounces or other units per container)*	Controlled Substance Content, *(Each uint)*	**FOR DEA USE ONLY** DISPOSTION	QUANTITY GMS.	MGS.
1	*2*	*3*	*4*	*5*	*6*	*7*
1						
2						
3						
4						
5						
6						
7						
8						
9						
10						
11						
12						
13						
14						
15						
16						

FORM DEA-41 (9-01) Previous edition dated 6-86 is usable. *See instructions on reverse (page 2) of form.*

Figure 4-14 DEA Sample Controlled Inventory Page.

Drug	Form	Drug	Form
_____ACTIQ 200 mcg	loz	_____ADDERALL XR 30 mg	cap
_____ACTIQ 400 mcg	loz	_____ALFENTAL 500 mcg 2 ml	amp
_____ACTIQ 600 mcg	loz	_____ALFENTAL 500 mcg 5 ml	amp
_____ACTIQ 800 mcg	loz	_____ALFENTAL 500 mcg 10 ml	amp
_____ACTIQ 1200 mcg	loz	_____ALFENTAL 500 mcg 20 ml	amp
_____ACTIQ 1600 mcg	loz	_____amphetamine sulfate 10 mg	tab
_____fentanyl citrate 200 mcg	loz	_____AMYTAL 30 mg	tab
_____fentanyl citrate 300 mcg	loz	_____AMYTAL 100 mg	tab
_____fentanyl citrate 400 mcg	loz	_____AMYTAL Sodium 65 mg	cap
_____ADDERALL 5 mg	tab	_____AMYTAL Sodium 200 mg	cap
_____ADDERALL 7.5 mg	tab	_____AMYTAL Sodium 250 mg	cap
_____ADDERALL 10 mg	tab	_____AMYTAL Sodium 500 mg	cap
_____ADDERALL 12.5 mg	tab	_____amobarbital 200 mg	cap
_____ADDERALL 15 mg	tab	_____amobarbital	pow
_____ADDERALL 20 mg	tab	_____ASTRAMORPH 0.5 mg/ml 2 ml	amp
_____ADDERALL 30 mg	tab	_____ASTRAMORPH 1 mg/ml 2 ml	amp
_____dextroamphetamine 5 mg	tab	_____ASTRAMORPH 4 mg/ml 2 ml	amp
_____dextroamphetamine 7.5 mg	tab	_____ASTRAMORPH 8 mg/ml 2 ml	amp
_____dextroamphetamine 10 mg	tab	_____ASTRAMORPH 10 mg/ml 2 ml	amp
_____dextroamphetamine 12.5 mg	tab	_____ASTRAMORPH 15 mg/ml 2 ml	amp
_____dextroamphetamine 15 mg	tab	_____ASTRAMORPH 15 mg/ml 2 ml	vial
_____dextroamphetamine 20 mg	tab	_____ASTRAMORPH 8 mg/ml 1 ml	vial
_____dextroamphetamine 30 mg	tab	_____ASTRAMORPH 10 mg/ml 1 ml	vial
_____ADDERALL XR 5 mg	cap	_____ASTRAMORPH 15 mg/ml 1 ml	vial
_____ADDERALL XR 10 mg	cap	_____ASTRAMORPH PF 5 mg/10 ml	amp
_____ADDERALL XR 15 mg	cap	_____ASTRAMORPH PF 10 mg/10 ml	amp
_____ADDERALL XR 20 mg	cap	_____ASTRAMORPH PF 10 mg/10 ml	vial
_____ADDERALL XR 25 mg	cap	_____AVINZA 30 mg	cap

Controlled Substance Record Retention

All pharmacies must maintain complete and accurate records on the purchase, dispensing, and disposition of all controlled substances. These records must be maintained for a minimum of 2 years according to federal law (state regulations take precedence if the records are to be maintained for a period greater than 2 years).

These records must be "readily retrievable." To be considered readily retrievable, the records must be kept by an automatic data processing system or electronic record-keeping system that can be separated from other records in a reasonable period. Second, the records must be easily identified through asterisking or highlighting the controlled substances.

The following records must be maintained by the pharmacy:

- DEA registration certificate
- Official Order Forms (DEA Form 222)
- Power of Attorney to sign DEA Form 222
- Invoices for Schedules II, III, IV, and V medications
- Initial and biennial inventories of controlled substances
- Report of Theft or Loss (DEA Form 106)
- Inventory of Drugs Surrendered for Disposal (DEA Form 41)
- Records of transfers of controlled substances between pharmacies

A pharmacy has three different options in filing prescriptions. All prescription records must be readily retrievable.

Option 1 (three separate files)

- A file for Schedule II drugs only.
- A file for Schedules III, IV, and V only.
- A file for all noncontrolled drugs.

Option 2 (two separate files)

- A file for Schedule II drugs only.
- A file for all other prescriptions (Schedules III, IV, V, and noncontrolled drugs). Schedules III, IV, and V must be stamped with a red "C."

Option 3 (two separate files)

- A file for all controlled prescriptions. Schedules III, IV, and V must be stamped with a red "C."
- A file for all noncontrolled prescriptions.

Theft of Controlled Substances

In the case of a robbery or theft of controlled substances, the pharmacy must notify the local police department, the DEA, and the state board of pharmacy. The pharmacy will complete a DEA Form 106 and send the original and a copy to the DEA. Refer to Figure 4-15. The pharmacy must retain a copy of the completed DEA Form 106 for its records. Information contained on a completed DEA Form 106 includes:

- Name and address of the pharmacy
- DEA registration number
- Date of theft
- Name and telephone number of the local police department
- Type of theft
- Identifying symbols or abbreviations used by the pharmacy
- List of controlled substances missing

Figure 4-15 Sample DEA Form 106.

REPORT OF THEFT OR LOSS OF CONTROLLED SUBSTANCES

Federal Regulations require registrants to submit a detailed report of any theft or loss of Controlled Substances to the Drug Enforcement Administration.
Complete the front and back of this form in triplicate. Forward the original and duplicate copies to the nearest DEA Office. Retain the triplicate copy for your records. Some states may also require a copy of this report.

OMB APPROVAL
No. 1117-0001

1. Name and Address of Registrants (include ZIP Code)

ZIP CODE ☐☐☐☐☐

2. Phone No. (Include Area Code)

3. DEA Registration Number
2. ltr. prefix ☐☐ 7 digit suffix ☐☐☐☐☐☐☐

4. Date of Theft or Loss

5. Principal Business of Registrant (Check one)
1 ☐ Pharmacy
2 ☐ Practitioner
3 ☐ Manufacturer
4 ☐ Hospital/Clinic
5 ☐ Distributor
6 ☐ Methadone Program
7 ☐ Other (Specify)

6. Country in which Registrant is located

7. Was Theft reported to Police?
☐ Yes ☐ No

8. Name and Telephone Number of Police Department (Include Area Code)

9. Number of Thefts or Losses Registrant has experienced in the past 24 months

10. Types of Theft or Loss (Check one and complete items below as appropriate)
1 ☐ Night break-in
2 ☐ Armed robbery
3 ☐ Employee pilferage
4 ☐ Customer theft
5 ☐ Other (Explain)
6 ☐ Lost in transit (Complete Item 14)

11. If Armed Robbery, was anyone:
Killed? ☐ No ☐ Yes (How many) ____________
Injured? ☐ No ☐ Yes (How many) ____________

12. Purchase value to registrant of Controlled Substances taken?
$

13. Were any pharmaceuticals or merchandise taken?
☐ No ☐ Yes (Est. Value)
$

14. IF LOST IN TRANSIT, COMPLETE THE FOLLOWING:

A. Name of Common Carrier

B. Name of Consignee

C. Consignee's DEA Registration Number

D. Was the carton received by the customer?
☐ Yes ☐ No

E. If received, did it appear to be tampered with?
☐ Yes ☐ No

F. Have you experienced losses in transit from this same carrier in the past?
☐ No ☐ Yes (How many) ____________

15. What identifying marks, symbols, or price codes were on the labels of these containers that would assist in identifying the products?

16. If Official Controlled Substances Order Forms (DEA-222) were stolen, give numbers.

17. What security measure have been taken to prevent future thefts or losses?

PRIVACY ACT INFORMATION

AUTHORITY: Section 301 of the Controlled Substances Act of 1970 (PL 91-513).
PURPOSE: Report theft or loss of Controlled Substances.
ROUTINE USES: The Controlled Substances Act authorizes the production of special reports required for statistical and analytical purposes. Disclosures of information from this system are made to the following categories of users for the purposes stated:
A. Other Federal law enforcement and regulatory agencies for law enforcement and regularly purposes.
B. State and local law enforcement and regulatory agencies for law enforcement and regulatory purposes.
EFFECT: Failure to report theft or loss of controlled substances may result in penalties under Section 402 and 403 of the Controlled substances Act.

In accordance with the Paper work Reduction Act of 1955, no person is required to respond to a collection of information unless it displays a ly valid OMB control number. The valid OMB control number for this collection of information is 1117-0001. Public reporting burden for this collection of information is estimated to average 30 minutes per response, including the time for reviewing instructions, searching existing data sources, gathering and maintaining the data needed, and completing and reviewing the collection of information.

FORM DEA - 106 (11-00) *Previous edition obsolete*

CONTINUE ON REVERSE

Mailing of Controlled Substances

Controlled substances may be mailed through the U.S. Postal Service if the following packaging standards are applied:

- The inner container of any parcel containing controlled substances is marked and sealed and is placed in a plain outer container or securely wrapped in plain paper.
- The inner container is labeled to show the name and address of the pharmacy.
- The outside wrapper does not indicate what the contents would be.

Tech Check

9. How many schedules are discussed in the Controlled Substance Act?(LO 4.4)
10. What is the maximum number of refills permitted for each schedule under the Controlled Substance Act?(LO 4.3c, 4.4)
11. Explain the different methods to file prescriptions.(LO 4.6)
12. Within what period must Schedules III to V prescriptions be filled?(LO 4.4)
13. How many times a year may a retail pharmacy destroy controlled substances?(LO 4.3)
14. You are a medical doctor and have applied for a DEA number; write a valid DEA number for yourself.(LO 4.3)

Federal Pharmacy Laws 1970–1979(LO 4.3c, d)

1970 – Poison Prevention Packaging Act (PPPA)
1970 – Occupational Safety and Health Act
1972 – Drug Listing Act
1976 – Medical Device Amendments

Poison Prevention Packaging Act of 1970

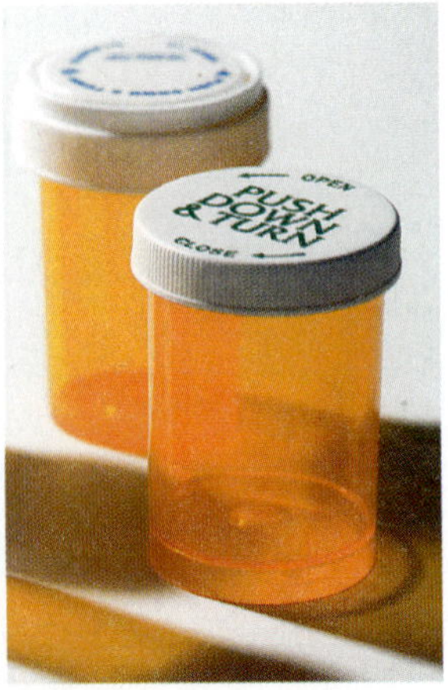

Figure 4-16 **Child-resistant containers.**

The Poison Prevention Packaging Act was enacted to reduce the accidental poisoning in children. The act requires that most OTC and legend drugs be packaged in child-resistant containers (Figure 4-16). These containers must be tested by the manufacturers to document they are child-resistant. In the test, children ranging from 42 to 51 months of age are unable to open within 5 minutes. If the child is unable to open the container, how to open the container is demonstrated to the child. The child is then given 5 minutes to open the container. If less than 20% of the children tested are able to open the container after the demonstration, it will be considered child resistant. Adults are also tested. They are given 5 minutes to open and close the container. If 90% of the adults are able to open and close it, the container is considered child resistant. A child-resistant container is one that cannot be opened by 80% of children younger than the age of 5, but can be opened by 90% of adults.

Exceptions

- Single-time dispensing of product in noncompliant container as ordered by the prescriber.
- Single-time or blanket dispensing of product in noncompliant container as requested by patient or customer in a signed statement. The signed statement must be stamped on the back of the original prescription and signed by the individual requesting the noncompliant container.
- One noncompliant size of the OTC product for patients who are elderly or disabled, provided that they contain the warning "This package for households without young children," or "Package not child resistant."
- Drugs dispensed to institutionalized patients if these are to be administered by an employee of an institution.
- Some of the medications not requiring child-resistant containers include:
    - Betamethasone with no more than 12.6 mg per package
    - Erythromycin Ethylsuccinate tablets in packages containing no more than 16 g
    - Inhalation aerosols
    - Mebendazole tablets with no more than 600 mg per package
    - Methylprednisolone tablets with no more than 85 mg per package
    - Oral contraceptives taken cyclically in the manufacturer's dispensing package
    - Pancrelipase preparations
    - Powdered anhydrous cholestyramine
    - Powdered colestipol up to 5 g per packet
    - Prednisone tablets with no more than 105 mg per package
    - Sodium fluoride tablets with no more than 264 mg of sodium fluoride per package
    - Sublingual and chewable isosorbide dinitrate, in dosages of 10 mg or less
    - Sublingual nitroglycerin tablets

Occupational Safety and Health Act of 1970

The Occupational Safety and Health Act of 1970 ensured a safe and healthful workplace for all employees. The law was developed to provide job safety and health standards for employees, maintain a reporting system for job-related injuries and illness, and reduce hazards in the workplace and to conduct audits to ensure compliance of the act. Its impact on pharmacy is addressed to air contaminants, flammable and combustible liquids, eye and skin protection, and hazard communication standard. This act requires usage of Material Safety Data Sheets (MSDS) to be provided with specific products. Because of the Occupational Safety and Health Act of 1970, we find Sharps containers in hospital pharmacies, and the usage of Universal Precautions and personal protective equipment (PPE).

Drug Listing Act of 1972

The purpose of the Drug Listing Act was to provide the FDA with the authority to compile a list of currently marketed medications in the United States.

Any drug company that manufactures or repackages medication in the United States must register with the FDA. Each drug is assigned a specific 11-digit number with three components separated by hyphens to identify it. This number is known as a **National Drug Code (NDC)** number.

The first five digits identify the manufacturer (labeler code), the next four digits identify the drug product (product code), and the final two digits represent the package size (packaging code). For example, the NDC number for Vytorin 10/40 manufactured by Merck Pharmaceuticals in a 90-tablet bottle is 66582-0313-54: 66582 identifies the drug manufacturer (Merck Pharmaceuticals), 0313 identifies the drug product (Vytorin 10/40), and 54 identifies the package. Some NDC numbers may have only only nine digits. A zero (0) preceding the labeling code and product code does not appear but is included in the NDC number. For example, the number would be in a (4-3-2) configuration. Four numbers (labeler code) with a zero in front, three numbers (produce code) with a zero in front and then two numbers (packaging code).

The following information is maintained by the FDA and is easily accessed.

- List of all drug products
- List of all drug products broken down by labeled indications or pharmacologic category
- List of all drugs by the manufacturer
- List of drug products' active ingredients
- List of drug products' inactive ingredients
- List of drug products containing a particular ingredient
- List of drug products recently marketed or remarketed
- List of discontinued drug products
- Labeling of all drug products
- Advertising of all drug products

This information enables the FDA to monitor all products marketed in the United States.

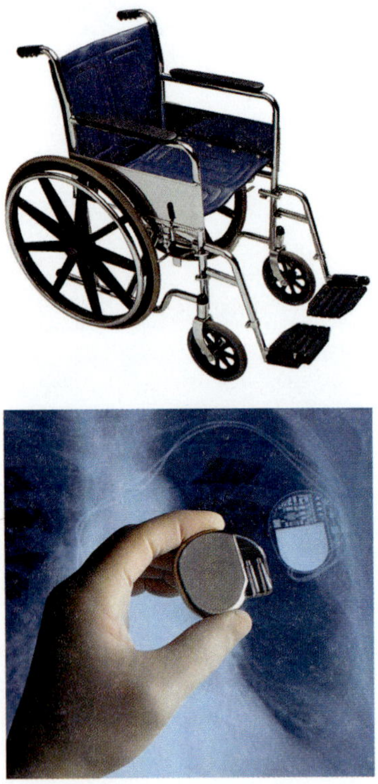

Figure 4-17 Medical devices.

National Drug Code (NDC) An 11-digit number identifying a particular medication. The first five digits identify the drug manufacturer, the next four digits represent a particular medication, and the last two digits identify the packaging of the product.

Medical Device Amendments of 1976

In 1976, medical devices were included under the Food, Drug and Cosmetic Act of 1938. A medical device is defined as any health care product that does not achieve its primary intended purposes by chemical action or by being metabolized. Medical devices include surgical lasers, wheelchairs, sutures, pacemakers, vascular grafts, intraocular lenses, and orthopedic pins (Figure 4-17). Other medical devices include diagnostic aids such as reagents and test kits for in vitro diagnosis of disease and other medical conditions such as pregnancy.

Tech Check

15. Why was the Poison Prevention Packaging Act enacted?(LO 4.3c)

16. Identify one medication that does not need to be placed in a child-resistant container.(LO 4.3c)

17. What are the three components of an NDC number?(LO 4.3d)

Federal Pharmacy Laws 1980–1999(LO 4.3 e, f, g)

1983 – Orphan Drug Act
1984 – Drug Price Competition and Patent Term Restoration Act
1987 – Prescription Drug Marketing Act (PDMA) of 1987
1987 – Omnibus Budget Reconciliation Act (OBRA-87) of 1987
1990 – Omnibus Budget Reconciliation Act (OBRA-90) of 1990
1994 – Dietary Supplement Health and Education Act (DSHEA)
1996 – Health Insurance Portability and Accountability Act (HIPAA) of 1996
1996 – Comprehensive Methamphetamine Control Act of 1996
1997 – FDA Modernization Act

Orphan Drug Act (ODA) of 1983

The Orphan Drug Act of 1983 was enacted to provide incentives for the drug manufacturers to develop medications to treat "rare diseases." A "rare disease" is a condition affecting less than 200,000 patients a year in the United States. There are between 5000 to 6000 rare diseases in the United States affecting over 25 million people. Many of these diseases are of genetic origin. These diseases are chronic, progressive, disabling, life-threatening, and have a negative impact on an individual's life. Many of these conditions have no treatment.

They have been defined as "orphaned" because the drug manufacturers have not developed medications due to the high cost of obtaining FDA approval and the manufacturer is unable to recoup its investment. A drug manufacturer will spend approximately $800 million to conduct the research and bring the product to market. The two largest categories of orphan drugs involve treatment for rare forms of cancer and metabolic disorders.

The following incentives resulted from the passage of the Orphan Drug Act:

- Sponsors are granted 7 years of marketing exclusivity after approval of its orphan drug product.
- Sponsors are granted tax incentives for clinical research.
- FDA's Office of Orphan Products Development encourages sponsors to conduct open protocols, allowing patients to be added to ongoing studies.
- Grants are available to defray costs of qualified clinical testing expenses incurred in connection with the development of orphan drugs.

Drug Price Competition and Patent Term Restoration Act of 1984

This act was enacted to facilitate the approval of generic medications while extending the **patent** protection for specific medications. A patent is an official document that confers the right or privilege to license. The act allowed for generic copies on a formerly approved new drug to be filed by

patent An official document conferring a right or privilege to license.

submitting an Abbreviated New Drug Application (ANDA). The ANDA process will be discussed in detail in Chapter 18. This action did not require a drug manufacturer to conduct animal and human studies on a drug product and therefore reduced the amount of time needed to bring a generic drug to market.

For the drug manufacturers of a patented drug, this legislation provided an extension of the patent life equal to the time required for the FDA to review the NDA, plus half of the time spent in the testing phase, up to a maximum of 5 years and not to exceed the usual 20-year patent term.

Prescription Drug Marketing Act of 1987

The Prescription Drug Marketing Act provides safeguards on the reliability of medication supplied in the United States. The act was intended to reduce the danger of adulterated, misbranded, and repackaged drugs being introduced into the market by secondary sources. It addressed issues involving reimportation, restricted sales, distribution of samples, and wholesale distribution.

The act prohibited the reimportation of drug products in the United States except by the drug manufacturer. It also prohibited the selling, trading, or purchasing of drug samples. The act prevented the resaling of medications purchased by a health care organization. Samples could be distributed only to medical practitioners licensed to prescribe medications. Because of this act, limits were imposed on prescription samples to prescribers and required a more accurate accounting of such medications. Finally, the act required drug manufacturers to maintain a list of their authorized wholesalers.

Omnibus Budget Reconciliation Act of 1987

The Omnibus Reconciliation Act of 1987 (OBRA-87) was enacted to protect the rights of the patient in long-term care facilities. This act gave the Centers of Medicare and Medicaid (CMS) the authority to enact key measures to reduce unnecessary costs and yet improve the quality of patient care in these facilities. Prior to this act, there were numerous patient treatment practices in place that may seem unethical today. OBRA-87 required that a patient's drug regimen be free of unnecessary drugs. An unnecessary drug is one that may eliminated or the dosage reduced for a given patient. An unnecessary drug may be a drug in an excessive dose being taken for an inappropriate period of time and without appropriate monitoring. For instance, the failure to provide liver function tests for specific medications might deem a medication unnecessary.

There was a time when patients in long-term care facilities were given antipsychotic medications when a diagnosis had not been indicated. These medications had become part of a standing order for all patients. OBRA-87 outlawed the prescribing of medications for affective disorder if a diagnosis had not been made and documented appropriately. Due to the adverse side effects of these medications, the CMS mandated that dosages be reduced if possible and other forms of therapy be used in conjunction with the medication. Other forms of therapy might include one-on-one therapy, group therapy, art therapy, or music therapy.

A major concern affecting pharmacy practice today is the number of prescription or medication errors. CMS regulations state that residents (patients) in a long-term care facility are free of significant errors. A prescription error is one where the strength is incorrect, administered at the wrong time or frequency, or administered incorrectly. For instance, promethazine is available in a 25-mg strength and can be administered orally, parenterally, or rectally. If the physician ordered promethazine 25 mg supp pr qid and the patient received promethazine 25 mg po qid, a medication error has occurred. Whose fault is it? What can be done to prevent this from happening again?

All long-term care facilities are required to provide both maintenance and emergency medications for their residents. Other areas addressed in this act include the proper labeling and storage of medications (controlled and non-controlled) in the facility. Infection control programs must be in place in the facility to prevent the spread of disease in the facility. Finally, both chemical and physical restraints are not to be used capriciously by the staff on patients. After reading about some of these provisions of the act, one can only imagine what was being done prior to 1987 in long-term care facilities.

Omnibus Budget Reconciliation Act of 1990 (OBRA-90)

The Omnibus Budget Reconciliation Act of 1990 (OBRA-90) required each state to develop and mandate drug utilization review (DUR) programs to enhance the quality of care to all patients covered by the Medicaid program. A drug utilization review program ensured that prescriptions are appropriate and medically necessary for the patient. Because of OBRA-90, pharmacists were required to perform drug utilization reviews and offer to counsel all patients on their medications as well as maintaining specific records.

The purpose of DUR is to identify potential medication therapy issues. DUR requires that the pharmacist screen the following:

- Therapeutic duplication
- Overutilization/underutilization of a medication
- Drug-disease contraindications
- Drug-drug interactions to include both prescription and OTC medications
- Incorrect duration of treatment
- Drug-allergy interactions
- Clinical abuse/misuse of medication

An offer to counsel all patients is mandated under OBRA-90. The information to be conveyed to the patient or their caregiver includes:

- The name and description of the medication
- The dosage form, route of administration, and duration of drug therapy
- Special directions and precautions for preparation, administration, and use by the patient
- Common severe side effects or adverse effects or interactions and therapeutic interactions that may be encountered
- Contraindications
- Techniques for self-monitoring of drug therapy
- Proper storage
- Refill information
- Action to be taken in the event of a missed dose

Finally, OBRA-90 required that pharmacy providers make a reasonable attempt to obtain, record, and maintain specific patient information. This patient information includes:

- Name, address, and telephone number
- Age and gender
- Significant disease state(s)
- Known allergies and/or drug reactions
- Comprehensive list of medication and relevant devices
- Pharmacist's comments about a particular individual's drug therapy

The original intent of this bill was to improve the quality of care Medicaid patients would receive. The failure for a pharmacist to comply with OBRA-90 may result in the loss of the pharmacy to participate in the Medicaid program. The intent of OBRA-90 has been extended to anyone receiving a prescription in the United States, whether or not one receives Medicaid benefits.

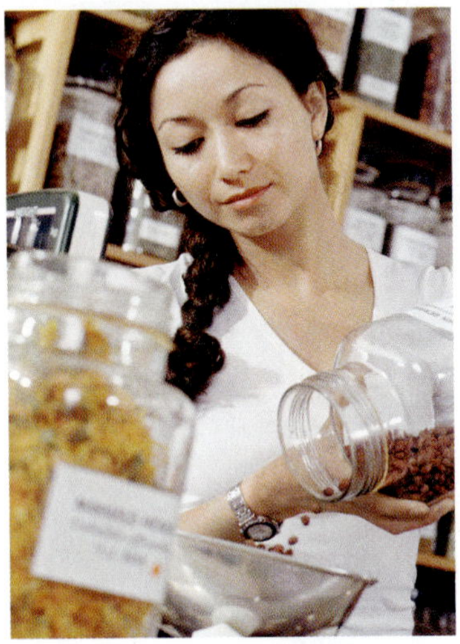

Figure 4-18 Herbal remedies store.

Dietary Supplement Health and Education Act of 1994 (DSHEA)

Because of consumer interest in various herbal dietary supplements and natural products, Congress felt it was important to regulate the labeling claims of these products (Figure 4-18). The products including vitamins, minerals, and amino acids are not considered drugs because they have not been submitted for review on a New Drug Application (NDA). Since an NDA has not been submitted, the FDA is unable to evaluate whether a product is safe and effective.

DSHEA forbids manufacturers or distributors of these products to make any advertising or labeling claims that use of the product can prevent or cure a specific condition. The products must contain the following disclaimer: "This product is not intended to diagnose, treat, cure or prevent any disease." The manufacturer may state how a product may benefit an individual with a specific deficiency.

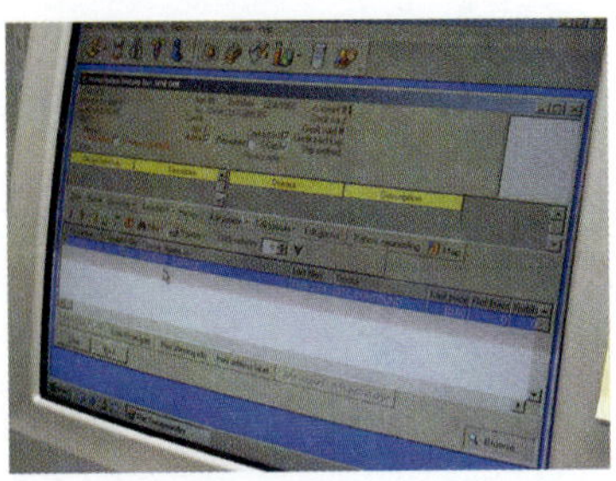

Figure 4-19 Electronic health records are Protected Health Information.

Protected Health Information (PHI) Individually identifiable health information transmitted or maintained in any form or medium.

Health Insurance Portability and Accountability Act of 1996 (HIPAA)

The ultimate goal of the Health Insurance Portability and Accountability Act of 1996 (HIPAA) is to protect a patient's **Protected Health Information (PHI)**. Any pharmacy that maintains a patient's health information in an electronic format or conducts financial and administrative transactions electronically must adhere to HIPAA (Figure 4-19).

It is the responsibility for each pharmacy to adopt policies and procedures relating to the protection of a patient's protected health information. A pharmacy must be consistent with handling all patients' protected health information. HIPAA provides important rights to all patients. These rights include:

- A right to access their information
- A right to seek details of the disclosure of their PHI
- A right to view a pharmacy's policies and procedures regarding their PHI

There are five essential components of the PHI to which a pharmacy must adhere. First, each pharmacy must take reasonable precautions to limit the use, disclosure of, and requests of PHI. A pharmacy must put into practice reasonable policies and procedures that limit how PHI is used, disclosed, and requested. The policy should be conspicuously posted.

Second, all individuals must be informed of the privacy practices of the pharmacy and this information must be provided to the patient on the date of the first prescription processed. It is the responsibility of the pharmacist to attempt to obtain written acknowledgment from the patient.

Third, a compliance officer must be appointed to ensure compliance with HIPAA. Fourth, all employees working in a pharmacy (pharmacists and pharmacy technicians) must receive training on HIPAA regulations. Finally, if a pharmacy discloses PHI to an individual or organization designated as a "business associate," it is the responsibility of the pharmacy to obtain written assurances that the information provided to the business associate will be used only for the purpose it was intended.

Security provisions went into effect in April 2005. These provisions must ensure that PHI is to remain confidential, whether by unauthorized access or intercepted during an electronic transmission. These standards affect the administrative, physical, and technical safeguards that a pharmacy must consider to protect the confidentiality, integrity, and availability of PHI.

Comprehensive Methamphetamine Control Act of 1996

The Comprehensive Methamphetamine Control Act was enacted to combat the growing methamphetamine problem in the United States. Two of the ingredients (pseudoephedrine and phenylpropanolamine) used in the production of methamphetamine are found in many common OTC cold medications. Pharmacies selling either of these ingredients must maintain specific records and provide reporting requirements as mandated under this act. Specific concerns for both pharmacists and pharmacy technicians include:

- The definition of retail distributor includes a grocery store, general merchandise store, or drug store, whose distribution of pseudoephedrine, phenylpropanolamine, or a combination of these two products is limited exclusively for personal use, both in the number and volume of sales, either to walk-in customers or in face-to-face transactions.
- A single transaction of pseudoephedrine and phenylpropanolamine are to be below 9 g or less than 3 g per package for legitimate medical use.

FDA Modernization Act of 1997

The FDA Modernization Act of 1997 was enacted to simplify FDA procedures and codify its current regulations. This act allowed patients with specific illnesses greater access to investigational medications. The act has speeded up the drug approval process and has encouraged the drug manufacturers to investigate pediatric uses of various medications. The FDA Modernization Act established methods to monitor the safety and effectiveness of drug products and began a program on the distribution of information on "off-label uses" of medications. This revision included more up-to-date definitions of drug, cosmetic, label, labeling, and new drug. In addition, the federal legend "Caution: Federal law prohibits dispensing without a prescription" was abbreviated to "Rx only."

Tech Check

18. Who may initiate the offer to counsel a patient?(LO 4.3f)

19. Who must counsel the patient?(LO 4.3f)

20. What type of conditions might an orphan drug treat?(LO 4.3e)

21. What is an example of a dietary supplement? (LO 4.3f)

22. What is PHI? Provide an example of it.(LO 4.3g)

23. What is the maximum amount of pseudoephedrine that may be purchased at a time?(LO 4.3g)

Federal Pharmacy Laws 2000–Present(LO 4.3h, i, 4.7)

2003 – Medicare Modernization Act
2004 – USP<797>
2004 – Isotretinoin Safety and Risk Management Act
2004 – Anabolic Steroid Control Act
2008 – Implementation of Medicaid Tamper Resistant Prescription Pad Law

Medicare Modernization Act of 2003

Prior to 2003, **Medicare** recipients had access to prescription drug benefits only in hospitals, nursing homes, and physicians' offices; they did not have access to outpatient facilities. The enactment of this act resulted in elderly people becoming eligible for either Medicare Part C (Medicare Advantage) or Medicare Part D (prescription drug plans). Medicare beneficiaries are now able to add a prescription component to their Medicare Part A coverage (hospitalization) and Medicare Part B coverage (physicians, home health care, and durable medical equipment).

Medicare Part D is a voluntary program that allows individuals to enroll during a 7-month window—3 months prior to their eligibility date, the month of their eligibility, or 3 months after their eligibility—otherwise they are able to enroll only in the last 1½ months of the calendar year during open season. One of the issues facing Medicare beneficiaries is which plan they should enroll in; individuals may have anywhere from 25 to 50 plans to chose from in their geographical area. All plans are required to cover at least two drugs in every therapeutic classification and all immunosuppressive, anticancer, antipsychotic, anticonvulsant, antidepressant, and antiretroviral medications.

Medicare Part D is overseen by the Centers for Medicare and Medicaid Services (CMS). The addition of a prescription benefit to Medicare provides beneficiaries with prescription benefits that were not available previously.

Medicare A program of the Social Security Administration, which provides medical care to the aged and disabled.

USP Chapter<797>

USP Chapter <797> (1), was enacted January 1, 2004, It set the first enforceable standards for sterile compounding. The intent of USP <797> is to provide procedural and practical requirements for safe compounding of sterile preparations. The requirements apply to all practice settings where sterile preparations are compounded. USP <797> contains many procedural training, and quality assurance requirements. Revisions to USP 797 were effective June 1, 2007, with compliance being ongoing.

USP <797>, the U.S. standard for sterile compounding, is important for several reasons:

- The Food, Drug and Cosmetic Act (and thus the FDA) recognizes the USP/NF (National Formulary) as the official compendia of U.S. drug standards. There are hundreds of USP drug standards and all standards numbered less than 1000 are enforceable by either individual state boards of pharmacy or the FDA. The FDA does not routinely inspect individual pharmacies but may intervene in the case of injuries, a death, or a complaint.
- USP/NF standards are often used as evidence of national standards in lawsuits.
- The Joint Commission (TJC) (formerly The Joint Commission Accreditation of Healthcare Organizations—JCAHO) has adopted these standards for use after July 1, 2004. TJC accreditation is the most universally recognized standard of U.S. health care system quality. TJC accreditation is required for reimbursement through the national Medicare program and almost all state Medicaid (welfare) programs.
- Many state boards of pharmacy are adopting USP <797> for their pharmacy inspections.

USP <797> standards are required for compounded products as well as any manufactured sterile product. The most important objective of USP Chapter <797> is to prevent harm to patients. This harm could occur when any of the of following occurs during compounding sterile products.

- Microbial contamination,
- Excessive bacterial endotoxins
- Variability in the intended strength of correct ingredients
- Unintended chemical and physical contaminants
- Ingredients of inappropriate quality

Steps that individuals and facilities must take to comply with the USP <797> guidelines include the following:

1. Educate yourself on the new standards
2. Determine CSP risk level
3. Complete revised gap analysis to determine level of current compliance
4. Develop action plan
5. Prioritize action items
6. Report gap analysis results and action plan to staff
7. Assign action plan items and timelines to specific employees
8. Document all action plan progress
9. Continually reassess for compliance

Isotretinoin Safety and Risk Management Act of 2004

Accutane (isotretinoin) is a very powerful medication used to treat acne. Unfortunately, the medication has been found to cause severe birth defects, induce spontaneous abortions, and produce adverse psychiatric effects to include depression, psychosis, suicidal ideation, suicide attempts, and suicide.

Because of this legislation, the following are now in place:

- Mandatory registry of all patients, practitioners, and pharmacists.
- Education of all practitioners and pharmacists on the risks associated with the drug, including birth defects and mental health risks.
- A requirement that Accutane and generics are prescribed only for severe recalcitrant nodular acne, the medical condition for which Accutane was approved, which is unresponsive to conventional therapy, including antibiotics. Accutane and its generic are often prescribed for mild acne or without trying other medications first.
- Monthly education of patients, both male and female, of the need to avoid pregnancy as completion of a survey to warn the patient of the adverse side effects. Patient visits will include one-on-one counseling, and patients or parents must sign an informed consent form.
- Certification of medical offices and clinics as treatment centers.
- No Internet, phone, or mail-order prescriptions.
- Thirty-day prescription allotments.
- Female patients required to have monthly pregnancy test and receive negative result before renewal of prescription.
- Appropriate blood testing during treatment and 30 days following treatment.
- Yearly evaluation of treatment centers to ensure compliance with program.
- Mandatory quarterly reporting of all adverse reactions and mandatory reporting within 15 days of all patient deaths associated with the drug.

Anabolic Steroid Control Act of 2004

On January 20, 2004, the act amended the Controlled Substances Act and replaced the existing definition of "anabolic steroid" with a new definition. The new definition altered the basis for all future administrative scheduling actions relating to the control of anabolic steroids as Schedule III medications by eliminating the requirement to prove muscle growth. This act increased the number of anabolic steroids to 59 substances. The amendment provided the requirements for handling substances as defined as anabolic steroids to include registration, security, labeling and packaging, inventory, record maintenance, prescriptions, disposal, importations and exportation, and criminal liability.

Medicaid Tamper Resistant Prescription Pad Law

As of April 1, 2008, physicians are required to adhere to the requirements of the Medicaid Tamper Resistant Prescription Pad Law. This piece of legislation applies to all handwritten prescriptions for covered outpatient drugs; drugs that are transmitted from the prescriber to the pharmacy verbally, by fax, or through e-prescribing are not impacted by the legislation. The law applies whenever Medicaid pays any portion of the cost of a prescription.

According to the act, a tamper-resistant prescription pad must contain at least one of three characteristics:

- One or more industry-recognized features designed to prevent unauthorized copying of a completed or blank prescription form
- One or more industry-recognized features designed to prevent the erasure or modification of information written on the prescription pad by the prescriber.
- One or more industry-recognized features designed to prevent the use of counterfeit prescription forms.

By October 1, 2008, a prescription pad must contain all three of the above characteristics to be considered tamper resistant. These regulations do not apply to any prescriptions presented to the pharmacy prior to April 1, 2008. If a pharmacy receives a prescription and there are questions whether the prescription meets the requirements of this act, the pharmacy staff may contact the prescriber's office for verification. The pharmacy may accept a faxed prescription from the physician's office until it has obtained tamper-resistant prescription pads.

A pharmacy may fill the prescription as an emergency prescription as long as it receives documentation from the prescriber's office within 72 hours. A prescription may be transferred from the original pharmacy to another pharmacy via a fax or telephone call. The second pharmacy does not need direct confirmation of the original prescription from the physician.

Tech Check

24. What Medicare part covers prescription medications purchased in a retail pharmacy?(LO 4.3h)

25. Which legislation allowed patients with specific diseases access to investigational medications?(LO 4.3e)

26. What did USP <797> set the first enforceable standards for?(LO 4.3h)

27. How many particles are permitted in 1 cubic foot to be considered an ISO Class 5?(LO 4.3h)

28. What conditions must be met for isotretinoin to be dispensed?(LO 4.3i)

29. How many refills are permitted on a prescription for isotretinoin?(LO 4.3i)

Regulatory Agencies(LO 4.8a, b, 4.9)

The Food and Drug Administration (FDA)

In 1938 the Food and Drug Administration (FDA) was formed to enforce the Food, Drug and Cosmetic Act of 1938. The FDA is responsible for protecting the public health by ensuring the safety, efficacy, and security of human and veterinary drugs, biological products, medical devices, our nation's food supply, cosmetics, and products that emit radiation. The FDA is also responsible for advancing the public health by helping speed innovations that make medicines and foods more effective, safer, and more affordable. The FDA also helps the public get the accurate, science-based information it needs to use medicines and foods to improve health.

Some of the agency's specific responsibilities include:

Biologics

- Product and manufacturing establishment licensing
- Safety of the nation's blood supply
- Research to establish product standards and develop improved testing methods

Cosmetics

- Safety
- Labeling

Drugs

- Product approvals
- OTC and prescription drug labeling
- Drug manufacturing standards

Foods

- Labeling
- Safety of all food products (except meat and poultry)
- Bottled water

Medical devices

- Premarket approval of new devices
- Manufacturing and performance standards
- Tracking reports of device malfunctioning and serious adverse reactions

Radiation-emitting electronic products

- Radiation safety performance standards for microwave ovens, television receivers, diagnostic x-ray equipment, cabinet x-ray systems (such as baggage x-rays at airports), laser products, ultrasonic therapy equipment, mercury vapor lamps, and sunlamps
- Accrediting and inspecting mammography facilities

Veterinary products

- Livestock feeds
- Pet foods
- Veterinary drugs and devices

Clinical Drug Studies

The FDA's goal of ensuring that all medications are safe and effective is accomplished through clinical studies. A clinical study is a research study using human beings to find treatments that work in people and new ways to improve their health. There are many different types of clinical trials, including those to study prevention options, new treatments or new ways to treat existing treatments, new screening and diagnostic techniques, and options for improving the quality of life for people who have serious medical conditions. A clinical study is conducted according to a plan called a protocol. A protocol describes what types of patients may enter the study, schedules of tests and procedures, drugs, dosages, and length of study, as well as the outcomes that will be measured.

Clinical trials may compare existing treatments to determine which is better. The current approved treatments are called the "standard treatments." Sometimes clinical trials are used to study different ways to use the standard treatments so they will be more effective, easier to use, and/or decrease side effects. A clinical study may be conducted to determine the best way to treat a specific population, which was not used in a previous clinical trial. Within recent years, drug manufacturers have been conducting an increased number of studies on the use of their medication on the pediatric population.

Monographs

A drug monograph is a component of a drug product label. The FDA-approved label is the official description of a drug product and includes indication (use of the drug); who should take it; adverse events (side effects); instructions for uses in pregnancy, children, and other population; as well as safety information for the patient. These labels are often found inside the drug packaging or attached to it. Information contained in a drug monograph includes:

- Description of a drug
- Clinical pharmacology
- Indications (uses for the drug)
- Contraindications (who should not take the drug)
- Warnings
- Precautions
- Adverse events (side effects)
- Drug abuse and dependence
- Dosage and administration
- Use in pregnancy; use in nursing mothers
- How the drug is supplied
- Safety information for the patient

Patient Package Inserts (PPIs)

A Product Package Insert (PPI) contains information for patients' understanding on how to safely use a drug product. The PPI is another example of a drug's labeling and therefore is regulated by the FDA. The FDA requires that a patient receive a PPI each time he or she receives specific medications. These products include hormones (estrogen, progesterone, and estrogen/progesterone combination products) and isotretinoin.

Good Manufacturing Practices (GMPs)

The Food, Drug and Cosmetic Act of 1938 established requirements that Good Manufacturing Practices (GMPs) are used in the practice of pharmacy. Good Manufacturing Practices consists of

- Obtaining information on GMP requirements
- Determining the appropriate quality system needed to control design, production, and distribution of the proposed device
- Designing products and processes
- Training employees

- Acquiring adequate facilities
- Purchasing and installing processing equipment
- Drafting the device master record
- Noting how to change the device master records
- Procuring components and materials
- Producing devices
- Labeling devices
- Evaluating finished devices
- Packaging devices
- Distributing devices
- Processing complaints and analyzing service and data repair
- Servicing devices
- Auditing and correcting deficiencies in the quality system
- Preparing for an FDA inspection

As one can see these practices are found in every step of the drug manufacturing process.

The FDA oversees the quality of drug products by reviewing the information submitted in applications as well as inspecting the physical facilities for adherence to requirements found under current Good Manufacturing Practices (GMPs). Good Manufacturing Practices consist of the following:

- Up-to-date concepts of risk management and quality system approaches are combined while continuing to ensure product quality.
- The latest scientific advances in pharmaceutical manufacturing and technology are used.
- Submission review program and the inspection program operate in a coordinated manner
- Regulation and manufacturing standards are applied consistently.
- Program management encourages innovation in pharmaceutical manufacturing.
- FDA resources are used both effectively and efficiently.

Within the past two decades numerous changes have occurred within the world of pharmacy, especially in pharmaceutical manufacturing. These changes include:

- Increased number of pharmaceutical products and a larger role of medicines in health care
- Decreased frequency of FDA manufacturing inspections due to a lower number of resources allocated for pharmaceutical manufacturing inspections
- FDA's gathering of experience with, and lessons learned from, various approaches to the regulation of product quality
- Advances in the pharmaceutical sciences and manufacturing technologies
- Application of biotechnology in drug discovery and manufacturing
- Advances in the science and management of quality
- Globalization of the pharmaceutical industry

Good Manufacturing Processes are extremely important to ensure that all drug products and medical devices are safe for the public.

The FDA works in conjunction with many other government regulatory agencies in areas related to the FDA. The Federal Trade Commission

(FTC) regulates all advertising excluding prescription drugs and medical devices. It is the FTC's responsibility to ensure that all advertising involving OTC medications is truthful and not misleading. The Bureau of Alcohol, Tobacco, Firearms and Explosives (ATF) is responsible for the labeling of alcohol and the amounts a hospital is able to purchase during a year. All questions regarding the reimbursement by either Medicaid or Medicare are addressed by the CMS.

Drug Enforcement Administration (DEA)

The Drug Enforcement Administration (DEA), www.justice.gov/dea/agency/mission.htm, mission statement reads as follows: The mission of the **Drug Enforcement Administration (DEA)** is to enforce the controlled substances laws and regulations of the United States. The DEA also brings to the U.S. criminal and civil justice system organizations and principal members of organizations involved in the growing, manufacture, or distribution of controlled substances appearing in or destined for illicit traffic in the United States. In addition, the agency recommends and supports nonenforcement programs aimed at reducing the availability of illicit controlled substances on the domestic and international markets.

In carrying out its mission as the agency responsible for enforcing the controlled substances laws and regulations of the United States, the DEA's primary responsibilities include:

- Investigation and preparation for the prosecution of major violators of controlled substance laws operating at interstate and international levels.
- Investigation and preparation for prosecution of criminals and drug gangs who perpetrate violence in our communities and terrorize citizens through fear and intimidation.
- Management of a national drug intelligence program in cooperation with federal, state, local, and foreign officials to collect, analyze, and disseminate strategic and operational drug intelligence information.
- Seizure and forfeiture of assets derived from, traceable to, or intended to be used for illicit drug trafficking.
- Enforcement of the provisions of the Controlled Substances Act as they pertain to the manufacture, distribution, and dispensing of legally produced controlled substances.
- Coordination and cooperation with federal, state, and local law enforcement officials on mutual drug enforcement efforts and enhancement of such efforts through exploitation of potential interstate and international investigations beyond local or limited federal jurisdictions and resources.
- Coordination and cooperation with federal, state, and local agencies, and with foreign governments, in programs designed to reduce the availability of illicit abuse-type drugs on the U.S. market through nonenforcement methods such as crop eradication, crop substitution, and training of foreign officials.
- Responsibility, under the policy guidance of the secretary of state and U.S. ambassadors, for all programs associated with drug law enforcement counterparts in foreign countries.

Drug Enforcement Administration (DEA) An agency of the Department of Justice whose mission is to enforce the controlled substance laws and regulations of the United States.

- Liaison with the United Nations, Interpol, and other organizations on matters relating to international drug control programs.
- Establishment of the quantities of specific controlled substances that can be manufactured during a year.

Occupational Safety and Health Administration (OSHA)

OSHA's mission is to ensure the safety and health of America's workers by setting and enforcing standards; providing training, outreach, and education; establishing partnerships; and encouraging continual improvement in workplace safety and health.

In pharmacy practice, OSHA has issued policies on hazard communication standards, hazardous drugs preparation, handling practices, hazardous drugs administration, hazardous drugs caregiving, disposal of hazardous drugs, storage of hazardous drugs, latex allergy, ergonomics, and workplace violence.

The Joint Commission (TJC) (formerly Joint Commission on Accreditation of Healthcare Organizations—JCAHO)

The major goal of The Joint Commission (TJC; formerly Joint Commission on Accreditation of Healthcare Organizations—JCAHO) is to improve the safety and quality of care provided to the public through the provision of health care accreditation and related services that support performance improvement in health care organizations.

TJC evaluates and accredits nearly 15,000 health care organizations and programs in the United States. An independent, not-for-profit organization, TJC is the nation's predominant standards-setting and accrediting body in health care. Since 1951, TJC has maintained state-of-the-art standards that focus on improving the quality and safety of care provided by health care organizations. TJC's comprehensive accreditation process evaluates an organization's compliance with these standards and other accreditation requirements. TJC accreditation is recognized nationwide as a symbol of quality that reflects an organization's commitment to meeting certain performance standards. To earn and maintain TJC's Gold Seal of Approval, an organization must undergo an onsite survey by a TJC survey team at least every 3 years laboratories must be surveyed every 2 years.)

TJC provides evaluation and accreditation services for the following types of organizations:

- General, psychiatric, children's, and rehabilitation hospitals
- Critical access hospitals
- Medical equipment services, hospice services, and other home care organizations
- Nursing homes and other long-term care facilities
- Behavioral health care organizations, addiction services
- Rehabilitation centers, group practices, office-based surgeries, and other ambulatory care providers
- Independent or freestanding laboratories

Table 4-2 Do Not Use List

Applies to all orders and all medication-related documentation that is handwritten (including free-text computer entry) or on preprinted forms.

Do Not Use	Potential Problem	Use Instead
U (unit)	Mistaken for "0" (zero), the number "4" (four) or "cc"	Write "unit"
IU (International Unit)	Mistaken for IV (intravenous) or the number 10 (ten)	Write "International Unit"
Q.D., QD, q.d., qd (daily) Q.O.D., QOD, q.o.d, qod (every other day)	Mistaken for each other Period after the Q mistaken for "I" and the "O" mistaken for "I"	Write "daily" Write "every other day"
Trailing zero (X.0 mg)* Lack of leading zero (.X mg)	Decimal point is missed	Write "X mg" Write "0.X mg"
MS MSO_4 and $MgSO_4$	Can mean morphine sulfate or magnesium sulfate Confused for one another	Write "morphine sulfate" Write "magnesium sulfate"
Additional Abbreviations, Acronyms, and Symbols (For Possible Future Inclusion in the Official "Do Not Use" List)		
Do Not Use	**Potential Problem**	**Use Instead**
> (greater than) < (less than)	Misinterpreted as the number "7" (seven) or the letter "L" Confused for one another	Write "greater than" Write "less than"
Abbreviations for drug names	Misinterpreted due to similar abbreviations for multiple drugs	Write drug names in full
Apothecary units	Unfamiliar to many practitioners Confused with metric units	Use metric units
@	Mistaken for the number "2" (two)	Write "at"
cc	Mistaken for U (units) when poorly written	Write "mL" or "milliliters"
µg	Mistaken for mg (milligrams) resulting in 1000-fold overdose	Write "mcg" or "micrograms"

**Exception: A "trailing zero" may be used only where required to demonstrate the level of precision of the value being reported, such as for laboratory results, imaging studies that report size of lesions or catheter/tube sizes. It may not be used in medication orders or other medication-related documentation.*

Source: **www.jointcommission.org, Copyright The Joint Commission, 2009, Reprinted with permission.**

As a result of the large number of prescription errors due to misinterpreting pharmacy abbreviations, TJC issued in May 2005 its official "Do Not Use List," which appears in Table 4-2. TJC has addressed the following issues affecting the practice of pharmacy: medication errors, locked medication cabinets, bar coding, and the IV admixture room.

State Boards of Pharmacy

Each state has a board of pharmacy that oversees pharmacy practice within that state. The board has the authority to determine the conditions for licensure of pharmacists, establish processes to investigate and discipline pharmacists, and set the conditions for pharmacy technicians to practice in the state. The composition of pharmacy boards and their members' terms is determined by the state.

National Association of Boards of Pharmacy (NABP)

The National Association of Boards of Pharmacy is composed of each state board of pharmacy. The NABP examines issues affecting pharmacy practice. However, it does not possess any regulatory authority.

Tech Check

30. What are the seven categories of products that the FDA oversees?(LO 4.8a)

31. Identify a medication for which a PPI must be given to a patient.(LO 4.8a)

32. Why are Good Manufacturing Practices important?(LO 4.8a)

Chapter Summary

Understanding the importance of laws, ethics, and regulatory agencies in the workplace, and their impact on the pharmacy practice, is vital to the pharmacy technician.

- Ethics are a moral philosophy of right versus wrong.
- The practice of pharmacy for both pharmacists and pharmacy technicians is guided by a code of ethics.
- There are many different types of laws: federal, state, criminal, and civil.
- Laws are established to protect society and likewise many different laws have been enacted in the pharmacy profession.
- In many situations, the enactment of pharmacy laws occurred after some tragedy involving medications in the United States took place.
- Every pharmacy technician needs to be familiar with federal and state laws affecting pharmacy practice.
- A pharmacy technician's failure to adhere to pharmacy laws may result in fines (both civil and criminal), suspension of the right to practice as a pharmacy technician, or even imprisonment.
- There are many different agencies, both federal and state, that oversee various aspects of pharmacy practice.

Chapter Review

Case Study Question

1. Is it good customer service to inform the patient of his daughter's prescription? Why or why not?(LO 4.2, 4.3g)

At Your Service Questions

1. Did the pharmacy technician handle the situation correctly?(LO 4.3c)
2. Why is this medication a controlled substance?(LO 4.3c)

Multiple Choice

Select the best answer.

1. Which of the following would be an example of adulteration?(LO 4.3a)
   a. Compounding a medication in a filthy environment
   b. Dispensing a medication without a label on the container
   c. Dispensing medications without a prescription
   d. All of the above

2. Which of the following would be an example of misbranding?(LO 4.3a)
   a. Dispensing a harmful medication to a patient
   b. Dispensing a medication without appropriate directions
   c. Failing to maintain a patient's information confidential
   d. All of the above

3. Which of the following is the federal legend that was required on prescriptions under the Durham-Humphrey Amendment?(LO 4.3b)
   a. Federal law prohibits the dispensing of this medication without a prescription
   b. Federal law prohibits the dispensing of this medication to anyone other than the intended individual
   c. Federal law prohibits the dispensing of this medication to any animal without a prescription from a veterinarian
   d. May be habit forming

4. Which amendment required that all medications be pure, safe, and effective?(LO 4.3b)
   a. Pure Food and Drug Act of 1906
   b. Food, Drug and Cosmetic Act of 1938
   c. Durham-Humphrey Amendment
   d. Kefauver-Harris Amendment

5. How many schedules are defined under the Controlled Substance Act of 1970?(LO 4.3c)
   a. Two
   b. Three
   c. Four
   d. Five

6. Which schedule of medication does *not* have a medical use in the United States and has the highest potential for abuse?(LO 4.3c)
   a. Schedule I
   b. Schedule II
   c. Schedule III
   d. Schedule IV

7. What is the minimum amount of time for controlled substance records to be retained according to federal law?(LO 4.3c)
   a. 6 months
   b. 1 year
   c. 2 years
   d. 7 years

8. How many times may a prescription for a controlled substance be transferred to another pharmacy?(LO 4.3c)
   a. One time
   b. Two times
   c. Three times
   d. Four times

9. Within what time period must a prescription for a Schedule IV medication be filled?(LO 4.3c)
   a. 1 week
   b. 1 month
   c. 6 months
   d. 1 year

10. What type of inventory must be taken every 2 years in a pharmacy?(LO 4.5)
    a. Biannual
    b. Biennial
    c. Initial
    d. Perpetual

11. What is the maximum number of refills a physician can authorize on a Schedule III medication?(LO 4.3c)
    a. One
    b. Two
    c. Five
    d. Twelve

12. Which of the following could *not* be a correct DEA number for Dr. Carolyn Adams?(LO 4.3c)
    a. AA1234563
    b. BA1234563
    c. CA1234563
    d. FA1234563

13. Which of the following medications does *not* need to be packaged in a child-resistant container because of the Poison Prevention Packaging Act of 1970?(LO 4.3c)
    a. Amoxicillin 250 mg/5 mL
    b. Cephalexin 500-mg capsules

c. Meperidine 50-mg tablets
d. Nitroglycerin

14. Which of the following is *not* a component of an NDC number?(LO 4.3d)
    a. Drug manufacturer
    b. Drug packaging
    c. Drug product
    d. Lot number

15. Which federal agency is responsible for ensuring that all drugs are pure, safe, and effective?(LO 4.8a)
    a. DEA
    b. FDA
    c. EPA
    d. ISMP

16. Which of the following is *not* a requirement of OBRA-90?(LO 4.3f)
    a. A drug utilization evaluation must be performed on each prescription
    b. A patient's information must be maintained confidential
    c. An offer to counsel a patient must be made
    d. Patient profiles must be maintained for all patients

17. Which pharmacy law protects a patient's private health information?(LO 4.3g)
    a. Pharmacy code of ethics
    b. OBRA-87
    c. OBRA-90
    d. HIPAA

18. Which of the following laws provided for prescription benefits to be paid to a retail pharmacy for Medicare patients?(LO 4.3h)
    a. CSA
    b. FDCA 1938
    c. PPPA
    d. MMA

19. Which right is *not* protected under HIPAA?(LO 4.3g)
    a. A right to access his or her information
    b. A right to seek details of the disclosure of his or her PHI
    c. A right to review a pharmacy's policies and procedures regarding PHI
    d. A right to review a pharmacy's pricing structure to ensure receiving the lowest possible price

20. How old must a person be to purchase an exempt narcotic?(LO 4.3c)
    a. 14 years of age
    b. 16 years of age
    c. 18 years of age
    d. There is no minimum age

Acronyms

Print the meaning of the following acronyms.

DEA ____________________
EPA ____________________
FDA ____________________
HIPAA ____________________
ISMP ____________________
NABP ____________________
OSHA ____________________
OTC ____________________
PHI ____________________
PPI ____________________
TJC ____________________

Critical Thinking Questions

1. Why should an individual be able to reimport prescriptions from Canada or another country into the United States?(LO 4.3e)

2. Identify medications that have gone from prescription status to OTC status within the past year.(LO 4.8)

HIPAA Scenario

Tommy, a 15-year-old Austin, Texas, high school student, is being treated for a sexually transmitted disease (STD). He is embarrassed and does not want his parents to know that he came to the hospital for care. When he comes to the pharmacy to pick up his antibiotic, he asks if you have to inform his parents about the reason for his visit. When he is told that it is not required that his parents be notified, he asks if any information will be given to his parents if they initiate questioning about the care he received today.

Discussion Questions(PTCB II. 73)

1. Is the pharmacy allowed to inform Tommy's parents about his treatment for an STD?
2. What is the law in your state for informing parents and guardians of the treatment of minors for STDs?

Internet Activities

1. Visit **www.fda.gov** and identify all medications that have been recalled in the past 3 months and the reason for the recall.(LO 4.8a)
2. Visit **www.jointcommission.org** and identify the standards affecting the practice of pharmacy.(LO 4.8b)
3. Visit the Web site of your state board of pharmacy and be prepared to discuss the content of that Web site with your classmates.(LO 4.9)

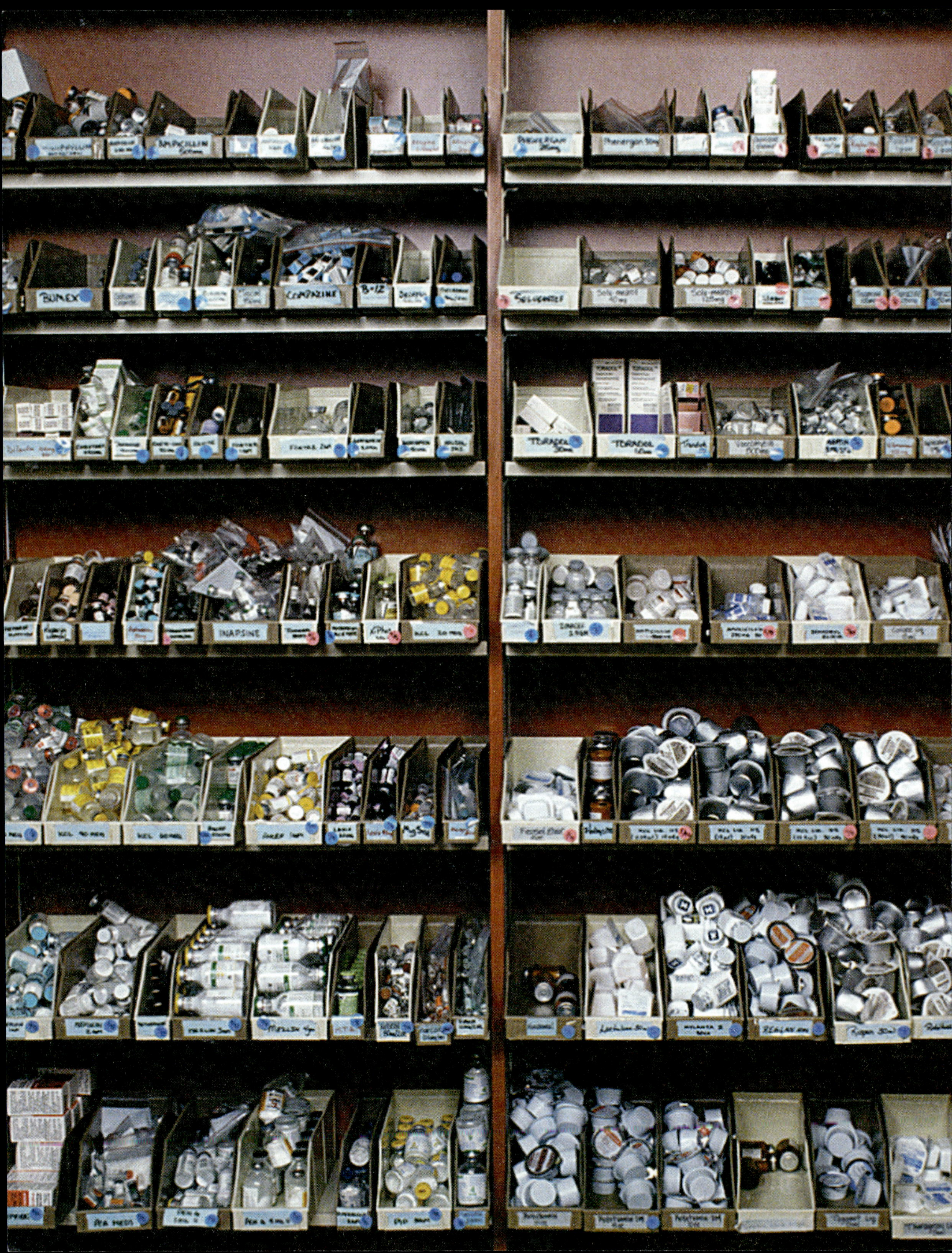
BUMEX
COMPAZINE
INAPSINE
TORADOL

Unit 2

Pharmacology and Medications

Chapter 5 Measurements and Calculations

Chapter 6 Introduction to Pharmacology

Chapter 7 Drug Classifications

Chapter 8 Over-the-Counter (OTC) Agents

Chapter 9 Complementary and Alternative Modalities

5 Measurements and Calculations

Key Terms

alligation
Arabic numbers
Clark's Rule
conversion factor
denominator
desired dose
diluent
dilution
dosage ordered
flow rate
international time (military time)
nomogram
numerator
percent
proportion
ratio
Roman numerals
Young's Rule

Learning Outcomes

Upon completion of this chapter, you will be able to:

5.1 Convert Roman numerals to the equivalent Arabic number.

5.2 Multiply and divide fractions.

5.3 Convert fractions to decimals, ratios, and percents.

5.4 Convert numbers to percents.

5.5 Distinguish between the various metric prefixes used in the practice of pharmacy.

5.6 Convert units between the metric, apothecary, avoirdupois, and household systems.

5.7 Convert temperatures between Celsius and Fahrenheit.

5.8 Convert time between the 12-hour and 24-hour clocks.

5.9 Interpret a written drug order.

5.10 Calculate the day's supply of a medication prescribed by a physician.

5.11 Identify on a drug label the drug name, form, dosage strength, route, manufacturer, and storage information.

5.12 Indicate the appropriate equipment for measuring the appropriate quantity of solids and liquids in the practice of pharmacy.

5.13 Convert the dosage ordered to the desired dose.

5.14 Convert the desired dose to the amount to administer.

5.15 Calculate the appropriate dose for a patient based upon age, weight, or body surface area.

5.16 Calculate the amount of drug of a given concentration to prepare a prescription yielding different concentrations.

5.17 Calculate the ending concentration of a preparation after diluting it with a diluent.

5.18 Calculate the correct quantities to be used in preparing a solution or semisolid using alligation.

5.19 Calculate the flow rate of an intravenous fluid.

5.20 Calculate the correct drop factor to be used for an intravenous infusion.

5.21 Calculate the number of drops per minute a patient will receive when given the flow rate and drop factor.

5.22 Explain the importance of calculations in the practice of pharmacy.

5.23 Demonstrate an understanding and application of proportions in pharmacy calculations.

5.24 Use dimensional analysis in performing pharmacy calculations.

5.25 Demonstrate an understanding of the application of international units and milliequivalents in pharmacy.

5.26 Interpret a prescription or medication order.

5.27 Reduce or enlarge a formula to meet the requirements of either a prescription or medication order.

5.28 Demonstrate an understanding of specific gravity and its application in compounding a product.

PTCB

In preparation for the certification examination, you should understand and perform activities associated with the following PTCB Knowledge Statement:

PTCB Knowledge Statement	*Domain I. Assisting the Pharmacist in Serving Patients*
	Knowledge of pharmaceutical and medical abbreviations and terminology (4)
	Knowledge of generic and brand names of pharmaceuticals (5)
	Knowledge of pharmacy calculations (50)
	Knowledge of measurement systems (51)

Case Study

You are filling a drug order that calls for 3.5 g of a medication. The medication comes in an oral suspension containing 100 mg of medication per 5 mL.

While reading this chapter, keep the following questions in mind.

1. How many milligrams of the medication does the order call for?(LO 5.6)
2. How many milliliters of the oral suspension would the patient need to take for each dose?(LO 5.6)
3. How many teaspoons of the oral suspension would the patient need to take for each dose?(LO 5.6)
4. Is the dosage ordered reasonable?(LO 5.6)

Introduction to Measurements and Calculations(LO 5.22)

The practice of pharmacy involves the preparation and dispensing of medication to the patient. It is the responsibility of the pharmacist to ensure that all pharmacy calculations are correct in preparing a patient's medication. The pharmacist must check all calculations the pharmacy technicians perform. Some of the areas involving pharmacy calculations include interpreting a prescription or medication order from a physician, compounding extemporaneous medications and IV admixtures, and calculating the correct dosage for a patient based upon age, weight, or body surface area and dispensing the correct quantity to the patient based on the physician's prescription and the insurance provider's requirements.

Although the pharmacy staff members do not administer medications to patients, their calculations must be correct for the nursing staff to accurately administer medications. "The Patient's Five Rights of Medication," which have been established by the Institute of Safe Medication Practice include:

1. Right patient
2. Right medication
3. Right strength/dose
4. Right route
5. Right time/frequency

In this chapter, you will focus on the right strength/dose (Right 3). You will learn the skills and techniques needed to accurately determine the correct strength and dose of a medication to be administered. These calculations will require you to use basic math skills and to be able to convert between commonly used measurement systems. As with most of the skills needed by a pharmacy technician, pharmaceutical calculations require that you pay attention to detail to ensure accuracy. Fortunately, learning a few basic skills will allow you to perform calculations accurately.

At Your Service

Mary Lock arrived at the pharmacy to pick up a prescription for her 3-year-old son, Brandon. The pharmacy technician looked for the completed prescription but could not find it with the others. The technician looked at the patient's profile to determine if a prescription had been filled for Brandon. She saw that a prescription for amoxicillin 250 mg/5 mL suspension had been ordered yesterday and it was waiting to be reconstituted.

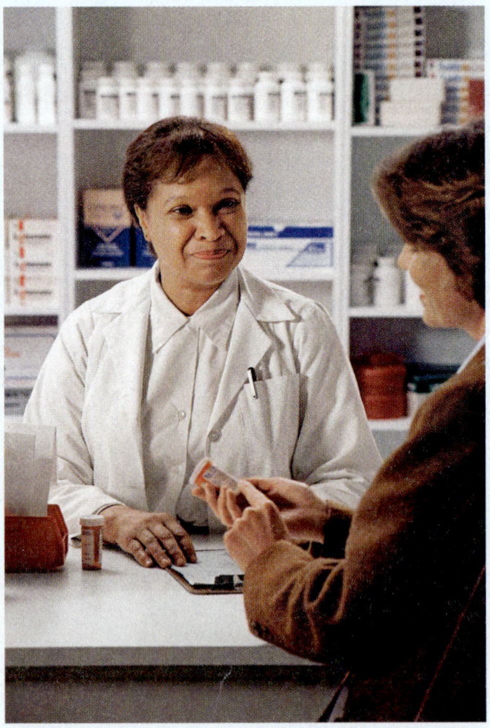

The pharmacy technician measured out the appropriate amount of distilled water, 88 mL, and showed it to the pharmacist before reconstituting it. She took the completed prescription order to Mary Lock and asked her if she had any questions for the pharmacist. Mary wanted to know if the dose was correct for Brandon based on his age and weight (45 pounds). Second, Mary asked why the prescription label said to take 1 teaspoon by mouth three times a day when the doctor had told her to give Brandon 5 milliliters of the medication three times a day.

While reading this chapter, keep the following questions in mind.

1. Was the dose appropriate for Brandon?(LO 5.15)
2. Was the amount of water added to the powder correct for the desired dose?(LO 5.16)
3. How would you explain to Mary the relationship between milliliters and teaspoons?(LO 5.6)

Numbering Systems (LO 5.1)

Two different numbering systems are used in pharmacy practice today, **Roman numerals** and **Arabic numbers**. A number is a total quantity, or amount of units. A numeral is a word or sign, or a group of words or signs, expressing a number. One must be able to translate Roman numerals into Arabic numbers before performing calculations and dispensing a medication.

Arabic Numbers

The Arabic system of numbers is a decimal system. It consists of 10 digits—zero through nine (0, 1, 2, 3, 4, 5, 6, 7, 8, and 9). The Arabic system is the most commonly used system in the practice of pharmacy.

Roman Numerals

In the Roman numeral system, letters are used to represent numerical values. Roman numerals are written as combinations of these letters, and can be written in either uppercase or lowercase letters. The building blocks of the Roman system are the letters I, V, X, L, C, D, and M. Only I, V, and X (which are equal to the Arabic numbers 1, 5, and 10) are needed to represent values from 1 through 30, which are the more commonly used Roman numerals today. Roman numerals are sometimes used when a prescriber writes quantities on a prescription or medication order (*See* Table 5-1).

In order to interpret a Roman numeral and translate it to the Arabic equivalent, you will need to follow the guidelines in the Caution box, "Interpreting Roman Numerals."

Table 5-1 Converting Roman Numerals

Roman Numeral*	Arabic Number	Roman Numeral	Arabic Number	Roman Numeral	Arabic Number
SS, $\overline{ss}$	$\frac{1}{2}$				
I, i	1	XI, xi	11	XXI, xxi	21
II, ii	2	XII, xii	12	XXII, xxii	22
III, iii	3	XIII, xiii	13	XXIII, xxiii	23
IV, iv	4	XIV, xiv	14	XXIV, xxiv	24
V, v	5	XV, xv	15	XXV, xxv	25
VI, vi	6	XVI, xvi	16	XXVI, xxvi	26
VII, vii	7	XVII, xvii	17	XXVII, xxvii	27
VIII, viii	8	XVIII, xviii	18	XXVIII, xxviii	28
IX, ix	9	XIX, xix	19	XXIX, xxix	29
X, x	10	XX, xx	20	XXX, xxx	30

*Roman numerals written with small letters are also correctly written with a line over the top; for example, iv and $\overline{iv}$ are both correct.

Arabic numbers The commonly used system of writing numbers using the 10 digits from zero through nine.

Roman numerals A system that uses the letters I, V, X, L, C, D, and M to represent numbers.

Caution

Interpreting Roman Numerals must be done carefully. Follow these guidelines:

- If a numeral appears twice in a row, count its value twice. If it appears three times in a row, count its value three times. (A Roman numeral should never be used more than three times in a row.)(LO 5.1)
- When a Roman numeral comes *between* two numerals with larger values, subtract the smaller numeral from the one to its right, then add the remaining values.(LO 5.1)
- If a numeral with a smaller value follows a numeral with a larger value, add their values.(LO 5.1)
- If a numeral with a larger value follows a numeral with a smaller value, subtract the smaller value from the larger one.(LO 5.1)

EXAMPLE

In the Roman numeral viii, the letter "i" appears three times in a row for a total value of three. This value is to be added to the value of five, represented by the letter "v," which gives us the Arabic value of eight. In the Roman numeral XIV, a smaller value (I) falls between two larger ones (X and V). Subtracting it from the value to its right leaves us with a value of four, which is then added to the remaining value (X), giving us an Arabic equivalent of 14.

Tech Check

Write the Arabic expression for the following Roman numerals:(LO 5.1)

1. I = _______

2. X = _______

3. XXX = _______

4. L = _______

5. C = _______

6. IV = _______

7. XX = _______

8. XL = _______

9. LX = _______

Mathematical Concepts(LO 5.2, 5.3, 5.4, 5.23, 5.24)

Fractions

numerator The value written in the top part of a fraction.

denominator The value written in the bottom part of a fraction.

A fraction consists of two parts—the **numerator,** which is the value on the top of the fraction, and represents parts of a whole. The **denominator,** which is the value in the bottom of the fraction, represents the whole. The denominator of a fraction can never have a value of zero. There are two

Table 5-2 Divisibility Tests of a Number

A number is divisible by	
2	if it ends in a 0, 2, 4, 6, or 8
3	if the sum of its digits is divisible by 3
4	if the last two digits make a number that is divisible by 4
5	if it ends in 0 or 5
6	if it is divisible by both 2 and 3
7	the number 7 has no simple test
8	if the last three digits make a number that is divisible by 8
9	if the sum of its digits is divisible by 9
10	if it ends in a zero

types of fractions: proper and improper fractions. A proper fraction is a fraction, where the numerator is less than the denominator. A proper fraction should always be reduced to its lowest terms, which means both the numerator and denominator do not have any common factors other than one. It is important to know if a number is divisible by another number to reduce a proper fraction to its lowest terms (refer to Table 5-2 for divisibility tests of a number).

An improper fraction is one where the numerator is greater than the denominator and should be converted to a mixed number.

In performing pharmacy calculations, it is important that a pharmacy technician is able to multiply and divide fractions. To multiply two fractions, simply multiply the numerators and then multiply the denominators. The answer should be reduced to lowest terms.

In order to multiply 2/3 by 3/5, first multiply the numerators ($2 \times 3 = 6$), and then multiply the denominators ($3 \times 5 = 15$). Therefore, $2/3 \times 4/5 = 6/15$, which both the numerator and denominator is divisible by 3 and the reduced answer is 2/5.

Division is the inverse operation of multiplication. To divide two fractions, multiply the first fraction by the reciprocal of the second fraction. The reciprocal is the fraction inverted or flipped upside down. The reciprocal of 2/3 is 3/2. The answer should be reduced to lowest terms.

EXAMPLES

In order to divide 1/4 by 2/3, first find the reciprocal of the second fraction (2/3), which is 3/2. Now multiply the two fractions together by multiplying the numerators (1×3) and then multiply the denominators (4×2). Therefore $1/4 \ / \ 2/3 = 3/8$.

Converting Fractions to Decimals

Because they are easier to enter into a calculator, decimals are often easier to work with than are fractions. In order to convert a fraction into a decimal, divide the numerator by the denominator.

EXAMPLE

To convert the fraction 5/8 into a decimal, you would divide the numerator (5) by the denominator (8): $5 \div 8 = 0.625$.

Converting a Number to a Percent

When converting a number to a percent, multiply the number by 100, and then add a percent sign to the resulting value. If the original value is a fraction, you should first convert it to a decimal.

EXAMPLE

To convert 3/5 to a percent, first convert it to a decimal ($3 \div 5 = 0.6$). Multiple the answer by 100 ($0.6 \times 100 = 60$), then add a percent sign to the answer (3/5 = 60%).

Ratio

A **ratio** compares two different numbers and is written in this format: a:b. This expression is read "a is to b." A ratio may be converted to a fraction by writing the first number in the ratio as the numerator and the second number in the ratio as the denominator. The ratio 1:2 could be converted to a fraction that would be expressed as 1/2. A ratio written as a fraction should always be reduced to lowest terms. In pharmacy practice a ratio may be used to express the strength of a substance.

Percent (%)

The expression **percent** means "parts per 100." A pharmacy technician looks at a bottle of medication on the pharmacy shelf and it states 10%, which means that it has 10 parts per 100 parts. A fraction can be converted to a percent by dividing the numerator by the denominator and multiplying the answer by 100. Refer to Table 5-3 for an equivalency of common fractions, ratios, decimals, and percents.

In the practice of pharmacy, *percent* is associated with many different dosage forms. The USP has established three different terms associated with the percentage of active ingredients contained within a solvent. These terms are:

- Percent weight-in-weight (w/w %)—the number of grams of solute dissolved in 100 gram of solvent, which can be found in solid and semisolid dosage forms. For instance, a 10% w/w ointment means that 10 gram of solute are contained in 100 gram of solid.
- Percent weight-in-volume (w/v %)—the number of grams of solute dissolved in 100 milliliters of solvent, which is used to describe the concentration of solutions, suspensions, or aerosols. A 0.9% w/v solution of sodium chloride indicates that 0.9 gram of sodium chloride is contained in 100 milliliters of solution (water).
- Percent volume-in-volume (v/v %)—the number of milliliters of solute dissolved in 100 milliliters of solvent, which can be found in a solution where a liquid is dissolved in a liquid. A 70% solution of isopropyl alcohol means that 70 milliliters of isopropyl alcohol are found 100 milliliters of solution.

ratio A comparison of two quantities having the same type of units.

percent Parts per 100.

Table 5-3 Equivalencies of Fractions, Ratios, Decimals, and Percents

Fractions	Ratios	Decimals	Percents
1/1000	1:1000	0.001	0.1%
1/500	1:500	0.002	0.2%
1/100	1:100	0.01	1%
1/50	1:50	0.02	2%
1/40	1:40	0.025	2.5%
1/30	1:30	0.033	3.3%
1/25	1:25	0.04	4%
1/15	1:15	0.067	6.7%
1/10	1:10	0.1	10%
1/9	1:9	0.111	11.1%
1/8	1:8	0.125	12.5%
1/7	1:7	0.143	14.3%
1/6	1:6	0.167	16.7%
1/5	1:5	0.2	20%
1/4	1:4	0.25	25%
1/3	1:3	0.333	33.3%
3/8	3:8	0.375	37.5%
2/5	2:5	0.4	40%
1/2	1:2	0.5	50%
3/5	3:5	0.6	60%
5/8	5:8	0.625	62.5%
2/3	2:3	0.667	66.7%
3/4	3:4	0.75	75%
4/5	4:5	0.8	80%
7/8	7:8	0.875	87.5%
8/9	8:9	0.889	88.9%

Proportion

A **proportion** is a comparison of two ratios that are equivalent. One can determine if the two ratios are equivalent through cross multiplication. Consider the example $3/6 = 4/8$. Cross multiply the numerator on the left side of the equation with the denominator on the right side of the equation ($3 \times 8 = 24$). Next, multiply the denominator on the left side of the equation with the numerator on the right side of the equation ($6 \times 4 = 24$). In this situation, the proportion is equivalent. As a pharmacy technician, the majority of your pharmaceutical calculations can be performed using proportions.

proportion An expression demonstrating that two ratios are equivalent.

You must make sure that the units of measurement expressed in the numerator of both sides of the equation are the same. In addition, the units of measurement expressed in the denominator of both sides of the equation must be the same or else they will need to be converted. If they are not, your answer will be incorrect. A discussion on conversion occurs later in the chapter.

Dimensional Analysis

Dimensional analysis (DA) is a calculation method that involves the logical sequencing and placement into an equation of all the arithmetical terms involved in the problem. Quantities and units are placed on one side of the equation in such a manner that all the units cancel out except the unit of measure of the desired answer. In using dimensional analysis, **conversion factors** (ratios of data) are added as necessary and individual terms inverted (to their reciprocals) to permit the cancellation of like units in the numerator(s) and denominator(s), leaving only the desired term(s) of the answer. An advantage of using dimensional analysis is the consolidation of multiple arithmetical steps to a single expression.

conversion factor A fraction made up of two values that are equal to one another but which are expressed in different units of measurement.

When using DA, the unknown value stands alone on one side of an equation. The conversion factor is placed on the other side of the equation, and the number being converted is placed over 1.

EXAMPLE

Consider the following example: How many fluid ounces are in 2 L if 1000 mL are in 1 L and 29.57 mL are in 1 fl oz?

Solution:

$$\frac{1\text{ fl oz}}{29.57\text{ mL}} \times \frac{1000\text{ mL}}{1\text{ L}} \times 2\text{ L} = 67.63\text{ fl oz}$$

Tech Check

10. Multiply the following fractions. When necessary, reduce the answer to lowest terms.(LO 5.2)

a. 2/3 × 1/8

b. 1/5 × 3/8

c. 1/4 × 3/4

11. Convert the following fractions to decimals. When necessary, round your answer to three places.(LO 5.3)

a. 7/8

b. 3/10

c. 2/3

12. Convert the following fractions to percents. When necessary, round the answer to two decimal places.(LO 5.3)

a. 3/16

b. 4/5

c. 1/3

13. Complete the following table.(LO 5.3)

Fraction	Ratio	Decimal	Percent
1/200			
			0.45%
	1:150		
		0.825	
	1:400		
		0.333	
			0.9%
4/5			
	1:2		
		0.0002	

14. What is meant by 25% (w/w)?(LO 5.34, 5.24)

15. How many milliliters of active ingredient are contained in 1000 mL of a 10% (v/v) solution?(LO 5.23, 5.24)

16. How many grams of active ingredient are contained in 1 lb (454 g) of 5% w/w ointment?(LO 5.23, 5.24)

17. How many grams of active ingredient are contained in a 3-mL solution that has an 0.83% (w/v) concentration?(LO 5.23, 5.24)

Pharmacy Units of Measurement(LO 5.5, 5.6, 5.12)

Metric System of Measurement

The metric system is the official system for weights and measures, as stated in the *United States Pharmacopeia* and *National Formulary.* The dosage of a solid or semi-solid drug is usually measured in milligrams and liquid medications are often measured in milliliters. There are times when a pharmacy technician will be required to calculate the correct dosage for patients based upon their weight; the dosage will be based upon milligrams of drug per kilogram of patient weight. The basic units of measurement in the metric system include the gram (g; for weight or mass), liter (L; for volume), and meter (m; for distance). The metric system uses prefixes based on multiples of 10 (refer to Table 5-4). As a pharmacy technician, it is

Table 5-4 Metric Prefixes

	Kilo-	Hecto-	Deka-	Base	Deci-	Centi-	Milli-	Micro-
Meaning	× 1000	× 100	× 10		/10	/100	/1000	/1000000
Abbreviation	k	h	da		d	c	m	mc
Weight	**kg**	hg	dag	g	dg	cg	**mg**	**mcg**
Volume	kL	hL	daL	L	dL	cL	**mL**	mcL
Length	km	hm	dam	m	dm	**cm**	mm	mcm

**Note:* Bold faced terms are more commonly used in pharmacy practice.

extremely important to know how to convert from a larger unit to a smaller unit and vice versa. When going from a larger unit to a smaller unit, you will multiply in multiples of 10 and going from a smaller unit to a larger unit, you will divide in multiples of 10.

EXAMPLE

Convert 15 g to milligrams

First, a gram (g) is larger than an milligram (mg). There are 1000 mg in 1 g. You may use a proportion in solving this problem:

$$\frac{1\text{ g}}{1000\text{ mg}} = \frac{15\text{ g}}{X\text{ mg}}$$

Cross multiply (1 g × X mg) and (1000 mg × 15 g):

$$(1\text{ g} \times X\text{ mg}) = (1000\text{ mg} \times 15\text{ g})$$

Divide both sides of the equation by 1 g to get the unknown number of mg:

$$\frac{(1\text{ g} \times X\text{ mg})}{1\text{ g}} = \frac{(1000\text{ mg} \times 15\text{ g})}{1\text{ g}}$$

$$\text{X} = 15{,}000\text{ mg}$$

Apothecary System of Measurement

The apothecary system of measurement is the traditional system of measuring and weighing ingredients in the practice of pharmacy. Although the system is rarely used today, a pharmacist or pharmacy technician may see a prescription or medication order where the prescriber has used it. The practice of pharmacy uses both the apothecary and metric system to measure out ingredients (Table 5-5). In both the apothecary and avoirdupois system, only the grain is the same.

Avoirdupois System of Measurement

The avoirdupois system is the system used by commerce in the United States and Britain. It is based upon a pound being equal to 16 ounces. This

Table 5-5 Apothecary Conversions

Apothecary Volume:
60 minims (m) = 1 fluid dram (ʒ)
8 fluid drams (480 minims) = 1 fluid ounce (fl oz)
16 fluid ounces = 1 pint (pt)
2 pints (32 fluid ounces) = 1 quart (qt)
4 quarts (8 pints) = 1 gallon (gal)
Apothecary Weight:
20 grains (gr) = 1 scruple (℈)
3 scruples (60 grains) = 1 dram (ʒ)
8 drachm (480 grains) = 1 ounce (oz)
12 ounces (5760 grains) = 1 pound (lb)

system along with the metric system is how products are purchased and sold in the United States (Table 5-6).

Household System of Measurement

The household or U.S. customary system is used for the patient to understand the quantity of medication to be taken at a particular time. Unlike the other systems we have studied, the household system is an approximate system of measurement (Table 5-7). An individual uses the utensils readily accessible in the home to administer medicine.

Table 5-6 Avoirdupois Conversions

Avoirdupois Weight:
437.5 grains (gr) = 1 ounce (oz)
16 ounces (7000 gr) = 1 pound (lb)

Table 5-7 Household Conversions

Household Volumes:
5 milliliters (mL) = 1 teaspoon (tsp)
3 teaspoons (tsp) = 1 tablespoon (tbsp)
2 tablespoons (tbsp) = 1 fluid ounce (fl oz)
8 fluid ounces (fl oz) = 1 cup
2 cups = 1 pint (pt)
2 pints (pt) = 1 quart (qt)
4 quarts (qt) = 1 gallon (gal)
Household Weights:
16 ounces (oz) = 1 pound (lb)

In various situations, the pharmacist or pharmacy technician may find that a conversion is needed to perform a pharmacy calculation. The *USP* has issued a table of exact equivalents for both weights and measures in the metric, apothecary, and avoirdupois systems. As a pharmacy technician, you will be required to memorize apothecary, avoirdupois, and household conversions. You can always solve these conversions by using proportions. Refer to Table 5-8 for these conversions.

There are specific tools used to measure both volumes and weights in pharmacy practice. The proper selection of the equipment chosen is based upon the desired precision of the measurement. Volumes are measured using either a cylindrical or conical graduate; small volumes may be measured using calibrated syringes or a pipette. Cylindrical graduates are calibrated using metric units, such as milliliters; conical graduates are calibrated in both metric and apothecary units. It is extremely important that the proper size graduate is chosen; the graduate should not contain more than five times the volume to be measured. If the graduate measures more than five times the desired volume, the possibility of a measuring error will increase.

Table 5-8 *USP* **Conversions for Weights and Measures**

Conversion Equivalents of Volume:
1 milliliter (mL) = 16.23 minims (m)
1 minim (m) = 0.06 mL
1 fluid drachm (fl ʒ) (dram) = 3.69 mL
1 fluid ounce (fl oz) = 29.57 mL
1 pint (pt) = 473 mL
1 gallon (U.S.) = 3785 mL
Conversion Equivalents of Weight:
1 gram (g) = 15.432 grains (gr)
1 kilogram (kg) = 2.20 pounds (lb)
1 grain (gr) = 0.065 gram (g) or 65 mg (can also be 60 mg)
1 ounce (oz - avoirdupois) = 28.35 grams (g)
1 ounce (oz) = 31.1 grams (g)
1 pound (avoirdupois) = 454 grams (g)
1 pound (apothecary) = 373.2 grams (g)
Other Equivalents:
1 oz (avoirdupois) = 437.5 grains (gr)
1 ounce (oz) = 480 grains (gr)
1 gallon (U.S.) = 128 fluid ounces (fl oz)
1 fluid ounce (fl oz) = 455 grains (gr)

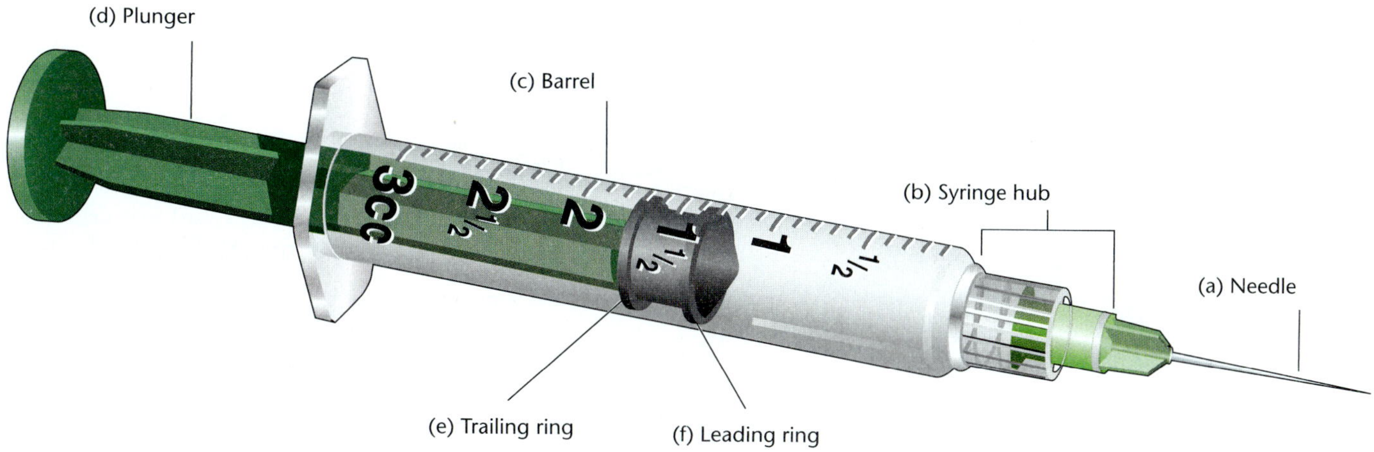

Figure 5-1 Parts of a standard syringe.

Many different types of balances and scales may be used in a pharmacy. Each type of scale or balance must meet specific standards that are established by the *USP* for sensitivity, capacity, and accuracy. Class A balances are used to weigh ingredients for the filling of prescriptions or small-scale compounding. Class A balances must have a sensitivity requirement of 6 mg or less and should not weigh less than 120 mg and not be able to weigh more than 120 g. Electronic balances are capable of weighing very small quantities such as 0.1 mg and often are self-calibrating with a digital readout. Electronic balances have the capability of weighing 60 to 120 g.

In hospitals, the pharmacy is responsible for preparing IV bags for patients upon receipt of a medication order from a physician. The pharmacy technician may be asked to reconstitute a vial of medication or prepare a medicated IV bag for a patient. The pharmacy technician will use a syringe in these preparations. He or she should select a syringe that contains no more than five times the volume being measured to ensure accuracy. Refer to Figure 5-1 for syringes used to prepare IVs.

Conversion Factors

It is often necessary to convert a measurement from one unit to another. We have already discussed conversions within the metric system. Now let us examine how to use the equivalents given in the above tables to convert units between different systems. A conversion factor is a fraction made up of two values that are equal to one another, but which are expressed in different units. Table 5-8 lists equivalents that can be used when writing conversion factors. The key to writing a conversion factor is to put the proper part of the equivalent into the numerator and denominator of the fraction. The following rule can be used when writing conversion factors from equivalents: *The part of the equivalent containing units that you want to convert from must go in the bottom of the conversion factor. The part containing units that you want to convert to must go in the top of the conversion factor.*

EXAMPLE

What conversion factor would you use to convert *from* pounds *to* kilograms?

1. Find the equivalent containing pounds and kilograms.

$$1 \text{ kg} = 2.2 \text{ lb}$$

2. Rewrite the equivalent as a fraction, putting the units you are converting from on the bottom and the units you are converting to on the top.

$$\frac{2.2 \text{ lb}}{1 \text{ kg}}$$

EXAMPLE

What conversion factor would you use to convert *from* milliliters *to* fluid ounces?

1. Find the equivalent containing milliliters and fluid ounces.

$$1 \text{ fl oz} = 30 \text{ mL}$$

2. Rewrite the equivalent as a fraction, putting the units you are converting from on the bottom and the units you are converting to on the top.

$$\frac{1 \text{ fl oz}}{30 \text{ mL}}$$

Using Conversion Factors

To use a conversion factor, multiply the number that is being converted by the numerator of the conversion factor, and divide the answer by the denominator of the conversion factor. You can then cancel the units that are the same in the numerator and denominator.

EXAMPLE

Convert 110 lb to kilograms

1. Find the equivalent containing pounds and kilograms.

$$1 \text{ kg} = 2.2 \text{ lb}$$

2. Rewrite the equivalent as a fraction, putting the units you are converting from on the bottom and the units you are converting to on the top.

$$\frac{1 \text{ kg}}{2.2 \text{ lb}}$$

3. Multiply the number being converted by the numerator of the conversion factor, while dividing by the denominator. Cancel any units found in both the numerator and denominator.

$$\frac{110 \cancel{\text{lb}} \times 1 \text{ kg}}{2.2 \cancel{\text{lb}}}$$

$$(110 \times 1 \text{ kg}) \div 2.2 = 50 \text{ kg}$$

$$110 \text{ lb} = 50 \text{ kg}$$

EXAMPLE

Convert 12.5 mL to teaspoons

1. Find the equivalent containing milliliters and teaspoons.

$$1 \text{ tsp} = 5 \text{ mL}$$

2. Rewrite the equivalent as a fraction, putting the units you are converting from on the bottom and the units you are converting to on the top.

$$\frac{1 \text{ tsp}}{5 \text{ mL}}$$

3. Multiply the number being converted by the numerator of the conversion factor, while dividing by the denominator. Cancel any units found in both the numerator and denominator.

$$\frac{12.5\ \cancel{\text{mL}} \times 1 \text{ tsp}}{5\ \cancel{\text{mL}}}$$

$$(12.5 \times 1 \text{ tsp}) \div 5 = 2.5 \text{ tsp}$$

$$12.5 \text{ mL} = 2.5 \text{ tsp}$$

Tech Check

18. How many milligrams are in 25 g? (LO 5.6)

19. How many milligrams are in 7.5 gr? (LO 5.6)

20. How many teaspoons are contained in 1 pt of solution? (LO 5.6)

21. A patient weighs 150 lb. How many kilograms does the patient weigh? (LO 5.6)

22. How many millilitres are $2\frac{1}{2}$ pt of syrup? (LO 5.6)

23. A patient is to receive 0.25 mg of medication. How many micrograms of medication is this? (LO 5.6)

24. How many grams are in 4 oz (wt)? (LO 5.6)

25. How many pounds does a 60 kg person weigh? (LO 5.6)

26. How many fluid ounces are equal to 75 mL? (LO 5.6)

27. How many gallons are equal to 4 L? (LO 5.6)

28. How many grams are equal to 500 mg? (LO 5.6)

29. A *Nitrostat* tablet contains 1/150 gr. How many milligrams are equal? (LO 5.6)

30. How many milliliters are equal to 6 fl oz? (LO 5.6)

31. A patient is to receive 5 gr of aspirin. How many milligrams are equal? (LO 5.6)

32. You have been asked to prepare 1/2 lb of an ointment for a dermatologist. How many grams should you prepare? (LO 5.6)

Other Units of Measurement(LO 5.7, 5.8, 5.11, 5.25)

International Units

The strength of some antibiotics (e.g., penicillin V and G, nystatin, and bacitracin), endocrine products (e.g., insulin), vitamins (e.g., vitamin A, vitamin D, and vitamin E), and biologicals (heparin) are based upon the activity of the drug and are known as "units." This form of measurement is approved by both the FDA and the *USP*.

Electrolytes

Electrolytes are salts that have the ability to conduct electrical charge when present in solution. Common electrolytes are sodium chloride, potassium chloride, magnesium sulfate, and calcium gluconate. Electrolytes are often prescribed in millimoles (mMol) and milliequivalents (mEq).

EXAMPLE

A physician has prescribed for a patient 30 mEq of potassium chloride 10% each morning. Potassium chloride is available as 20 mEq/15 mL. How many milliliters will the patient need to take each morning?

Solution: The problem can be solved using proportions.

$$\frac{20 \text{ mEq}}{15 \text{ mL}} = \frac{30 \text{ mEq}}{\text{X mL}}$$

Cross multiply:

$$(20 \text{ mEq} \times X \text{ mL}) = (15 \text{ mL} \times 30 \text{ mEq})$$

Divide both sides of the equation by 20 mEq

$$\frac{(20 \text{ mEq} \times X \text{ mL})}{20 \text{ mEq}} = \frac{(15 \text{ mL} \times 30 \text{ mEq})}{20 \text{ mEq}}$$

$$X = 22.5 \text{ mL}$$

Temperature Measurements

The practice of pharmacy requires that medications be stored at the proper temperature in order for the patient to obtain the maximum effect of the medication. The *USP-NF* has established specific terms to correspond with the storage of medications:

- Cold—Any temperature not exceeding 8°Celsius (46°Fahrenheit)
- Cool—Any temperature between 8 and 15°C (46 and 59°F)
- Room Temperature—Any temperature between 15 and 30°C (59 and 86°F)
- Warm—Any temperature between 30 and 40°C (86 and 104°F)
- Excessive Heat—Any temperature greater than 40°C (104°F)

Pharmacy technicians must be able to convert between the Fahrenheit and Celsius systems of measuring temperatures to make sure that medications are being stored at the proper temperature. This can be done by using the following equation:

$$9C = 5F - 160$$

where °C represents Celsius and °F stands for Fahrenheit.

Time Conversions

Many health care facilities, such as hospitals, express time using a 24-hour clock instead of using the more conventional 12-hour clock, which requires the designation of either "am" or "pm." A traditional 12-hour clock is a potential source for errors in administering medication. On the 12-hour clock, each time occurs twice a day. For example, 10:00 occurs both in the morning (10:00 am) and at night (10:00 pm) If the abbreviation indicating morning or night is not clearly marked, the patient could receive medication at the wrong time.

The 24-hour clock (referred to as **international time**, sometimes called **military time**) avoids this opportunity for error. Each time occurs only once a day. In international time, 10:00 am is written as 1000, whereas 10:00 pm is written as 2200 and is read as 22 hundred hours.

When you write the time using a 12-hour clock, you separate the hour from the minutes by a colon, then add am or pm to indicate if the time is before or after noon. When you write the time using a 24-hour clock, you use a four-digit number with no colon and is read as 10 hundred hours. The first two digits represent the hour; the last two digits, the minutes. Follow the guidelines in the Caution box below.

Caution

Always write International Time correctly. Follow these guidelines:

1. The first two digits represent the number of hours since midnight.(LO 5.8)
   a. If the time is between midnight and 1:00 am, the first two digits are 00.
   b. 1:00 am through 9:00 am require the addition of a 0 before the hour (written 0100 through 0900).
   c. You must add 12 to the conventional hour for times that occur after noon (example: 3:00 pm becomes 1500).
   d. Midnight can be written as either 0000 or 2400.
2. The last two digits represent the number of minutes past the hour.(LO 5.8)

Table 5-9 shows the appropriate conversion between a 12-hour clock and a 24-hour clock.

Tech Check

33. What temperature is 75°F equal to in the Celsius system?(LO 5.7)

34. What temperature is 32°C equal to in the Fahrenheit system?(LO 5.7)

35. What time is 3:00 pm equivalent to using a 24-hour clock?(LO 5.8)

international time (military time) Time based on the 24-hour clock.

Table 5-9 24-Hour Clock Versus 12-Hour Clock

International Time (Military Time)	12-Hour Clock
0000 or 2400	12:00 am
0100	1:00 am
0200	2:00 am
0300	3:00 am
0400	4:00 am
0500	5:00 am
0600	6:00 am
0700	7:00 am
0800	8:00 am
0900	9:00 am
1000	10:00 am
1100	11:00 am
1200	12:00 pm
1300	1:00 pm
1400	2:00 pm
1500	3:00 pm
1600	4:00 pm
1700	5:00 pm
1800	6:00 pm
1900	7:00 pm
2000	8:00 pm
2100	9:00 pm
2200	10:00 pm
2300	11:00 pm

Dosage Calculations (LO 5.13, 5.14, 5.15)

There will be times when a physician will prescribe a medication and the pharmacy does not have the strength prescribed. After informing the pharmacist of the situation, you may be required to calculate the correct dose for the patient. To determine the **desired dose,** you must know the **dosage ordered** and the dose on hand. The dosage ordered will be found on the physician's prescription or medication order, while the dose on hand will be found on the label of the medication.

As previously stated, the desired dose must have the same units as the dose on hand. If the dosage ordered has the same units as the dose on hand, then the desired dose is the same as the dosage ordered. If the dosage ordered is in different units than the dose on hand, however, it will be necessary to convert the dosage ordered to a desired dose.

desired dose The amount of drug to be administered at a single time.

dosage ordered The amount of drug to be administered and the frequency it is to be given.

Determining the Desired Dose

EXAMPLE

A drug order reads 5 gr of aspirin daily. The drug label indicates 325 mg tablets. The desired dose, in milligrams, needs to be calculated from the dosage ordered, which is in grains.

In this example, units need to be converted from one system to another. Earlier in the chapter, you learned how to write and use conversion factors that allowed you to do this. In this situation, you need to find an equivalent that contains milligrams and grains. (If you do not remember this equivalent, refer to Table 5-8.)

1. Find the equivalent containing milligrams and grains.

$$1 \text{ gr} = 65 \text{ mg}$$

2. Rewrite the equivalent as a fraction, putting the units you are converting from on the bottom and the units you are converting to on the top.

$$\frac{65 \text{ mg}}{1 \text{ gr}}$$

3. Multiply the number being converted by the numerator of the conversion factor, while dividing by the denominator. Cancel any units found in the numerator and denominator.
4.

$$\frac{5\ \cancel{\text{gr}} \times 65 \text{ mg}}{1\ \cancel{\text{gr}}}$$

$$(5 \times 65 \text{ mg}) \div 1 = 325 \text{ mg}$$

Therefore, 5 gr is equal to 325 mg.

The desired dose is 325 mg.

EXAMPLE

A patient presents a prescription at the pharmacy to receive 150 mg of Zantac Syrup in each dose. How many milliliters should the patient take?

Recall that conversion factors were made up of two values that were equivalent but expressed in different units. According to the label, there are 75 mg of the drug in every 5 mL of the syrup. The dosage unit (Q) is 5 mL, and the dose on hand (H) is 75 mg. For Zantac syrup, 5 mL = 75 mg. These two values are equivalent to one another, which means that they can be used to make a conversion factor. If the desired dose (D) for a patient is 150 mg, we can find the amount to administer (A) by converting from mg of Zantac to mL of Zantac syrup.

1. According to the drug label, 5 mL = 75 mg.
2. Rewrite the equivalent as a fraction, putting the units you are converting from on the bottom and the units you are converting to on the top.

$$\frac{5 \text{ mL}}{75 \text{ mg}}$$

3. Multiply the number being converted by the numerator of the conversion factor, while dividing by the denominator. Cancel any units found in the numerator and denominator.

$$\frac{150\ \cancel{\text{mg}} \times 5\ \text{mL}}{75\ \cancel{\text{mg}}}$$

$$(150 \times 5\ \text{mL}) \div 75 = 10\ \text{mL}$$

Therefore, 150 mg is equal to 10 mL.

The amount to administer is 10 mL.

Because calculations of the amount to be administer or dispense always involve converting from the desired dose to the amount to dispensed, the following formula can be used:

$$A = \frac{D \times Q}{H}$$

where

D = desired dose—this is the dose ordered changed to the same unit of measure as the dose on hand
H = dose on hand—the amount of drug contained in each unit
Q = dosage unit—how the drug will be administered, such as tablets or milliliters
A = amount to dispense (unknown).

In this formula, the desired dose (D) must first be calculated from the dosage ordered. (Recall that if the dosage ordered is already in the same units as the dose on hand, no calculation is needed.) The dosage unit (Q) and the dose on hand (H) are found on the drug label. The amount to be administered or dispensed (A) is the unknown.

EXAMPLE

A drug order reads 375 mg of cephalexin suspension every 8 hours. Referring to the drug label in Figure 5-2, find the amount to administer.

1. Find Q and H on the drug label.

   Q = 5 mL

   H = 250 mg

2. Calculate the desired dose from the dosage ordered.

   Since the dosage ordered (375 mg) and the dose on hand (250 mg) are already in the same units, no calculation is needed.

   D = 375 mg

3. Calculate the amount to be administered or dispensed (A).

$$A = \frac{D \times Q}{H}$$

$$A = \frac{375\ \cancel{\text{mg}} \times 5\ \text{mL}}{250\ \cancel{\text{mg}}}$$

$$A = (375 \times 5 \text{ mL}) \div 250$$

$$A = 7.5 \text{ mL}$$

The amount to be administered is 75 mL.

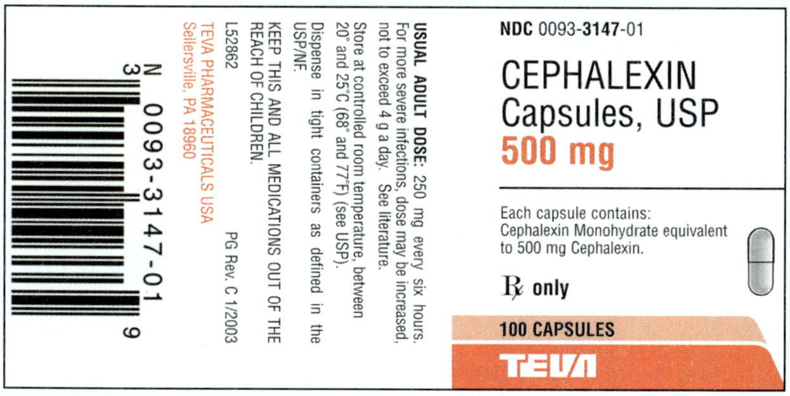

Figure 5-2 Cephalexin.

EXAMPLE

A drug order reads 120 mg of Tigan injected intramuscularly every 8 hours as needed for nausea. Referring to the drug label in Figure 5-3, find the amount to administer.

1. Find Q and H on the drug label.

$$Q = 1 \text{ mL}$$

$$H = 100 \text{ mg}$$

2. Calculate the desired dose from the dosage ordered.

   Since the dosage ordered (120 mg) and the dose on hand (100 mg) are already in the same units, no calculation is needed.

   D = 120 mg

Figure 5-3 Tigan.

3. Calculate the amount to be administered or dispensed (A).

$$A = \frac{D \times Q}{H}$$

$$A = \frac{120 \cancel{\text{mg}} \times 1 \text{ mL}}{100 \cancel{\text{mg}}}$$

$$A = (120 \times 1 \text{ mL}) \div 100$$

$$A = 1.2 \text{ mL}$$

The amount to be administered is 1.2 mL.

Pediatric Dosing

Children require different amounts of medication than adults. These doses are affected by the individual's age, weight, body surface area, organ development, sex, and disease state. An individual's age is broken down into one of several categories.

Neonatal: birth to 1 month of age
Infancy: 1 month to 1 year of age
Early childhood: 1 year to 5 years of age
Late childhood: 6 years to 12 years of age
Adolescence: 13 years to 17 years of age

To calculate the appropriate dosage for children, one of several methods may be used. **Young's Rule** uses age as a guide; **Clark's Rule** utilizes weight as the determining factor; milligram per kiligram uses weight in terms of kiligrams for a patient and body surface area (BSA) uses both height and weight as the basis for choosing a dose.

$$\text{Young's Rule} = \frac{\text{Age of child (expressed in years)}}{\text{Age of child (in years)} + 12} \times \text{Adult dose}$$

$$\text{Clark's Rule} = \frac{\text{Weight of child (expressed in pounds)}}{150} \times \text{Adult dose}$$

Body Surface Area

Body surface area (BSA) is a method used to calculate dosages based on the height (expressed in centimeters and inches) and weight (expressed in kilograms and pounds) of an individual. As a pharmacy technician, you will notice that no two individuals are the same in body composition whether they are an adult or a child. A disease may cause an individual to lose weight and certain medications may cause an individual to gain weight. The use of BSA is more accurate than using either age or weight but is slightly more difficult to calculate. The BSA is expressed in square meters (m^2). A **nomogram** is used in the calculation. The BSA is calculated by locating the weight and height of a patient on the nomogram and drawing a straight line between these two points. The BSA for a patient is found where the line intersects the BSA column. Refer to Figure 5-4 for an example of a child's nomogram, and refer to figure 5-5 for an example of an adult nomogram.

All three of the previously mentioned methods require the adult dose and the given parameter to be provided to the practitioner to calculate the appropriate dose. The adult dose may be measured in milligrams, milliliters, units, milliequivalents, or even tablets.

Young's Rule A method of calculating a child's dose based upon the child's age and the recommended adult dose of a particular drug.

Clark's Rule A method of calculating a child's dose based upon the child's weight and the recommended adult dose of a particular drug.

nomogram A chart using the weight and height of a patient to calculate the correct dose for the patient.

Tech Check

36. A 3-year-old child is prescribed amoxicillin. If the adult dose is 250 mg, how many milligrams should the child receive?(LO 5.15)

37. A 65-lb male is prescribed cephalexin. If the adult dose is 500 mg, how many milligrams should the patient receive?(LO 5.15)

38. An adult patient weighs 98 lb and is 5′1″ tall. Using the nomogram, find the patient's BSA. The dose of vincristine ordered by the physician is 10 mg/m2 per day. What is the dose in mg? (Refer to nomogram.)(LO 5.15)

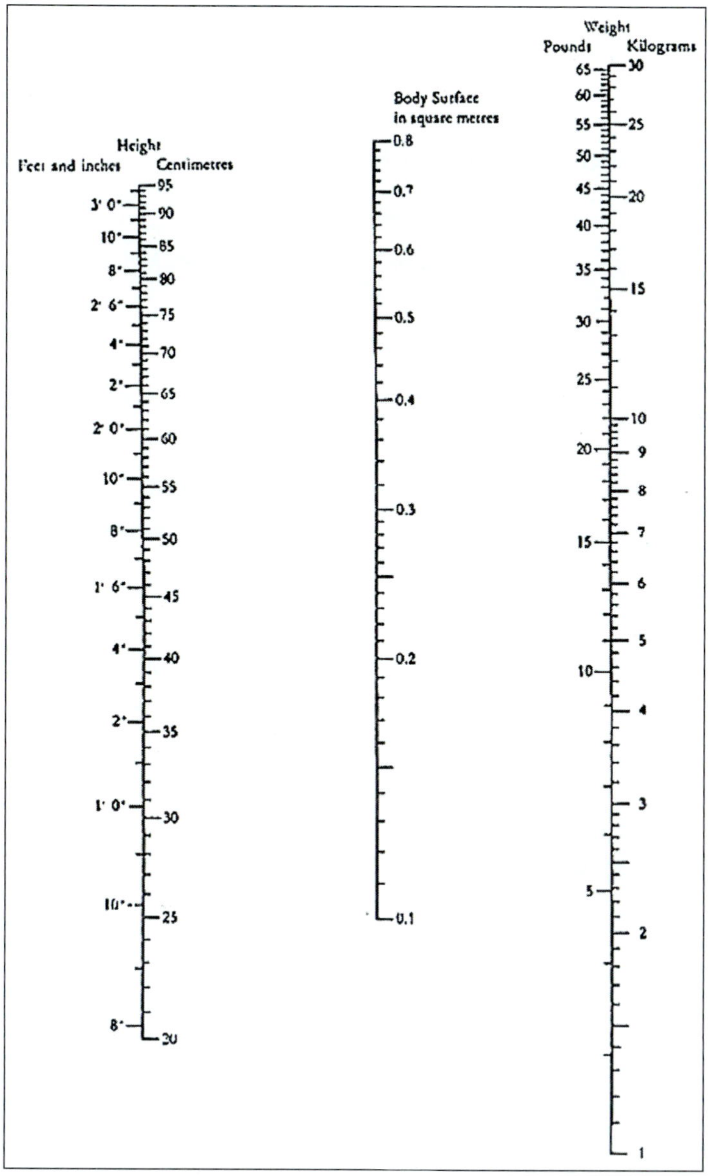

Figure 5-4 **Children's nomogram.**

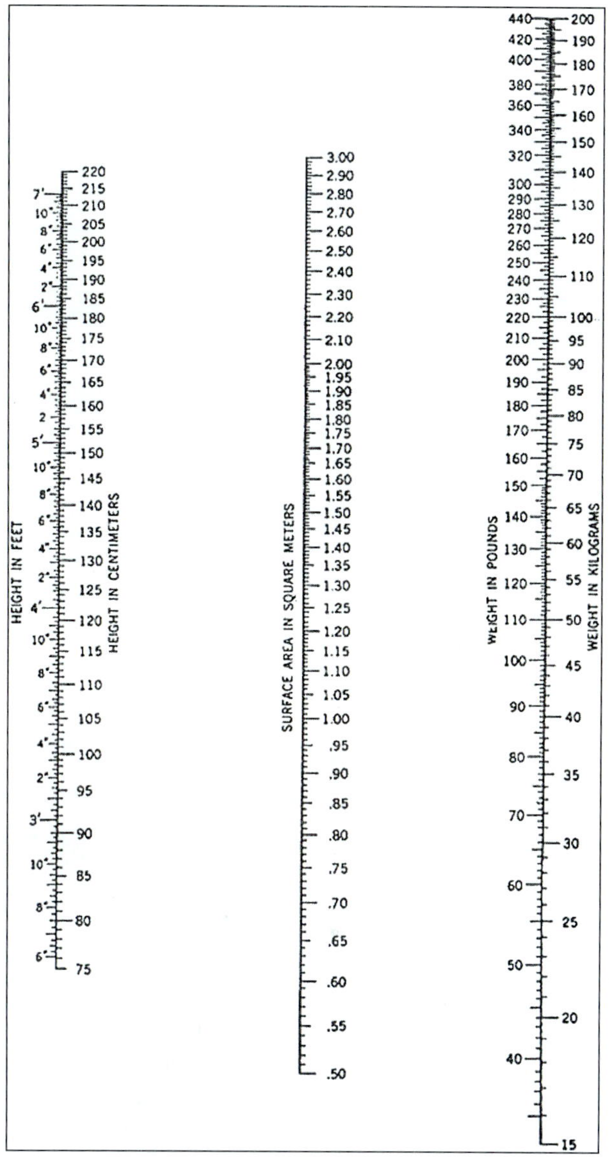

Figure 5-5 **Adult's nomogram.**

Physician's Orders and Prescriptions (LO 5.9, 5.10, 5.26)

Pharmacy Abbreviations

Physicians use abbreviations when writing orders. Memorize the commonly used ones and have available a complete list of those accepted at your facility. Approved abbreviations vary among facilities. You may encounter either uppercase or lowercase letters as well as orders with or without punctuation. You may also notice slight differences in the way that abbreviations are spelled. Some physicians use lowercase Roman numerals, such as *ii*, to indicate numbers. You may also see these numerals with a line over them, such as $\overline{ii}$. Physicians may also put a line over general and frequently used abbreviations, such as *a, ac, c, p,* and s when the abbreviations are lowercase.

Table 5-10 lists some commonly used abbreviations. Please note that an institution (hospital or HMO) may use different abbreviations for these terms, or may use periods after them.

Table 5-10 Commonly Used Pharmacy Abbreviations

General Abbreviations			
Abbreviation	**Meaning**	**Abbreviation**	**Meaning**
aq	water	**p̄, p**	after
aq dist	distilled water	**q, q., q̄**	every
a, ā	before, ante	**qs**	quantity sufficient
aa, āā	of each	**R**	take
BP	blood pressure	**s̄**	without
c, c̄	with	**sig. s**	write on label
disp	dispense	**ss, s̄s̄**	one-half
et	and	**sys**	Systolic
iss, ĪSS	one and one-half	**tbs, T**	tablespoon
NKA	no known allergies	**tsp, t**	teaspoon
NKDA	no known drug allergies	**ut dict, ud**	as directed
NPO, n.p.o.	nothing by mouth		
Form of Medication			
Abbreviation	**Meaning**	**Abbreviation**	**Meaning**
cap, caps	capsule	**MDI**	metered-dose inhaler
comp	compound	**sol, soln.**	solution
dil.	dilute	**SR**	slow-release
EC	enteric-coated	**supp.**	suppository
elix.	elixir	**susp.**	suspension
ext.	extract	**syr, syp.**	syrup
fld., fl	fluid	**syr**	syringe
gtt, gtts	drop, drops	**tab**	tablet
H	hypodermic	**tr, tinct, tinc.**	tincture
LA	long-acting	**ung, oint**	ointment
liq	liquid		
Route (Where to Administer)			
Abbreviation	**Meaning**	**Abbreviation**	**Meaning**
ad, A.D., AD*	right ear	**od, O.D., OD**	right eye
as, A.S., AS*	left ear	**os, O.S., OS**	left eye
au, A.U., AU*	both ears	**ou, O.U., OU**	both eyes

(Continued)

Table 5-10 Commonly Used Pharmacy Abbreviations *(Continued)*

Route (How to Administer)			
Abbreviation	**Meaning**	**Abbreviation**	**Meaning**
GT	gastrostomy tube	**NG, NGT, ng**	nasogastric tube
IVPB	intravenous piggyback	**NJ**	nasojejunal tube
IVSS	intravenous soluset	**per**	per, by, through
ID	intradermal	**po, p.o., PO,P.O.**	by mouth; orally
IM, I.M.	intramuscular	**R, P.R., p.r.**	rectally
IV, I.V.	intravenous	**sub-q, Sub-q**	subcutaneous, beneath the skin
IVP	intravenous push	**SL, sl**	sublingually, under the tongue
KVO, TKO	keep vein open	**top, TOP**	topical, applied to skin surface
Frequency			
Abbreviation	**Meaning**	**Abbreviation**	**Meaning**
a.c., ac, AC, $\overline{\text{ac}}$	before meals	**qam, q.a.m.**	every morning
ad. lib, ad lib	as desired, freely	**qpm, o.n., q.n.**	every night
b.i.d., bid, BID	twice a day	**q.h., qh**	every hour
b.i.w.	twice a week	**q. ___ hrs, q ___ h**	every ___ hours
h, hr	hour	**qhs, q.h.s.**	every night, at bedtime
LOS	length of stay	**q.i.d., qid, QID**	4 times a day
min	minute		
non rep	do not repeat	**rep**	repeat
n, noc, noct	night	**SOS, s.o.s.**	once if necessary, as necessary
od	every day	**stat**	immediately
p.c., pc, PC, $\overline{\text{pc}}$	after meals	**t.i.d., tid, TID**	3 times a day
p.r.n., prn, PRN	when necessary, when required, as needed		

Figure 5-6 Prescription order form.

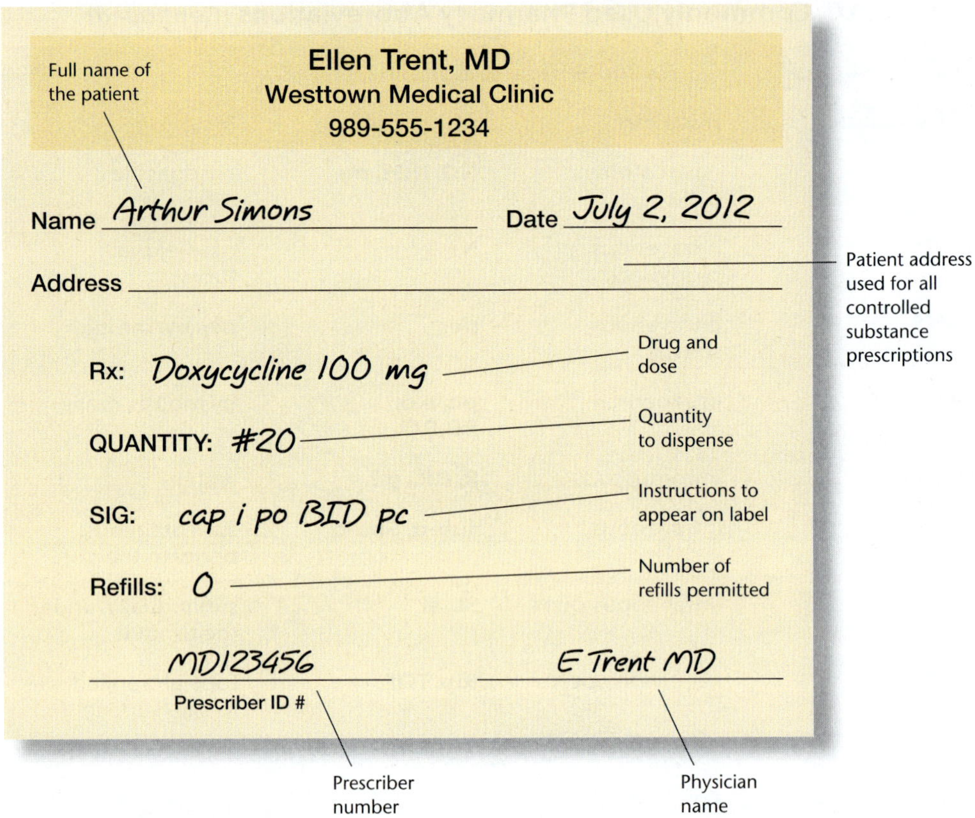

Prescription Order

A prescription order is a medication order on a prescription blank to be filled at an ambulatory or outpatient facility such as a retail pharmacy. Most prescription orders may be transmitted to the pharmacist via telephone order or facsimile order from the physician's office or brought in to the pharmacy by the patient or the patient's representative. In some situations, a prescription order may be transmitted electronically to the pharmacy from the physician's office.

The components of a prescription include (Figure 5-6):

- Prescriber's information, which includes the physician's name, office address, and office telephone number, and may include an office fax number (if a physician is prescribing a controlled substance, it must contain the physician's DEA number)
- Name and home address of the patient (superscription)
- Date the prescription was written (superscription)
- Medication prescribed that includes the strength and quantity (inscription)
- Dispensing directions to the pharmacist (subscription)
- Directions for the patient (signa and/or transcription)
- Refill and labeling information
- Physician's signature

Medication (Drug) Order

A medication order is a written request from a physician on a physician's order form for a patient in an inpatient facility. Drug orders must contain the following information: the name of the patient, the name of the drug,

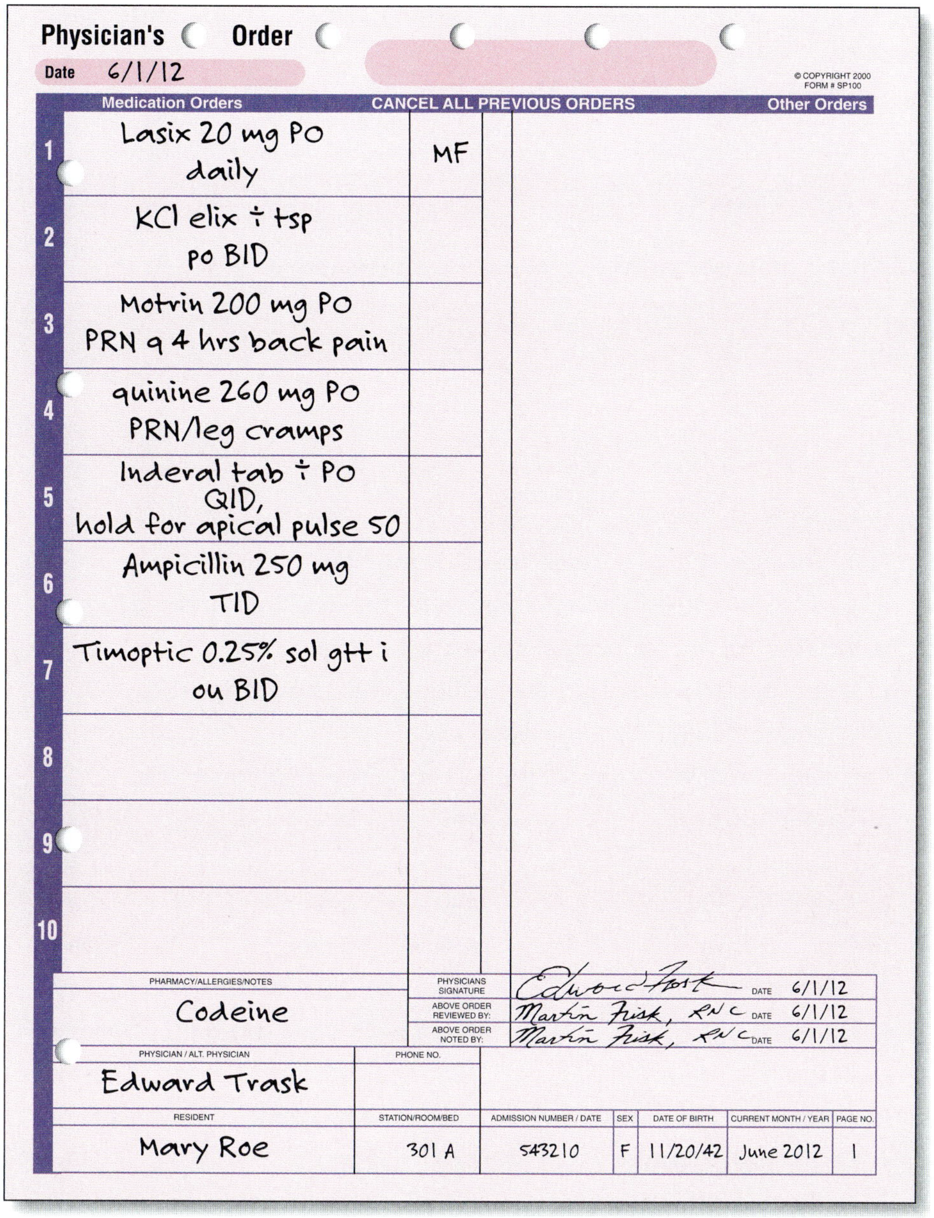

Physician's Order

Date 6/1/12

© COPYRIGHT 2000 FORM # SP100

	Medication Orders		CANCEL ALL PREVIOUS ORDERS / Other Orders
1	Lasix 20 mg PO daily	MF	
2	KCl elix $\dot{\bar{\text{i}}}$ tsp po BID		
3	Motrin 200 mg PO PRN q 4 hrs back pain		
4	quinine 260 mg PO PRN/leg cramps		
5	Inderal tab $\dot{\bar{\text{i}}}$ PO QID, hold for apical pulse 50		
6	Ampicillin 250 mg TID		
7	Timoptic 0.25% sol gtt i ou BID		
8			
9			
10			

PHARMACY/ALLERGIES/NOTES: Codeine

PHYSICIANS SIGNATURE: Edward Trask DATE 6/1/12

ABOVE ORDER REVIEWED BY: Martin Fisk, RNC DATE 6/1/12

ABOVE ORDER NOTED BY: Martin Fisk, RNC DATE 6/1/12

PHYSICIAN / ALT. PHYSICIAN: Edward Trask

PHONE NO.

RESIDENT	STATION/ROOM/BED	ADMISSION NUMBER / DATE	SEX	DATE OF BIRTH	CURRENT MONTH / YEAR	PAGE NO.
Mary Roe	301 A	543210	F	11/20/42	June 2012	1

Figure 5-7 Physician's order form.

the dose of the drug, the route of administration, and the frequency of administration. They may also include additional instructions, such as to be given after meals, or when needed for pain. Figure 5-7 shows an example of a physician's order form.

Days Supply

In pharmacy practice today, pharmacy technicians must be able to calculate the correct days supply for each prescription they fill. This is especially important because of the restrictions imposed by managed-care and for customer service. The majority of managed care prescription plans will pay for only a 30-day supply of medication. If a pharmacy dispenses more than the allowed days supply and a managed-care provider audits the pharmacy, the pharmacy may be required to reimburse the managed-care provider and therefore will lose money.

To calculate a day's supply of a medication, the following equation can be used:

Days supply = Total quantity dispensed/Total quantity taken per day

Tech Check

39. What is the meaning of the following abbreviations?(LO 5.26)

g

mL

ac

pc

stat

40. What is a "signa"?(LO 5.26)

41. Refer to Figure 5-8 to answer the following:(LO 5.26)

a. What is the route of administration for the first drug ordered?

b. What is missing from the second drug order?

c. What special instructions are included with drug order #5?

d. What is missing from drug order #5?

42. Calculate the days supply for the following prescriptions:(LO 5.10)

a. Zantac 150 mg	#60	1 bid	Days
b. Augmentin 500 mg	#42	1 tid	Days
c. Ampicillin 500 mg	#40	1 qid	Days
d. Prozac 20 mg	#60	1 q am	Days
e. Tylenol #3	#30	1-2 q 4-6 h prn pain	Days
f. Humulin N U-100	10 mL	35 units sub-q qd	Days
g. Ortho Tri-Cyclen	#28	1 qd	Days
h. Amoxicillin 250 mg	#30	1 cap q8h	Days
i. Cephalexin 250 mg	#28	1 qid	Days
j. Hydrochlorothiazide 50 mg	#15	1/2 tab every other day	Days

Drug Labels(LO 5.11)

Drug labels include information that you will need when calculating dosages. Included on the label you will find the generic name of the drug, the name and location of the manufacturer, the lot or batch number, the dosage strength and dosage form, quantity, expiration date, and storage conditions. On brand name drugs you will also find the companies' trade name for the medication. The route of administration may also be included, although it is not normally included for oral dosage forms such as tablets and capsules. Figure 5-8 shows an example of a typical label for an oral medication.

The information that you are most likely to need from the label when filling a drug order includes the name (either trade or generic), dosage strength, and dosage form. You should always check the expiration date as well. If you are repackaging a portion of the container, the new container

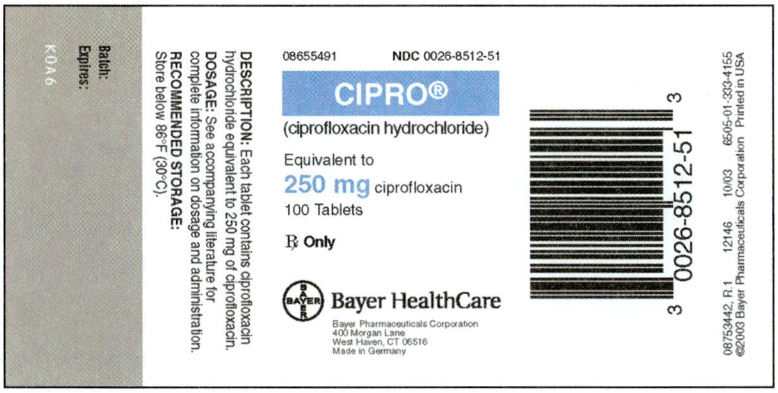

Figure 5-8 **Label for oral medication.**

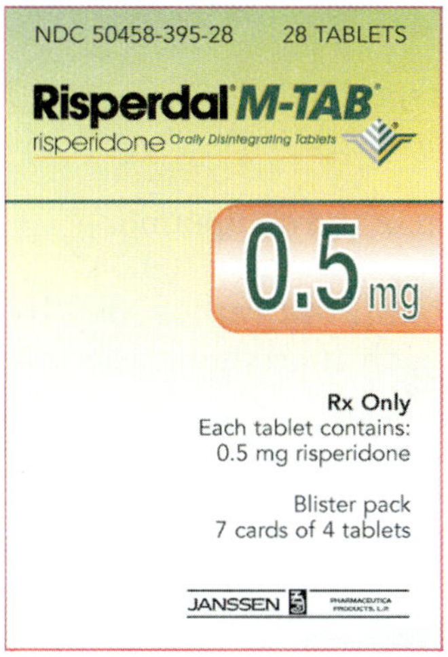

Figure 5-9 **Drug label, Risperdal.**

will need to include either the trade name of the drug or the generic name plus manufacturer. Other information may also be required, depending on the nature of the order.

Tech Check

Refer to the label shown in Figure 5-9.

43. What is the generic name of the medication?(LO 5.11)

44. Who is the manufacturer of the medication?(LO 5.11)

45. What is the dosage strength of the medication?(LO 5.11)

46. How many tablets are in the package of the drug pictured in figure 5-9?(LO 5.11)

Compounding(LO 5.16, 5.17, 5.18, 5.27, 5.28)

Reducing and Enlarging a Formula

Pharmacy technicians may find that they must compound a product that is either greater or less than the original quantity prescribed. During this process, the proportions of medications must be maintained. If a formula specifies a total quantity, we may determine how much of each ingredient is needed to prepare a different total quantity by using this formula:

$$\frac{\text{Total quantity in formula (as specified)}}{\text{Total quantity of formula as desired}} = \frac{\text{Quantity of an ingredient (as specified) in formula}}{\text{X}}$$

Where X = quantity of an ingredient for the quantity of the formula desired.

For instance, a formula for a compound weighing 100 g contains 20 g of ingredient A. How many grams of the ingredient are needed to make 500 g of the compound? The problem can be solved by using the above-mentioned proportion:

$$\frac{\text{100 g (formula specified)}}{\text{500 g (formula desired)}} = \frac{\text{20 g of ingredient A (specified)}}{X \text{ g (ingredient A needed)}}$$

X = 100 g of ingredient A is needed to make 500 g of the compound.

Sometimes formulas do not specify a total amount, but rather may be expressed in parts. To calculate the quantities of each ingredient, the following equation may be used:

$$\frac{\text{Total number of parts in formula (as specified)}}{\text{Number of parts of an ingredient (as specified)}} = \frac{\text{Total quantity of formula (as desired)}}{X \text{ (quantity of an ingredient)}}$$

Dilution

Dilution is the process by which one prepares a mixture of a lower strength or concentration by adding an inert ingredient **(diluent)** to the original product. There are four variables in a dilution problem:

- Initial strength or concentration that can be expressed as a percent (percentage), a fraction (mg/mL), or a ratio. It is important to remember our previous definitions of w/w %, w/v %, and v/v %.
- Initial volume (liquid) or initial weight (solid or semi solid)
- Final strength, which can be expressed as a percent (%), a fraction (mg/mL), or a ratio.
- Final volume (liquid) or final weight (solid or semisolid).

Several observations can be noted in a dilution problem between these variables. First, the initial strength is always greater than the final strength in a dilution problem. Second, the final volume (or final weight) is greater than the initial volume (or initial weight). Finally, the sum of the initial volume (or initial weight) and the amount of diluent added will equal the final volume (or final weight). One can use the following equation for a dilution problem.

$$\text{Initial vol. (IV)} \times \text{Initial strength (IS)} = \text{Final vol. (FV)} \times \text{Final strength (FS)}$$

Let us look at the following example.

dilution The process of reducing the strength of a substance through the addition of an inert substance.

diluent An inert substance that reduces the strength of a substance.

EXAMPLE

A patient brings into the pharmacy a prescription for 1 L of a 30% isopropyl alcohol solution. The pharmacy stocks 70% isopropyl alcohol. How much of the 70% solution will the pharmacy technician use? How much diluent will the pharmacy technician use?

Let us look at what we know. What is the initial strength? 70%. What is the final concentration of the prescribed drug? 30%. How much are we to prepare? One liter (1000 mL). Since we have identified three of the four components of the equation, we can now calculate the quantity of 70% isopropyl alcohol needed for this preparation.

$$\text{Initial volume (IV)} \times (70\%) = (1000\text{ mL}) \times (30\%)$$

$$\text{Initial volume} = \frac{(1000\text{ mL}) \times (30\%)}{70\%}$$

Initial volume = 428.57 mL or 428.6 mL of 70% isopropyl alcohol is needed.

The second part of the question asks how much diluent will need to be added to prepare this solution. The amount of diluent to be added can be calculated by subtracting the initial volume from the final volume (Final volume − Initial volume = Amount of diluent to be added).

1000 mL − 428.6 ml = 571.4 mL of diluent

If the problem we just completed had the strengths expressed in either the form of a fraction or ratio, we could convert these strengths to percents as was discussed earlier in the chapter. One thing to remember is that the initial and final strength must be expressed in the same format.

Occasionally in the practice of pharmacy, the pharmacist or pharmacy technician may be asked to prepare a product that is more concentrated than the initial strength. This can be done by one of two means—evaporation of the liquid or by adding solute to the compound. Refer to Table 5-11 for hints in solving dilution problems. The previous formula can be used, but the following differences will occur:

- The final strength will be greater than the initial strength.
- The initial volume or weight will be greater than the final volume or weight.
- The initial volume or weight will be equal to the sum of the amount of diluent added and the final volume or weight.

Alligation Method

An **alligation** is an arithmetical method of solving problems that involve the mixing of solutions or mixtures of solids processing different percentage strengths and is utilized in pharmacy when a pharmacist or pharmacy technician is compounding either a solution or a solid. The strength being prepared is different from what they have on the shelf. In this situation,

Table 5-11 Hints in Solving Dilution Problems

1. The initial strength is always greater than the final strength in a dilution problem.
2. The final volume (or final weight) is greater than the initial volume (or initial weight).
3. The sum of the initial volume (or initial weight) and the amount of diluent added will equal the final volume (or final weight).

alligation An arithmetical method of solving problems that involves mixing solutions or mixtures of solids possessing different percentage strengths.

they have at least two different concentrations on the shelf—one that is greater than the desired concentration, and one that is less than the desired concentration. For example, a pharmacist receives an order to prepare 4 oz of a 10% solution using both a 25% and 5% solution. How much of each of these should the pharmacist use?

Step 1: Draw a tic-tac-toe table.

Step 2: Place the highest concentration in the upper left-hand corner, the lowest concentration in the lower left-hand corner, and the desired concentration in the middle.

25%		
	10% (4 oz)	
5%		

Step 3: Subtract the desired concentration from the highest concentration and place that number in the lower right-hand corner and express the answer as parts. Next, subtract the lowest concentration from the desired concentration, place that number in the upper right-hand corner, and label it as parts.

25%		5 parts
	10% (4 oz)	
5%		15 parts

Step 4: Total the number of parts: 5 + 15 parts = 20 parts.

Step 5: Set up a proportion using the parts of the highest and lowest concentration and the total quantity to be prepared.

$$25\%: \frac{5 \text{ parts}}{20 \text{ parts}} \times 4 \text{ oz} = 1 \text{ oz of } 25\% \text{ needed}$$

$$5\%: \frac{15 \text{ parts}}{20 \text{ parts}} \times 4 \text{ oz} = 3 \text{ oz of } 5\% \text{ needed}$$

Step 6: Check your work by adding the amounts of each concentration to see if they equal the amount to be compounded.

Specific Gravity

Specific gravity is defined as a ratio that compares the weight of a substance to an equal volume of a substance chosen as a standard (water). Mathematically, it can be written:

$$\text{Specific gravity} = \frac{\text{Weight of substance}}{\text{Weight of an equal volume of water}}$$

If a substance has a specific gravity of less than 1 that means the substance is lighter than water. If a substance has a specific gravity greater than 1 the substance is heavier than water. A pharmacy technician may need to use specific gravity when compounding a medication. Refer to Table 5-12 for specific gravity of various substances.

Table 5-12 Specific Gravity of Substances

Agent	Specific Gravity
Isopropyl alcohol	0.71
Alcohol	0.81
Liquid petrolatum	0.87
Water	1.00
Polysorbate 80	1.08
Polyethylene glycol 400	1.13
Glycerin	1.25
Syrup	1.31
Hydrochloric acid	1.37

Tech Check

47. Calculate the quantity of each ingredient required to make 480 mL of calamine lotion.(LO 5.27)

a. Calamine 80 g

b. Zinc oxide 80 g

c. Glycerin 20 g

d. Bentonite magma 250 mL

e. Calcium hydroxide topical solution qs 1000 mL

48. Calculate the following quantities of each ingredient required to make 1 lb (454 g) of the following ointment.(LO 5.27)

a. Coal tar 5 parts

b. Zinc oxide 10 parts

c. Hydrophilic ointment 50 parts

49. You receive a prescription to prepare 80 mL of a 0.5% boric acid solution. On the pharmacy shelf, you have 2.5% boric acid solution. How much of the 2.5% solution will you use and how much diluent?(LO 5.16)

50. A patient presents the pharmacy with a prescription for 120 mL of a 6% potassium chloride solution. Your pharmacy stocks only 20% potassium chloride solution. How much of the 20% solution will you use and how much diluent?(LO 5.16, 5.17)

51. You have received a medication order to prepare 30 mL of a 2:10 atropine solution for a physician. The pharmacy stocks a 2:8 solution of atropine. How many milliliters of a 2:8 solution will you use?(LO 5.16)

52. A patient presents you with a prescription for 60 mL of a 0.5% Zantac solution. How many milliliters of a 1.0% Zantac solution would you use?(LO 5.16)

53. What is the specific gravity of 100 mL of glycerin that weighs 125 g?(LO 5.28)

Intravenous Applications (LO 5.19, 5.20, 5.21)

Flow Rates

Pharmacists and pharmacy technicians do not administer injections, but they need to be able to interpret the physicians' orders for IV infusions and admixtures. The pharmacy staff may be called upon to assist nursing personnel in their calculations involving these dosage forms. Both pharmacists and pharmacy technicians must be able to calculate accurately the needs of patients when supplies are sent to nursing stations. It is the responsibility of the pharmacy staff to ensure that a patient's IV solution arrives prior to the designated time for it to be infused.

A rate is an infusion rate, synonymous with IV **flow rate**, is one of the ways prescribers in institutional pharmacies express the quantities of IV fluids needed by patients. These rates can be expressed in the following manner:

mL/h	milliliters per hour
gtts/min	drops per minute
X mL over *Z* h	milliliters over a number of hours
mg/min	milligram per minute (actual quantity of drug)

The formula for calculating a rate of infusion is:

Rate of infusion (R) =Volume of fluid to be infused (V)/Infusion time (T)

Any medication order must have two of the three parameters (R, V, or T) provided to calculate the missing parameter. The following are examples of the three basic relationships needed to master these calculations.

Calculating rate of infusion: Infuse 2 L normal saline (NS) over 24 hours. What is the rate in mL/h?

R = V/T, R = 2000 mL/24 h

R = 83 mL/h

Calculating time of infusion: 1 L D5W is to be infused at the rate of 125 mL/h. How long will the infusion last? How many 1 L IV bags will be needed in 1 day?

Infusion time:

R = V/T
125 mL/h = 1000 mL/T h
Cross multiply and solve for T
T × 125 = 1000 mL
T = 1000 mL/125 mL/h
T = 8 h

Number of bags for 1-day supply: 1 day = 24 h

From the above calculation, it takes 8 hours to infuse 1 L (1000 mL) = 1 bag. One can calculate the number of bags needed in 24 hours by using a proportion method.

8 h: 1 bag: 24: X bags

X = 24/8 = 3 bags

flow rate A comparison of two measurements with different types of units. In the practice of pharmacy, one of the units compared is time.

Time of supply: IV infusions are administered in institutions using military time, thus 0000 (12 midnight) to 2400 hr (12 midnight the following day). Medical administration records will indicate what times medications are to be administered. In providing IV infusions at the right time, the pharmacy staff must be able to calculate what period an IV infusion is to be provided and what quantity to provide to meet the needs of the patient.

EXAMPLE

A 1000 mL IV solution is to run at the rate of 120 mL/h starting at 0800 hours. When will the infusion end?

Step 1: Calculate the number of hours it will take the IV infusion to run using the formula:

R = V/T

120 mL/h = 1000 mL/T

T = 8.33 h.

Converting 0.33 h to minutes gives

0.33 h × 60 min = 20 min

T = 8 h 20 min

Step 2: Starting at 0800 hr and running the IVF at the rate provided, the IV fluid will run out at 08.00 + 8 h 20 min = 1620 hours (or 4:20 pm).

Calculating volume of infusion: An IV fluid is running at 150 mL/h. How many 1-L bags will be needed in 2 days?

R = V / T

In this case T = 2 days = 48 h

150 = V / 48

V = 150 × 48 = 7200 mL

1 bag = 1000 mL, 7200 mL = 7200/1000 bags = 7.2 1-L bags

Pharmacy will supply 8 bags!

Administration Sets and the Drop Factor

Many times IV infusion rates are written in drops per minute (gtts/min) rather than in milliliters per hour (mL/hr). This introduces a new factor to our general equation and depends on the equipment selected by the nursing staff to administer the infusion. *This factor does not change the rate of infusion. It only expresses the rate in a different unit.*

The drop factor (DF), as it is commonly known, converts the volume delivered in milliliters to drops when a specific size of IV administration set is selected. An administration set, for example, with a DF of 10 converts each milliliter of IV fluid administered to 10 gtts. The three most common administration sets are those with a DF of 10 gtts/mL, 15 gtts/mL, and 60 gtts/mL (this administration set is also referred to as a microdrip or minidrip set). Each sterile pack of an administration set will always have its DF printed on the pack. Selecting the required set is therefore not a problem. After converting mL to drops with the DF, the time of infusion is then converted to minutes from hours.

EXAMPLE

An IV infusion is running at 83 mL/h. What is the rate in drops per minute when using a 15 gtts/mL administration set?

$$83 \text{ mL/h} = X \text{ gtts/min}$$

First, convert mL to drops using the DF for the admin set.

$$83 \text{ mL} = (83 \times 15) \text{ drops}$$

Then use the smaller period, minutes, so that both sides of the equation are expressed in the same units:

$$(83 \text{ mL} \times 15 \text{ gtts/mL})/60 \text{ min} = X \text{ gtts/min}$$

$$X = 20.7 \text{ gtts/min; Approx. } 21 \text{ gtts/min}$$

Please note the above IV fluid at the rate of 83 mL/h is the same as running the IV fluid at the rate of 21 gtts/min.

Calculating the Drop Factor

Sometimes nurses have to determine the size of administration set (DF) to select based on a doctor's prescription. For example, if the nursing staff were instructed to infuse 1 L NS at the rate of 42 gtts/min over 24 hours, what DF should be used? Using the formula of R = V/T, the rate has been provided as drops per minute. The rate, in milliliters per hour, can also be determined using the volume and time of infusion given:

$$R = 1000 \text{ mL/24 h}$$

$$1000 \text{ mL/24 h} = 41.7 \text{ mL/h}$$

Since the DF only converts milliliters per hour to drops per minute, the two rates must be equal. Therefore,

$$41.7 \text{ mL/h} = 42 \text{ gtts/min}$$

Convert mL to drops by multiplying by the DF and convert hours to minutes by multiplying by 60, giving the following:

$$41.7 \times \text{DF}/1 \text{ h} \times 60 \text{ min} = 42 \text{ gtts/min}$$

$$\text{DF} = 42 \times 60/41.7 = \text{Approx. } 60 \text{ gtts/mL}$$

$$\text{DF} = 60 \text{ gtts/mL (the microdrip) is the answer.}$$

Infusions Containing Medications

The calculation of the rate at which a medication is administered via an IV fluid is one of the most important duties of an institutional pharmacy staff. The flow rate, or quantity of drug given over a period, can be calculated in the same manner using the same mathematical relationships stated in the previous examples.

EXAMPLE

5000 units heparin in 1 L NS is administered over 12 hours using a microdrip administration set. How many units of heparin is the patient receiving every minute?

Step 1: Calculate the rate in milliliters per hour:

1000 mL/12 h = 83.3 mL/h

5000 units heparin in 1000 mL NS

is 5 units/mL NS

The patient will be receiving 83.3 mL × 5 units heparin per hour based on the rate calculated in milliliters per hour above. Therefore, the patient is receiving 416.5 units/h.

Step 2: Calculate the number of units/min:

Units/min = 416.5/60 min = 6.94 units/min or 7 units/min

Tech Check

54. 1 L NS is to be administered over 24 hours. The administration set to be used has a drop factor of 15 gtts/mL. What is the rate of infusion in milliliters per hour? (LO 5.19)

55. Calculate the infusion rate in milliliters per hour and drops per minute for 1 L NS administered over 10 hours using an administration set that is calibrated at 60 gtts/mL. (LO 5.19)

56. 500 mL of NS is to be run at a rate of 125 mL/hr using a drop factor of 15 gtts/mL. Calculate the infusion in drops per minute. How many bags will be needed for 2 days? (LO 5.19)

Chapter Summary

Pharmacy calculations are performed in all pharmacy practices. Calculations are used to determine the appropriate dosage for a patient, to calculate the correct quantities in compounding medications, and to figure out the correct days supply of medication being billed to an insurance provider. It is extremely important that pharmacy technicians check their calculations three times before they ask the pharmacist to recheck them. A miscalculation may have a significant impact on a patient's recovery and could even be fatal.

It is important to remember the following:

- Pharmacy technicians encounter both Arabic numbers and Roman numerals every day when they are processing prescription and medication orders.
- A medication's strength can be expressed as a fraction, ratio, or percent. Often a pharmacy technician may be required to convert a strength from one form to another form when preparing an order.
- Pharmacy practice has utilized many different systems of measurement (apothecary, avoirdupois, metric, and household systems) throughout the years. Pharmacy technicians must be able to convert from one system to another based upon the physician's order.
- Drug literature may express the storage conditions of a particular medication in either Celsius or Fahrenheit temperatures.
- Pharmacy technicians must be able to interpret a prescription/medication order properly to ensure the patient is receiving the correct drug in the proper strength at the correct time.
- Third-party providers may place limits on the

quantity of medication that can be dispensed at a particular time and therefore the proper days supply is calculated for reimbursement.

- Calculating the correct dosage of a medication can be affected by the patient's age, weight, height, or body surface area.
- Compounding a medication requires the pharmacy technician to calculate the correct quantities of each ingredient to prepare the medication as ordered by the physician.
- In a hospital setting, pharmacy technicians use calculations in determining the number of IV bags to be sent to the patients' floor at the correct time.
- The practice of pharmacy utilizes mathematics every day.

Chapter Review

Case Study Questions

1. How many milligrams of the medication does the order call for?(LO 5.6)
2. How many milliliters of the oral suspension would the patient need to take for each dose?(LO 5.6)
3. How many teaspoons of the oral suspension would the patient need to take for each dose?(LO 5.6)
4. Is the dosage ordered reasonable?(LO 5.6)

At Your Service Questions

1. Was the dose appropriate for Brandon?(LO 5.15)
2. Was the amount of water added to the powder correct for the desired dose?(LO 5.16)
3. How would you explain to Mary Lock the relationship between milliliters and teaspoons?(LO 5.16)

Multiple Choice

1. What is the Arabic number represented by XXIV?(LO 5.1)
   a. 26
   b. 35
   c. 14
   d. 24
2. 4/5 × 3/5 is equal to
   a. 12/5
   b. 7/5
   c. 7/25
   d. 12/25
3. 21/25 is equal to
   a. 0.75
   b. 0.48
   c. 0.84
   d. 0.43
4. 3/8 is equal to
   a. 375%
   b. 37.5%
   c. 3.75%
   d. 0.375%
5. 40 g is equal to
   a. 40,000 kg
   b. 400 cg
   c. 400 mg
   d. 40,000 mg
6. 4 teaspoons is equal to
   a. 20 mL
   b. 15 mL
   c. 10 mL
   d. 5 mL

7. Eight fluid ounces is equal to
   a. 16 teaspoons
   b. 240 mg
   c. 240 mL
   d. 24 tablespoons
8. Which of the following pairs has the same time correctly written two different ways?(LO 5.8)
   a. 1430 and 4:30 pm
   b. 0000 and 2400
   c. 5:00 am and 500
   d. 0000 and noon
9. It is now 10:00 pm What time will it be in 6 1/2 hours?(LO 5.8)
   a. 1630
   b. 1650
   c. 0430
   d. 0450
10. A drug order reads 1.5 mL IM qid. How many milliliters will be needed for 1 day?(LO 5.10)
    a. 3 mL
    b. 4.5 mL
    c. 0.6 mL
    d. 6 mL
11. A drug order reads 300 mg twice a day. The medication comes in 150-mg tablets. What is the desired dose?(LO 5.13)
    a. 600 mg
    b. 300 mg
    c. 2 tablets
    d. 4 tablets

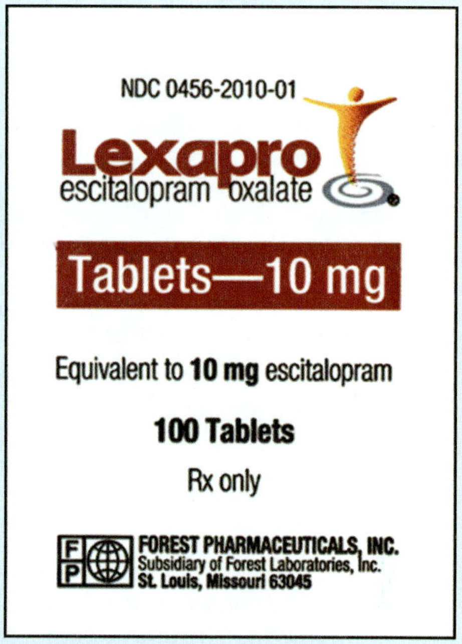

12. Referring to the label above, which of the following is false?(LO 5.11)
    a. The medication should be refrigerated.
    b. The usual dose is one tablet daily.
    c. The generic name is escitalopram oxalate.
    d. The trade name is Lexapro.

Applying Pharmacy Calculations

Solve the following pharmacy calculations.

1. The pharmacist receives a prescription for a patient for potassium phosphate 4.4 mEq/mL. The physician has prescribed the patient to receive 25 mEq with each dose. How many milliliters will the patient receive as a dose?(LO 5.23, 5.25)
2. A patient is to receive 220,000 units of Nystatin Oral Suspension for each dose. Nystatin is available as a 100,000 units/mL suspension. How many milliliters will the patient receive with each dose?(LO 5.23, 5.25)
3. From the following formula for hydrophilic petrolatum, calculate the quantities of each ingredient to make 1 pound of product.(LO 5.27)

Stearyl alcohol	3 parts
White wax	8 parts
White petrolatum	86 parts

4. From the following formula, calculate the quantities required to make 1 gallon of phenobarbital elixir.(LO 5.27)

Phenobarbital	4 g
Orange oil	0.25 mL
Certified red color	qs
Alcohol	200 mL
Propylene glycol	100 mL
Sorbitol solution	600 mL
Water, to make	1000 mL

5. If 500 tablets contain 1.5 g of active ingredient, how many grams of ingredient will be needed to produce 1375 tablets?(LO 5.27)
6. The temperature in the pharmacy refrigerator is 15°C, what is the temperature in Fahrenheit?(LO 5.7)
7. If an IV solution fluid is adjusted to deliver 20 mg of medication to a patient per hour,

how many milligrams are delivered per minute?(LO 5.19)

8. The pharmacy receives the following prescription:(LO 5.10)

   Premarin 0.625 mg #100
   1 tab qd

   How many days will the prescription last?

9. A patient brings in the following prescription:(LO 5.10)

   Atrovent Inhalation Solution 0.02% 2.5 mL* 25 vials.
   One vial qid

   How many days will the prescription last?

10. A patient weighs 84 lb and is receiving ampicillin at a rate of 100 mg/kg/day. What is the total daily dose in grams?(LO 5.15)

11. Calculate the dose for a child 6 years of age with an adult dose of 100 mg.(LO 5.15)

12. A 45-lb child is to receive 5 mg of phenytoin per kilogram of body weight daily as an anticonvulsant. How many milliliters of a pediatric phenytoin suspension containing 30 mg per 5 mL should the child receive?(LO 5.15)

13. A patient has a BSA of 1.94. The physician orders a daily dose of 900 mg/m2 of methotrexate for the patient. What is the daily dose, in milliliters, if the concentration of methotrexate is 25 mg/mL?(LO 5.15)

14. If a potassium chloride elixir contains 20 mEq of potassium ions in each 15 mL of elixir, how many milliliters will provide 25 mEq of potassium ions to each patient?(LO 5.25)

15. A patient is using Lantus Insulin (100 units/mL) and is to use 25 units. How many milliliters will the patient inject?(LO 5.25)

16. A patient is to receive 2000 units of heparin. Heparin is available as 5000 units/mL. How many milliliters do you prepare for the patient?(LO 5.25)

17. From the following formula, calculate the quantity of each ingredient required to make 454 g of powder:(LO 5.27)

Calcium carbonate	5 parts
Magnesium oxide	1 part
Sodium bicarbonate	4 parts
Bismuth subcarbonate	3 parts

18. A prescription is written for a mouthwash consisting of the following:(LO 5.27)

Diphenhydramine elixir	170 mL
Lidocaine viscous	50 mL
Nystatin suspension	200 mL
Erythromycin ethyl succinate suspension	52 mL
Cherry syrup	28 mL

   How much of each ingredient should be used in preparing 1 gallon of the suspension?(LO 5.27)

19. A substance weighs 200 g/100 mL. What is the specific gravity?(LO 5.28)

20. The dose of a certain antibiotic is 5 mg per kg of body weight. How many milligrams should be used for a person weighing 145 lb?(LO 5.15)

21. The order is for morphine 3 mg. The label reads morphine 1/10 gr/mL. How many milliliters would you give?(LO 5.6)

22. If a prescription reads Theophylline Elixir 80 mg/15 mL, what is the dose in teaspoonfuls if the required dose is 120 mg?(LO 5.6)

23. The average adult dose of amoxicillin is 500 mg tid. If the child is 4 years old and 45 lb, what would the dose be for this child using both Young's Rule and Clark's Rule?(LO 5.15)

24. The usual pediatric dose of cefazolin sodium is 25 mg/kg/day divided equally into three doses. What would be the single dose in milligrams for a child weighing 44 lb?(LO 5.15)

25. Insulin is available in a concentration of 100 units/mL. A patient order reads 0.8 unit/kg/day in divided doses. The patient weighs 102 lb. How many milliliters should the patient receive each day?(LO 5.25)

26. How many grams of amino acid are contained in 500 mL of 9.5% solution?(LO 5.27)

27. You need to prepare 4 oz of a 2% zinc oxide ointment. How many grams of zinc oxide powder will be needed to prepare this ointment?(LO 5.16)

28. You want to make 2 fl oz of a 6% potassium chloride solution and you have in stock a 20% solution. How many milliliters of the 20% solution will you need?(LO 5.16)

29. A prescription reads cefaclor 250 mg/5 mL. The directions read 375 mg bid × 10 days. What is the dose in teaspoons?(LO 5.6)

30. The order calls for quart of a 5% Lugol's solution and you have in stock 15% Lugol's solution. How many millilitres of the 15% Lugol's solution are needed to fill this order?(LO 5.16, 5.17)

31. You are asked to prepare 50 mL of a 1:100 Rifampin suspension and you have in stock a 1:20 Rifampin suspension. How many milliliters of the 1:20 suspension will you need?(LO 5.16, 5.17)

32. A pharmacist has weighed out 3 g of coal tar and has given it to the pharmacy technician to compound a 1% ointment. What will be the weight of the final product?(LO 5.16,17)
33. You are asked to prepare 60 mL of a 0.5 mg/mL Zantac solution and you have in stock a 1 mg/mL solution. How many milliliters of the 1 mg/mL solution will you use?(LO 5.16, 5.17)
34. You have a 70% solution and a 15% solution, and you are asked to make 480 mL of a 30% solution. What parts of each strength will be used and what will be the final volume of each needed for the prescription?(LO 5.16, 5.17)
35. How much 10% and 60% dextrose solution should be mixed to make 2 L of a 40% dextrose solution?(LO 5.18)
36. Prepare 2 L of a 1/8% solution from a 10% stock solution. How much water was added?
37. You are asked to prepare 500 mL of D10W. You have available to use sterile water and D20W. How many milliliters of each will you use?(LO 5.18)
38. A prescription is written for Dilantin 5% in zinc oxide qs 120 g. How many Dilantin 50-mg tablets are needed to prepare this compound?(LO 5.16)
39. A prescription is written for salicylic acid 1%, menthol 1/4% in triamcinolone 0.1% cream. How much salicylic acid powder should be used if the prescription is for 240 g?(LO 5.9, 5.16)
40. You need to prepare 16 fl oz of potassium bromide 250 mg/mL. How many grams of potassium bromide should you weigh?(LO 5.6, 5.16)
41. A prescription is written for a mouthwash containing the following:(LO 5.26, 5.27)

Diphenhydramine elixir	170 mL
Lidocaine viscous	50 mL
Nystatin suspension	200 mL
Erythromycin ethyl succinate suspension	52 mL
Cherry syrup to make 500 mL mouthwash	28 mL

How much lidocaine viscous would be needed if you needed to prepare only 100 mL of the mouthwash?(LO 5.9, 5.20, 5.27)

42. A 500-mL bag of TPN runs at 60 gtts/min using a microdrip administration set.
    a. How long will the infusion run?(LO 5.19)
    b. If the infusion was started at 1300 hr, when will the infusion be completed?(LO 5.8, 5.19)
43. A patient is to receive 1000 units of heparin per hour from a 250 mL 1/2 NS containing 25,000 units heparin. At what rate in millimeters per hour should the solution be administered?(LO 5.19)
44. Augmentin 500 mg in 200 mL NS is administered over 1 hour q8h. With an admin set calibrated at 10 gtts/mL calculate(LO 5.20,5.21, 5.26)
    a. the rate in gtts/min.
    b. the milligrams of Augmentin per day.
45. You are asked to prepare a 100-mL piggyback containing 250 mg of drug A. The drug is to be infused over 1/2 hour using a kit that delivers 30 gtts/mL. What is the rate in drops per minute?(LO 5.21)
46. If a 1000 mL bag of 0.9% sodium chloride solution is run at 100 mL/hr, how long will the bag last?(LO 5.19)
47. How many milliliters of IV fluid will a patient receive if infused at the rate of 120 mL/h over 3 1/2 hours?(LO 5.x)
48. A patient is to receive 30 mEq potassium chloride in 1000 mL NS at the rate of 125 mL/h. How many milliequivalents per hour will the patient be receiving?(LO 5.19, 5.25)
49. What will be the rate in drops per minute if a patient receives 1 L IVF over an 8-hour period (use the conversion factor of DF = 15 gtts/mL)(LO 5. x)
50. 1000 mL of Lactated Ringers Solution is to be given every 8 hours.(LO 5.10, 5.19, 5.21)
    a. How many 1000-mL bags should be given each day?
    b. How many milliliters per hour will the patient receive?
    c. How many milliliters per minute will the patient receive?
    d. How many drops per minute will the patient receive using a 15 gtts/mL kit?

Critical Thinking Questions

1. Which of the following methods (using age, weight, or body surface area) is the most accurate in calculating the correct dose for a patient and why?(LO5.15)
2. Visit a local pharmacy and select an OTC medication. Identify on the label the following information: drug name, dosage form, dosage strength, route of administration, and the proper storage conditions of the medication.(LO5.11)
3. While working in a pharmacy, interpret a prescription or medication order, and calculate the days supply for the prescription.(LO 5.9, 5.10)

HIPAA Scenario

Janet Brown works at a pharmacy in downtown Kansas City. On Monday she received a fax from another pharmacy containing prescription information on a patient. Janet placed the fax on the counter in the staff break area because she did not know who requested it. The fax had no header and when Janet called the pharmacy that sent the fax, the secretary there did not know who requested the information either. She told Janet, "Someone from your pharmacy asked for it. I don't remember who." Janet left the fax in the break area and eventually forgot about it.

Discussion Questions (PTCB II. 73)

1. Should Janet have done anything differently? If so, what?
2. What consequences could occur based upon Janet's actions?
3. Is there anything that the secretary at the other pharmacy could have done differently?

Internet Activities

Go to the Web site **http://rxlist.com/** to find the information needed to answer the following questions.

The physician has ordered Lasix 60 mg po stat for an adult patient suffering from edema.

1. What is the generic name of Lasix?(LO 5.11)
2. In what strengths are Lasix tablets available?(LO 5.11)
3. Which strength would you administer to the patient and how many tablets would you need to give?(LO 5.13)

The physician has ordered ranitidine 600 mg po bid.

1. What is the trade name of ranitidine?(LO 5.11)
2. You have 150-mg tablets available. What is the amount to administer for one dose? Does this seem reasonable to you?(LO 5.13)

Introduction to Pharmacology

6

Learning Outcomes

Upon completion of this chapter, you will be able to:

6.1 Differentiate between the following terms: *pharmacology, pharmacokinetics, pharmacy,* and *toxicology*.

6.2 Discuss the principles affecting pharmacokinetics.

6.3 Explain the processes (absorption, distribution, metabolism, and elimination) involved in pharmacokinetics.

6.4 Explain the factors affecting the absorption of a drug.

6.5 Explain the issues affecting the distribution of a drug in the body.

6.6 Explain the factors affecting the metabolism of a drug in the body.

6.7 Explain the factors affecting the elimination of a drug in the body.

6.8 Identify factors affecting the selection of a proper dosing schedule for a medication.

6.9 Discuss the function of a dose-effect curve and factors that may change the shape of it.

6.10 Differentiate among hyperreactivity, hyporeactivity, supersensitivity, tolerance, tachyphylaxis, and idiosyncrasy.

6.11 Identify factors that modify the effects of medication.

6.12 Explain the meaning of "mechanism of action" as it applies to pharmacy.

6.13 Explain the selective action of drugs including drug receptors and site of action.

6.14 Compare and contrast the various routes of administration for medication.

6.15 Differentiate between bioavailability and bioequivalence.

6.16 Define a drug and the various names given to a drug.

6.17 Identify and explain the terminology associated with pharmacology.

6.18 Differentiate between the various types of side effects.

6.19 Distinguish between the two types of addiction.

6.20 Explain the effect medications can have on pregnancy and the pregnancy codes developed by the FDA.

Key Terms

absorption
acid
active transport
ADME process
adverse effect
affinity
agonist
antagonism
antagonist
base
bioavailability
brand name
chemical name
competitive antagonist
diffusion
drug
drug contraindication
drug-disease contraindication
ED50
efficacy
enteral administration
generic name
half-life (t1/2)
hepatic
LD50
loading dose

Key Terms

maintenance dose
mechanism of action
parenteral administration
passive transport
pharmacokinetics
potency
potentiation
prophylactic dose
receptor site
side effect
site of action
therapeutic index (TI)
toxic effects

Case Study

Andrew was assisting the pharmacist in the pharmacy one day when he noticed they were filling many prescriptions for Werdna, a new anticoagulant for patients with artificial heart valves. Werdna is available as an oral tablet and a subcutaneous injection. Andrew noticed that the dosage for Werdna varied from patient to patient regardless of weight, height, age, or sex. He was extremely perplexed because patients who weighed more than the other patients did not necessarily require more medication than those patients who weighed less. He noticed the amount prescribed orally was greater than the amount prescribed subcutaneously. He asked the pharmacist to explain why the dosing varied significantly. The pharmacist explained that the pharmacokinetics of the medication affected the dosage prescribed by the physician.

While reading this chapter, keep the following question in mind:

1. What factors affect the absorption, distribution, metabolism, and elimination of the drug?(LO 6.4, 6.5, 6.6, 6.7)

PTCB

In preparation for the certification examination, you should understand and perform activities associated with the following PTCB Knowledge Statements:

PTCB Knowledge Statement — *Domain I. Assisting the Pharmacist in Serving Patients*

- Knowledge of therapeutic equivalence (6)
- Knowledge of drug interactions (12)
- Knowledge of effects of patient's age (14)
- Knowledge of pharmacology (16)
- Knowledge of common and severe side effects or adverse effects, allergies, and therapeutic contraindications associated with medications (17)
- Knowledge of drug indications (18)
- Knowledge of drug stability (52)

PTCB Knowledge Statement — *Domain II. Maintaining Medication and Inventory Control Systems*

- Knowledge of bioavailability standards (8)

Introduction to Pharmacology(LO 6.16)

A **drug** is defined as any chemical agent that affects living processes. Drugs are prescribed and administered to prevent, diagnose, treat, or cure a disease. Medications are derived and produced from a variety of sources. These include plants (digoxin, quinine, and codeine), animals (Premarin), and minerals (silver nitrate). A medication may be made synthetically (acetaminophen) or through biotechnological processes (erythropoietin).

A medication may have multiple names and they include:

- **Chemical name,** which is a description of the chemical structure of a drug. A chemical name is an extremely long name that contains short syllables and numbers. The chemical name for the antibiotic Zithromax is

drug Any chemical agent that affects living processes.

chemical name Description of the chemical structure of a drug.

(2R,3R,4R,5R,8R,10R,11R,12S,13S,14R)-13-[(2,6-dideoxy-3-C-methyl-3-O-methyl-a-L-ribo-hexopyranosyl)oxy]-2-ethyl-3,4,10-trihydroxy-3,5,6,8,10,12,14-heptamethyl-11[(3,4,6,-trideoxy-3-(dimethylamino)-B-D-xylo-hexopyranosy)]-1-oxa-6-azacyclopentadecan-15-one.

- **Generic name** (nonproprietary name) is the name given to a drug by its drug manufacturer. It is also referred to as the United States Adopted Name (USAN). The generic name is not protected under trademark law. Generic names begin with lowercase letters. (*Note:* Often doctors capitalize the first letter of the name even if it is a generic drug.) The generic name for Zithromax is azithromycin.
- **Brand name** (proprietary or trade name) is assigned by the drug manufacturer and is protected under trademark law. Only the drug manufacturer is permitted to use the trade name. All brand names will have a generic and chemical name but not all generic names will have a brand name. Trade names begin with uppercase (capital) letters. The brand name for azithromycin is Zithromax.

Terms Associated with Pharmacology (LO 6.1, 6.8, 6.10, 6.12, 6.13, 6.17)

Pharmacology is a science that deals with the knowledge of:

- History of a drug
- Source of a drug
- Physical and chemical properties of a drug

generic name The nonproprietary name given to a drug by its drug manufacturer.

brand name The proprietary or trade name assigned by the drug manufacturer and protected under trademark law.

At Your Service

One of your patients, Mary Smith, brings in her prescription of naproxen to be refilled at your pharmacy. During her visit she informs you that she has been experiencing stomach problems, such as heartburn, after taking the medication. In addition, she mentions that she becomes extremely tired when taking her medicine. The patient asks you if she is taking her medication properly and informs you she is taking it on an empty stomach like she does with her other prescription medications.

While reading this chapter, keep the following question in mind.

1. Is this a side effect of naproxen and what should she do? (LO 6.11)

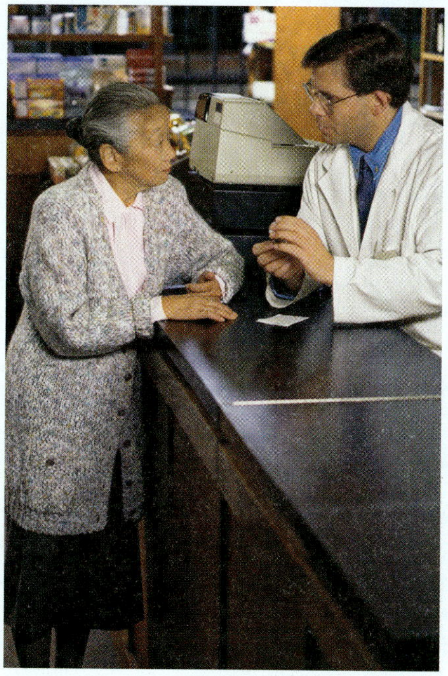

- Compounding of a drug
- Biochemical and physiological effects of a drug
- Mechanisms of action of a drug
- Absorption, distribution, biotransformation, and excretion of a drug
- Therapeutic use of a drug

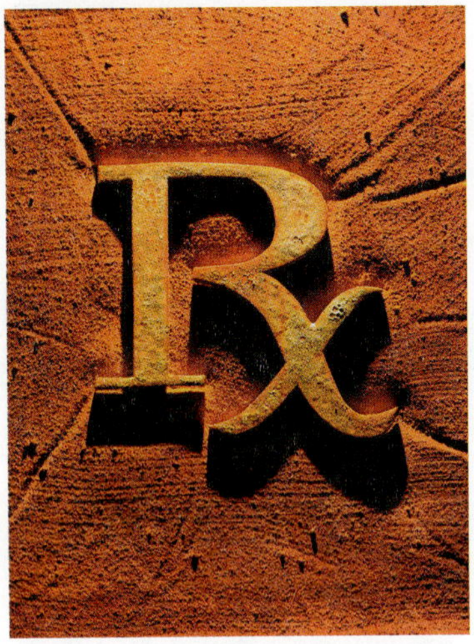

Pharmacology requires an individual to understand how the human body works. The human body wishes to maintain a level of homeostasis (balance) throughout it at all times. It must be able to communicate with the cells, tissues, organs, and body systems in order to maintain homeostasis. This is accomplished by having a "messenger" produced by the cell and sent to other cells in the human body through extracellular liquids. Examples of these messengers in the body include histamine and prostaglandin.

These messengers communicate to specific cells known as a "target cells." Each target cell possesses receptors, which are molecules located on the cell and that bind with specific molecules. The body has a multitude of receptors that perform many different functions. This interaction is referred to as specificity. An analogy of this relationship can be described as a key and a lock, where only a specific key can open a particular lock.

Every medication possesses specific actions and produces an effect on a specific condition. Many drugs can produce multiple effects on the body. A drug is usually described by its most prominent effect or by the action thought to be the basis of the effect. The intended effect of a drug is referred to as its therapeutic effect. The therapeutic effect of a drug that is used for a specific purpose is known as the indication of a drug. A **drug contraindication** is a condition when a drug is not indicated and should not be prescribed. A **drug-disease contraindication** is one where the administration of a drug should be avoided because it may worsen the patient's condition.

An undesired effect of a drug can be classified as a **side effect, adverse effect,** or **toxic effect.** A side effect is not necessarily harmful and is accepted by an individual. Common side effects include nausea, vomiting, headaches, constipation, and diarrhea. An adverse effect is a side effect that occurs for a longer period than a side effect and is more intense. Examples of an adverse effect include mental confusion, tachycardia (rapid heartbeat), or difficulty in urinating. Often adverse effects can be reduced by lowering the drug dosage for the patient.

Toxic effects are more serious than either side or adverse effects. They may be extremely dangerous and may become fatal if they continue in an individual. Many drugs can cause toxic effects if the dosage of the drug is excessive; this includes acetaminophen. The **LD50,** lethal dose 50, is a test performed to determine a drugs safety, and refers to the lethal dose of a drug that will kill 50% of the animals it is tested on. The LD50 is used in predicting the safety of a drug.

The **ED50** is the amount of drug needed to produce one-half of the maximum response. This ratio indicates the relative safety of a drug.

The **therapeutic index (TI)** is a ratio of the lethal dose 50 (LD50) compared to the effective dose 50 (ED50).

If the LD50 were 500 mg and the ED50 were 25 mg, the therapeutic index would be expressed as:

$$\text{TI} = \text{LD50}/\text{ED50} = 500\text{ mg}/25\text{ mg} = 20$$

drug contraindication Condition when a drug is not indicated and should not be prescribed.

drug-disease contraindication Condition when administration of a drug should be avoided because it may worsen the patient's condition.

side effect Drug effect other than the therapeutic effect that is undesirable but not harmful.

adverse effect A physical effect that occurs for a longer period than a side effect and is usually more intense.

toxic effect More serious than either a side or adverse effect. It may be extremely dangerous and may become fatal if it continues in an individual.

LD50 Lethal dose 50—lethal dose of a drug that will kill 50% of the animals it is tested on.

therapeutic index (TI) Ratio of lethal dose 50 (LD 50) compared to the effective dose 50 (ED50).

ED50 Effective dose 50—amount of drug needed to produce one-half of the maximum response.

This ratio indicates that 20 times the amount of the drug is needed to produce a lethal effect in 50% of the animals tested as needed to produce a therapeutic effect in 50% of the animals tested.

A drug will not provide the same effect in all patients, and a patient may not experience the same effect (both desired and undesired effects) every time he or she takes the medication. Specific terms are used to refer to patients who are sensitive or resistant to a drug or experience an unusual effect of the drug.

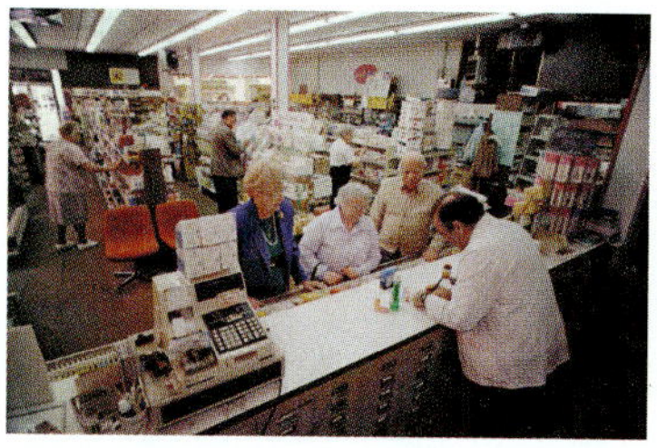

- Hyperreactivity—when a patient experiences the desired effect at a low dosage
- Hyporeactivity—when a patient experiences the desired effect only at high dosages
- Supersensitivity—increased sensitivity to a drug resulting in denervation
- Tolerance—a decreased sensitivity to a drug because of exposure to the drug
- Tachyphylaxis—tolerance that develops after a few doses of the drug has been taken
- Idiosyncrasy—an unusual effect of a drug regardless of the intensity or the dosage

Other terms are used in the subject of pharmacology, and it is important to have an understanding of them. The **site of action** of a drug refers to the place in the body where the drug produces its effect. In some situations, the site of effect may not be known. **Mechanism of action** describes how a drug produces its effect and sometimes the drug is classified by this means. For instance, a selective serotonin reuptake inhibitor (SSRI) is used in the treatment of depression. SSRI describes its mechanism of action and the term is given to those drugs that act in the same manner.

The **receptor site** identifies the exact cell site on a specific cell where a drug produces its effect. Many drug receptor sites have been identified, but some have not. A drug that binds to a specific receptor and produces a specific drug action is known as an **agonist.** An agonistic drug will produce a predictable therapeutic action. An agonist possess two key properties—affinity and efficacy. **Affinity** refers to the ability of a drug to bind to the cell structure. **Efficacy** refers to how successful a drug is able to produce its effect.

An **antagonist** is a drug that does not bind to a specific site. It is sometimes referred to as a "blocking agent" because it prevents a drug from producing its effect. Antagonists interact selectively with the receptors. A **competitive antagonist** is a drug that competes for a specific site on a cell that an agonist is attempting to use. Some medications may produce their effect by interacting with chemically nonspecific membrane lipids. Other drugs may work with enzymes, transport proteins, and nucleic acids. Others may act without any direct interaction of the cell. Naloxone is an example of a drug used for its antagonistic properties in the treatment of a drug overdose caused by certain pain medications. The drug (agonist or antagonist) with the greatest number of receptor sites will produce the effect. Refer to Figure 6-1 (p. 174).

site of action Place in the body where the drug produces its effect.

mechanism of action Explanation of how a drug produces its effects.

receptor site Identifies the exact cell site on a specific cell where a drug produces its effect.

agonist Drug that binds to a specific receptor and produces a specific drug action.

affinity A drug's ability to bind to the cell structure.

efficacy Describes how successful a drug is able to produce its effect.

antagonist A drug that does not bind to a specific site.

competitive antagonist A drug that competes for a specific site on a cell that an agonist is attempting to use.

potency A measure of the strength or concentration of a drug to produce a specific effect.

Medication Dosing

Potency refers to a measure of the strength or concentration of a drug to produce a specific effect. The potency of a drug is affected by the absorption,

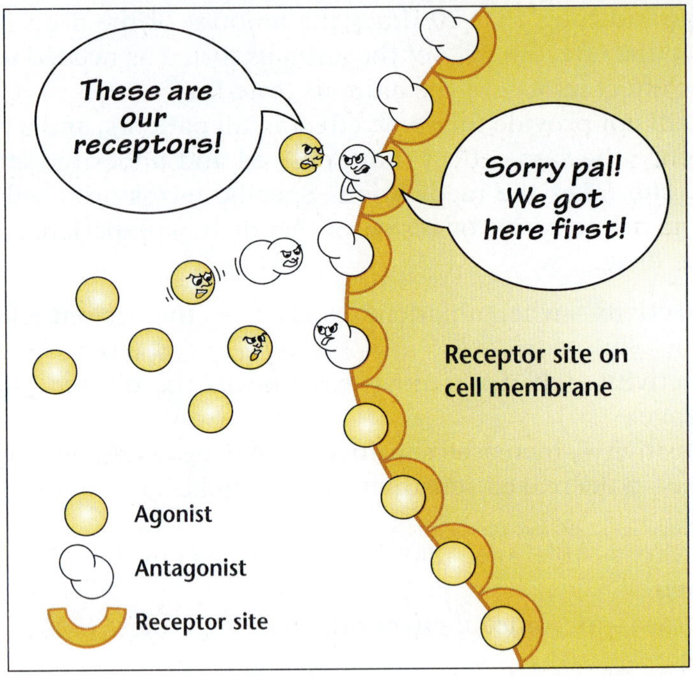

Figure 6-1 Competitive antagonism.

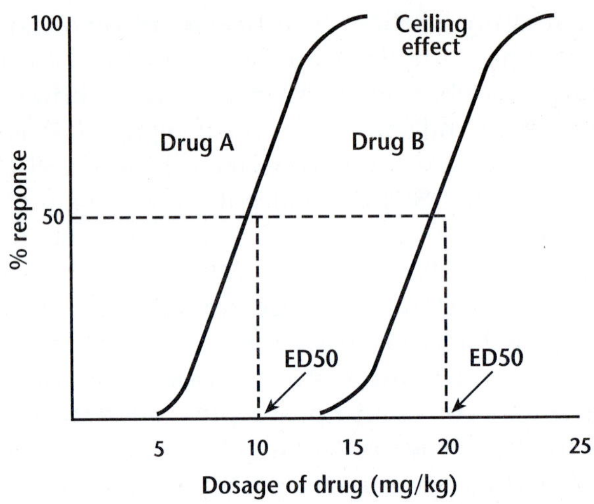

Figure 6-2 Dose-response curve.

distribution, metabolism, and elimination of the drug and the ability of the drug to bind with its receptors. A drug's potency is unimportant because it makes little difference whether the effective dose of a drug is 1 mg or 100 mg but rather that it is administered in proper dosage. Studies have not shown that the more potent of two drugs is necessarily superior to the other one. A low potency is a drawback only if the effective dose is so large that it is awkward to administer to the patient.

The response of a drug is affected by the amount of drug (dose) given to a patient to produce a therapeutic effect under stable conditions. The dose-effect relationship commonly occurs after taking one dose of the medication. The relationship between a dose and its response can be plotted as a graph and is referred to as a dose-response curve, which is shown in Figure 6-2 comparing two different drugs.

The dose-response is proportional to the amount of the dose. As the dose increases, the amount of the response will increase. Conversely, if the dose is reduced the response will decrease. The ceiling effect of a drug is the amount of drug that will not produce an additional response. Often a dose above the ceiling effect may produce undesirable side effects, adverse effects, or possibly toxic effects. Drugs within the same drug classification may be more potent than other drugs and will require a smaller dosage to produce the ceiling effect. An example of this occurs with the HMG CoA reductase inhibitors where pravastatin 40 mg produces the same effect as simvastatin 20 mg as does atorvastatin 10 mg.

A time-response curve is used to illustrate the relationship between the plasma concentration of a drug and the time to obtain the concentration. A time-response curve will show the:

- Onset of action (the first observable effects of a drug)
- Duration of action (the length of time a drug continues to produce an affect)
- Termination of the action of the drug (where the effect is no longer observed)

Figure 6-3 depicts a time-response curve.

The effect of a single dose of medication may be characterized by the time it takes for an effect to be observed, the amount of time to obtain the maximum effect of a drug, and its duration of effect. Differences in the rate of absorption can occur due to different routes of administration or dosage forms. This can have a significant impact on the drug concentration and its affect. As the dosage of a drug is increased, the amount of time for the effect to be observed is reduced and the peak effect is increased without a change in the time of peak effect.

A **loading dose** is a larger initial dose compared to the subsequent doses. Loading doses are used to obtain a therapeutic response quicker for a patient than would normally be expected. A physician may feel that it is best for the patient to obtain a therapeutic level of the medication quicker and may prescribe a loading dose for the patient. A Z-Pak (azithromycin) is an example of a medication that begins with a loading dose. The patient takes 2 pills as a single dose on day 1 and then 1 pill as a single dose on days 2 through 5.

A **maintenance dose** is a dose that is given after the loading dose to maintain a therapeutic concentration of the drug in the body. A maintenance dose is a smaller dose compared to the loading dose. The dosing is calculated based upon the amount of drug needed to maintain an appropriate drug level within the therapeutic range. A **prophylactic dose** is one that given to prevent a situation from developing. The most common example of a prophylactic dose is prescribing 2 g of amoxicillin prior to a visit to the dentist or giving a dose of IV antibiotics before surgery. Both are done to prevent an infection.

loading dose Larger initial dose compared to the subsequent doses.

maintenance dose Dose given after the loading dose to maintain a therapeutic concentration of the drug in the body.

prophylactic dose Dose given to prevent a situation from developing.

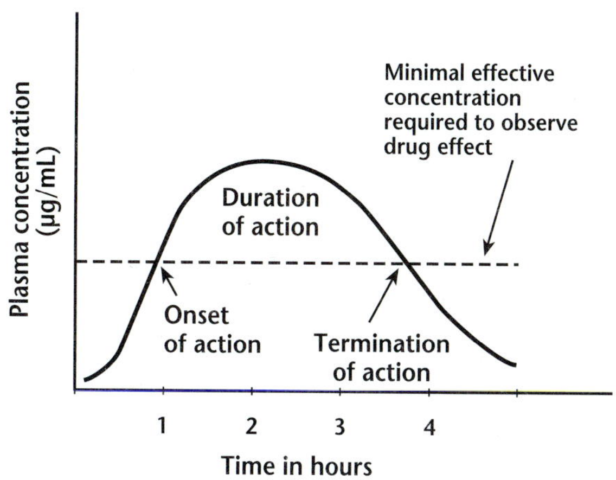

Figure 6-3 Time-response curve.

Tech Check

1. What term refers to the intended effect of a drug?(LO 6.17)
2. What type of drug blocks the effect of another drug?(LO 6.17)
3. What term refers to how a drug works?(LO 6.17)
4. What terms refers to the strength or concentration of a drug?(LO 6.17)
5. What are three terms used to describe undesired effects of a drug?(LO 6.17)

Pharmacokinetics(LO 6.2)

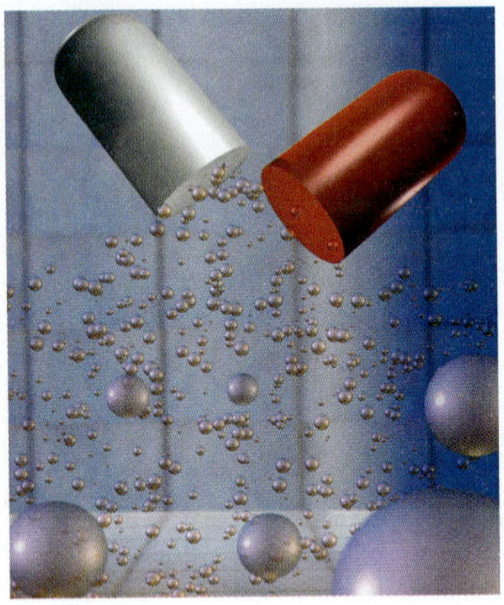

Pharmacokinetics is the study of the absorption, distribution, metabolism, and elimination of drugs, sometimes referred to as the **ADME process.** Figure 6-4 depicts the movement of a drug within the body using both enteral and parenteral routes of administration. The dosage of a medication is the amount of medicine administered at one time that will determine the concentration of a drug at its sites of action and the intensity of its effects.

Several pharmacokinetic principles affect the proper dosing of a medication for a patient. These pharmacokinetic principles are based upon models and include:

- The body is considered a single compartment. The distribution of a drug within this compartment is assumed uniform. However, there are times when a two-compartment model is used resulting in the opposite.
- Absorption and elimination of a specific drug is assumed constant. In other words, the amount of the drug present is eliminated at a constant rate per unit of time.
- The rate of elimination is affected by the **half-life (t1/2).** Half-life is defined as the amount of time for one-half of the drug present to be eliminated from the body. A drug's half-life is independent of the drug concentration or the dosage. After approximately four half-life cycles, this process is 93.75% complete.

These principles are used in selecting and adjusting a drug's dosage schedule and interpreting the serum concentrations of medications in the blood, serum, or plasma. This information supplements clinical monitoring and provides a guide for proper dosing. Some of the factors that affect pharmacokinetics include:

- The physiochemical properties of a drug molecule and its membranes
- Drug characteristics, such as its molecular size and shape
- The lipid solubility of the ionized and nonionized forms of the drug
- Drug interactions with other drugs
- Drug interactions with food
- Changes in the cardiovascular, renal, or hepatic functions
- Delay in observing the effect of the drug

The cell membrane is a thin layer of lipid material interspersed with small, water-filled channels. Protein like substances are found on both

pharmacokinetics Study of the absorption, distribution, metabolism, and elimination of drugs.

ADME process Absorption, distribution, metabolism, and elimination.

half-life (t1/2) Amount of time for one-half of the drug present to be eliminated from the body.

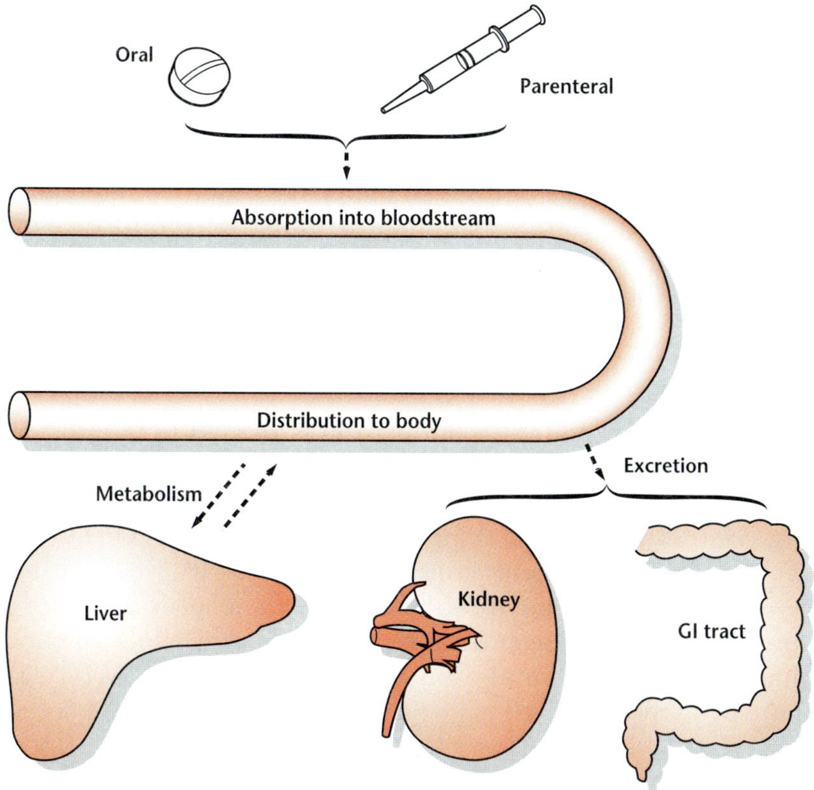

Figure 6-4 Movement of a drug in the body.

sides of the lipid material. These substances may or may not allow a drug to cross this membrane easily due to the chemical nature of the drug.

Most drugs are weak **acids** or **bases** and are present in solution as both ionized and unionized substances. The unionized portion is lipid soluble and can readily cross the cell membrane. The ionized form has difficulty crossing the lipid membrane because of its low lipid solubility or due to its size. An acidic medication is unionized when it is in an acidic environment ($pH < 7$) and will be readily absorbed, but an acidic drug in an alkaline environment ($pH > 7$) will take longer to be absorbed. A basic medication is normally unionized when it is in an alkaline environment. Basic medications are absorbed better in an acidic environment. The choice of the route of administration will be affected whether a drug is acidic or basic.

If a patient experiences a drug overdose, the antidote selected will depend on whether the drug is acidic or basic. The drug needs to be in an ionized form for it to be eliminated. The pH of the urine will need to be adjusted to promote a drug's excretion. Acidic drugs need to be eliminated in alkaline urine and an alkaline drug needs to be eliminated in acidic urine.

Passive transport is the most common method for a drug to cross a membrane. This method requires no energy for this process to occur. The drug's molecules penetrate the aqueous channels of the membrane or dissolve in the membrane. Both nonpolar lipid soluble compounds and polar water-soluble compounds can cross this barrier. **Diffusion** is the process in which a substance goes from a higher to a lower concentration. The transfer of the drug is affected by the lipid solubility of the substance. Diffusion occurs faster when there is a large difference between these two concentrations. If the difference between the two concentrations is small, it will take longer for the drug to cross this membrane.

acid Substance that yields hydrogen atoms when dissolved in water. It has a pH less than 7.

base Substance that yields hydroxide atoms when dissolved in water. It has a pH greater than 7.

passive transport Most common method for a drug to cross a membrane.

diffusion Process in which a substance goes from a higher to a lower concentration.

Active transport is a selective process and requires energy to take place, where a substance goes from a lower to a higher concentration. This process involves the usage of specific proteins to occur.

A drug's effect on the body is affected by its concentration in the blood or plasma. This is extremely important when certain medications are prescribed. Medications used to prevent epilepsy (Dilantin), bipolar disease (lithium), and blood clotting (Coumadin) must be monitored properly especially when pharmacokinetic variations occur with patients receiving the same medication. Other situations requiring close monitoring involve patients possessing an impaired renal or hepatic function when aminoglycosides (Vancocin or Garamycin) are prescribed for bacterial infections.

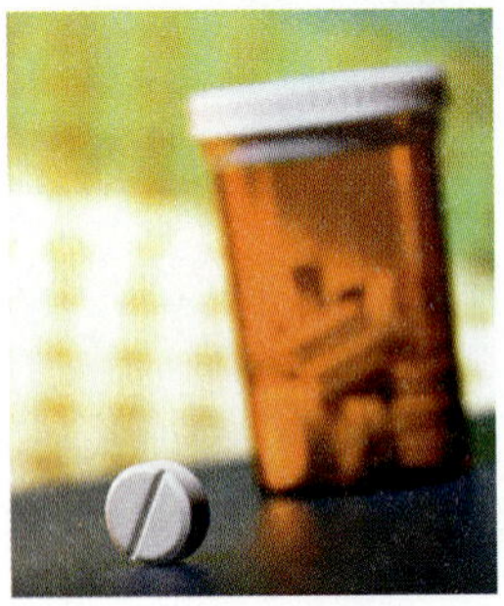

The amount of drug found in the plasma is related to the pharmacokinetic processes of absorption, distribution, metabolism, and elimination, which are discussed later in chapter. These pharmacokinetic processes are occurring continuously while a patient is taking the medication. These processes measure the plasma concentration of a drug over a period of time, the onset of action, the duration of action, the termination of action, the minimum effective concentration, the maximum effective concentration, which becomes the minimum toxic concentration (MTC), and the therapeutic drug range.

Tech Check

6. What are the components of the ADME process?(LO 6.2)
7. What process occurs when a drug goes from a higher to a lower concentration?(LO 6.2)
8. In what form must a drug occur for it to be eliminated from the body?(LO 6.2)

Absorption(LO 6.3, 6.4, 6.14, 6.15)

Absorption is the process by which a drug enters the bloodstream. Oral medications require the drug to be absorbed from the digestive system from either the stomach or intestine. The drug enters the bloodstream where it is taken to the liver to be metabolized by enzymes. A drug must be absorbed before it can produce its effect. Medications administered intravenously enter the bloodstream immediately.

Many factors affect the absorption of the drug. These factors include:

- Solubility—Drugs dissolved in aqueous solutions are more rapidly absorbed than those in oily vehicles.
- Disintegration—Solid drugs are affected by their dissolution rate with their absorption. The conditions found at the site of absorption, such as pH of the acid, can slow down this rate. Some insoluble substances may not be absorbed. The dosage form of a drug will affect its disintegration rate (i.e., a capsule breaks down quicker than a tablet).
- Concentration—The concentration of the drug can affect its absorption; the higher the concentration the more rapid the absorption.

active transport Selective process that requires energy to take place, where a substance goes from a lower to higher concentration.

absorption Process by which a drug enters the bloodstream.

- Blood flow to the site of absorption—Increased blood flow brought about by massage or local application of heat will improve blood circulation. Vasoconstrictors, shock, or trauma may slow down absorption.
- Absorbing surface area—The larger the surface area the greater the absorption.

Route of Administration: Enteral Versus Parenteral

Oral administration is the most common method of **enteral administration** of a medication. Enteral administration requires the use of the digestive system. It is generally the safest, most convenient, and most economical route of administration for the patient. There are several disadvantages of the oral route, which include a variable and sometimes incomplete absorption rate for specific drugs. Medications administered orally may require up to an hour before absorption occurs, resulting in a delayed onset of action. The medication may irritate the stomach wall of the patient causing the patient to vomit. A drug may be destroyed by enzymes found in the stomach or the acidity of the stomach. Certain drugs may bind to specific types of food and therefore it maybe extremely difficult for the drug to be absorbed by the body. For example, some tetracyclines may bind to dairy products and the absorption is impacted. Finally, the liver may metabolize certain medications before they gain access to the circulatory system.

Sublingual medications, which are placed under the tongue such as nitroglycerin, are rapidly absorbed from the oral mucosa. A higher concentration of the drug will be found in the bloodstream quicker than if it travels through the digestive tract. More of the drug is available for metabolism because it does not undergo a breakdown by the digestive juices of the stomach.

Rectal medications are classified as enteral dosage form. These medications may be used if the possibility of vomiting occurs or the patient is unconscious. A therapeutic response is often seen within 15 to 30 minutes. The absorbed drug does not pass through the liver before it enters systemic circulation. Some disadvantages of rectal medications include an irregular or incomplete absorption of the drug.

Parenteral administration results in a quicker response because the absorption process is avoided. The process is more rapid and predictable than oral administration, and the prescriber is able to order a more accurate dose for a patient using parenteral administration. This route of administration provides a positive alternative to oral administration if the patient is unconscious, uncooperative, or is unable to take a medication orally. There are several disadvantages of parenteral medications: Strict asepsis must be maintained to prevent infection from occurring; the patient may experience pain or discomfort when an injection is administered; special skills are required for a patient to administer an injection; parenteral medications are more expensive than oral medications; and finally, if an error is made by administering the wrong drug or an incorrect dose of the drug, it is more difficult to reverse the effects of the drug than an oral dose.

Parenteral medications are delivered outside of the gastrointestinal system. There are many routes by which a drug may be administered parenterally using a syringe. These include:

- Intravenous (into the vein)
- Subcutaneous (under the skin)

enteral administration Oral administration of a drug.

parenteral administration Medications delivered outside of the gastrointestinal system.

- Intramuscular (into the muscle)
- Intra-arterial (into the artery)
- Intrathecal (into the spinal cord)
- Intraperitoneal (into the peritoneal cavity)

Other parenteral methods not using a syringe include medications inhaled into the lungs, applied topically to the skin, or instilled in the eyes and ears.

An individual receiving an intravenous medication may begin to experience the effect of the drug within a minute. This route of administration is extremely beneficial in emergencies. The possibility of adverse effects is greater when intravenous solutions are used. Intravenous solutions should be injected slowly. Not all solutions are suitable for intravenous administration, especially if the solution contains insoluble substances. Examples of intravenous medications include IV fluids, such as dextrose 5% in water (D5W), nutrient supplements, and certain antibiotics.

Drugs administered subcutaneously (under the skin) provide a prompt absorption rate of aqueous solutions. The onset of action is within a few minutes of the injection. Medications inactivated by the gastrointestinal tract may find this route as an appropriate route of administration. Subcutaneous injections do not permit large volumes to be injected into the body. Insulin is an example of a medication administered subcutaneously.

Aqueous drugs administered intramuscularly are absorbed promptly into the body but not as quickly as an IV solution. The onset of action is within several minutes. Intramuscular medications are suitable if a small volume is administered or if the substance is oily. Intramuscular medications may also interfere with the results of certain diagnostic tests. Both narcotics and antibiotics may be administered intramuscularly.

Some medications may be injected directly into an artery (intra-arterial) to produce a localized effect on a particular organ or tissue. The medicine's effect is observed within 1 minute. An injection into an artery requires greater care than other parenteral injections. This route of administration may be used with antineoplastic and diagnostic agents.

Some medications are administered into the spinal cord (intrathecal) when a local or rapid effect of drugs is desired in either the meninges or the cerebrospinal column. The onset of action is within several minutes of the administration. Examples of medications administered into the spinal cord include Lidocaine or antibiotics for central nervous system (CNS) infections.

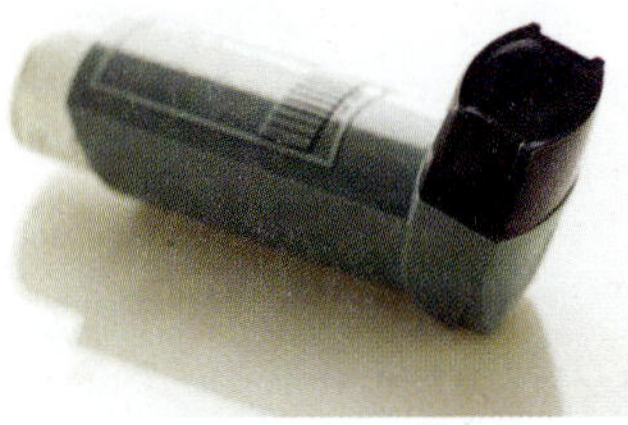

The treatment of respiratory conditions may require the pulmonary absorption of medications in the lungs. The pulmonary absorption of a drug results in effects being noticed almost instantaneously due to the large surface area of respiratory tract and its absorption into the bloodstream. Nebulizers and inhalers are examples of two dosage forms that require pulmonary absorption of the drug. Inhalation therapy may provide a local effect at the site of action. Some of the disadvantages of inhalation products are the difficulty in regulating the dose; patients experiencing problems in administering the dose; and gases irritating the pulmonary lining.

Topical medications can be applied to either the skin or mucous membranes. These areas include the mucosa membranes of the conjunctiva (eye), nasopharynx, vagina, colon, urethra, and the urinary bladder.

The skin acts as a protective barrier for the body and therefore very few medications are capable of penetrating the intact skin. The absorption of medications is proportional to their lipid solubility because the epidermis acts as a barrier to lipids. Unlike the epidermis, the dermis is freely permeable to many solutes and more prone to systemic absorption. Suspending the drug in an oily vehicle and rubbing the topical agent into the skin improves the absorption of the active ingredient. Unfortunately, systemic toxicity may occur for local anesthetics.

Bioavailability

Bioavailability refers to the rate and extent to which an active drug is absorbed into the body. Particle size can affect the disintegration and dissolution of a drug product. The bioavailability of a drug can be affected by differences in drug formulation, route of administration, factors affecting gastrointestinal absorption, and different dosage forms from various manufacturers. In addition, different lot numbers may result in differences in bioavailability. The Food and Drug Administration (FDA) requires bioavailability testing on all drugs.

Some of the terms used when discussing bioavailability include:

- Chemically equivalent—meeting the chemical and physical standards established by governmental or regulatory agencies.
- Biologically equivalent—yielding similar concentrations in the blood and tissues.
- Therapeutically equivalent—producing the same therapeutic effect.

The *USP* established therapeutic equivalent codes for medications and are found in Table 6-1 (p. 182). A drug may be chemically equivalent but not biologically or therapeutically equivalent.

Tech Check

9. Which route of administration produces the quickest effect?(LO 6.14)
10. What three terms are used to describe bioavailability?(LO 6.15)
11. What bioavailability classification is given to a drug that does not have bioavailability problems?(LO 6.15)
12. What are three advantages of a drug administered enterally?(LO 6.14)
13. What are three parenteral routes of administration?(LO 6.14)

Distribution(LO 6.3, 6.5)

After a drug is absorbed into the bloodstream, it may be distributed into the interstitial, cellular, or transcellular fluids. The distribution of the drug is affected by the drug itself, cardiac output, and blood flow. In many situations the drug uses the process of passive or simple diffusion, where the drug goes from a higher to a lower concentration. Medications that are lipid soluble are able to readily cross various membranes found throughout the body and distribute throughout all fluids.

Medications are distributed promptly from the blood into the heart, brain, liver, and kidney, but it takes longer for them to be distributed in

bioavailability Rate and extent to which an active drug is absorbed into the body.

Table 6-1 ***USP* Therapeutic Equivalent Codes**

Type A Codes: Drug products that the FDA considers to be therapeutically equivalent to other pharmaceutically equivalent products—that is, drug products for which:
1. There are no known or suspected bioequivalence problems. These are designated AA, AB AN, AO, AP, or AT depending on their dosage form.
AA—Products in conventional dosage forms not presenting bioequivalence forms
AB—Products meeting necessary bioequivalence requirements
AN—Solutions and powder for aerosolization
AO—Injectable oil solutions
AP—Injectable aqueous solutions an in certain instances, intravenous nonaqueous solutions
AT—Topical solutions
2. Actual or potential bioequivalence problems have been resolved with adequate in vivo or in vitro evidence supporting bioequivalence. These are designated AB.
Type B Codes: Drug products that the FDA at this time considers not to be therapeutically equivalent to other pharmaceutically equivalent products—that is, drug products for which actual or potential bioequivalence problems have not been resolved by adequate evidence of bioequivalence. Often the problem is with specific dosage forms rather than with active ingredients. They are designated BC, BD, BE, BN, BP, BR, BS, BT, BX, or B (asterisk).
B*—Drug products requiring further FDA investigation and review to determine therapeutic equivalence
BC—Extended-release dosage forms (capsules, injectables, and tablets)
BD—Active ingredients and dosage forms with documented bioequivalence problems
BE—Delayed-release oral dosage forms
BN—Products in aerosol-nebulizer drug delivery systems
BP—Active ingredients and dosage forms with potential bioequivalence problems
BR—Suppositories or enemas that deliver drugs for systemic absorption
BS—Products having standard deficiencies
BT—Topical products with bioequivalence issues
BX—Drug products for which the data are insufficient to determine therapeutic equivalence

muscle or fat. If a drug does not cross specific membranes, the drug may become limited to specific sites of action. Some medications may build up in specific tissues resulting in a higher concentration and therefore the effect of the drug may be prolonged.

Passage of Drugs into and Across Cells

A medication is capable of crossing a cell membrane and entering into the cell. Several factors affect the ability of a medication to cross a membrane, including their protein-binding ability, the water coefficient, and changes of the pH of the two different fluids. If one raises or lowers the pH of the two substances, different effects will be observed. Nonelectrolytes enter a cell by the process of diffusion and the effect is proportionate to their lipid solubility.

The distribution of drugs in the CNS is restricted to the cerebrospinal fluid. Drugs that are either ionized and/or lipid insoluble are largely excluded from the brain. Nonionized forms of weak acids and bases are restricted, but they are able to enter the brain because of the high cerebral blood flow and their high lipid solubility.

Many drugs bind to plasma proteins, such as albumin and globulin that circulate throughout the body. These proteins assist in regulating the osmotic pressure found in the blood and help transport important substances throughout the body. The extent of a drug's affinity for binding to plasma proteins is dependent on the characteristics of the drug. For example, warfarin is 90% protein bond. A drug binding to plasma proteins may limit its concentration in tissues and at the site of action. Binding will limit the glomerular filtration by the kidney but does not limit its renal secretion or metabolism in the liver. Many lipid-soluble drugs are stored in the neutral fat of the body. These drugs may be present in the body fat several hours after administration, but take a long time to be released because of the limited blood supply.

The liver, kidney, and brain receive the greatest amount of blood in the body. As a result, they receive the greatest amount of the drug that has been administered. On the other hand, some tissues (such as fat tissue) receive a smaller quantity of blood and if the drug is water soluble, it will not be stored in the fat cells.

Reservoirs and Redistribution

Reservoirs are areas within the body where a drug may accumulate. The drug will be released into the body when plasma concentrations of the drug decrease. Plasma proteins, fat, extracellular areas, and cellular areas are used as reservoirs. Many drugs accumulate in muscle and other cells in higher concentrations than in extracellular fluids. If the intracellular concentration is high and the binding is reversible, the tissue involved may represent a sizeable drug reservoir. The liver may store large quantities of some drugs. Lipid-soluble drugs may be stored in the natural fat found in the body. An obese person will store a larger supply of a drug due to increased fat content.

A drug's effect normally ends during its metabolism, but there are times when a drug may be redistributed from its site of action to another site. Redistribution becomes an important factor when lipid-soluble drugs act on the brain or the cardiovascular system when administered intravenously or through inhalation. A drug's effect occurs quickly as it reaches its site of action but decreases rapidly. The drug may continue to remain in the body but will be at concentration that is below what is needed to produce an effect.

Placental Transfer of Drugs

Many drugs are capable of crossing the placental barrier and may cause congenital birth defects in the fetus. These drugs cross the placenta by simple diffusion. A lipid-soluble, nonionized drug is capable of entering the fetus's blood from the mother. A fetus is exposed to every drug that a

Table 6-2 Drugs and Their Associated Birth Defects

Drug	Birth Defect
androgens	Masculinization of female fetus
carbamazepine	Craniofacial and fingernail deformities
estrogen	Feminization of male fetus
lithium	Cardiac defects
phenytoin	Craniofacial and limb deformities, growth retardation
retinoic acid	Craniofacial, cardiac, and CNS defects
Tetracycline	Dental birth defects
warfarin	Facial, cartilage, and CNS defects

woman takes during her pregnancy. Some of the medications that may cause birth defects are found in Table 6-2.

Tech Check

14. What factors affect drug absorption in the body?(LO 6.5)

15. Which organs receive the greatest amount of blood in the body?(LO 6.5)

16. What is an example of a drug that may cause a birth defect?(LO 6.5)

17. What three factors affect a drug's distribution?(LO 6.5)

Metabolism(LO 6.3, 6.6)

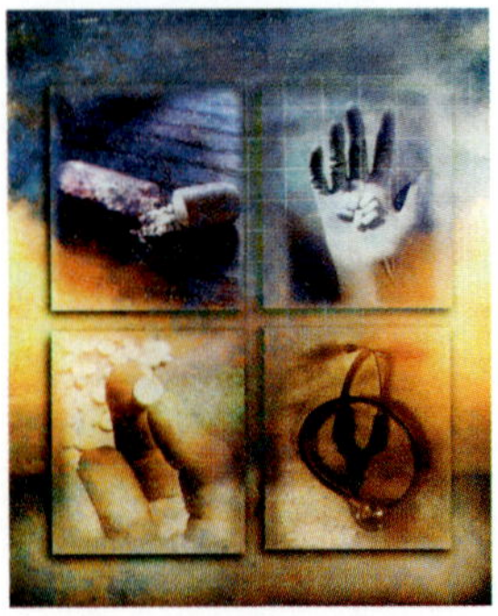

Metabolism (biotransformation) is the process of converting a drug to a state of activity or inactivity where it may be eliminated by the body. A drug is inactivated by metabolism. The processes for converting a drug are based upon chemical reactions (synthetic or nonsynthetic) that involve a drug's metabolism. Synthetic reactions are known as conjugation because they involve a coupling between the drug and its metabolite. Nonsynthetic reactions involve the processes of oxidation, reduction, or hydrolysis. These processes result in a change in activity or inactivation of the drug. The liver is responsible for the metabolism of drugs in the body.

Hepatic Microsomal Drug-Metabolizing System

The **hepatic** microsomal drug metabolizing system involves enzyme systems found in the hepatic endoplasmic reticulum that may speed up the conjugation or the oxidation of the drug. The hepatic blood flow will affect the metabolism of a drug by the liver. This system converts lipid-soluble drugs to a water-soluble drug form. A water-soluble form of a drug can be eliminated by the kidneys. A lipid-soluble drug is frequently reabsorbed into the bloodstream. Many drugs are inactivated by metabolism but a few are converted into pharmacologically active metabolites. An example would be the conversion of prednisolone to prednisone in the body. Some drugs can increase the activity of microsomal enzymes.

hepatic Referring to the liver.

Two unique situations—enzyme induction and enzyme induction—may occur within this system. Enzyme induction is the process where a medication stimulates the system by increasing the number of enzymes within a system. In this situation, the rate of the metabolism of a drug will increase and its duration of action will decrease. Some drugs can inhibit the drug microsomal-metabolizing enzyme resulting in enzyme inhibition. Enzyme inhibition slows down a drug's metabolism and therefore increases the length and intensity of a drug.

When a drug is administered orally and is absorbed into the bloodstream, it is carried to the liver before it is distributed throughout the body. Many drugs are converted as they pass through the liver resulting in a process known as first-pass metabolism. First-pass metabolism reduces the amount of active drug in the body.

Tech Check

18. What is the purpose of metabolism?(LO 6.6)

19. What term refers to the process where a medication stimulates the metabolism of a drug by increasing the number of enzymes?(LO 6.6)

20. What process metabolizes a drug in the liver?(LO 6.6)

21. What organ is responsible for metabolism?(LO 6.6)

Elimination(LO 6.7)

A drug can be eliminated from the body unchanged or as a metabolite of the original drug. The kidney is extremely important in the elimination of a drug and its metabolites. The renal elimination of drugs consists of three distinct processes: glomerular filtration, active tubular secretion, and passive tubular reabsorption. During glomerular filtration, blood is filtered through the kidney resulting in the filtered substances being reabsorbed into the blood, active tubular secretion, and passive tubular reabsorption. The filtration process is dependent on a substance's protein-binding ability and its glomerular filtration rate.

In the proximal renal tubule, tubular secretion occurs and ions are pulled out of the nephrons and transported back to the blood. This transport system may be bidirectional and some drugs are both secreted and reabsorbed. Multiple systems may be working during the elimination process depending on the specific drug substance.

Passive reabsorption occurs in the proximal and distal tubules. During tubular reabsorption, various mechanisms transport sodium ions into circulation. During this phase, substances responsible for the sodium reabsorption and maintaining acid-base balance in the body exchange potassium ions for sodium ions. The pH of the urine will affect whether a drug is excreted or reabsorbed.

After the oral administration of a drug, some of the drug passes unabsorbed through the gastrointestinal (GI) tract. This unabsorbed drug may be eliminated in the feces. The enterohepatic (intestinal) pathway allows specific fat-soluble drugs to enter the intestines through the biliary tract. Once the drug is released into the intestines, a metabolite is excreted in the

Table 6-3 Drug Classifications and Examples of Drugs Found in Breast Milk

Drug Classification	Examples
Antibiotics	Ampicillin, erythromycin, penicillin, streptomycin, sulfa drugs, and tetracycline
Antiepileptics	Phenytoin, primidone
Antithyroid drugs	Thiouracil
Bipolar agents	Lithium
CNS stimulants	Nicotine
Narcotic analgesics	Codeine, methadone, morphine
Sedative-hypnotics	Barbiturates and chloral hydrate
Tranquilizers	Chlorpromazine

bile and is reabsorbed into the blood. Drugs that follow this pathway have a longer duration of action because of the repeated recycling of the drug.

A few medications are eliminated by the lungs. These medications are converted to a product that can be replaced from the blood in the respiratory tract. Some drugs and their metabolites can be found in breast milk. Some of the drug classifications and examples that can be eliminated in breast milk are found in Table 6-3. Drugs may also be found in the sweat and saliva, but in extremely small amounts.

Tech Check

22. Which organ is responsible for eliminating most drug products?(LO 6.7)

23. What is an example of a drug that can be found in breast milk?(LO 6.7)

24. What are the three processes that occur during renal elimination?(LO 6.7)

Dosing Considerations(LO 6.8, 6.9, 6.11)

Many factors may modify the effects of a particular drug. A physician must consider them when prescribing a medication to a patient. Some patients may not take the medication according to the instructions provided by the physician, referred to as nonadherence (noncompliance). Nonadherence may be intentional or unintentional. Several reasons that affect nonadherence include the patient, the patient's illness, and the drug regimen.

Age

During the first 12 months of a neonate's life, the infant's organs are continuing to develop. It is not until after the first year that the organs are completely developed. The drug dosage for very young infants is affected by differences in the relative volumes of body fluid compartments, reduced binding of drugs to plasma proteins, a not fully developed renal function system, and incomplete development of the blood-brain barrier. Children younger than 12 require specific dosing of medication due to two important variables: organ development and body size. Second, the amount of medication to produce a therapeutic effect on a child is less than that of an adult due to the weight, height, and body surface area (BSA). Doses need to be properly calculated to produce the proper therapeutic effect.

On the other hand, persons who are elderly may respond to medications differently due to their ability to inactivate or excrete drugs from the body and having other disease states. Liver and kidney function decreases as we age. Elderly people (older than 70 years of age) take disproportionately more medications than young adults do. This creates an opportunity for improved pharmaceutical care and increased medication monitoring of this population.

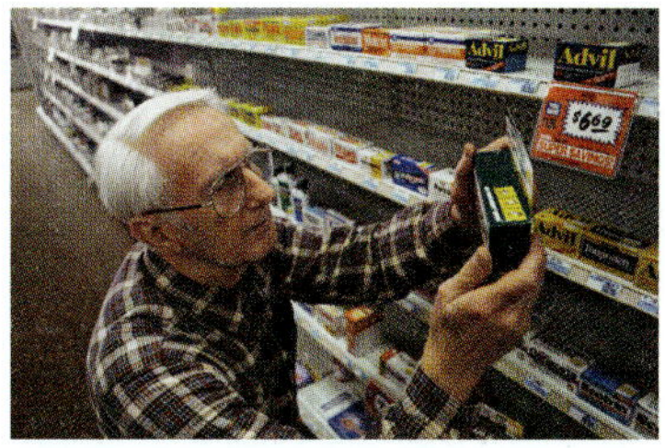

Body Size

The dosage prescribed for a patient should be adjusted for individuals, who are unusually lean or obese. In addition, special consideration should be made for patients who may be dehydrated or having edema.

Sex

Studies have demonstrated that women are more vulnerable to the effects of certain medications than men due to their smaller body size. Hormones also may have an impact on various medications. In addition, body fat varies between males and females.

Timing of Administration

The timing of medication administration may influence the dosage, especially with oral medications. Medication absorption is optimal for most drugs when the stomach is empty, but some drugs are absorbed better if they are taken with food. In addition, some medications may irritate the stomach, which may influence a patient's compliance in taking the medication.

Tolerance

Tolerance may be acquired with certain medications, especially with those classified as controlled substances. There are several different types of tolerance: cross tolerance, pharmacokinetic tolerance, and pharmacodynamic tolerance. Cross tolerance occurs when the effects of pharmacologically related drugs must be increased to maintain the same effect. Pharmacokinetic tolerance occurs with induced synthesis of hepatic microsomal enzymes in a drug's metabolism. Pharmacodynamic tolerance is affected by neuronal adaptation.

Other Factors Affecting Drug Dosing

Other factors affecting drug dosing include:

- The rate and degree of absorption are affected by the route of administration.
- A patient's dosage should be adjusted for patients who have either an impaired hepatic or renal system or both.

- Certain pathological (disease) factors may affect how a particular drug acts on the body.
- Physiological factors such as water and electrolyte balance, acid-base status, and body temperature may influence how a drug acts within the body.
- Genetic factors may contribute to the normal inconsistency of a drug's effect especially in a drug's metabolism.

Drug Interactions

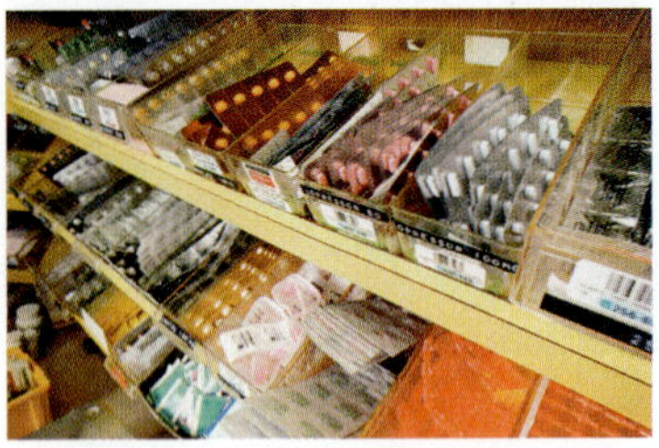

Whenever a patient is taking more than one drug the possibility of a drug interaction is present. An enzyme known as cytochrome P-450 is found in the liver. This enzyme has been identified to be active in the biotransformation of many drugs. Grapefruit contains substances that inhibit cytochrome P-450 found in the intestines. This inhibition results in more of the drug being absorbed into the bloodstream. Food has demonstrated the ability to interact with the actions of drugs. For instance, dairy products consumed before taking tetracycline results in a process known as chelation, where the dairy product binds to the tetracycline and reduces the amount absorbed by the body.

Various terms are used when discussing drug interactions and include *addition, synergism, potentiation,* and *antagonism*. Addition is the combined effect of two drugs. It is equal to the sum effects of each drug taken alone. Synergism is a drug interaction where the combined effect of two drugs if taken together is greater than the sum of their parts. The combined effect is more intense or longer in duration than the sum of their individual effects. Drugs used for their synergistic effect are usually prescribed together. An example of a synergistic effect would be a patient taking a CNS depressant and consuming alcohol at the same time. The combination of these two substances may cause increased sedation, respiratory depression, or impaired motor function, which if excessive could lead to death.

Potentiation is the process where one drug increases the potency or strength of another medication and the effect is greater than the effect of each drug prescribed alone. An example of potentiation involves dispensing Phenergan with Demerol. The Phenergan will act to prolong the effect of Demerol.

Antagonism is the process where a drug blocks the effects of a medication. In the situation of a drug overdose of a narcotic such as morphine, the drug Narcan (naloxone) may be prescribed to counteract the effects of the morphine.

potentiation The process where one drug increases the potency or strength of another medication and the effect is greater than the effect of each drug prescribed alone.

antagonism The process where a drug blocks the effects of a medication.

Tech Check

25. What are three things that can affect a patient's dosing?(LO 6.8, 6.9)

26. What is an example of a drug interaction?(LO 6.11)

27. What type of effect results when two medications are taken and the combined effect is greater than the sum of the two effects?(LO 6.11)

Side Effects(LO 6.18, 6.19)

No drug is free from side effects (adverse effects). At times, these effects may be small; other times it may be fatal to an individual. Side effects may appear promptly or they may take time to appear. Some side effects occur only in some patients or only in combination with other drugs. Other times the side effect may be controlled by adjusting the dosage of the drug. At times, an undesired effect of a drug for one patient may become the desired effect for another patient. An example of this is Benadryl. Benadryl may be prescribed for a patient who is experiencing an allergic reaction but the patient begins to experience drowsiness. In another situation, a patient has been hospitalized and is having difficulty falling a-sleep; the physician may prescribe Benadryl due to its side effect of drowsiness.

Allergic Responses (Hypersensitivity)

Even though the likelihood of an individual experiencing an allergic reaction to a drug is low, it is possible. There is a need for a safe method of detecting a susceptible patient before prescribing and administering the drug.

Drug allergies can take a wide range of forms resulting immediately or be being delayed for a period. Examples of allergic responses include:

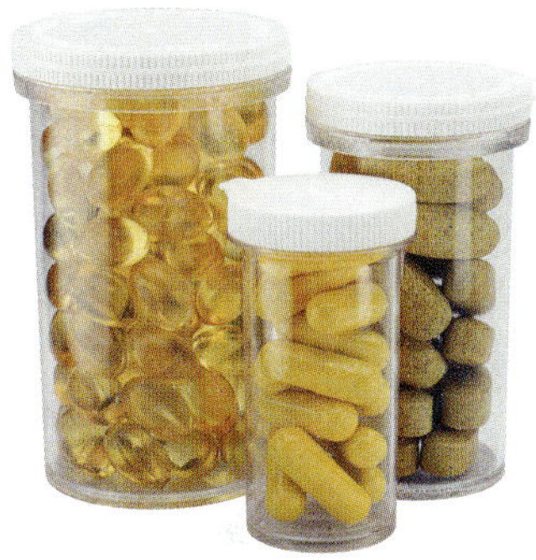

- Anaphylactic reactions
- Asthma
- Fever
- Mild rashes
- Rhinitis
- Urticaria

An anaphylactic reaction is an adverse drug effect that may be fatal to an individual. If an individual experiences this type of reaction, he or she may have trouble breathing because the trachea begins to close. Examples of medications that may produce anaphylactic reactions include penicillin and sulfa medications.

Hepatoxicity and Nephrotoxicity

Many drugs are concentrated in the liver and kidney; damage to these organs by an adverse effect of drug is not uncommon. Some drugs may cause hepatoxicity and nephrotoxicity as a result of a drug allergy. Certain drugs may cause jaundice. A medication may interfere with bilirubin metabolism in the body—damage to the kidneys may result in glomerulopathy, glomerulonephritis, and tubular necrosis. In some situations hypotension or hypertension may occur.

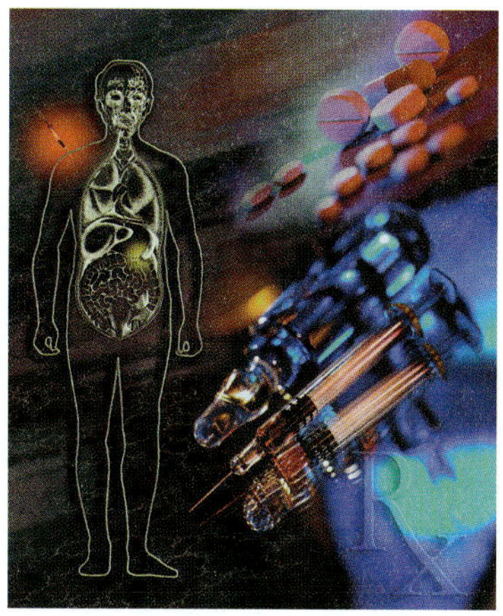

Drug Dependence (Drug Addiction)

Any drug that alters mood or perception has the potential to be abused and is potentially capable of producing drug dependence. Examples of drugs that have a potential for abuse include opioids, sedatives, alcohol, amphetamines, CNS stimulants, cocaine, "crack" cocaine, heroin, and marijuana. A common characteristic of drug dependence is psychological dependence, which is a craving that requires periodic or chronic administration of the drug for pleasure or relief of pleasure. Physical dependence causes physical

Table 6-4 FDA Pregnancy Categories

Pregnancy Category A	Drug studies in pregnant woman have not demonstrated risk to the fetus.
Pregnancy Category B	Drug studies have not been performed in pregnant women; animal studies have not demonstrated fetal risk.
Pregnancy Category C	Either drug studies have not been performed in pregnant women or animals or, if drug studies have been tested on animals the tests have revealed some teratogenic potential but the risk to the fetus is unknown.
Pregnancy Category D	Drug studies have revealed adverse risk to the fetus. The benefit-to-risk ratio of the drug must be established before use during pregnancy.
Pregnancy Category X	Drug studies have revealed teratogenic effects in women and/or animals. Fetal risk clearly outweighs benefit. Drug is contraindicated in pregnancy.
Pregnancy Category NR	Drugs have not yet been rated by the FDA.

symptoms to appear when the administration of the drug is stopped. These symptoms are referred to as withdrawal or abstinence syndrome. Drug abuse refers to a situation where a medication is repeatedly taken for non-medical purpose.

Tech Check

28. What are two types of addiction?(LO 6.19)

29. What type of drug response may be fatal?(LO 6.18)

30. What organ is affected by nephrotoxicity?(LO 6.18)

Pregnancy(LO 6.20)

When a woman takes a medication during her pregnancy, the unborn fetus is exposed to the drug. Both absorption and distribution of a drug occur in the fetus using the same processes as they do in the mother. The fetus is at greatest risk during the first trimester of pregnancy. Teratogens are medications that may produce an adverse effect on the fetus to include birth defects and growth retardation.

The FDA has established categories identifying the possibility of a drug producing adverse effects on a fetus based upon drug testing. Refer to Table 6-4 for a description of these categories.

All unnecessary medication should be avoided during pregnancy. Medications not known to be reasonably safe on the basis of long usage should be avoided by women of child-bearing age.

Tech Check

31. What pregnancy category indicates that drug studies in pregnant women have not indicated harm to the fetus?(LO 6.20)

32. What pregnancy category is contraindicated in pregnant women?(LO 6.20)

Chapter Summary

Understanding the basics of pharmacology in the workplace is vital to the pharmacy technician. Important points to know are:

- Drugs can be made from plants, animals, minerals, made synthetically, or through biotechnology.
- Drugs may have three names: a chemical, generic, and brand name.
- Pharmacology is the science involving the study of drugs; the physical and chemical properties; biochemical and physiological properties; the absorption, distribution, metabolism, and elimination of a drug; and the therapeutic use of a drug.
- Drugs affect the receptors on a cell to produce an effect.
- Pharmacokinetics is the study of the absorption, distribution, metabolism, and elimination of a drug.
- Both the liver and the kidneys play important roles in the pharmacokinetics of a drug.
- Bioavailability tests are required for all drugs.
- Variations in a patient's age, weight, size, sex, and physical condition may affect the response a drug produces in the body.
- Medications are tested by the FDA to determine any potential adverse effects on a pregnant woman and her fetus.

Chapter Review

Case Study Question

1. What factors affect the absorption, distribution, metabolism, and elimination of the drug?(LO 6.4, 6.5, 6.6, 6.7)

At Your Service Question

1. Is this a side effect of naproxen and what should she do?(LO 6.11)

Multiple Choice

Select the best answer.

1. Which of the following is a possible source of a medication?(LO 6.16)
   a. Animal
   b. Plant
   c. Synthetic
   d. All of the above
2. Which of the following may affect the absorption of a drug?(LO 6.4)
   a. Drug concentration
   b. Drug dissolution
   c. Drug solubility
   d. All of the above
3. Which of the following does *not* affect the distribution of a drug?(LO 6.5)
   a. The drug itself
   b. Blood flow
   c. Cardiac output
   d. Renal output
4. Which of the following does *not* affect the ability of a drug to cross into and across cells?(LO 6.5)
   a. pH of the fluid
   b. Protein binding
   c. Route of administration
   d. Water coefficient
5. How many half-life cycles does it take a drug to be eliminated from the body?(LO 6.2)
   a. 1
   b. 2
   c. 3
   d. 4
6. What pregnancy category reveals that drug studies in women have *not* demonstrated a risk to the fetus?(LO 6.20)
   a. Pregnancy Category A
   b. Pregnancy Category B
   c. Pregnancy Category C
   d. Pregnancy Category X

7. Which of the following factors affects absorption of a drug (may select more than one)?(LO 6.4)
   a. Concentration
   b. Dissolution
   c. Solubility
   d. All of the above
8. Which of the following is considered a parenteral route requiring a syringe?(LO 6.14)
   a. Intramuscular
   b. Intravenous
   c. Subcutaneous
   d. All of the above
9. What FDA equivalency code indicates that a drug meets the necessary bioequivalence requirements?(LO 6.15)
   a. AA
   b. AB
   c. B
   d. BD
10. Which of the following is used to measure a drug's safety?(LO 6.2)
    a. ED50
    b. LD50
    c. SSRI
    d. TI
11. Which of the following medications is capable of crossing the placental barrier and causing a potential birth defect?(LO 6.20)
    a. Estrogen
    b. Phenytoin
    c. Tetracycline
    d. All of the above
12. Which of the following medications may be found in breast milk?(LO 6.20)
    a. Codeine
    b. Lithium
    c. Nicotine
    d. All of the above
13. Which of the following does *not* affect the effects of a drug?(LO 6.8)
    a. Body weight
    b. FDA classification
    c. Rate of elimination
    d. Volume of distribution
14. What type of toxicity affects the liver?(LO 6.7)
    a. Hepatoxicity
    b. Nephrotoxicity
    c. Pulmonary toxicity
    d. None of the above
15. Which of the following drug interactions occurs when the combined effects of two drugs if taken together is equal to the sum of their parts?(LO 6.10)
    a. Additive effect
    b. Antagonism
    c. Potentiation
    d. Synergism
16. Which of the following terms refers to how well a drug agent accomplishes its goal?(LO 6.17)
    a. Affinity
    b. Agonist
    c. Antagonist
    d. Efficacy
17. Which of the following is *not* a disadvantage of an oral dosage form?(LO 6.14)
    a. The absorption process is more rapid and predictable.
    b. Certain oral medications may bind to various food products.
    c. Certain oral drugs may be destroyed by digestive enzymes.
    d. The liver may metabolize the drug before it reaches the circulatory system.
18. Which of the following is *not* a parenteral route of administration?(LO 6.14)
    a. Inhalation
    b. Intramuscular
    c. Intravenous
    d. Sublingual
19. Which of the following is *not* an example of renal excretion?(LO 6.7)
    a. Active tubular secretion
    b. Active glomerular reabsorption
    c. Glomerular filtration
    d. Passive tubular reabsorption
20. Which of the following medications do *not* require a physician's monitoring?(LO 6.7)
    a. Coumadin
    b. Dilantin
    c. Lithium
    d. Keflex

Matching

Match the word to its definition.

_____ 1. A substance that blocks a receptor site preventing a drug from producing its therapeutic effect

_____ 2. A ratio comparing the lethal dose of a drug to its effective dose

_____ 3. The study of the absorption, distribution, metabolism, and elimination of a drug

_____ 4. Having a pH less than 7

_____ 5. The strength or concentration of a drug to produce a specific effect

_____ 6. How a drug produces its effect

_____ 7. A brand name drug

_____ 8. The use of a drug

_____ 9. An unusual effect of a drug regardless of its intensity or dosage

_____10. A decreased sensitivity to a drug

_____11. An injection into a vein

_____12. The amount of time required for one-half of the drug to be eliminated from the body

_____13. A dose used to obtain a therapeutic dose sooner

_____14. Possessing an electrical charge

15. Generic name

a. Acid
b. Antagonist
c. Half-life
d. Idiosyncrasy
e. Indication
f. Intravenous
g. Ionized
h. Loading dose
i. Mechanism of action
j. Nonproprietary name
k. Pharmacokinetics
l. Potency
m. Proprietary name
n. Therapeutic index
o. Tolerance

Critical Thinking Questions

1. A patient picks up a prescription from the pharmacy and begins to read the drug monograph that accompanies the prescription. He or she becomes disturbed after reading the side effects associated with the prescription. How would you handle the situation? What would you say to the patient?[LO 6.18]

2. A 180-lb man is picking up a prescription for Coumadin for both his wife (110 lb) and himself. He notices the strength for his prescription is for 2.5 mg each day and his wife's prescription is 7.5 mg every day. He is perplexed at the differences in the dosing on the prescription and asks if a mistake was made. You check the original prescriptions the man presented to the pharmacy and the prescriptions were filled correctly. How would you explain this situation to the man regarding the dosing?[LO 6.2]

3. A pregnant woman is having an antibiotic prescription filled for a respiratory infection. She did not mention to her physician that she was pregnant. What would you do to find out if the prescription is safe for her to take? Where would you find the information?[LO 6.20]

4. A diabetic patient is purchasing strips for his glucometer. He mentions to you that because of the cost of the test strips, he is testing his blood only every other day. What would you do after hearing the patient's statement?[LO 6.9]

5. A customer presents a prescription for Wellbutrin XL 150 mg. The physician has approved the use of a generic product. The patient is surprised that the cost of the prescription is 65% less than the brand name product. The patient wants to know if it is the same drug. What type of testing occurs to ensure that it will provide the same results as the brand name?[LO 6.15]

HIPAA Scenario

Paul is a pharmacy technician who was recently hired to work in a small retail pharmacy. His friends stop by occasionally to chat with him when they shop at the store. One day his friend Sam asks him if he can refill his wife's prescription for her pain medication. When Paul asks Sam for the name of the medication, Sam tells him that it is Tylenol with codeine #3. Paul checks the wife's profile, sees a prescription for acetaminophen with codeine #3, and processes the refill for Sam. Later in the day, Sam calls the pharmacy and informs the pharmacist the wrong medication was dispensed to him and the medicine is not controlling the pain. The pharmacist speaks to Sam and informs him the generic medication was dispensed. Two days later, Sam's wife calls in a refill for the same medication. After several minutes Paul learns that Sam's wife never received the refill he gave to Sam. Afraid to admit that he allowed Sam to refill the prescription without any authorization from his spouse, Paul goes to his supervisor for help.

Discussion Questions(PTCB II. 73)

1. How would you explain to Sam the difference between a brand name drug and the generic drug?
2. What factors could affect how the medication works in the body?
3. Could someone have an addiction in this situation and if so, what type?

Internet Activities

1. Visit **www.fda.gov** and identify 10 medications that have recently been approved to be available as a generic drug.(LO 6.16)
2. Visit **www.fda.gov** and find information on adverse event reporting. What type of information is required when filling out this form?
3. Visit your state board of pharmacy's Web site and review the regulations regarding generic drug substitution. What conditions must be met in dispensing generic medications in your state?(LO 6.15)
4. Visit **www.fda.gov** and identify medications that have had medical and clinical pharmacology review conducted.(LO 6.1)

7

Drug Classifications

Learning Outcomes

Upon completion of this chapter, you will be able to:

7.1 Define the term *classification*.

7.2 List the reasons drug classifications are important to pharmacy technicians.

7.3 Differentiate between agonists and antagonists.

7.4 Define and describe the role of neurotransmitters as they relate to drug action.

7.5 Classify medications or agents given a particular organ, system, or function.

7.6 Define *controlled substances*.

7.7 Identify drugs categorized as controlled substances.

Key Terms

adverse effects
central nervous system (CNS)
contraindication
controlled substance
dosage form
indication
interaction
receptor

PTCB

In preparation for the certification examination, you should understand and perform activities associated with the following PTCB Knowledge Statement:

PTCB Knowledge Statement

Domain I. Assisting the Pharmacist in Serving Patients

Knowledge of generic and brand names of pharmaceuticals (5)
Knowledge of therapeutic equivalence (6)
Knowledge of signs and symptoms of disease states (10)
Knowledge of drug indications (18)

Case Study

Thomas Brown, CPhT, is the pharmacy technician at ABC Pharmacy, an independent pharmacy. Mr. Lee is a new customer who came in with the following new prescription:

Peter J. Collins, M.D.
3321 W. 5th Street
Anytown, USA

Name: Nelson Lee Date: October 14, 2012

Address: 342 Elm Avenue Anytown, USA

Rx: Augmentin® 875 mg

SIG: One tablet every 12 hours for 10 days. #20

Refills: 0

P. Collins, M.D.

Mr. Lee tells Thomas that he is being treated for an infection, and that he hopes this medication works because he is currently taking amoxicillin 500 mg and it is not working. Mr. Lee also tells Thomas that he is planning on continuing to take the amoxicillin, as that is a prescription written by another doctor and was filled at another pharmacy 3 days ago.

While reading this chapter, keep the following questions in mind:

1. As a pharmacy technician, why is this situation significant to Thomas?(LO 7.2)
2. What should Thomas say to Mr. Lee?(LO 7.2, 7.5)
3. What should Thomas say to the pharmacist?(LO 7.2)

Introduction to Drug Classifications(LO 7.1)

Medications are classified based upon therapeutic use, drug family, and/or mechanism of action. Through understanding drug classification, the pharmacy technician is able to identify medications of the same therapeutic class, family, or mechanism of action as belonging to the same category. Medications are identified in this manner, which facilitates the technician's understanding of drug action and therapeutic use.

Drug classifications are important because they help the technician understand the clinical uses, **adverse effects,** and potential **interactions** of medications. By understanding the medications in a given category, a technician may help prevent a medication error due to drug class duplication (two drugs with similar actions administered to the same patient), recognize a potential drug-drug interaction, or identify a potential **contraindication** for the use of a particular drug. For example, if a patient's profile contains information that the patient is allergic to a particular drug, the pharmacy technician should be able to recognize any medication belonging to the class of drugs to which the patient is allergic. The technician in this case is contributing to safe medication use for the patient through his or her knowledge of drug classification.

adverse effects Negative nontherapeutic effects associated with medication use.
interaction Event occurring as a result of two or more agents being used together.
contraindication Situation in which a particular drug should not be used.

At Your Service

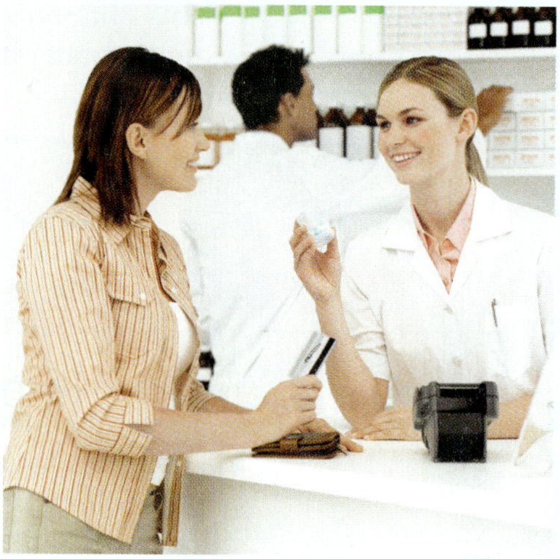

Cynthia is a pharmacy technician in a busy chain drugstore pharmacy. Mrs. Jones is a regular customer who has had a prescription for Tri-Norinyl (an oral contraceptive) filled at the pharmacy where Cynthia works for the past 6 months. This month when Mrs. Jones came in for her regular refill of Tri-Norinyl, she mentioned to Cynthia in passing that she had received another prescription while visiting her cousin in another state. Cynthia asked Mrs. Jones about the prescription. Mrs. Jones explained that as she had a severe toothache, she visited a dentist while out of state who prescribed an antibiotic. Cynthia was concerned because she knows there is a drug interaction between some antibiotics and oral contraceptives.

While reading this chapter, keep the following questions in mind.

1. As a pharmacy technician, why should Cynthia be concerned about Mrs. Jones's statements?(LO 7.5)
2. What should Cynthia say to Mrs. Jones?(LO 7.2)
3. If you were Cynthia, what actions would you take?(LO 7.2, 7.5)

Drug Classifications(LO 7.1, 7.2)

Basically, drug classifications are ways of grouping similar or like drugs into a category. Drug categories may be based upon mechanism of action (e.g., 3-hydroxy-3-methyl-glutaryl-CoA [HMG-CoA] reductase inhibitors), disease, or condition for which the medication is intended (e.g., osteoporosis medications), site of action in the body (e.g., gastrointestinal medications), drug-**receptor** interaction (e.g., antihistamines), general effect (e.g., antibiotics), or drug family (e.g., cephalosporins). Using the various methods of classification, a single drug may have more than one drug classification. For example, diazepam is a benzodiazepine (family), sedative-hypnotic (general effect), and a gamma amino butyric acid (GABA) agonist (mechanism of action). The Food and Drug Administration (FDA) has a role in the classification of drugs, as it is the agency responsible for approving medications for specific **indications.** Patients themselves play a role in drug categorizations as they often understand and describe the classifications of medications in the simplest terms (e.g., pain medication or heart medication). It is important for the pharmacy technician to be able to communicate effectively in the pharmacy to discern between the more common classification terms used by the patient and the more technical terms used by the pharmacist. The pharmacy technician will in many cases serve as a type of translator for the patient. For example, if the patient calls

receptor Specific site of drug or chemical action.

indication Purpose for which a specific medication is approved for use.

the pharmacy asking for a refill of blood pressure pills, the pharmacy technician should be able to recognize diuretics and angiotensin-converting enzyme (ACE) inhibitors listed in the patient's profile as being agents that can lower blood pressure.

This chapter explores drug classifications starting with the physiologic system where pharmacologic agents exhibit activity. The agents are further subcategorized by either mechanism of action, family, or drug-receptor interaction, whichever is most commonly employed.

Central Nervous System Medications (LO 7.3, 7.4, 7.5, 7.6, 7.7)

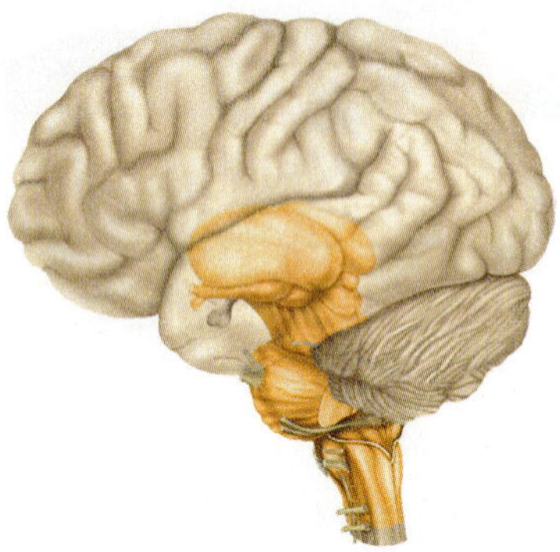

Figure 7-1 The CNS includes the brain and spinal cord.

The **central nervous system (CNS)** consists of the brain and the spinal cord (Figure 7-1). Medications affecting the CNS are numerous and range from medications to cause sleep (hypnotic agents) to agents that relieve pain.

The following list identifies the agents that will be covered in this section:

- Sedative-hypnotic agents
- Psychiatric medications
    - Antipsychotic agents
    - Antidepressants
    - Psychomotor stimulants
- Agents for movement disorders
    - Anticonvulsant agents
    - Anti-Parkinson agents
- Anesthetics
    - General anesthetics
    - Local anesthetics
- Muscle relaxants
- Analgesics
    - Narcotic analgesics
    - Nonnarcotic analgesics
    - Nonsteroidal anti-inflammatory agents
    - Antigout medications

Sedative-Hypnotic Drugs

Sedative-hypnotic agents are employed in the management of various conditions including but not limited to anxiety, insomnia, and induction or are used as adjuncts to anesthesia. The term *sedative* refers to the relaxing properties of a medication, whereas the term *hypnotic* refers to the ability of the agent to induce sleep. Alcohol is a commonly used "sedative-hypnotic" agent in that it is a CNS depressant. Individuals self-medicate with alcohol to induce relaxation or "calm nerves." Antihistamines that cause drowsiness through inhibiting acetylcholine (an excitatory neurotransmitter) are often used as over-the-counter (OTC) sedative-hypnotic agents.

Antianxiety agents or anxiolytics are sedative agents that are employed in the management of anxiety, a generalized sense of fear or doom. Anxiolytics tend to have a shorter half-life than the hypnotic agents, in order to render the patient relaxed but not overly sleepy. Hypnotic agents have longer

central nervous system (CNS) Brain and the spinal cord.

half-lives and are therefore used to induce sleep, not just relaxation. The majority of sedative-hypnotic agents are **controlled substances,** which are agents that have the potential for physical and psychological dependence and abuse. Controlled substances are classified by schedules I, II, III,IV, or V, and as such, have restrictions with dispensing and adverse drug reactions of abuse, dependence, and tolerance.

Psychiatric Medications

Antipsychotic medications are employed in the management of mental disorders such as schizophrenia, but may also be used to manage nausea, agitation, or as adjuncts to anesthesia. The specific neurotransmitters that are blocked by the antipsychotic medications are dopamine or serotonin. These agents work by blocking dopamine or serotonin receptors in the CNS. Other terms for antipsychotic agents are *neuroleptic agents* and *major tranquilizers*.

Generally, antidepressants are used to manage the symptoms associated with depression. Some of these agents are also employed in the management of nocturnal enuresis, chronic neuropathic pain, premenstrual syndrome (PMS), smoking cessation, and obsessive-compulsive disorders. The antidepressants consist of several main subcategories:

- Tricyclic antidepressants (TCAs)
- Selective serotonin reuptake inhibitors (SSRIs)
- Serotonin-norepinephrine reuptake inhibitors (SNRIs)
- Monoamine oxidase inhibitors (MAOIs)
- Miscellaneous (agents with mechanisms of action different from those mentioned)

Lithium is a mood-stabilizing agent employed in the management of bipolar affective disorder (BAD). It is not considered an antidepressant, antipsychotic, or a sedative-hypnotic. It is also an example of a "legend drug," requiring a prescription but without a specific classification. Serum levels must be checked regularly while a patient is on lithium, as elevated serum levels are associated with toxicity. Lithium is marketed under several trade names including Eskalith, Lithonate, Lithane, Lithobid, and Lithotabs.

Psychomotor stimulants are agents that exhibit excitatory effects on the CNS. These agents include anorexiants for weight loss, amphetamines for attention deficit hyperactivity disorder (ADHD) and narcolepsy, and miscellaneous agents including caffeine, nicotine, and cocaine. All of the amphetamines and anorexiants are controlled substances, and therefore have abuse potential.

Psychomimetics (drugs of abuse) are illegal agents used recreationally by individuals. Use of these agents is dangerous as there is no standardization of the amount of drug in a **dosage form** nor is there any guarantee of the purported contents of the dosage form. These agents include CNS stimulants, depressants, and hallucinogens. It is important for the pharmacy technician to remember that prescription drugs may be abused as well as illegal street drugs.

Common illicit drugs of abuse include:

- Cocaine (powder and crystallized forms)
- Heroin
- Lysergic acid diethylamide (LSD)
- MDMA (Ecstasy)
- Methamphetamine

controlled substance Pharmacologic agent included in Schedules I, II, III, IV, or V, which has potential for physical and/or psychological dependence and abuse.

dosage form Vehicle into which a drug is incorporated to enable administration.

Agents for Movement Disorders

Antiepileptic agents are also called anticonvulsant drugs or seizure medications. Generally, these agents work by depressing the CNS or by decreasing the spread of the focus of the stimulus. Anticonvulsants have also been employed in the management of chronic pain and bipolar affective disorder.

Parkinson's disease is a progressive movement disorder due to lack of dopamine or inactivity of dopamine in the CNS. Anti-Parkinson's drugs may increase the dopamine level in the CNS (Levodopa), increase dopamine access to its receptor sites (dopamine agonists), interfere with the metabolism of dopamine in the CNS (monoamine oxidase [MAO] inhibitors and catechol-0-methyltransferase [COMT] inhibitors), or decrease relatively high activity of acetylcholine (anticholinergics).

Anesthetic Agents (Local and General)

Local anesthetics may be employed to minimize pain perception in surgical procedures while maintaining consciousness of the patient. These agents may also be used in topical forms to alleviate pain due to sunburn, dental procedures, hemorrhoids, and muscle aches.

General anesthetics are agents that are employed to cause a loss of consciousness for surgical procedures. These agents may be administered via intravenous or gaseous routes, and are often used with other medications to maintain surgical anesthesia.

Muscle Relaxants

Muscle relaxants are used in the management of acute muscle injury resulting from muscle injuries. Although these agents are not controlled substances, they have been known to cause drowsiness, and may impair ability to drive.

Analgesics

An analgesic agent is one that relieves pain. Narcotic analgesics are controlled substances, related to opium, that relieve pain and have abuse potential. Many of the narcotic analgesics contain a nonopioid analgesic (e.g., acetaminophen) in combination with an opioid analgesic (codeine). Aside from abuse potential, dependence, and tolerance, these agents also cause euphoria, dry mouth, urinary retention, and constipation.

Nonsteroidal anti-inflammatory drugs (NSAIDs) are used for conditions to provide alleviation of pain mediated by inflammation (e.g., rheumatoid arthritis). These agents work by inhibiting the activity of prostaglandins, which are mediators of inflammatory pain.

Gout is an inflammatory condition caused by elevated uric acid levels in the bloodstream. The uric acid may crystallize to form painful sites of inflammation. Agents used to manage gout consist of anti-inflammatory agents like the NSAIDs, agents to decrease uric acid production in the body (allopurinol), agents to increase uric acid excretion (probenecid, sulfinpyrazone), and anti-inflammatory agents (colchicine, NSAIDs).

Table 7-1 identifies pharmacologic agents that exhibit activity in the CNS that were discussed in the previous section.

Table 7-1 CNS Agents

Sedative-Hypnotic Agents			
Antihistamines diphenhydramine (Benadryl) hydroxyzine pamoate (Vistaril) hydroxyzine HCl (Atarax) midazolam (Versed)	**Barbiturates** pentobarbital (Nembutal) secobarbital (Seconal)	**Benzodiazepines** alprazolam (Xanax) estazolam (ProSom) flurazepam (Dalmane) quazepam (Doral) temazepam (Restoril) triazolam (Halcion)	**Miscellaneous** chloral hydrate (Aquachloral) esopiclone (Lunesta) zaleplon (Sonata) zolpidem (Ambien, Ambien CR)
Psychiatric Medications			
Antidepressants ***MAOI*** phenelzine (Nardil)	**Antipsychotics** aripiprazole (Abilify) chlorpromazine (Thorazine) clozapine (Clozaril) fluphenazine (Prolixin, Permitil) haloperidol (Haldol) loxapine (Loxitane) mesoridazine (Serentil) molindone (Moban) olanzapine (Zyprexa) perphenazine (Trilafon) prochlorperazine (Compazine) risperidone (Risperdal) thioridazine (Mellaril) thiothixene (Navane) trifluoperazine (Stelazine) ziprasidone (Geodon)	**Miscellaneous** bupropion (Wellbutrin, Wellbutrin SR)	
SNRIs mirtazapine (Remeron) nefazodone (Serzone) trazodone (Desyrel) quetiapine (Seroquel) venlafaxine (Effexor) desvenlafaxine (Pristiq)	**SSRIs** citalopram (Celexa) escitalopram (Lexapro) fluoxetine (Prozac, Sarafem) fluvoxamine (Luvox) paroxetine (Paxil) sertraline (Zoloft)	**TCAs** amitriptyline (Elavil) desipramine (Norpramin) doxepin (Sinequan) imipramine (Tofranil) nortriptyline (Aventyl, Pamelor)	**Psychomotor Stimulants** amphetamine sulfate (various) benzphetamine (Didrex) dextroamphetamine (Dexedrine) diethylpropion (Tenuate) mazindol (Mazanor, Sanorex) methamphetamine HCl (Desoxyn) phendimetrazine tartrate (Bontril PDM) phentermine HCl (Adipex-P, Ionamin) sibutramine (Meridia)
Agents for Movement Disorders			
Anticonvulsants carbamazepine (Tegretol) clonazepam (Klonopin) diazepam (Valium) ethosuximide (Zarontin) fosphenytoin (Cerebyx) gabapentin (Neurontin) lamotrigine (Lamictal) levetiracetam (Keppra) lorazepam (Ativan) oxcarbazepine (Trileptal) phenobarbital (various) phenytoin (Dilantin)	**Anti-Parkinson's Agents** amantadine (Symmetrel) benztropine mesylate (Cogentin) bromocriptine (Parlodel) carbidopa/levodopa (Sinemet) entacapone (Comtan) pergolide (Permax) pramipexole (Mirapex)		

(Continued)

Table 7-1 CNS Agents *(Continued)*

Agents for Movement Disorders contd...			
Anticonvulsants primidone (Mysoline) tiagabine (Gabitril) topiramate (Topamax) valproic acid (Zonegran) zonisamide (Depakene, Depakote)	**Anti-Parkinson's Agents** ropinirole (Requip) selegiline (Eldepryl) tolcapone (Tasmar)		
Anesthetics			
General Anesthetics diazepam (Valium) enflurane (Ethrane) etomidate (Amidate) halothane (Fluothane) isoflurane (Forane) ketamine (Ketalar) lorazepam (Ativan) methohexital (Brevital) midazolam (Versed) nitric oxide (INOmax) propofol (Diprivan) sevoflurane (Sevorane, Ultane) thiopental (Pentothal)	**Local Anesthetics** benzocaine/antipyrine (Auralgan) bupivacaine (Marcaine) capsaicin (Capsin, Zostrix) dibucaine (Nupercainal) lidocaine (Xylocaine, Lidocaine) pramoxine (Anusol, Proctofoam)		
Muscle Relaxants			
baclofen (Lioresal) carisoprodol (Soma) chlorzoxazone (Paraflex, ParafonForte DSC) cyclobenzaprine (Flexeril) dantrolene (Dantrium) diazepam (Valium) metaxalone (Skelaxin) methocarbamol (Robaxin) orphenadrine (Norflex)			
Analgesics			
Narcotic Analgesics acetaminophen with codeine (Tylenol No. 1, 2, 3, or 4) alfentanil (Alfenta) aspirin with codeine (Empirin No. 1, 2, 3, or 4) buprenorphine (Buprenex) butorphanol (Stadol) codeine (various) dezocine (Dalgan) fentanyl (Sublimaze, Duragesic, Actiq System) hydrocodone and acetaminophen (Lorcet, Vicodin) hydrocodone and aspirin (Lortab ASA) hydrocodone and ibuprofen (Vicoprofen) hydromorphone (dilaudid) levorphanol (Levo-Dromoran) meperidine (Demerol) methadone (Dolophine)	**Nonnarcotic Analgesics** acetaminophen (Tylenol) aspirin (various) tramadol (Ultram) tramadol/acetaminophen (Ultracet)	**Nonsteroidal Anti-Inflammatory Agents** diclofenac (Cataflam, Voltaren) diflunisal (Dolobid) etodolac (Lodine) fenoprofen (Nalfon) flurbiprofen (Ansaid) ibuprofen (Motrin) indomethacin (Indocin) ketoprofen (Orudis, Oruvail) ketorolac (Toradol) meloxicam (Mobic) nabumetone (Relafen) naproxen (Aleve, Anaprox, Naprosyn) oxaprozin (Daypro) piroxicam (Feldene) sulindac (Clinoril) tolmetin (Tolectin)	**Antigout Agents** allopurinol (Zyloprim, Lopurin) colchicine (various) colchicine/probenecid (Colbenemid) probenecid (Benemid) sulfinpyrazone (Anturane)

(Continued)

Table 7-1 CNS Agents *(Continued)*

Analgesics contd...		
Narcotic Analgesics morphine (Duramorph, MS Contin, Oramorph SR) nalbuphine (Nubain) oxycodone (OxyContin) oxycodone and acetaminophen (Percocet, Tylox) oxycodone and aspirin (Percodan, Percodan-Demi) oxymorphone (Numorphan) pentazocine (Talwin) propoxyphene (Darvon) propoxyphene and acetaminophen (Darvocet-N-100) propoxyphene and aspirin (Darvon Compound-65, Darvon-N with Aspirin)		

Tech Check

1. List three anticonvulsant medications.(LO 7.5)
2. List three medications employed in the management of pain.(LO 7.5)
3. Define *analgesic*.(LO 7.5)

Cardiovascular System Medications(LO 7.5)

The cardiovascular system consists of the heart, arteries, and veins (Figure 7-2). Medications affecting the cardiovascular system include cardiac glycosides for heart failure, antiarrhythmic medications, antianginal medications, and antihypertensive medications.

Heart failure occurs when the heart is unable to pump blood effectively enough to meet the body's demands. Patients in heart failure often need multiple medications to manage their condition. Certain medications used in heart failure (vasodilators, ACE inhibitors, and diuretics) may also be used to manage hypertension. Drugs that have positive inotropic effects (cardiac glycosides and other positive inotropes) increase the force of the myocardial contraction, causing the heart to work more efficiently. Vasodilators allow for improved blood circulation to all areas of the body.

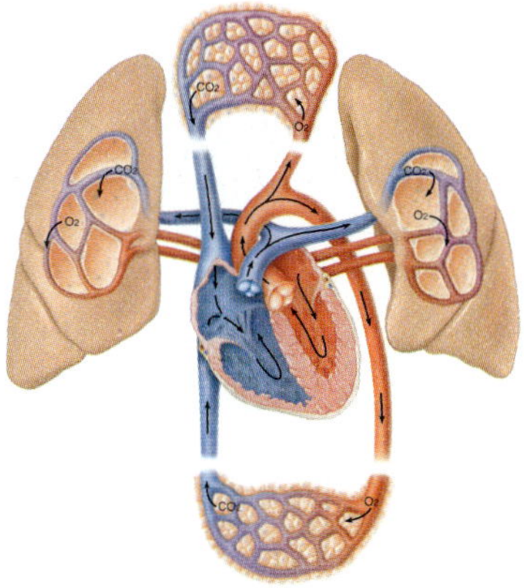

Figure 7-2 Cardiovascular System.

Antiarrhythmic Medications

Antiarrhythmic medications affect the electrical conduction system of the heart. These medications have various mechanisms of action including sodium channel blockade, beta adrenergic blockade, potassium channel blockade (prolonging repolarization), and calcium channel blockade.

Antianginal Medications

Antianginal medications relieve pain associated with chest pain due to inadequate myocardial oxygen supply. Immediate release sublingual

Table 7-2 Cardiovascular System Agents

Heart Failure Medications	Antiarrhythmic Medications	Antianginal Medications
Cardiac Glycosides digoxin (Lanoxin) **Positive Inotropic Agents** amrinone (Inocor) milrinone (Primacor) **Vasodilators** hydralazine (Apresoline) minoxidil (Loniten) nitroprusside* (Nipride)	**Class I** disopyramide (Norpace) lidocaine (Xylocaine) flecainide (Tambocor) mexiletine (Mexitil) procainamide (Pronestyl, Procan) quinidine (Quinidex, Quinaglute) **Class II** esmolol (Brevibloc) **Class III** amiodarone (Cordarone, Pacerone) dofetilide (Tikosyn) ibutilide (Corvert) sotalol (Betapace) **Class IV** verapamil (Calan, Isoptin) **Miscellaneous** adenosine (Adenocard) atropine (various) digoxin (Lanoxin)	isosorbide dinitrate (Isordil, Sorbitrate, Dilatrate-SR) isosorbide mononitrate (Ismo, Imdur) nitroglycerin (Nitrostat, Nitrolingual, Nitro-Bid, Nitrodisc, Transderm-Nitro)

*Dilates both arteries and veins.

dosage forms manage acute angina, whereas longer-acting tablets and capsules provide management for predictable anginal attacks. These agents share similar activity with the vasodilator agents. It is important to note that the dosage form determines use for nitroglycerin. Sublingual tablets and spray are for acute angina, whereas the patch would be used to manage hypertension.

Table 7-2 identifies agents for heart failure, antiarrhythmic agents, and antianginal agents.

Tech Check

4. Which agent is a cardiac glycoside?(LO 7.5)
5. Identify three antiarrhythmic medications.(LO 7.5)
6. Which forms of nitroglycerin are used in the management of acute angina that is associated with a heart attack?(LO 7.5)

Renal/Vascular System Medications(LO 7.5)

The renal system is also known as the urinary system and consists of the kidneys, ureters, urinary bladder, and the urethra (Figure 7-3). The renal system plays an important role in the ADME process; refer to chapter 6 to review the ADME process.

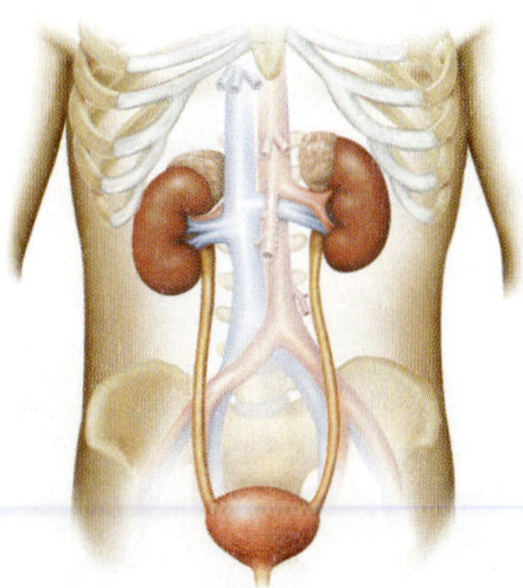

Figure 7-3 Renal System.

Diuretics

Diuretics are agents that decrease blood volume through increasing urinary volume (Figure 7-3). They are employed in the management of congestive heart failure, hypertension, glaucoma, renal failure, and kidney stones. A patient who is taking a thiazide or a loop diuretic may also require potassium supplementation, as these agents cause an increase in urinary elimination of potassium.

Antihypertensive Agents

Antihypertensive agents are various categories of medications used to reduce blood pressure. As blood pressure equals cardiac output multiplied by peripheral vascular resistance, most antihypertensives are designed to reduce either cardiac output and/or peripheral vascular resistance. A patient may need to take a few medications from different antihypertensive drug categories in order to manage blood pressure effectively.

Antihyperlipidemic Agents

Antihyperlipidemic agents are drugs used to decrease plasma lipids and cholesterol. High cholesterol levels increase the risk of coronary artery disease, heart attacks, and stroke. Various agents work by decreasing the absorption of fats from the gastrointestinal system, increasing the activity of fat metabolizing enzymes, and decreasing the production of cholesterol by the liver.

Hematologic Agents

Hematologic agents consist of anticoagulants, antiplatelet agents, antithrombotic agents, and hematopoietic stimulants. Anticoagulants interfere with blood clotting through inhibition of various factors in the clotting cascade. Antiplatelet agents interfere with platelet adhesion and aggregation. Antithrombotic (thrombolytic) agents are drugs that are used to lyse or destroy existing blood clots. Hematopoietic stimulants are pharmacologic agents used to increase red or white blood cells.

Dietary Supplements

Dietary supplements are employed in the management of anemia and other disorders of the blood. Table 7-3 (p. 206) contains a list of the most common agents. Refer to Chapter 9 for more information on the dietary supplements.

Tech Check

7. Agents that decrease blood volume through increasing urinary volume are ______. (LO 7.5)
8. List four categories of antihypertensive agents. (LO 7.5)
9. Enoxaparin, heparin, and warfarin are categorized as ______. (LO 7.5)
10. Pravastatin, niacin, and cholestyramine may be employed in the management of ______. (LO 7.5)

Table 7-3 Renal and Vascular Agents

Diuretics	Antihypertensives	Hematologic Agents	Lipid-Lowering Agents	Antianemic Dietary Supplements
Loop bumetanide (Bumex) furosemide (Lasix) torsemide (Demadex) **Potassium-Sparing** amiloride (Midamor) spironolactone (Aldactone) triamterene (Dyrenium) **Thiazide** chlorothiazide (Diuril) chlorthalidone (Hygroton) hydrochlorothiazide (HydroDIURIL) indapamide (Lozol) metolazone (Zaroxolyn) **Diuretic Combinations** hydrochlorothiazide/ amiloride (Moduretic) hydrochlorothiazide/ spironolactone (Aldactazide) hydrochlorothiazide/ triamterene (Dyazide, Maxzide)	**Alpha-1 Adrenergic Blockers** doxazosin (Cardura) prazosin (Minipress) terazosin (Hytrin) **Angiotensin-Converting Enzyme Inhibitors** benazepril (Lotensin) captopril (Capoten) enalapril (Vasotec) fosinopril (Monopril) lisinopril (Prinivil, Zestril) moexipril (Univasc) erbumine perindopril (Aceon) quinapril (Accupril) ramipril (Altace) trandolapril (Mavik) **Angiotensin Receptor Blockers** candesartan (Atacand) eprosartan (Teveten) irbesartan (Avapro) losartan (Cozaar) telmisartan (Micardis) valsartan (Diovan) nisoldipine (Sular) **Centrally Acting Agents** clonidine (Catapres, Catapres TTS) methyldopa (Aldomet) **Beta Adrenergic Blockers** acebutolol (Sectral) atenolol (Tenormin) betaxolol (Kerlone) bisoprolol (Zebeta) carteolol (Cartrol) carvedilol (Coreg) labetalol (Normodyne, Trandate) metoprolol (Lopressor, Toprol XL) nadolol (Corgard) penbutolol (Levatol) pindolol (Visken) propranolol (Inderal) timolol (Blocadren) nebivolol (Bystolic) **Calcium Channel Blockers** amlodipine (Norvasc) diltiazem (Cardizem, Diltia XT, Dilacor, Cartia XT, Tiazac) felodipine (Plendil) isradipine (DynaCirc) nicardipine (Cardene) nifedipine (Procardia, Procardia XL, Adalat, Adalat CC) nimodipine (Nimotop) verapamil (Calan, Isoptin, Verelan) **Vasodilators** hydralazine (Apresoline) minoxidil (Loniten)	**Anticoagulants** ardeparin (Normiflo) argatroban (Acova) bivalirudin (Angiomax) dalteparin (Fragmin) enoxaparin (Lovenox) fondaparinux (Arixtra) heparin (various) lepirudin (Refludan) tinzaparin (Innohep) warfarin (Coumadin) **Thrombolytic Agents** alteplase (Activase) aminocaproic acid (Amicar) anistreplase (Eminase) aprotinin (Trasylol) danaparoid (Orgaran) dextran 40 (Rheomacrodex) reteplase (Retavase) streptokinase (Abbokinase) tenecteplase (TNKase) urokinase (Streptase, Kabikinase) **Antiplatelet Agents** abciximab (ReoPro) aspirin (various) clopidogrel (Plavix) dipyridamole (Persantine) dipyridamole/aspirin (Aggrenox) eptifibatide (Aggrastat) ticlopidine (Ticlid) tirofiban (Integrilin) **Hematopoietic Stimulants** darbepoetin alfa (Aranesp) epoetin alfa (Epogen, Procrit) filgrastim (Neupogen) oprelvekin (Neumega) pegfilgrastim (Neulasta) sargramostim (Prokine, Leukine)	**Bile Acid Binding Resins** cholestyramine (Questran, LoCholest) colestipol (Colestid) **HMG-CoA Reductase Inhibitors** atorvastatin (Lipitor) fluvastatin (Lescol) lovastatin (Mevacor, Altocor) pravastatin (Pravachol) simvastatin (Zocor) rosuvastatin (Crestor) **Fibric Acid Derivatives** clofibrate (Atromid-S) fenofibrate (Tricor) gemfibrozil (Lopid) **Miscellaneous** ezetimibe (Zetia) niacin (Niaspan, Nicobid)	cyanocobalamin (Vitamin B_{12}) (various) ferrous Gluconate (Fergon) ferrous sulfate (various) folic acid (various) iron dextran (DexFerrum, InFeD) iron sucrose (Venofer)

Respiratory System Medications(LO 7.5)

The respiratory system moves air in and out of the lungs. This process is called ventilation, respiration, or breathing. The system functions to deliver oxygen to the bloodstream and remove carbon dioxide from the blood (See Figure 7-4)

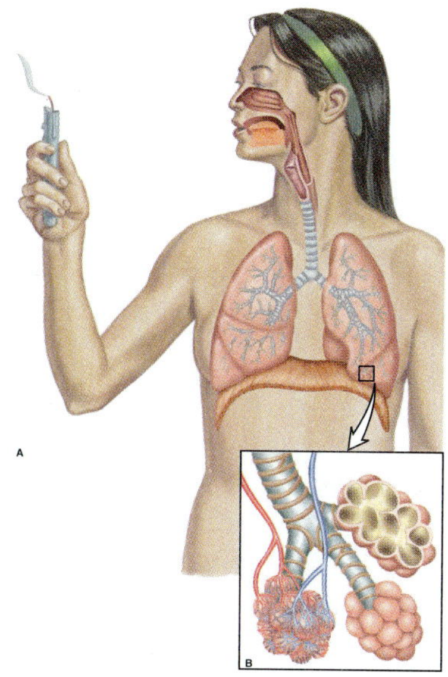

Figure 7-4 Respiratory System.

Antihistamines

Antihistamines block histamine receptors, inhibiting the allergic response and reducing symptoms like runny nose, watery eyes, and sneezing. These agents are also employed in the management of allergies and anaphylaxis. Newer antihistamines such as desloratadine, loratadine, fexofenadine, and cetirizine are formulated to cause less drowsiness than older agents such as chlorpheniramine, diphenhydramine, and hydroxyzine.

Bronchodilators

Bronchodilators are employed in the management of asthma and other respiratory diseases like emphysema and chronic bronchitis. Many of the respiratory inhalants, like the corticosteroids, enhance the effects of the bronchodilators by reducing inflammation.

Agents demonstrating activity in the respiratory system are listed in Table 7-4.

Table 7-4 Respiratory System Agents

Respiratory Agents	
Antihistamines	**Respiratory Inhalants**
astemizole (Hismanal)	acetylcysteine (Mucomyst)
azelastine (Astelin)	beclomethasone (Beconase, Vancenase, Beclovent, Vanceril)
cetirizine (Zyrtec)	beractant (Survanta)
chlorpheniramine (Chlor-Trimeton)	budesonide (Rhinocort, Pulmicort)
clemastine fumarate (Tavist)	calfactant (Infasurf)
cyproheptadine (Periactin)	colfosceril Palmitate (Exosurf Neonatal)
desloratadine (Clarinex)	cromolyn sodium (Intal, Nasalcrom)
diphenhydramine (Benadryl)	dexamethasone (Dexacort Turbinaire)
fexofenadine (Allegra)	flunisolide (AeroBid, Nasalide, Nasarel)
hydroxyzine HCl (Atarax)	fluticasone (Flovent, Flonase)
hydroxyzine pamoate (Vistaril)	fluticasone propionate/salmeterol (Salmeterol Xinafoate)
loratadine (Claritin, Alavert)	xinafoate (Advair Diskus)
Bronchodilators	nedocromil (Tilade)
albuterol (Proventil, Ventolin, Volmax)	tiotropium (Spiriva)
albuterol/Ipratropium (Combivent)	triamcinolone (Azmacort, Nasacort, Nasacort AQ)
aminophylline (various)	ciclesonide (Alvesco)
bitolterol (Tornalate)	**Miscellaneous Agents**
epinephrine (Adrenalin, Sus-Phrine, EpiPen)	dornase alfa (Pulmozyme)
formoterol (Foradil)	montelukast (Singulair)
ipratropium (Atrovent)	omalizumab (Xolair)
isoproterenol (Isuprel)	zafirlukast (Accolate)
levalbuterol (Xopenex)	zileuton (Zyflo)
metaproterenol (Alupent, Metaprel)	
pirbuterol (Maxair)	
salmeterol (Serevent, Serevent Diskus)	
terbutaline (Brethine, Bricanyl)	
theophylline (Theolair, Somophyllin, Theo-Dur, Slo-Phyllin, Uniphyl)	

Tech Check

11. List three antihistamine agents.(LO 7.5)

12. List four bronchodilator agents.(LO 7.5)

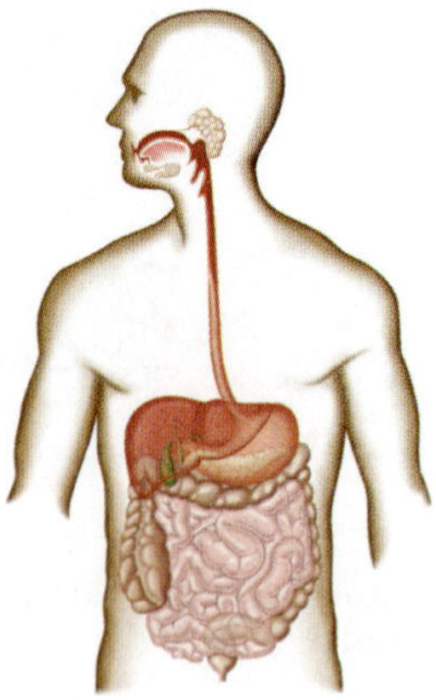

Figure 7-5 Gastrointestinal System.

Gastrointestinal System Medications(LO 7.5)

Agents used to treat gastrointestinal conditions are numerous (Figure 7-5). Common maladies affecting the gastrointestinal tract are:

- Nausea
- Vomiting
- Diarrhea
- Constipation
- Peptic ulcer disease
- Inflammatory bowel disease

H2 Blockers

Histamine 2 receptor antagonists (also known as H2 blockers) decrease gastric acid secretion into the stomach by blocking the histamine receptors on the parietal cells. These agents are all available OTC and by prescription, meaning there is a great risk for medication duplication. They are used to treat peptic ulcer disease.

Proton Pump Inhibitors

Proton pump inhibitors are medications that interfere with the sodium-potassium ATPase pump on the parietal cell in the gastrointestinal tract. These agents are effective at decreasing the production and secretion of gastric acid, reducing acidity. Inhibitors of the proton pump are employed in the management of hyperacidity disorders, gastroesophageal reflux disease (GERD), duodenal ulcers, and erosive esophagitis.

Antacids

Antacids are drugs used to neutralize the acid in the stomach. Generally, these agents are not absorbed into the systemic circulation, but have their primary activity in the stomach.

Antiemetic Agents

Antiemetic agents decrease nausea and vomiting by various mechanisms (e.g., increasing peristalsis [metoclopramide] or by suppressing the emesis center in the CNS [prochlorperazine]). Other agents in this category suppress the activity of serotonin, which is thought to have role in nausea and vomiting.

Antidiarrheal Agents

Antidiarrheal agents may work by decreasing peristalsis (loperamide) or by increasing bulk in the stools (kaolin-pectin).

Laxatives and Cathartics

Laxatives and cathartics are agents that work to cause defecation. These agents cause defecation by increasing bulk in the stools and surfactant action, by increasing peristalsis, and by altering the osmotic concentration gradient.

Miscellaneous Gastrointestinal Agents

Miscellaneous gastrointestinal agents are employed in a variety of conditions including inflammatory bowel disease, spastic colon, and hemorrhoids. Sucralfate (Carafate) is an aluminum salt that binds to necrotic ulcer tissue to speed healing. This agent is available as a tablet and as an oral suspension, and requires an acidic environment to effectively bind to ulcer tissue.

Table 7-5 lists the common gastrointestinal agents discussed in this section.

Table 7-5 Gastrointestinal System Agents

Agents for Ulcer Disease and GERD			
Antacids	**Histamine 2 Receptor Blockers**	**Proton Pump Inhibitors**	**Antiemetics**
alginic acid/aluminum hydroxide/magnesium trisilicate (Gaviscon) aluminum hydroxide (Amphojel, AlternaGEL) aluminum hydroxide/ magnesium hydroxide (Maalox) aluminum hydroxide/ magnesium hydroxide/ simethicone (Mylanta, Mylanta II, Maalox Plus) aluminum hydroxide, magnesium trisilicate (Gaviscon, Gaviscon-2) calcium carbonate (Tums, Alka-Mints) magaldrate (Riopan)	cimetidine (Tagamet, Tagamet HB) famotidine (Pepcid, Pepcid AC) nizatidine (Axid, Axid NR) ranitidine (Zantac, Zantac 75)	esomeprazole (Nexium) lansoprazole (Prevacid) omeprazole (Prilosec, Prilosec OTC) pantoprazole (Protonix) rabeprazole (AcipHex)	aprepitant (Emend) chlorpromazine (Thorazine) dimenhydrinate (Dramamine) dolasetron (Anzemet) dronabinol (Marinol) droperidol (Inapsine) granisetron (Kytril) metoclopramide (Reglan) meclizine (Antivert) ondansetron (Zofran) palonosetron (Aloxi) prochlorperazine (Compazine) promethazine (Phenergan) scopolamine (Transderm-Scop) thiethylperazine (Torecan) trimethobenzamide (Tigan)
Antidiarrheals			
bismuth subsalicylate (Pepto-Bismol) diphenoxylate/atropine (Lomotil) kaolin-pectin (Kaodene, Kaopectate, Parepectolin) lactobacillus (Lactinex) octreotide (Sandostatin) paregoric (camphorated tincture of opium) (various)			
Laxatives and Cathartics			
bisacodyl (Dulcolax) docusate calcium (Surfak) docusate potassium (Dialose) docusate sodium (Colace) glycerin (various)			

(Continued)

Table 7-5 Gastrointestinal System Agents *(Continued)*

Laxatives and Cathartics contd...			
lactulose (Chronulac, Cephulac, Enulose) magnesium citrate (various) polyethylene glycol electrolyte solution (GoLYTELY, Colyte) psyllium (Metamucil, Serutan, Effer-Syllium) sodium phosphate (Visicol)			
Miscellaneous Agents			
balsalazide (Colazal) dicyclomine (Bentyl) hyoscyamine (Anaspaz, Cystospaz, Levsin) hyoscyamine/atropine/scopolamine/phenobarbital (Donnatal) infliximab (Remicade) mesalamine (Rowasa, Asacol, Pentasa) misoprostol (Cytotec) olsalazine (Dipentum) propantheline (Pro-Banthine) sulfasalazine (Azulfidine) tegaserod maleate (Zelnorm) sucralfate (Carafate)			

Tech Check

13. Agents decreasing nausea and vomiting are called ______.(LO 7.5)

14. Agents increasing the frequency of defecation are classified as ______.(LO 7.5)

15. List three proton pump inhibitors.(LO 7.5)

16. Agents that neutralize stomach acid are classified as ______.(LO 7.5)

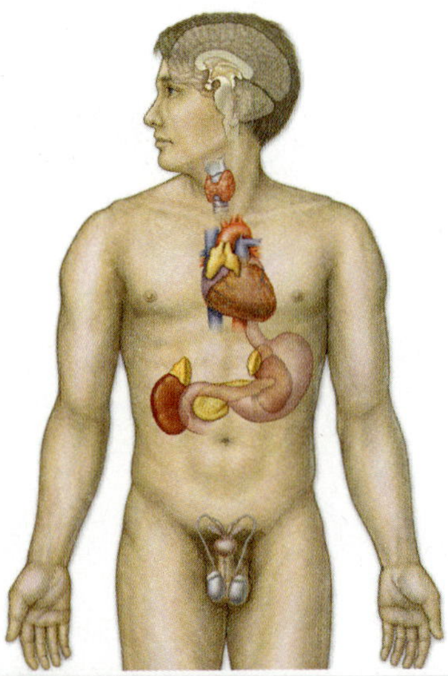

Figure 7-6 Endocrine System.

Endocrine System Medications(LO 7.5)

The endocrine system, along with the nervous system, regulates the body. The endocrine system excretes chemical substances directly into the blood stream (Figure 7-6).

Adrenal Steroids

Adrenal steroids are available in various dosage forms and have multiple uses. Indications include adrenal cortical insufficiency, allergic states, dermatologic diseases, and respiratory diseases. These agents are also known as the glucocorticoids.

Gonadal Hormones and Oral Contraceptives

Oral contraceptive agents may contain a progestin only or a combination of an estrogen and a progestin. They can also be divided in to monophasic and multiphasic products.

Thyroid Medications

The thyroid gland secretes hormones that mediate metabolic processes throughout the body. Hypothyroidism occurs when the thyroid gland does not secrete adequate hormone. Synthetic hormone supplementation is the treatment of choice. Hyperthyroidism occurs when the thyroid gland secretes too much thyroid hormone. Antithyroid agents decrease thyroid hormone synthesis and/or secretion.

Osteoporosis Agents

Agents used in the management of osteoporosis include a range of drugs from mineral and vitamin supplements to the bisphosphonates (agents that decrease the resorption of bone).

Antidiabetic Agents

Diabetes mellitus is an endocrine disorder of impaired carbohydrate metabolism. Agents used to manage this disorder include oral agents with various mechanisms of action and insulins with varying durations of action.

Insulins may be mixed by the patient in the syringe or may be acquired in premixed formulations to decrease the number of injections needed daily.

Examples of combination insulins are:

- Humulin 70/30
- Humulin 50/50
- Novolin 70/30
- Humalog Mix

Tocolytic and Oxytocic Agents

Tocolytic agents are used to prevent preterm labor through decreasing uterine motility. Oxytocic agents enhance uterine motility, causing labor to progress at a more rapid pace. This process is called labor induction.

Table 7-6 identifies the endocrine system agents.

Table 7-6 Endocrine System Agents

Adrenal Steroids			
betamethasone (Celestone) cortisone (Cortone Acetate) dexamethasone (Decadron, Dexone, Dalalone) hydrocortisone (Cortef, Hydrocortone, Solu-Cortef) methylprednisolone (Medrol, Solu-Medrol, Depo-Medrol) dexamethasone (Decadron, Dexone, Dalalone) prednisone (Orasone, Liquid Pred) triamcinolone (Aristocort, Kenalog)			

(Continued)

Table 7-6 Endocrine System Agents *(Continued)*

Gonadal Hormones and Oral Contraceptives		
Hormonal Supplementation Agents esterified estrogens (Estratab, Menest) esterified estrogens/ methyltestosterone (Estratest) estradiol (Estrace) estradiol, transdermal (Estraderm, Climara, Vivelle) estrogen, conjugated (Premarin) estrogen, synthetic conjugated (Cenestin) estrogen, conjugated/ medroxyprogesterone (Prempro, Premphase) estrogen, conjugated/ methyltestosterone (Premarin with Methyltestosterone) ethinyl estradiol (Estinyl, Feminone) norethindrone acetate/ ethinyl estradiol (Fem HRT)	**Parenteral Hormonal Contraceptives** estradiol cypionate/ medroxyprogesterone acetate (Lunelle) ethinyl estradiol/ levonorgestrel (Preven) etonorgestrel/ethinyl estradiol (Nuvaring) ethinyl estradiol/ norelgestromin (Ortho-Evra) levonorgestrel (Norplant) medroxyprogesterone (Depo-Provera)	**Oral Contraceptive Agents** ***Combination Monophasic*** ethinyl estradiol/desogestrel (Alesse 21, 28, Apri 28, Desogen 28, Kariva 28, Mircette, Ortho-Cept 28) ethinyl estradiol/drospirenone (Yasmin 28) ethinyl estradiol/ethynodiol diacetate (Demulen 1/35, Demulen 1/50, Zovia 1/35E, Zovia 1/50E) ethinyl estradiol/levonorgestrel (Aviane 28, Lessina 28, Levlen 28, Levlite 28, Levora 28, Nordette 21, 28, Portia 28) ethinyl estradiol/norethindrone (Brevicon 28, Estrostep 28, Junel Fe 1/20, Junel Fe1.5/30, Loestrin Fe 1.5/30, Loestrin Fe 1/20, Microgestin Fe 1/20, Microgestin Fe 1.5/30, Modicon, MonoNessa, Necon 0.5/35, Necon 1/35, Nortrel 0.5/35, Nortrel 1/35, Norinyl 1/35, Ortho-Novum 1/35 28, Ovcon 35, Ovcon 50) ethinyl estradiol/norgestrel (Cryselle 28, Lo/Ovral 21, Lo/Ovral 28, Low-Ogestrel 28, Ogestrel 28, Ovral 21, 28) ethinyl estradiol/norgestimate (MonoNessa, Ortho-Cyclen 28, Sprintec 28) mestranol/norethindrone (Necon 1/50, Norinyl 1/50, Ortho-Novum 1/50 28) ***Combination Multiphasic*** ethinyl estradiol/desogestrel (Cyclessa 28, Velivet) ethinyl estradiol/levonorgestrel (Enpresse 28, Tri-Levlen 28, Triphasil 21, 28, Trivora-28) ethinyl estradiol/norethindrone (Necon 10/11 21, 28, Necon 7/7/7, Nortrel 7/7/7, Ortho-Novum 10/11, Ortho-Novum 7/7/7, Tri-Norinyl 21,28) ethinyl estradiol/norgestimate (Ortho Tri-Cyclen 21, 28, Ortho Tri-Cyclen lo 21, 28, Tri-Nessa 28, Tri-Sprintec) ***Progestin Only*** Norethindrone (Camila, Errin, Jolivette 28, Micronor, Nor-QD, Nora-BE 28) norgestrel (Ovrette)

(Continued)

Table 7-6 Endocrine System Agents *(Continued)*

Thyroid Medications			
Antithyroid Agents methimazole (Tapazole) potassium iodide (Lugol's Solution, SSKI, Thyro-Block) propylthiouracil (various)	**Thyroid Supplements** dessicated thyroid (various) levothyroxine (Synthroid, Levoxyl, Levothroid) liothyronine (Cytomel, Triostat) liotrix (Thyrolar)		
Bisphosphonates			
alendronate sodium (Fosamax) etidronate disodium (Didronel) pamidronate disodium (Aredia) risedronate sodium (Actonel) tiludronate sodium (Skelid)			
Antidiabetic Agents			
Oral Antidiabetic Agents ***Alpha-Glucosidase Inhibitors*** acarbose (Precose) miglitol (Glyset) ***Biguanide*** metformin (Glucophage) ***Meglitinide*** nateglinide (Starlix) repaglinide (Prandin) ***Sulfonylureas*** chlorpropamide (Diabinese) glimepiride (Amaryl) glipizide (Glucotrol) glyburide (DiaBeta, Micronase, Glynase) tolazamide (Tolinase) tolbutamide (Orinase) ***Thiazolidinediones*** pioglitazone (Actos) rosiglitazone (Avandia)	**Injectible N insulin Agents** ***Incretin-Mimetic*** exenatide (Byetta)	**Amylinomimetic** pramlintide (Symlin)	**Insulins** ***Ultra Rapid Acting*** insulin aspart (NovoLog), insulin glulisine (Apidra), insulin lispro (Humalog), inhaled insulin (Exubera) ***Rapid Acting*** Regular Iletin II, Humulin R, Velosulin, Novolin R ***Intermediate Acting*** NPH Iletin II, Lente Iletin IIHumulin N, Novolin L ***Long Acting*** Ultralente, Humulin L, insulin glargine (Lantus)
Tocolytics and Oxytocics			
Tocolytic Agents ritodrine (Yutopar) magnesium sulfate (various) terbutaline (Brethine)	**Oxytocic Agents** oxytocin (Pitocin, Syntocinon) ergonovine maleate (Ergotrate) methylergonovine maleate (Methergine)		

Tech Check

17. Classify the following agents:(LO 7.5)

a. glyburide

b. ortho-evra

c. propylthiouracil

d. alendronate

e. humulin 70/30

Anti-Infective Medications(LO 7.5)

Antimicrobial Agents

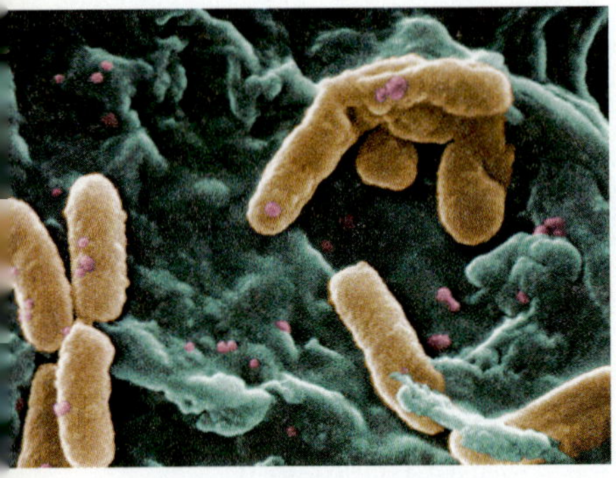

Figure 7-7 Pseudomonas aeruginosa bacteria.

Antimicrobial agents generally refer to medications used to manage infections caused by bacteria (gonorrhea, bacterial otitis media) (Figure 7-7). Antiviral agents are pharmacologic agents specifically used to treat infections caused by viruses (common cold, herpes). Antifungal agents are used in the eradication of infections caused by fungi (athlete's foot, ring worm).

Antimicrobial agents consist of several subcategories of agents. Bactericidal antibiotics are agents that kill bacteria through various mechanisms (lysis of cell wall, or inhibition of DNA gyrase). Bacteriostatic antimicrobial agents inhibit bacterial cell proliferation and eventually eradicate the bacteria. Subcategories of antimicrobial agents include:

- Aminoglycosides
- Beta lactams
- Fluoroquinolones
- Macrolides
- Sulfonamides
- Tetracyclines
- Various miscellaneous agents

Aminoglycosides are agents that inhibit protein synthesis. These agents are not acid-stable, which means that they are not absorbed through the gastrointestinal tract. Neomycin oral solution or tablets may be used in preparation for bowel surgery, but with negligible absorption into the circulation. Hence, administration of these agents is topical (ophthalmic or dermatologic) or intravenous.

Beta lactams encompass a very large category and include the penicillins, cephalosporins, carbapenems, carbacephems, and monobactams.

Beta-lactam antibiotics share a common molecular structure, the beta-lactam ring. Lysis of this ring renders the antimicrobial agent ineffective. Beta-lactam antibiotics are divided into various subcategories, penicillins, cephalosporins, carbapenems, carbacephems, and monobactams. Penicillins and cephalosporins are further divided into various categories based upon antimicrobial spectrums.

Cephalosporins are beta-lactam antibiotics that are divided into generations based upon the time of their development and antimicrobial spectrum. They are the only antimicrobial agents that are subdivided into generations.

Fluoroquinolones are antimicrobial agents with bactericidal activity through inactivation of DNA gyrase, the enzyme that gives DNA its double helix formation. These agents are contraindicated in pregnancy and can be administered to individuals younger than 18 years of age only if they have been diagnosed with cystic fibrosis.

Macrolides are bacteriostatic antibiotics employed in the management of various infections, principally respiratory infections.

Ketolides were designed to overcome antimicrobial drug resistance. Currently, there is only one available agent in this category in the United States.

Sulfonamides are bacteriostatic antimicrobial agents, and are employed against a variety of infections from otitis media to urinary tract infections.

Tetracyclines are antimicrobial agents that are bacteriostatic. As agents for insoluble complexes with minerals (calcium, magnesium, and aluminum), they should not be taken with dairy products, antacids, and multiple vitamins containing minerals. They are also contraindicated in pregnant patients, lactating patients, and pediatric patients.

Some antimicrobial drugs have distinctive mechanisms of action and cannot be grouped into one category or family. They are categorized in Table 7-7 as miscellaneous antimicrobial agents.

Antifungal Agents

Antifungal agents are reserved for use against fungal infections, which most commonly occur in the skin, nails, and scalp.

Antiviral Agents

Antiviral agents are used to manage viral infections. Viral infections are often difficult to manage as viruses are obligate parasites (they do not have their own cell walls) and must use the host's cells to survive.

Antiretroviral Agents

Antiretrovirals are employed in the management of human immunodeficiency virus (HIV). These agents are subdivided into categories based upon the mechanism of action of the drug.

Antiprotozoal Agents

Protozoal infections are common in underdeveloped countries where sanitary conditions and control of vectors of disease are poor. As travel to these areas is common, the protozoal infections are not limited to certain areas.

Antihelmintic Agents

Helminthic (worm) infections in humans may involve one of the following three major groups of infections: nematodes, trematodes, and cestodes.

Table 7-7 Infectious Disease Agents

Antibacterial Agents			
Aminoglycosides amikacin (Amikin) gentamycin (Garamycin) neomycin (various) streptomycin (various) tobramycin (Nebcin)	**Penicillins** amoxicillin (Polymox, Amoxil) amoxicillin/clavulanate (Augmentin) ampicillin (Amcill, Omnipen) cefprozil (Cefzil) dicloxacillin (Dynapen) mezlocillin (Mezlin) nafcillin (Nallpen) oxacillin (Bactocill, Prostaphlin) penicillin G, aqueous (Pentids) penicillin G, benzathine (Bicillin) penicillin G, procaine (Wycillin) penicillin V (PenVee-K, Veetids) piperacillin (Pipracil) piperacillin/tazobactam (Zosyn) ticarcillin (Ticar) ticarcillin/ potassium clavulanate (Timentin)	**Carbapenems** ertapenem (Invanz) imipenem-cilastatin (Primaxin) meropenem (Merrem)	**Fluoroquinolones** ciprofloxacin (Cipro) gatifloxacin (Tequin) levofloxacin (Levaquin, Quixin) lomefloxacin (Maxaquin) moxifloxacin (Avelox) norfloxacin (Noroxin) ofloxacin (Floxin, Ocuflox) sparfloxacin (Zagam) trovafloxacin (Trovan)
Sulfonamides sulfisoxazole (Gantrisin) sulfacetamide (Bleph-10) sulfamethoxazole/ trimethoprim (Bactrim, Septra)	**Cephalosporins** cefadroxil (Duricef, Ultracef) cefazolin (Ancef , Kefzol) cephalexin (Keflex, Keftabs) cephradine (Velosef) cefaclor (Ceclor) cefmetazole (Zefazone) cefonicid (Monocid) cefotetan (Cefotan) cefoxitin (Mefoxin) cefprozil (Cefzil) cefuroxime (Ceftin) cefdinir (Omnicef) cefditoren (Spectracef) cefixime (Suprax) cefoperazone (Cefobid) cefotaxime (Claforan) cefpodoxime (Vantin) ceftazidime (Fortaz) ceftibuten (Cedax) ceftizoxime (Cefizox) ceftriaxone (Rocephin) cefepime (Maxipime)	**Carbacephem** loracarbef (Lorabid)	**Macrolides** azithromycin (Zithromax) clarithromycin (Biaxin) dirithromycin (Dynabac) erythromycin (EES, E-mycin) erythromycin/sulfisoxazole (Eryzole, Pediazole)
Ketolide telithromycin (Ketek)	**Tetracyclines** doxycycline (Doryx, Vibramycin, Vibra-Tabs) demeclocycline (Declomycin) minocycline (Arestin, Dynacin, Minocin)	**Glycylcycline** tigecycline (Tygacil)	**Miscellaneous** clindamycin (Cleocin, Cleocin-T) fosfomycin (Monurol) linezolid (Zyvox) metronidazole (Flagyl, Metrogel)

(Continued)

Table 7-7 Infectious Disease Agents *(Continued)*

Antibacterial Agents contd...			
			quinupristin-dalfopristin (Synercid) tinidazole (Tindamax) vancomycin (Vancocin)
Antifungal Agents			
amphotericin B (Fungizone) amphotericin B cholesteryl (Amphotec) amphotericin B lipid (Abelcet) amphotericin B liposomal (AmBisome)	caspofungin (Cancidas) clotrimazole (Lotrimin, Mycelex) econazole (Spectazole) fluconazole (Diflucan) griseofulvin (Fulvin, Grifulvin)	itraconazole (Sporanox) ketoconazole (Nizoral) miconazole (Monistat) nystatin (Mycostatin)	oxiconazole (Oxistat) sertaconazole (Ertaczo) terbinafine (Lamisil) voriconazole (VFEND)
Antiviral Agents			
acyclovir (Zovirax) adefovir (Hespera) amantadine (Symmetrel) atazanivir (Reyataz) cidofovir (Vistide) famciclovir (Famvir)	foscarnet (Foscavir) ganciclovir (Cytovene, Vitrasert) interferon alfa-2b/ribavirin (Rebetron) oseltamivir (Tamiflu)	palivizumab (Synagis) peg interferon alfa 2a (Pegasys) penciclovir (Denavir) ribavirin (Virazole) rimantadine (Flumadine)	valacyclovir (Valtrex) valganciclovir (Valcyte) zanamivir (Relenza)
Antiretroviral Agents			
abacavir (Ziagen) amprenavir (Agenerase) delavirdine (Rescriptor) didanosine (Videx) efavirenz (Sustiva) emtricitabine (Emtriva)	enfuvirtide (Fuzeon) etravirine (Intelence) fosamprenavir (Lexiva) indinavir (Crixivan) lamivudine (Epivir)	lopinavir/ritonavir (Kaletra) nelfinavir (Viracept) nevirapine (Viramune) ritonavir (Norvir) saquinavir (Fortovase, Invirase)	stavudine (Zerit) tenofovir (Viread) zalcitabine (Hivid) zidovudine (Retrovir) zidovudine/lamivudine (Combivir)
Antiprotozoal Agents			
chloroquine (Aralen) mefloquine (Larium) metronidazole (Flagyl)	nitazoxanide (Alinia) paromomycin (Humatin) pentamidine (Pentam)	pyrimethamine (Daraprim, Fansidar) primaquine (various)	quinacrine (various) quinine (various)
Antihelmintic Agents			
ivermectin (Stromectol) mebendazole (Vermox)	praziquantel (Biltricide)	pyrantel pamoate (Mintezol)	thiabendazole (Antiminth, Pin-X)
Antiseptics and Disinfectants			
Antiseptics acetic acid chlorhexidine ethanol hexachlorophene hydrogen peroxide isopropanol merbromin potassium permanganate povidone-iodine salicylic acid silver sulfadiazine undecylenic acid triclocarban	**Disinfectants** benzalkonium chloride cetylpyridinium chloride formaldehyde halazone nitromersol thimerosal sodium hypochlorite (household bleach)		

Antihelmintic therapy is aimed at antagonizing the metabolic processes of the parasite.

Antiseptics and Disinfectants

Disinfectants antagonize bacterial growth on inanimate objects, such as instruments and equipment. Antiseptics reduce bacterial growth on both animate and inanimate objects and are often incorporated into soaps and cleansers. Preservatives have disinfectant properties, but the primary purpose of these agents is to maintain the effectiveness of drugs and vaccines.

See Table 7-7 for a listing of infectious disease medications.

Tech Check

18. List three macrolide antibiotics.(LO 7.5)

19. Categorize each of the following:(LO 7.5)

- **a.** Amoxicillin
- **b.** Cefaclor
- **c.** Doxycycline

20. List four antiretroviral agents:(LO 7.5)

21. Classify each of the following:(LO 7.5)

- **a.** Benzalkonium chloride
- **b.** Povidone-iodine
- **c.** Halazone
- **d.** Isopropanol

Antineoplastic Medications(LO 7.5)

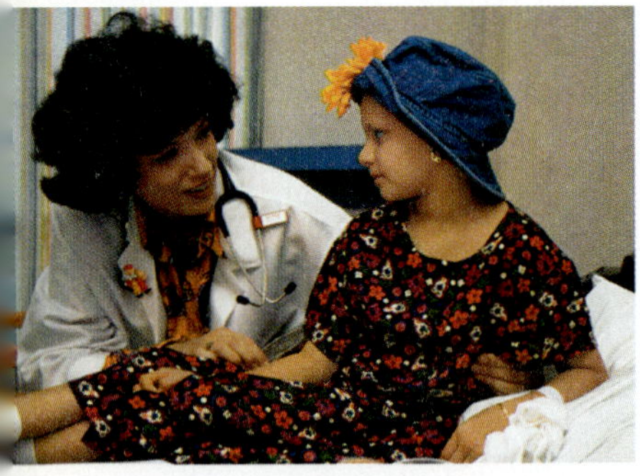

Figure 7-8 Doctor with cancer patient.

Antineoplastic agents are employed in the chemotherapy of cancer (Figure 7-8). They may also be employed for short-term therapy in the management of severe cases of Crohn's disease, psoriasis, or rheumatoid arthritis. Toxicities associated with use of the antineoplastic agents are severe, such as myelosuppression.

Antineoplastics can be divided into the following main categories:

- Alkylating agents
- Antibiotics
- Antimetabolites
- Hormones
- Mitotic inhibitors

There are additional antineoplastic agents with mechanisms of action that do not fit into the above categories. All of the categories can be found in Table 7-8.

Table 7-8 Antineoplastic Agents

Alkylating Agents

- altretamine (Hexalen)
- busulfan (Myleran, Busulfex)
- carboplatin (Paraplatin)
- carmustine (BiCNU, Gliadel)
- chlorambucil (Leukeran)
- cisplatin (Platinol)
- cyclophosphamide (Cytoxan, Neosar)
- ifosfamide (Ifex, Haloxon)
- mechlorethamine (Mustargen)
- melphalan (Alkeran)
- procarbazine (Matulane)
- streptozocin (Zanosar)
- triethylenetriphosphamide (Thio-Tepa, Tespa)

Antibiotics

- bleomycin sulfate (Blenoxane)
- dactinomycin (Cosmegen)
- daunorubicin (Daunomycin, Cerubidine)
- epirubicin (Ellence)
- idarubicin (Idamycin)
- mitomycin (Mutamycin)

Antimetabolites

- cytarabine (Cytosar-U)
- cytarabine Liposome (DepoCyt)
- floxuridine (various)
- fludarabine phosphate (Fludara)
- fluorouracil (Adrucil)
- gemcitabine (Gemzar)
- mercaptopurine (Purinethol)
- methotrexate (Folex, Rheumatrex)
- 6-thioguanine (Tabloid)

Hormonal Agents

- abarelix (Plenaxis)
- anastrozole (Arimidex)
- bicalutamide (Casodex)
- estramustine (Estracyt, Emcyt)
- exemestane (Aromasin)
- fluoxymesterone (Halotestin)
- flutamide (Eulexin)
- fulvestrant (Faslodex)
- goserelin (Zoladex)
- seuprolide (Lupron, Viadur, Eligard)
- levamisole (Ergamisol)
- megestrol acetate (Megace)
- nilutamide (Nilandron)
- tamoxifen (Nolvadex)
- triptorelin (Trelstar Depot, Trelstar LA)

Mitotic Inhibitors

- etoposide (VePesid)
- vinblastine (Velban, Velbe)
- vincristine (Oncovin, Vincasar PFS)
- vinorelbine (Navelbine)

Miscellaneous Agents

- aldesleukin (Proleukin)
- aminoglutethimide (Cytadren)
- L-asparaginase (Elspar, Oncaspar)
- bacillus Calmette Guérin (TheraCys, Tice BCG)
- bevacizumab (Avastin)
- bortezomib (Velcade)
- cladribine (Leustatin)
- dacarbazine (DTIC)
- docetaxel (Taxotere)
- gefitinib (Iressa)
- gemtuzumab ozogamicin (Mylotarg)
- hydroxyurea (Hydrea, Droxia)
- imatinib (Gleevec)
- irinotecan (Camptosar)
- letrozole (Femara)
- leucovorin (Wellcovorin)
- mitotane (Lysodren)
- mitoxantrone (Novantrone)
- paclitaxel (Taxol)
- pemetrexed (Alimta)
- rasburicase (Elitek)
- thalidomide (Thalomid)
- topotecan (Herceptin)
- trastuzumab (Hycamtin)

Tech Check

22. The five main categories of antineoplastic agents discussed in this chapter are _____.(LO 7.5)

23. Toxicities associated with antineoplastic agents are _____.(LO 7.5)

Immune System Medications(LO 7.5)

Immune system medications affect the functioning of the immune system to either stimulate its activity or to decrease its activity (Figure 7-9).

Immunomodulators stimulate the body's own defense system to combat various diseases. Immunosuppressive agents decrease the immune system's activity to minimize its reactivity to organ transplants (reducing risk of organ rejection) or to chemotherapy. Table 7-9 lists immune system medications.

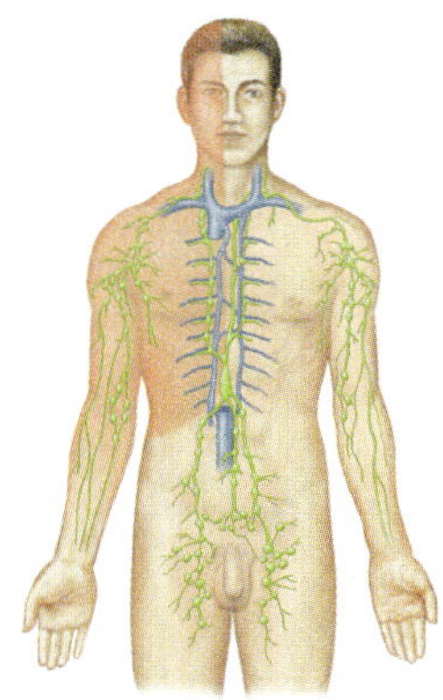

Figure 7-9 Immune System.

Table 7-9 Immune System Agents

Immunomodulators	Immunosuppressive Agents
adalimumab (Humira)	azathioprine (Imuran)
anakinra (Kineret)	basiliximab (Simulect)
etanercept (Enbrel)	cyclosporine (Sandimmune, NePO)
interferon alfa (Roferon-A, Intron A)	daclizumab (Zenapax)
interferon alfacon-1 (Infergen)	lymphocyte Immune Globulin (Atgam)
interferon beta-1b (Betaseron)	muromonab-CD3 (Orthoclone OKT3)
interferon gamma-1b (Actimmune)	mycophenolate Mofetil (CellCept)
peg interferon alfa-2b (PEG-Intron)	sirolimus (Rapamune)
	tacrolimus (Prograf, Protopic)

Tech Check

24. Define *immunomodulator*.(LO 7.5)

25. Define *immunosuppressant*.(LO 7.5)

26. List three immunomodulators.(LO 7.5)

27. List three immunosuppressants.(LO 7.5)

Dermatologic, Ophthalmic, and Otic Medications(LO 7.5)

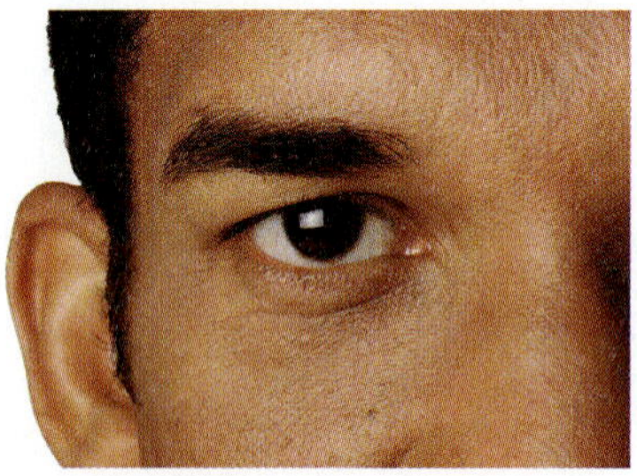

Figure 7-10 Medications are used to treat the skin (dermatologic), eye (ophthalmic), and ear (otic).

Dermatologic refers to the skin. Ophthalmic refers to the eye. Otic refers to the ear. Various medications in different forms are used to treat these three locations of the body (see Figure 7-10).

Dermatologic Agents

Dermatologic agents are applied to the surface of the skin to treat a variety of conditions. As previously mentioned in this chapter, antibiotics, antifungals, and antivirals are not interchangeable with respect to the pathogens they antagonize. Other conditions specific to dermatologic preparations are the antipsoriatics, trichogenics, moisturizers, and anti-parasitics. Preparations for the skin, eyes, and ears are all considered to be topical. Table 7-10 identifies common dermatologic, ophthalmic, and otic preparations.

Ophthalmic Agents

Ophthalmic agents are various medications reserved for use in the eye. Glaucoma is an ophthalmic condition that must be treated with pharmacologic agents to reduce intraocular pressure. Other types of ophthalmic preparations include:

- Antiallergy agents
- Antibacterial agents
- Antifungal agents
- Anti-inflammatory agents
- Antiviral agents
- Miscellaneous agents (including agents for dry eyes, ophthalmic decongestants, and diagnostic agents)

Otic Preparations

Otic (ear) preparations are available in liquid dosage forms, either as solutions or suspensions. These agents must never be instilled into the eyes as sterility, tonicity, and pH may be incompatible with the eyes.

Table 7-10 Dermatologic, Ophthalmic, and Otic Agents

Dermatologic Agents

Agents for Wart Removal
imiquimod (Aldara)
podophyllin (Condylox)

Anti-Acne Agents
adapalene (Differin)
azelaic acid (Azelex)
tretinoin (Retin-A)
tazarotene (Tazorac)

Antifungal Agents
amphotericin B (Fungizone)
ciclopirox (Loprox)
butenafine (Mentax)
econazole (Spectazole)
haloprogin (Halotex)
ketoconazole (Nizoral)
miconazole (Monistat)
naftifine (Naftin)
nystatin (Mycostatin)
oxiconazole (Oxistat)
sulconazole (Exelderm)
terbinafine (Lamisil)
tolnaftate (Tinactin)

Antipruritics
doxepin, topical (Zonalon)
pramoxine (Tronothane)

Antivirals
acyclovir (Zovirax)
penciclovir (Denavir)

Corticosteroids
alclometasone dipropionate (Aclovate)
amcinonide (Cyclocort)
betamethasone dipropionate (Diprosone)
clobetasol propionate (Temovate)
desonide (DesOwen)
fluocinolone (Synalar)
fluocinonide (Lidex)
flurandrenolide (Cordran)
halcinonide (Halog)
halobetasol propionate (Ultravate)
hydrocortisone (Hytone)
mometasone furoate (Elocon)
triamcinolone acetonide (Aristocort)

Analgesics
triethanolamine salicylate (Aspercreme)
capsaicin (Zostrix)

Antibacterials
bacitracin (Baciguent)
bacitracin/polymyxin B (Polysporin)
bacitracin/neomycin/polymyxin B (Neosporin)
clindamycin (Cleocin)
erythromycin (A/T/S, EryDerm, Erycette)
gentamicin (Garamycin, G-Mycitin)
metronidazole (MetroGel)
mupirocin (Bactroban)
neomycin sulfate (Myciguent)

Antiparasitics
crotamiton (Eurax)
lindane (Kwell)
permethrin (Nix, Elimite)

Antipsoriatics
anthralin (Anthra-Derm)
calcipotriene (Dovonex)
pimecrolimus (Elidel)
tacrolimus (Prograf, Protopic)
tazarotene (Tazorac)

Emollient Agents
lactic acid/ammonium hydroxide Lac-Hydrin)

Local Anesthetics
dibucaine (Nupercainal)
lidocaine (Xylocaine)

Ophthalmic Agents

Anti-Allergy Agents
cromolyn sodium (Opticrom)
emedastine (Emadine)
ketotifen (Zaditor)
lodoxamide (Alomide)
olopatadine (Patanol)
pemirolast (Alamast)
rimexolone (Vexol)
naphazoline/pheniramine acetate (Naphcon A)

Anti-Inflammatory Agents
dexamethasone (AK-Dex, Decadron)
ketorolac (Acular)

Agents for Glaucoma
acetazolamide (Diamox)
apraclonidine (Iopidine)
betaxolol (Betoptic)
brimonidine (Alphagan)
brinzolamide (Azopt)
carteolol (Cartrol, Ocupress)
dipivefrin (Propine)
dorzolamide (Trusopt)
dorzolamide/ Timolol (Cosopt)
echothiophate Iodine (Phospholine Ophthalmic)
latanoprost (Xalatan)
levobunolol (Betagan)
methazolamide (Neptazane)
pilocarpine (Pilocar, Pilopine HS Gel)
timolol (Timoptic)

Antifungal
natamycin (Natacyn)

Antiviral
trifluridine (Viroptic)

Antibiotics
bacitracin (AK-Tracin)
bacitracin/polymyxin B (AK Poly Bac, Polysporin Ophthalmic)
bacitracin/neomycin/polymyxin B (AK Spore, Neosporin Ophthalmic)
bacitracin/neomycin/polymyxin B/hydrocortisone (AK Spore HC, Cortisporin)
ciprofloxacin, ophthalmic (Ciloxan)
erythromycin, ophthalmic (Ilotycin)
gentamicin, ophthalmic (Garamycin, Genoptic, Gentacidin, Gentak)
neomycin/dexamethasone (Neo-Dex Ophthalmic, NeoDecadron Ophthalmic)
neomycin/polymyxin B/ dexamethasone (Maxitrol)
neomycin/polymyxin B/prednisolone (Poly-Pred Ophthalmic)
ofloxacin (Ocuflox)
silver Nitrate (Dey-Drop)
sulfacetamide (Bleph-10, Cetamide, Sodium Sulamyd)
sulfacetamide/prednisolone (Blephamide)
tobramycin (TobraDex)
tobramycin/dexamethasone (AKTob, Tobrex)

Miscellaneous Agents
artificial tears (Tears Naturale)
cyclopentolate (Cyclogyl)

Otic Preparations

acetic acid/aluminum acetate (Otic Domeboro)
benzocaine/antipyrine (Auralgan)
ciprofloxacin, otic (Cipro HC Otic)
neomycin/colistin/hydrocortisone (Cortisporin TC Otic Drops)
neomycin/colistin/thonzonium (Cortisporin TC Otic Suspension)
neomycin/polymyxin/hydrocortisone (Cortisporin Otic)
polymyxin B/hydrocortisone (Otobiotic Otic)
triethanolamine (Cerumenex)

Tech Check

28. List three antifungal dermatologic agents.(LO 7.5)

29. Which dermatologic agent is an anti-acne and an antipsoriatic agent?(LO 7.5)

30. What type of dermatologic agent is permethrin?(LO 7.5)

31. Name the ophthalmic antifungal agent.(LO 7.5)

32. List three ophthalmic antibiotic agents.(LO 7.5)

Chapter Summary

The proper classification of medications enables the pharmacy technician to function more effectively as a paraprofessional with the licensed pharmacist. Important points to know are:

- Drug classifications are ways of grouping similar or like drugs into a category that may be based upon mechanism of action, physiologic system, or symptoms.
- By understanding drug classification, the pharmacy technician is able to identify medications of the same therapeutic class, family, or mechanism of action as belonging to the same category, which may assist the pharmacist in providing better care with fewer risks.
- Controlled substances are pharmacologic agents included in Schedules I, II, III, IV, or V, which have potential for physical and/or psychological dependence and abuse.
- Codeine, morphine, and alprazolam are examples of controlled substances.

Chapter Review

Case Study Questions

1. As a pharmacy technician, why is this situation significant to Thomas?(LO 7.2)
2. What should Thomas say to Mr. Lee?(LO 7.2, 7.5)
3. What should Thomas say to the pharmacist?(LO 7.2)

At Your Service Questions

1. As a pharmacy technician, why should Cynthia be concerned about Mrs. Jones's statements?(LO 7.5)
2. What should Cynthia say to Mrs. Jones?(LO 7.2)
3. If you were Cynthia, what actions would you take?(LO 7.2, 7.5)

Multiple Choice

Select the best answer.

1. Which of the following medications is not a controlled substance?(LO 7.7)
   a. Diazepam (Valium)
   b. Methylphenidate (Ritalin)
   c. Carbamazepine (Tegretol)
   d. Zolpidem (Ambien)
2. An agent that causes, initiates, or enhances a specific physiologic effect through pharmacologic means is called a(n) ________ (LO 7.3)
   a. agonist.
   b. antagonist.
   c. antidote.
   d. antihistamine.

3. A situation in which a particular drug should not be used under any circumstances is called a(n) ________(LO 7.2)
   a. adverse effect.
   b. indication.
   c. precaution.
   d. contraindication.
4. Which of the following is *not* a neurotransmitter?(LO 7.4)
   a. Acetylcholine
   b. Bromocriptine
   c. Dopamine
   d. Serotonin
5. The method by which a drug exerts its effects is called ________(LO 7.2)
   a. adverse effects.
   b. indication.
   c. mechanism of action.
   d. contraindication.

Matching

Match the agent with its appropriate classification according to system or category.(LO 7.5)

_______ 1.	Omeprazole	a. Central nervous system
_______ 2.	Phenobarbital	b. Endocrine system
_______ 3.	Albuterol	c. Cardiovascular system
_______ 4.	Amiodarone	d. Gastrointestinal system
_______ 5.	Irbesartan	e. Respiratory system
_______ 6.	Paroxetine	
_______ 7.	Insulin	
_______ 8.	Enflurane	
_______ 9.	Enoxaparin	
_______10.	Medroxyprogesterone	

Match the agent with its appropriate classification according to system or category.(LO 7.5)

_______11.	Lamivudine	a. Antibiotic
_______12.	Itraconazole	b. Antiviral
_______13.	Cefaclor	c. Antineoplastic
_______14.	Cyclophosphamide	d. Antiretroviral
_______15.	Ciprofloxacin	e. Antifungal
_______16.	Vidarabine	
_______17.	Terbinafine	
_______18.	Vincristine	
_______19.	Acyclovir	
_______20.	Efavirenz	

Critical Thinking Questions

Mr. Simons has called the pharmacy requesting a refill of his cholesterol medication. You know Mr. Simons is a regular customer and you immediately access his medication profile in the pharmacy computer system. The following list of medications is contained in the patient's profile:

Rx #	Medication	Strength	Qty	Last Fill	Original Fill	Refills
22145	Timoptic solution	0.25%	5	10/10/2012	1/15/2012	1
24432	Zocor tablet	20 mg	30	9/3/2012	6/1/2012	2
25901	Amoxicillin	250 mg	30	7/25/2012	7/25/2012	0
26211	Lasix tablet	40 mg	30	8/19/2012	9/19/2012	3
26212	Slow-K	8 mEq	30	8/19/2012	9/19/2012	3

You indicate to Mr. Simons that you have accessed his medication profile. He says that since you already have it available, is it possible for him to get a refill on his "water" pills.

1. Which of the medications is the cholesterol medication Mr. Simons is requesting?(LO 7.5)
2. Provide more technical terms to classify Zocor.(LO 7.5)
3. Which of the following medications is the "water" pill?(LO 7.5)
4. Which of the following medications should be dispensed with the water pill for potassium supplementation?(LO 7.5)

HIPAA Scenario

Margaret Sanchez is a patient of Dr. Foster, a cardiologist in a busy private practice. Dr. Foster needs information from Margaret's pharmacy on the number of times she has refilled her medication for hypertension, so he can evaluate any adverse affects or contraindications for other medication he has prescribed for Margaret.

Lindsay McCallum, Margaret's niece, is a pharmacy technician intern at the pharmacy Margaret uses for all of her prescriptions. Lindsay also knows Dr. Foster's medical assistant, Tricia. Tricia confided to Lindsay that she has had a difficult time getting the necessary information from Margaret's pharmacy.

Lindsay wants to help, so she told Tricia to call the pharmacy and pretend to be Margaret's insurance provider seeking information in order to process a claim. When Tricia called the pharmacy, Lindsay transferred the call to the pharmacist on duty. The unsuspecting pharmacist provided Tricia with Margaret's information.

Discussion Questions (PTCB II.73)

1. Since Tricia was seeking medication information on Margaret, which could have a direct affect on her current cardiac treatment, has she broken any laws by using the method in which she obtained the information for Dr. Foster?
2. Should Lindsay and Tricia be disciplined since they were seeking a means to a "legitimate end"?

Internet Activities

1. Go to **www.rxlist.com.** Click on the most recent "Top 200 Drugs." Print out the list and attempt to classify as many as possible without looking them up. Research with a partner any medications you could not classify.(LO 7.2, 7.5)
2. Go to **www.fda.gov.** Click on "Product Approvals." On the site, enter the key words "new drug approvals" in the search. Choose a new product approval from the list and present the drug to the class. In your presentation, include the date of the FDA approval, the trade and generic names of the agent, the classification or category of the agent, and the therapeutic use for the agent.(LO 7.5)

Over-the-Counter (OTC) Agents

8

Learning Outcomes

After completing this chapter, you will be able to:

8.1 Discuss *over-the-counter (OTC)* agents.

8.2 Identify the legal requirements for OTC agents.

8.3 Differentiate between OTC and prescription agents.

8.4 Differentiate between OTC drugs and dietary supplements.

8.5 Identify categories of OTC medications.

8.6 Classify OTC agents.

8.7 Explain the common diagnostic agents/kits that are available OTC.

Key Terms

analgesic
antipyretic
broad spectrum
emesis
excipient
mydriasis
over-the-counter (OTC)
vasoconstriction
xerostomia

PTCB

In preparation for the certification examination, you should understand and perform activities associated with the following PTCB Knowledge Statement:

PTCB Knowledge Statement

Domain I. Assisting the Pharmacist in Serving Patients

Knowledge of drug interactions (12)
Knowledge of effects of patient's age (14)
Knowledge of nonprescription (OTC) formulations (28)

Case Study

Jack gets all of his prescriptions filled at Best Service Pharmacy where Peggy has been a technician for 5 years. She knows that Jack takes medications for high blood pressure that are often changed, because his blood pressure has been difficult to control. Today, Jack came in coughing and sneezing. He indicated that he caught a "bug" from his nephew, Chris. He wanted to purchase some over-the-counter (OTC) cough and cold preparations at the same time he came to pick up his prescriptions. He picked up a bottle of Nyquil for purchase.

While reading this chapter, keep the following questions in mind:

1. What are the contraindications of taking the cold medication along with medication for high blood pressure?(LO 8.5, 8.6)
2. How should Peggy handle this situation?(LO 8.2)

Introduction to OTC(LO 8.1, 8.2, 8.3, 8.5)

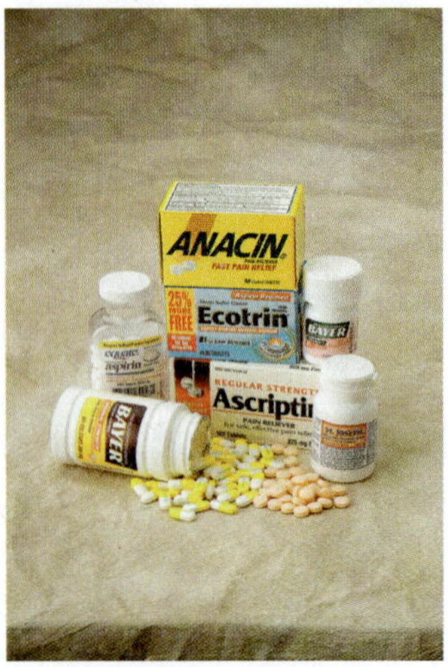

Figure 8-1 Over-the-counter aspirin.

Medications that are approved by the Food and Drug Administration (FDA), but for which access is not controlled by a prescription, are known as **over-the-counter (OTC)** or nonprescription medications (Figure 8-1). Although these agents are deemed safe enough to be purchased without a prescription, the competent pharmacy technician must have a clear understanding of the types and pharmacology of OTC agents as well as which populations of patients should avoid particular agents. The sale of some OTC agents, like pseudoephedrine, may be governed by additional state regulations (such as Oklahoma) regarding the sale of items containing this agent. The purpose of this chapter is to familiarize the pharmacy technician student with the types of agents that are part of the 100,000 agents approved by the FDA and available without prescription.

Consumerism has been defined as the promotion of the consumers' interests and as movements or policies aimed at regulating the products, services, methods, and standards of manufacturers, sellers, and advertisers in the interests of the buyer. The rise in consumerism and the increasing age of the population in the United States have resulted in an increase in the use of nonprescription agents. The FDA is the agency that is responsible for consumer protection with respect to prescription and nonprescription drugs, as well as medical devices, food, dietary supplements, and vaccines.

Although nonprescription agents are safe and effective, there are special populations of patients, or consumers, who by virtue of their age should discuss OTC drug use with their physician prior to taking a medication. Warnings are often included on the medication label to indicate whether an agent should be employed in a particular group of patients. In addition, there may be restrictions with OTC medication use in patients due to various illnesses or conditions. Restrictions for use may result from an interaction between the pharmacokinetic profile of the drug with the age of the patient, an interaction between the agent and the disease or condition, or an interaction between prescription agents the patient is likely taking and the OTC agent. A critical interaction may occur between a

over-the-counter (OTC) Agent or product available without a prescription, also nonprescription.

excipient Inactive ingredient incorporated into a dosage form.

patient's condition and an **excipient**, which is an inactive ingredient in an OTC agent. For example, diabetic patients requiring OTC cough syrups are well advised to use a sugar-free and alcohol-free preparation. In any case, the pharmacy technician should be aware of the potential interactions and alert the pharmacist. The most common groups of patients with medication restrictions are:

- Children
- Diabetics
- Hypertensive patients
- Nursing mothers
- Pregnant women
- Older patients

The pharmacy technician should also be aware that some OTC agents have the potential for abuse. The technician should be concerned and notify the pharmacist when a customer tries to purchase large quantities of one medication or medications with the same or similar active ingredients, especially cough and cold preparations. In some states, the purchase of pseudoephedrine-containing preparations is restricted by state law to reduce the illegal manufacturing of methamphetamine.

The Combat Methamphetamine Epidemic Act of 2005 has been incorporated into the Patriot Act signed by President Bush on March 9, 2006. The act limits OTC sales of cold medicines that contain the ingredient pseudoephedrine, which is commonly used to make methamphetamine. The amount of pseudoephedrine that an individual can purchase at one time is limited and individuals may be required to present photo identification to purchase products containing pseudoephedrine. In some states, stores are required to keep personal information about purchasers for at least 2 years.

Other OTC agents found to have abuse potential include dextromethorphan and sedating antihistamines like diphenhydramine. In some cases, the agent of abuse is not the active ingredient, but an excipient (inactive ingredient), like alcohol. Obviously, if visual indicators of impairment are apparent, such as slurred and or incoherent speech, it would be prudent to alert the pharmacist prior to the sale of nonprescription agents to such a patient. An example of this abuse is the "methamphetamine epidemic" we face on a daily basis. This problem started with ephedrine, then pseudoephedrine. This is one of the most destructive epidemics that exists today.

Legal Requirements for OTC Agents (LO 8.2, 8.6)

Safety

It is important to note that OTC agents are evaluated by the FDA on the basis of safe and efficacious use without a prescriber's oversight. Although a medication may be deemed safe in general, the patient must be able to understand the appropriate use of the medication (Figure 8-2). This usually involves reading, understanding, and following the directions on the label. Table 8-1 identifies information included on the nonprescription drug label.

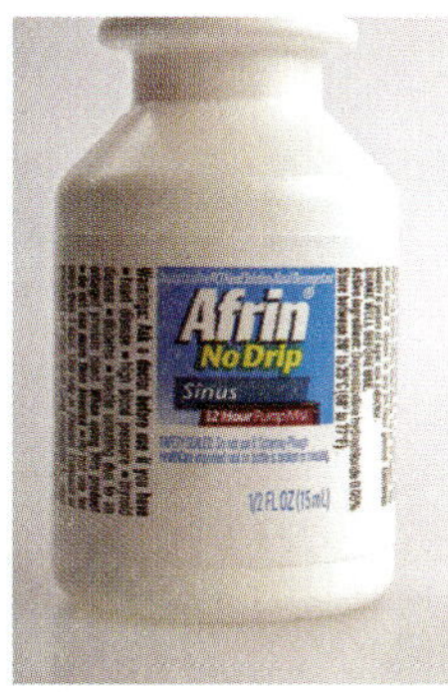

Figure 8-2 Nonprescription drug label.

At Your Service

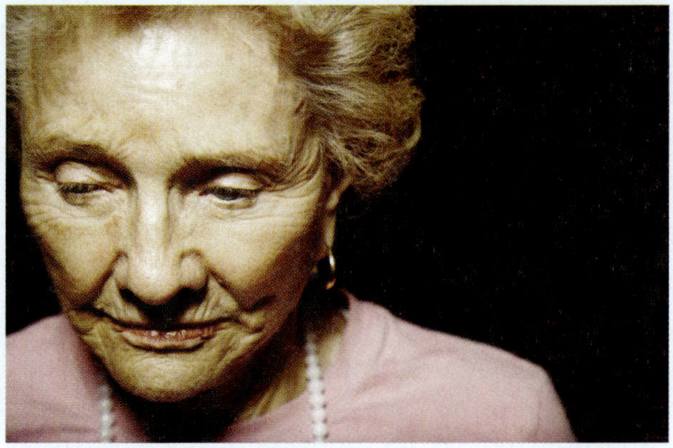

Mrs. Quincy is 75 years old. Although she is retired, she has an active lifestyle including volunteer work, lawn bowling, and babysitting her three grandchildren. She has diabetes, glaucoma, and frequently complains of not being able to sleep at night. Mrs. Quincy has seasonal allergies but did not want to go to her doctor for a prescription. She wants to purchase something to help stop her watering eyes and sneezing.

While reading this chapter, keep the following questions in mind.

1. What type or category of nonprescription medication is Mrs. Quincy requesting?(LO 8.5)
2. Why should she speak to the pharmacist prior to taking anything OTC for her allergies?(LO 8.6)
3. As a pharmacy technician, what do you tell this patient?(LO 8.2)

Table 8-1 Drug Product Label Information

Description of the drug
Clinical pharmacology
Indications (uses for the drug)
Contraindications (who should not take the drug)
Warnings
Precautions
Adverse events
Drug abuse and dependence
Dosage and administration
Use in pregnancy, use in nursing mothers
Use in children and older patients
How the drug is supplied
Safety information for the patient

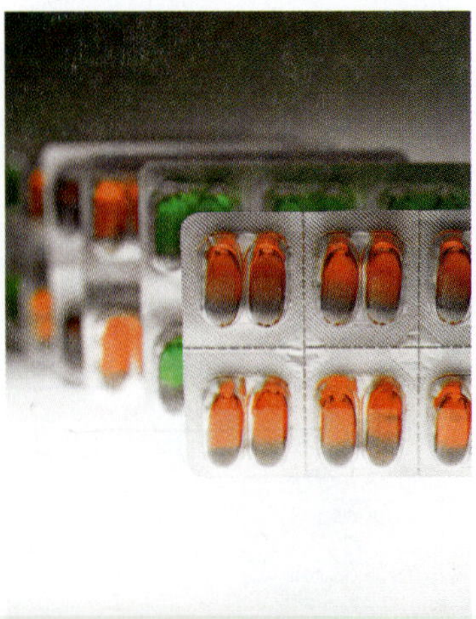

Figure 8-3 Tamper resistant packaging.

Packaging

Tamper-evident packaging is designed to alert the medication user that a product or package has been compromised or opened (Figure 8-3). Although product tampering cannot always be prevented, the consumer should inspect packages previous to purchase. The pharmacy technician should be aware of types of tamper-evident packaging used on commonly purchased agents to help prevent the sale of such items, and to work to prevent tampering in the pharmacy. Patients may sometimes open boxes and containers in an effort to see what a medication looks like. Although not malicious, this constitutes tampering and must be prevented. Some types of tamper-evident packaging include shrink-wrap, glued box tops, and multiple layers of plastic wrapping or packaging.

Child-resistant packaging is designed to prevent children from opening medications and potentially taking them. Child-resistant packaging may include safety caps (Figure 8-4), which may be difficult for some adults to open. The safety caps may be removed with the patient's consent; however, all medications should be kept out of the reach of children.

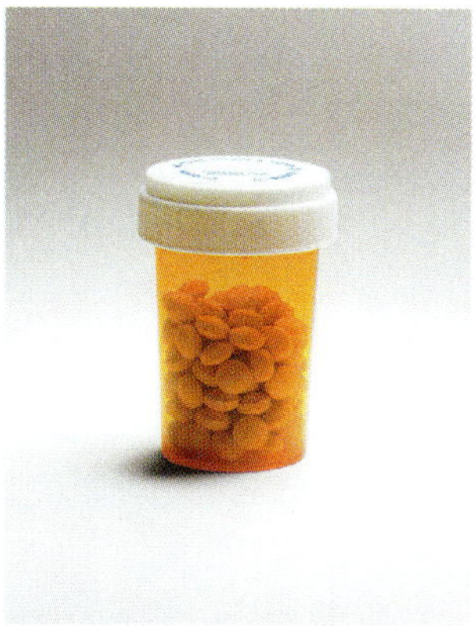

Figure 8-4 **Safety caps.**

Transitioning

Prescription agents that are judged to be safe for OTC use may be transitioned from prescription only to either prescription or OTC. When a medication becomes available as an OTC agent, it may initially be available at a lower strength than the prescription strength. The FDA oversees the process of transitioning prescription-only preparations to OTC available status. First, the drug sponsor submits data supporting the transition to the FDA. Next, an OTC advisory committee and other consultants review the data. As a result of this review, a recommendation report is developed. If the advisory committee and consultants agree, a proposed monograph is developed and public comment is invited. The final monograph is prepared and reviewed. The last step in the process is the publication of the final monograph in the *Federal Register* and in the Code of Federal Regulations. Table 8-2 lists agents that were previously available as prescription only and are now available without prescription.

Table 8-2 **Nonprescription Agents Previously Available as Prescription Only**

Nonprescription Agent	Prescription Agent
Advil, Motrin IB (ibuprofen 200 mg)	Motrin (ibuprofen 400 mg, 600 mg, 800 mg)
Alavert, Claritin (loratidine 5mg)	Claritin (loratadine 10 mg)
Alli (orlistat 60mg)	Xenical (orlistat 120 mg)
Axid NR (nizatidine 75 mg)	Axid (nizatidine 150 mg)
Pepcid AC (famotidine 10 mg, 20 mg)	Pepcid (famotidine 20 mg, 40 mg)
Prilosec-OTC (omeprazole 20mg)	Prilosec (omeprazole 20 mg, 40 mg)
Tagamet HB (cimetidine 200 mg)	Tagamet (cimetidine 400 mg, 600 mg, 800 mg)
Zyrtec (cetirizine HCl 10mg)	Zyrtec (cetirizine HCl 5 mg, 10 mg)
Zantac75 (ranitidine 75 mg)	Zantac (ranitidine 150 mg, 300 mg)

Tech Check

1. Which organization oversees the process of transitioning prescription-only preparations to OTC available status?(LO 8.2)
2. Identify information listed on the nonprescription drug label.(LO 8.2)
3. What is the nonprescription agent for Pepcid?(LO 8.3, 8.6)

Types of OTC Agents(LO 8.4, 8.5, 8.6, 8.7)

The following types of OTC agents will be highlighted in this chapter:

- Analgesics and antipyretic agents
- Central nervous system agents
- Gastrointestinal system agents
- Genitourinary system agents
- Integumentary system agents
- Ophthalmic agents
- Oral/dental care agents
- Otic agents
- Respiratory system agents
- Miscellaneous agents

Analgesic and Antipyretic Agents

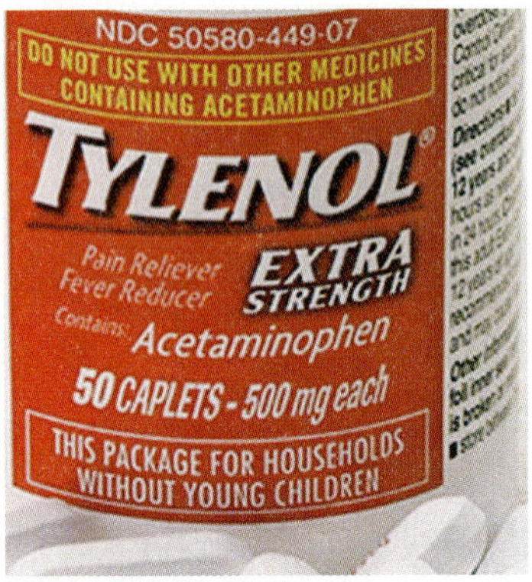

Figure 8-5
Acetaminophen.

Analgesic agents are medications used to relieve pain. Analgesic agents, like aspirin and ibuprofen, also exert anti-inflammatory and antipyretic activity. **Antipyretics** are fever-reducing agents. Pain relievers work by inhibition of cyclo-oxygenase (COX) to decrease prostaglandin synthesis (aspirin and nonsteroidal anti-inflammatory drugs, or NSAIDs)) or through raising the pain threshold (acetaminophen) (Figure 8-5). The following agents are pain relievers:

- Aspirin
- Acetaminophen
- Ibuprofen
- Ketoprofen
- Naproxen

Caution

A single dose of aspirin daily (81 to 325 mg) is used to exert antiplatelet effects. The antiplatelet effect of aspirin reduces the risk of heart attacks and strokes through inhibition of platelet aggregation and adhesion. The pharmacist should be notified if a patient is taking any dose of aspirin with antiplatelet or anticoagulant agents, as well as some herbal supplements.

Refer to Chapters 7 and 9 for more background regarding interactions between these agents.

analgesic An agent that relieves pain.

antipyretic An agent that reduces fever.

Common adverse drug reactions associated with aspirin and nonsteroidal anti-inflammatory agents include nausea, vomiting, and epigastric (stomach) distress. Some gastrointestinal symptoms may be alleviated by administering the agents with food or are enteric coated. Aspirin formulations that are enteric coated reduce the potential irritation aspirin can cause to the stomach. Aspirin and NSAIDs should not be used in a patient who has peptic ulcer disease or gastroesophageal reflux disease (GERD) because these agents may exacerbate or worsen the symptoms of the diseases.

Acetaminophen is associated with few adverse drug reactions (nausea, vomiting, hypersensitivity). However, it is associated with hepatic toxicity in the event of an overdose (more than 4 g daily) and/or in combination with alcohol or in patients taking medications requiring extensive hepatic metabolism. The pharmacy technician should encourage patients to read labels of nonprescription agents that contain acetaminophen assess how much is being taken daily. It is also important to educate patients not to take more than one acetaminophen containing preparation at a time to avoid overdose of the drug.

Caution

Aspirin should not be used as a fever-reducing agent in pediatric patients due to the risk of the development of Reye's syndrome (potentially fatal hepatic encephalopathy).

Pain relievers are available in oral and topical dosage forms (see Table 8-3). For example, acetaminophen is available as an elixir, suspension, suppository, powder, chewable tablet, tablet, and caplet. External analgesics, commonly called counterirritants, are generally used for short-term management of local pain. Agents from this category exhibit pharmacologic effects by stimulating nerve endings to decrease sensitivity to pain, through the depletion of substance-P (a pain mediator), or by inhibition of prostaglandins (Figure 8-6). The primary adverse drug reaction associated with the use of topical analgesics is skin irritation.

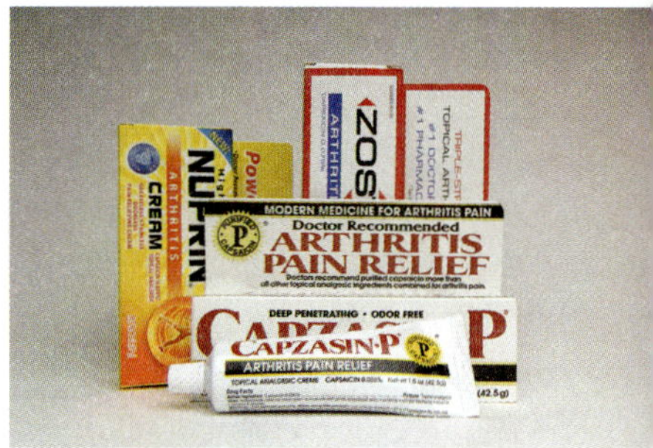

Figure 8-6 Topical analgesics.

Table 8-3 Common Nonprescription Analgesics

Internal Agents		
Brand Name	**Active Ingredient**	**Dosage Form**
Advil	ibuprofen	Suspension, tablet
Aleve	naproxen	Tablet
Bayer Aspirin	aspirin	Tablet
Tylenol	acetaminophen	Capsule, chewable tablet, elixir, suspension, tablet
External Agents		
Brand Name	**Active Ingredient**	**Dosage Form**
Absorbine Jr. Extra Strength	menthol	Solution
Flex-All Ultra Plus Gel	menthol, methyl salicylate, camphor	Gel
Zostrix	capsaicin	Cream

The following agents exert analgesic activity through topical application:

- Camphor
- Capsaicin
- Capsicum oleoresin
- Eucalyptus oil
- Menthol
- Methyl nicotinate
- Methylsalicylate
- Trolamine salicylate

Tech Check

4. Which of the internal agents discussed is used for its antiplatelet, analgesic, and anti-inflammatory properties?(LO 8.5, 8.6)

5. Which internal agent is associated with liver failure at high doses and when combined with alcohol?(LO 8.6)

Central Nervous System Agents

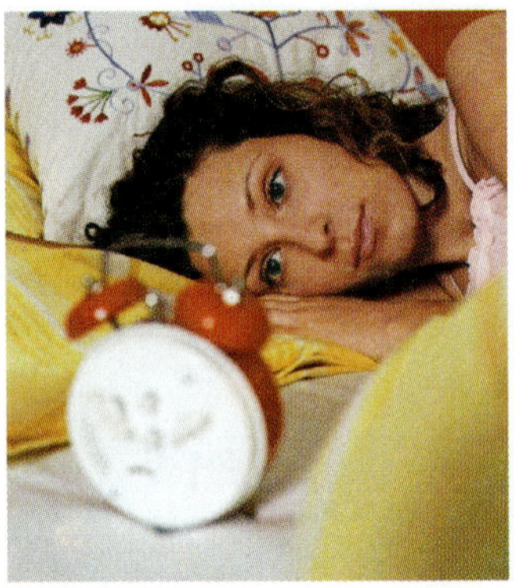

Figure 8-7 Patient with insomnia.

Central nervous system agents available as nonprescription drugs are used for insomnia and motion sickness. Insomnia is defined as the inability to sleep. OTC sleep aids utilize the anticholinergic effects of antihistamines to produce drowsiness (Figure 8-7). Common antihistamine agents incorporated into sleep agents are diphenhydramine and doxylamine.

The pharmacy technician should be aware that these agents may interact with other sedative-hypnotics, narcotic analgesics, and alcohol to cause excessive drowsiness. In addition, their anticholinergic effects limit their use in patients with glaucoma, prostatic hypertrophy, gastrointestinal obstruction, and patients taking other preparations with anticholinergic effects. Nonprescription antihistamines like Claritin (loratadine) are not incorporated into sleep aids because the anticholinergic effect of drowsiness is not as pronounced as in diphenhydramine and doxylamine. Table 8-4 identifies common nonprescription agents for insomnia.

Caution

Always read the package label. It is possible that agents with the same brand name contain different active ingredients.

Table 8-4 Agents for Insomnia

Brand Name	Active Ingredient
Nytol	diphenhydramine
Sominex	diphenhydramine
Unisom Nighttime Sleep Aid	doxylamine
Unisom Sleepgels	diphenhydramine

Agents for motion sickness work by decreasing the cholinergic activity in the inner ear, an area responsible for the sense of balance and equilibrium. These agents also have anticholinergic activity and therefore may relieve the nausea associated with motion sickness, but they may also cause drowsiness. Agents for motion sickness include:

- Bonine (meclizine)
- Dramamine (dimenhydrinate)

As agents for motion sickness demonstrate anticholinergic activity, adverse drug reactions associated with these agents include blurred vision, drowsiness, dry mouth, and lethargy.

Tech Check

6. Patients taking OTC sleep aids should be advised to avoid combining them with __________. (LO 8.5)

7. Adverse drug reactions associated with anticholinergic drugs include __________. (LO 8.6)

Gastrointestinal System Agents

Keeping in mind that the gastrointestinal tract starts at the mouth and ends at the anus (Figure 8-8), there are many types of agents available to treat the various maladies that affect the gastrointestinal tract.

In addition to agents for indigestion or upset stomach, the following subcategories of agents will be discussed in this section:

- Antidiarrheals
- Antiemetics
- Antiflatulents
- Antihemorrhoidal preparations
- Laxatives

Table 8-5 categorizes common nonprescription gastrointestinal agents.

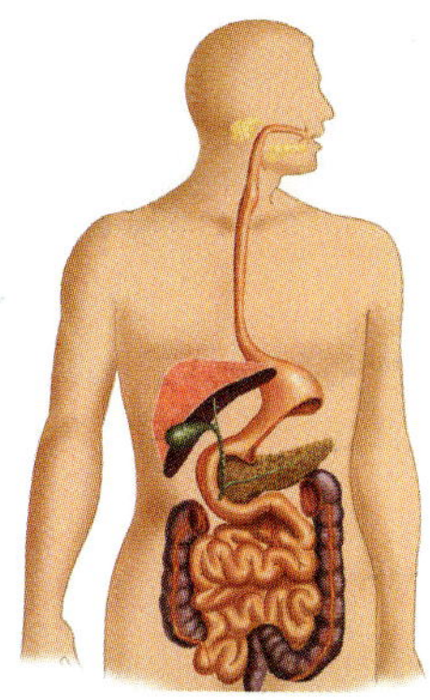

Figure 8-8 The gastrointestinal tract.

Agents for Indigestion—Antacids

Antacids are not extensively absorbed and work by increasing gastric pH (decreasing gastric acidity). Antacids usually contain two or more agents that are combined for their additive pharmacologic effects and their opposing adverse drug effects. For example, Maalox (Figure 8-9) contains a combination of magnesium hydroxide (which often causes diarrhea) and aluminum hydroxide (which may cause constipation) because they both exhibit antacid effects.

Histamine 2 receptor blockers (cimetidine, famotidine, nizatidine, ranitidine) decrease gastric pH through decreasing acid secretion from the parietal cells. Proton pump inhibitors (omeprazole) decrease gastric acidity by inhibiting the movement of hydrogen içons (components of hydrochloric acid) into the stomach. Prior to 2005, omeprazole (Prilosec) was available as prescription only. All of the histamine-2 (H^2) receptor blockers were previously prescription only. These agents are used for heartburn, upset stomach, and symptoms of ulcer disease.

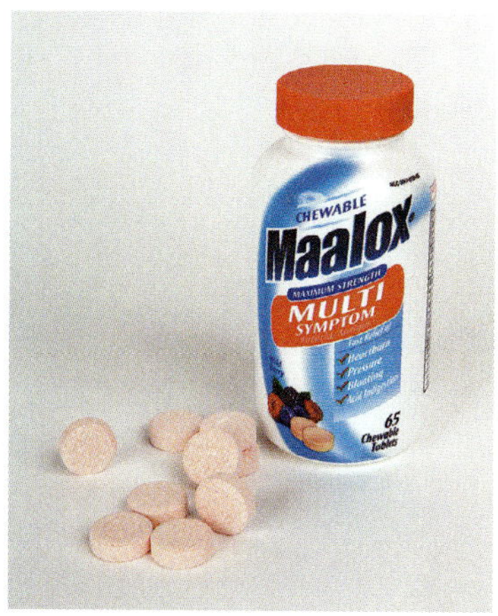

Figure 8-9 Maalox.

Table 8-5 Common Gastrointestinal Agents

Category	Brand Name	Active Ingredient	Dosage Form
Agents for Indigestion	Maalox	aluminum hydroxide, magnesium hydroxide	Liquid, tablet
	Mylanta Double Strength	aluminum hydroxide, magnesium hydroxide, simethicone	Liquid, tablet
	Pepcid AC	famotidine	Tablet
	Zantac 75	ranitidine	Tablet
Antidiarrheals	Imodium AD	loperamide	Liquid, tablet
	Kaopectate	attapulgite	Liquid, tablet
	Pepto-Bismol	bismuth subsalicylate	Liquid, tablet
Antiemetics	Emetrol	phosphorated carbohydrate solution	Liquid
	Pepto-Bismol	bismuth subsalicylate	Liquid, tablet
Antiflatulents	Gas-X	simethicone	Tablet
	Mylicon drops	simethicone	Solution
Antihemorrhoidals	Anusol	pramoxine, zinc oxide, mineral oil	Ointment
	Fleets Pain Relief Pads	pramoxine, glycerin	Moistened pad
	Preparation H	Glycerin, shark liver oil, lanolin	Cream, ointment, suppositories
Laxatives	Carter's Little Pills	bisacodyl	Tablet
	Colace	docusate sodium	Capsule, solution, syrup
	Ex-Lax	sennosides	Chewable tablet, tablet
	Metamucil	psyllium	Powder

Antidiarrheals

Nonprescription antidiarrheals work by either decreasing peristalsis (loperamide) or by increasing the bulk of the stools (kaolin-pectin). Loperamide should not be used if the patient has an intestinal parasite or bacterial poisoning (e.g., salmonella or botulism). Patients may also wish to take electrolyte replacement products (Figure 8-10) like Gatorade or Pedialyte to combat dehydration and malnutrition as a result of diarrhea.

Antiemetics

Antiemetic agents suppress the sensitivity of the gag center in the central nervous system. By raising the threshold for vomiting, **emesis** is decreased. The agents for motion sickness have antiemetic properties as they suppress the stimulation of the emesis center. Other antiemetics are carbohydrate-dense suspensions that decrease gastrointestinal upset and propensity to develop nausea and vomiting.

emesis Vomiting.

The pharmacy technician should be aware that syrup of ipecac, an emesis agent to be used in the event of some poisoning, is available as a nonprescription agent. It is important to note, however, that syrup of ipecac should not be used indiscriminately and is therefore not an appropriate agent to employ in all types of poisonings or in poisonings involving corrosive agents.

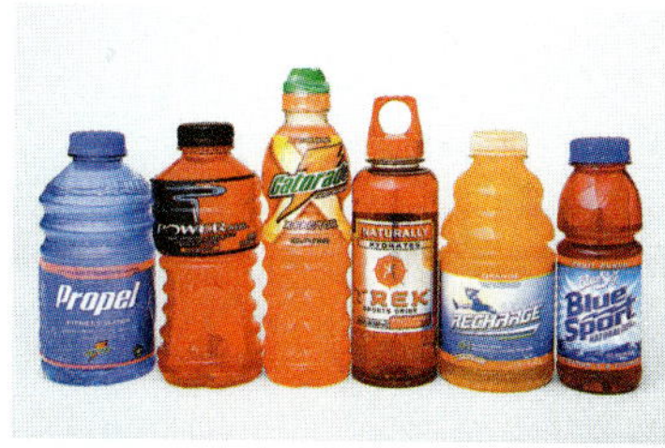

Figure 8-10 Electrolyte drinks.

Antiflatulents

Antiflatulent agents—for example, simethicone—may be used separately or may be combined with antacids. Antiflatulent agents decrease surface tension of gas bubbles in the stomach to decrease bloating, belching, and flatulence.

Antihemorrhoidals

Antihemorrhoidal preparations are available in multiple topical forms (creams, foams, wipes, suppositories) and often contain active ingredients that are antipruritic (anti-itching) and/or local anesthetics to reduce irritation and pain. Patients should consult a physician prior to starting therapy with aspirin or nonsteroidal anti-inflammatory agents or if there is increased bleeding resulting from inflamed hemorrhoids.

Laxatives

Laxatives (or cathartics) are used to increase defecation. There are several categories of laxatives available without prescription. Categories or types of laxatives are based upon their mechanisms of action, and are described as follows:

- Bulk-forming—increase the bulkiness of stool aiding in defecation
- Emollient—increase moisture in stool composition
- Osmotic—attract water into the lumen of the colon resulting in catharsis
- Stimulants—increase movement of matter through the gastrointestinal tract by stimulating peristalsis
- Stool softeners—surfactants that decrease surface tension easing defecation

Caution

Laxatives should not be used if the patient is experiencing nausea, vomiting, and/or abdominal pain.

Tech Check

8. List at least three agents for indigestion.(LO 8.6)

9. What is the name of the agent that is used to induce emesis?(LO 8.6)

10. What subcategory of laxatives increases moisture in stool composition (LO 8.6)

Genitourinary System Agents

Nonprescription genitourinary system medications are primarily limited to agents for candida infections, genital itching, urinary tract analgesics, and contraceptive agents. A major concern is that although these agents may be available without a prescription, the patient may have a condition

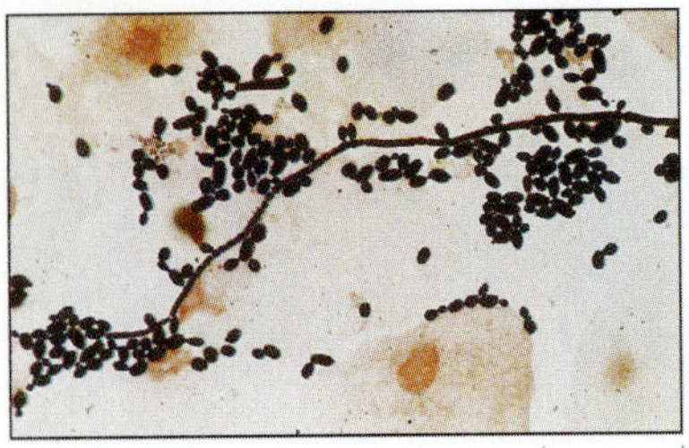

Figure 8-11 Candida albicans.

that may require seeing a physician. The pharmacy technician should alert the pharmacist if he or she witnesses a patient attempting to make multiple purchases of these types of items.

Nonprescription agents for candida (yeast) infections are limited to topical application, and vaginal creams or suppositories (Figure 8-11). Female patients often ask about these agents to manage a condition that is commonly known as a "yeast" infection. These preparations are available in 1- to 7-day treatment regimens. Active ingredients are butoconazole, clotrimazole, miconazole, or tioconazole. It is critical that the patient follows all instructions carefully and reports to her physician should her symptoms remain unresolved. Genitourinary products for male patients are for what is commonly called "jock itch" or tinea cruris. Antifungal preparations are available in aerosol sprays and powders. None of these agents is indicated for sexually transmitted infections (STIs).

Agents for genital itching are creams, gels, or wipes that are available to ease vaginal dryness and or itching. These agents are palliative only, and are not designed to treat or cure any infection or condition.

Patients seeking relief from urinary tract irritation may ask for products containing phenazopyridine. These products are urinary tract analgesics but have no antimicrobial properties. They also contain an azo dye, which means that the products it can discolor urine and other body fluids to a reddish-orange color.

Contraceptives

OTC contraceptive agents are limited to spermicides (nonoxynol-9) that are incorporated into a dosage form or vehicle for administration. Dosage forms include foams, gels, vaginal suppositories, and films. Nonoxynol-9 is also incorporated into the lubricant for condoms, but should not be used in sensitive individuals. Instructions must be followed carefully for optimal spermicidal activity. Most importantly, a spermicide is inadequate protection against transmission of STIs and human immunodeficiency virus (HIV).

Refer to Table 8-6 for common nonprescription genitourinary agents.

Integumentary System Agents

The integumentary (dermatologic) system involves more than just the skin, but also hair and nails. As such, the majority of dosage forms for these types of agents are applied topically and include creams, shampoos, gels, ointments, lotions, powders, liniments, and soaps. Patients should be aware that these products are intended for external use only, and may cause considerable health risks if they are ingested or applied to mucus membranes. It is important to note that agents that are applied to the skin to relieve muscle/joint pain are not considered integumentary system agents even though it is the means by which they are administered. Table 8-7 (p. 237) identifies common integumentary system agents available without prescription.

The following list identifies conditions for which nonprescription topical agents are available:

- Acne
- Alopecia
- Bacterial infections
- Corns, calluses, and warts

Table 8-6 Common Genitourinary Agents

Category	Brand Name	Active Ingredient	Dosage Form
Agents for Vaginal Candidiasis	Femcare	clotrimazole	Suppository
	Monistat 7	miconazole	Cream, suppository
	Vagistat-1	tioconazole	Ointment
Agents for Tinea Cruris	Cruex	Undecylenic acid-zinc undecylenate	Aerosol powder, cream
Urinary Tract Analgesics/ Antiseptics	Azo-Standard	phenazopyridine	Tablet
Agents for Vaginal Dryness	Gynecor	hydrocortisone	Cream
	Vagisil	benzocaine, resorcinol	Cream
Contraceptive Agents	Encare	nonoxynol-9	Suppository
	Ortho Options	nonoxynol-9	Foam
	Delfen Foam		
	Vaginal Contraceptive Film (VCF)	nonoxynol-9F	film

- Dandruff
- Dermatitis
- Fungal infections
- Parasitic infestations
- Sunburn/sunscreen

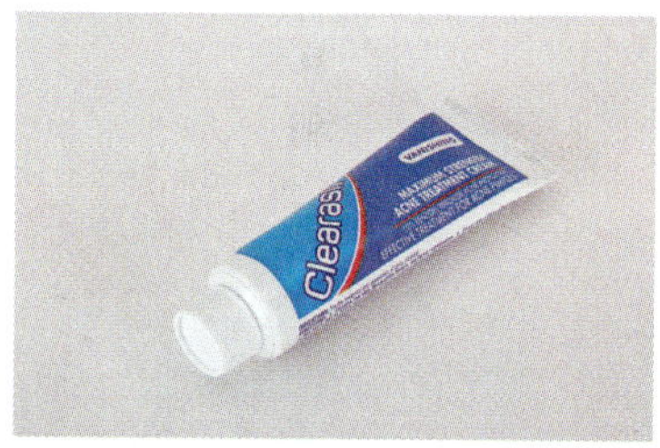

Figure 8-12 Acne medication.

Anti-Acne Agents

Anti-acne products are available in several dosage forms including soaps, gels, applicator pads, and creams (Figure 8-12). The most common active ingredient used in anti-acne products is benzoyl peroxide. Patients using this agent for the first time should be referred to the pharmacist for counseling, as it may cause skin irritation, particularly at higher concentrations. Benzoyl peroxide has been associated with redness, peeling, and stinging upon application.

Alopecia Agents

Alopecia is defined as loss of hair or baldness. Rogaine (minoxidil) is applied to areas where hair growth is desired. Hair growth as a result of using this agent is reversible. In addition, patients should be cautioned to apply this agent only to areas where more hair growth is desirable.

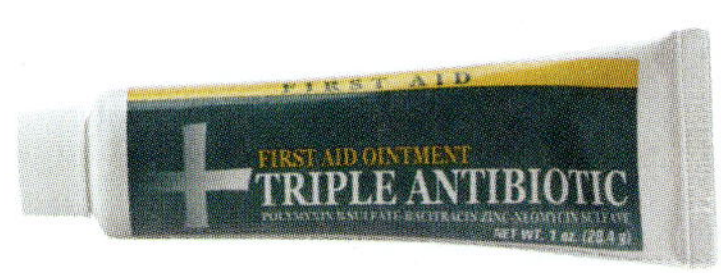

Figure 8-13 Antibiotic ointment.

Antibacterial Agents

Antibacterial agents are used to decrease the risk of development of infections as a result of surface scratches or scrapes (Figure 8-13). Multiple antibiotics are combined in one dosage form (typically or cream or ointment)

Table 8-7 Common Integumentary System Agents

Category	Brand Name	Active Ingredient	Dosage Form
Acne	Clearasil	salicylic acid	Cream, pad
	Fostex	benzoyl peroxide	Soap
	Oxy Balance	benzoyl peroxide	Gel
Alopecia	Rogaine	minoxidil	Lotion
Antibacterials	Bacitracin	bacitracin	Ointment
	Neosporin	bacitracin, neomycin, polymyxin B	Ointment
	Polysporin	bacitracin, polymyxin B	Ointment, powder
Corns, Calluses, Warts	Compound W	salicylic acid	Gel, liquid, medicated disc
	Duofilm	salicylic acid	Liquid
	Duofilm Patch for Kids	Salicylic acid	Medicated disc
Dandruff	Head & Shoulders	pyrithione zinc	Shampoo
	Ionil T Plus	coal tar	Shampoo
	Selsun Blue	selenium sulfide	Shampoo
Dermatitis	Benadryl Extra Strength	diphenhydramine, zinc acetate	Cream, gel, spray, stick
	Caladryl	calamine, pramoxine	Cream, lotion
	Cortaid	hydrocortisone	Cream, ointment
Antifungals	Desenex	undecylenic acid-zinc undecylenate	Ointment, powder, spray powder
	Dr. Scholl's Athletes Foot	tolnaftate	Aerosol, powder, spray powder
Pediculosis	Nix	permethrin	Creme rinse
	Rid	pyrethrins, piperonyl butoxide	Shampoo
Sunscreens, Sunburn Agents	Americaine	benzocaine	Aerosol
	Solarcaine Aloe	lidocaine, aloe	Cream, gel, spray

to provide for **broad-spectrum** antibacterial coverage. Topical antibacterial agents are not effective against deeper infections, such as cellulitis or folliculitis. Patients with these infections should be referred to a physician.

Corn, Callus, and Wart Removal Agents

Agents for the removal of corns, calluses, or warts primarily employ the use of salicylic acid, which softens and hydrates keratin aiding in the removal of the raised and/or hardened skin. Salicylic acid should not be applied to broken or irritated skin, and should be applied only to the corn, callous, or wart.

Anti-Dandruff Agents

Dandruff is a condition of increased epidermal cell proliferation resulting in the shedding of "flakes." Pyrithione zinc, selenium sulfide, salicylic acid, sulfur, and tar derivatives are incorporated into shampoos to reduce cell

broad spectrum Exhibits activity against a wide variety of bacteria.

proliferation and turnover. Patients using these shampoos should take care to avoid shampoo contact with the eyes, and should be instructed to rinse the hair thoroughly after using.

Dermatitis Agents
Dermatitis is defined as inflammation and itching of the skin. Contact dermatitis is itching and inflammation as a result of contact with an irritant (jewelry, poison ivy, detergents). The corticosteroids are used to decrease irritation and itching through the inhibition of the inflammatory response. Corticosteroids are also called glucocorticoids, and are not to be used on broken or infected skin. The corticosteroids may also be employed as a component in the management of psoriasis (a dermatologic condition characterized by rapid cell turnover resulting in shiny, silver scales and pinpoint bleeding). Other types of agents employed against dermatitis include antihistamines (diphenhydramine) and local anesthetics (benzocaine).

Antifungals
Fungal infections—like athlete's foot, ringworm, and jock itch—are common (Figure 8-14). Topical antifungal agents such as clotrimazole and miconazole primarily affect the synthesis of ergosterol, a necessary constituent of fungal cell membranes.

Without ergosterol, fungal cell membranes cannot contain the components of the cell, causing cell death. Tolnaftate is used to interfere with the proper growth of fungal cells, and is used to prevent and treat tinea pedis (athlete's foot). Undecylenic acid is incorporated into powders, ointments, or solutions to retard fungal cell growth. Although there are topical agents for nail fungus (tinea unguium), patients who may have the condition should be referred to a physician as systemic treatment may be required.

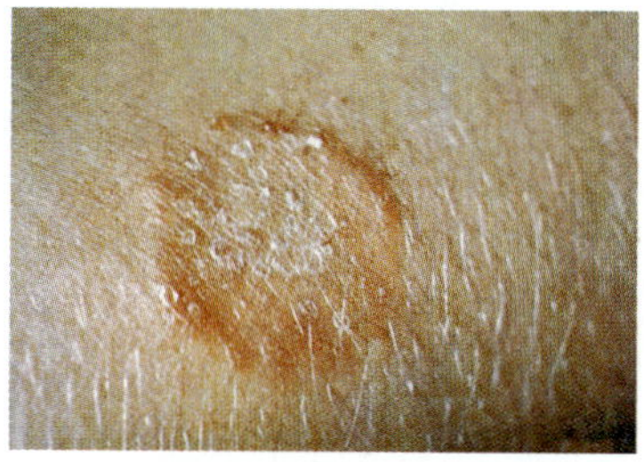

Figure 8-14 **Ringworm on skin surface.**

Pediculosis
Pediculosis is defined as a parasitic infestation with lice (Figure 8-15), which may be transmitted through physical contact with a person with lice or through inanimate articles (clothing, linens, combs, brushes). Agents used to manage these infestations—permethrin and pyrethrum extract—cause paralysis and death in the lice through interfering with their neuronal membranes. Due to the risk of neurological damage, these agents should not be used in patients younger than 2 years of age.

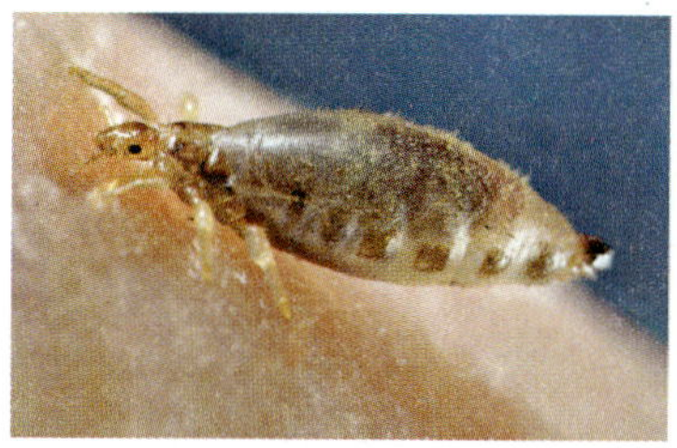

Figure 8-15 **Female body louse, *Pediculus humanus var. corporis*.**

Sunscreens
Sunscreens work by absorbing or blocking ultraviolet light. Agents for sunburn (skin sensitivity and irritation as a result of sun overexposure) employ the use of local anesthetics, corticosteroids, analgesics, and aloe vera to reduce local pain and tenderness. Patients are well advised to avoid subsequent excessive exposure to sunlight to allow for healing of the affected areas. If the sunburn is around the eyes or is severe and over a large part of the body, patients should consult a physician.

Tech Check

11. Identify the agent that is used for hair loss.(LO 8.6)

12. Identify an appropriate agent to use for head lice.(LO 8.6)

13. Individuals using corn or wart removal agents should avoid _____.(LO 8.5)

Ophthalmic Agents

Although there are several categories of nonprescription agents designed for ophthalmic administration, there are common precautions that must be observed when administering any agent that is administered in the eye (Figure 8-16).

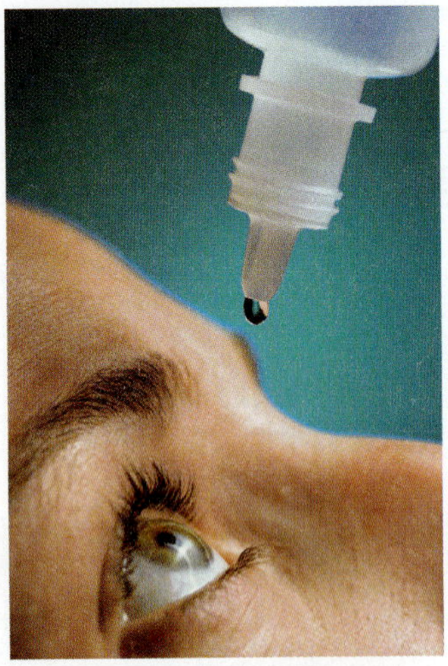

Figure 8-16 **Eye drops.**

1. The manufacturer's expiration date should be adhered to as long as the package seal is not broken. Once the seal is broken and the first drops are administered, the medication should be discarded after 30 days.
2. Hands should be washed prior to administration to avoid contaminating the drops and irritating the eyes.
3. The tip of the dropper or applicator should not touch the eye, eyelid, or eyelashes during administration to decrease the risk of contamination. The cap should be replaced immediately after medication administration.
4. Ophthalmic preparations should not be used if the medication changes color or becomes cloudy.
5. Patients should see a physician if there is a foreign object in the eye, if there has been chemical exposure to the eyes, if the eyes have been scratched or scraped, or if the eyes have been infected.
6. Patients who wear contact lenses should contact their eye health professional prior to using eye drops not designed for use with contact lenses.

In addition to products for contact lenses, the categories of ophthalmic medications available without prescription are:

- Antihistamines
- Artificial tears and ophthalmic lubricants
- Decongestants

Ophthalmic Antihistamines

Ophthalmic antihistamines are used to manage allergy symptoms such as tearing and itching of the eyes by blocking the histamine response. It is important to keep in mind that these agents are not curative, but manage symptoms only. Antazoline and pheniramine are ophthalmic antihistamines that may be combined with ophthalmic decongestants in eye drops to provide relief from allergy-related symptoms while reducing redness.

Artificial Tears and Ophthalmic Lubricants

Artificial tears and ophthalmic lubricants are used to relieve the symptoms of dry eyes. Artificial tears are designed to mimic the effects of natural tears as tear production is decreased. Ophthalmic lubricants are designed to increase viscosity of the patient's own tears. Glycerin, carboxymethylcellulose, and hydroxyethyl cellulose are examples of agents incorporated into ophthalmic products to increase the viscosity of tears. Some lubricants are available in an ophthalmic ointment form to provide for longer-lasting lubricant activity.

Ophthalmic Decongestants

Ophthalmic decongestants are agents that reduce the appearance of redness in the eyes. They work by constricting conjunctival blood vessels through alpha adrenergic receptor stimulation. Patients should be cautioned that if symptoms persist for more than 72 hours, they should consult a physician. Rebound redness of the eye may result from prolonged or excessive use of

Table 8-8 Common Ophthalmic Agents

Category	Brand Name	Active Ingredient	Dosage Form
Artificial Tears/ Ophthalmic Lubricants	Artificial Tears	sodium chloride, hydroxypropyl methylcellulose	Drops
	Cellufresh	sodium chloride, carboxymethylcellulose	Drops
	Lacri-Lube S.O.P.	white petrolatum, mineral oil	Ointment
Decongestants	Allerest	naphazoline	Drops
	Murine Tears Plus	tetrahydrozoline	Drops
	Visine	tetrahydrozoline	Drops
Decongestant-Antihistamine Combinations	Naphcon-A Solution	naphazoline, pheniramine maleate	Drops
	Vasocon A	naphazoline, antazoline	Drops

these agents. Patients with glaucoma should consult a physician prior to using them. Common ophthalmic decongestants are:

- Naphazoline
- Oxymetazoline
- Phenylephrine
- Tetrahydrozoline

Adverse drug reactions associated with the nonprescription ophthalmic agents are primarily limited to transient tingling and blurred vision. The ophthalmic decongestants may also cause **mydriasis** or pupil dilation. Table 8-8 identifies common nonprescription ophthalmic agents.

Tech Check

14. What type of ophthalmic agent is most often incorporated into an ointment?(LO 8.6)

15. What type of agent should be used in patients with seasonal allergies?(LO 8.5, 8.6)

Oral/Dental Care Agents

Most of the agents available as nonprescription agents for oral and dental care are for relief of symptoms, and are not designed to treat a specific disease. OTC agents include canker and cold sore preparations, and agents for sensitive teeth, toothache and oral pain, and **xerostomia** (dry mouth).

Canker and Cold Sore Agents

Agents for canker and cold sores are primarily local anesthetics designed to help relieve the pain and irritation resulting from the lesion. There is no cure for either type of lesion, but nonprescription agents are designed to speed

mydriasis Dilation of the pupil.

xerostomia Dry mouth.

healing and relieve pain. Agents are available in lip balms, ointments, and oral rinses. Local anesthetics—for example, benzocaine, dyclonine, lidocaine, and tetracaine—are used to decrease the sensitivity to pain. Carbamide peroxide or hydrogen peroxide may be incorporated into mouth rinses to cleanse lesions inside the mouth resulting in decreased inflammation and pain.

Sensitive Teeth

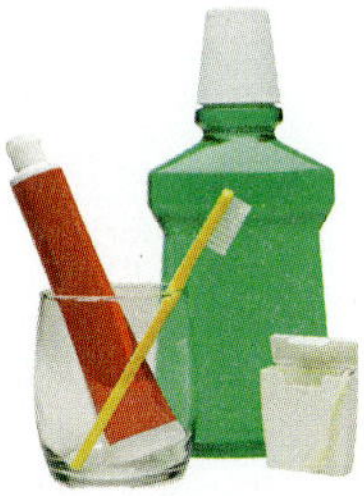

Figure 8-17 Dental products.

Individuals with sensitive teeth may have pain or an overly intense feeling of heat or cold depending upon the type of items they may be ingesting at the time. Fluorides form a protective coating over the enamel to reduce the risk of cavities, while potassium nitrate and strontium chloride are thought to reduce the transmission of pain. These items are available as toothpastes and mouthwashes. Pregnant patients should consult a physician prior to using any of these products (Figure 8-17).

Toothache and Oral Pain

Toothache and other types of oral pain, such as teething, are primarily managed with local anesthetics (benzocaine and dyclonine) and counterirritants (camphor, menthol, and phenol). While local anesthetics cause numbness and work by decreasing sensitivity to pain, counterirritants cause tingling through the stimulation of nerve endings.

Xerostomia

Patients with xerostomia, or dry mouth, do not produce adequate saliva due to decreased salivary gland activity. Dry mouth may be the result of treatment with drugs that exhibit anticholinergic effects. Agents for dry mouth incorporate viscosity-increasing agents like carboxymethylcellulose and hydroxyethyl cellulose into dosage forms to serve as saliva substitutes.

Adverse drug reactions with the oral and dental care agents are uncommon; however, patients may experience hypersensitivity or allergy to any of the ingredients incorporated into the dosage forms. It is critical that patients not experiencing relief of symptoms contact a physician or pharmacist for assistance. Table 8-9 outlines common oral care products.

Otic Agents

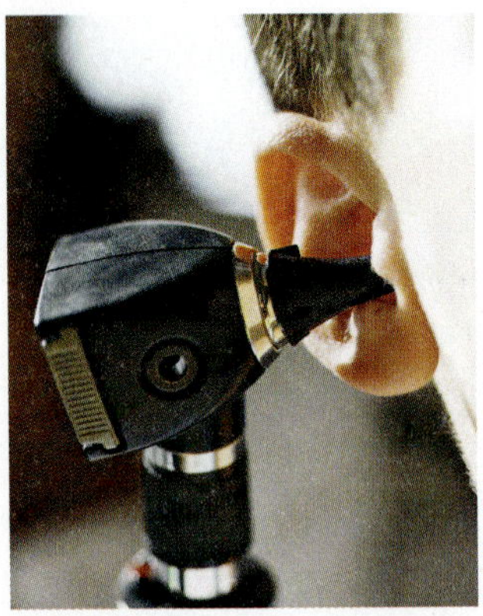

Figure 8-18 Examination of child's ear using otoscope.

Nonprescription agents for the ear are limited to ceruminolytics (ear wax removal agents) and agents to remove water from the ear through evaporation. Neither of these types of agents is appropriate to use in the event of a suspected ear infection or ear drum perforation. Patients should be referred to the pharmacist or physician in the event of a suspected ear infection (Figure 8-18).

Table 8-10 identifies common nonprescription otic agents.

Respiratory System Agents

Available nonprescription medications for the respiratory system are primarily cough, cold, and flu medications (Figure 8-19). Agents in these categories are designed to manage the symptoms of viral infections. Patients may exhibit any number of symptoms when experiencing a cold or flu, therefore OTC preparations often contain a number of active ingredients to manage specific symptoms. It is critical that the patient read the label to

Table 8-9 Common Oral Care Products

Category	Brand Name	Active Ingredient	Dosage Form
Canker and Cold Sores	Campho-Phenique Cold Sore	camphor, phenol	Gel
	Gly-Oxide Liquid	carbamide peroxide	Solution
	Orabase	benzocaine	Gel
	Zilactin	benzyl alcohol	Gel
Sensitive Teeth	Aquafresh Sensitive	potassium nitrate, sodium fluoride	Gel
	Sensodyne	potassium nitrate, sodium fluoride	Gel
Toothache and Oral Pain	Anbesol	benzocaine, camphor, phenol	Gel, liquid
	Blistex	camphor, phenol	Ointment
	Orajel	benzocaine	Gel
Dry Mouth	Salivart	sodium carboxymethylcellulose	Solution

Table 8-10 Otic Agents

Brand Name	Active Ingredient	Dosage Form
Debrox	carbamide peroxide	Liquid
Swimear	isopropyl alcohol	Liquid

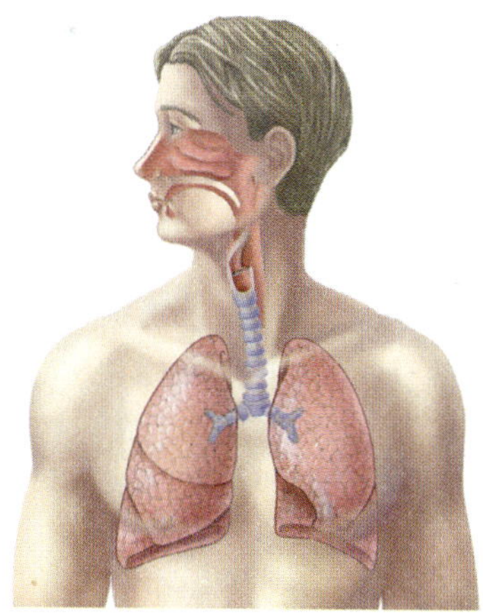

Figure 8-19 Respiratory system.

determine which active ingredients are incorporated into the cough, cold, and flu medication; several of the agents may interact with other drugs or worsen specific diseases or health conditions.

The types of active ingredients often contained in cough, cold, and flu preparations are:

- Analgesics
- Antihistamines
- Antitussives
- Oral decongestants
- Nasal decongestants
- Expectorants

Analgesics

Analgesics are pain relievers that are often incorporated into cough, cold, and flu preparations to relieve the pain and fever commonly associated with viral infections. Patients experiencing viral upper respiratory tract infections may complain of headache, body aches and pains, and sore throat. Analgesic agents incorporated into cough, cold, and flu preparations are acetaminophen and ibuprofen. These agents were discussed in greater detail earlier in this chapter (Figure 8-20).

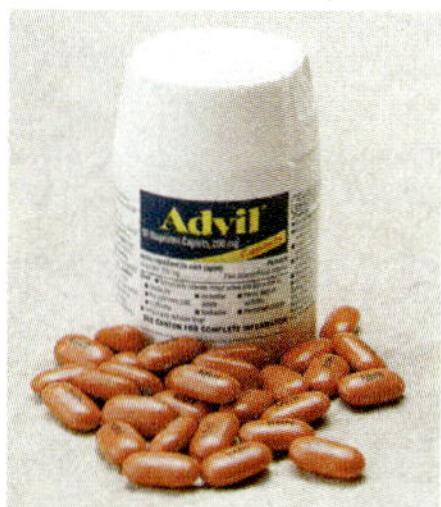

Figure 8-20 Analgesic pain reliever.

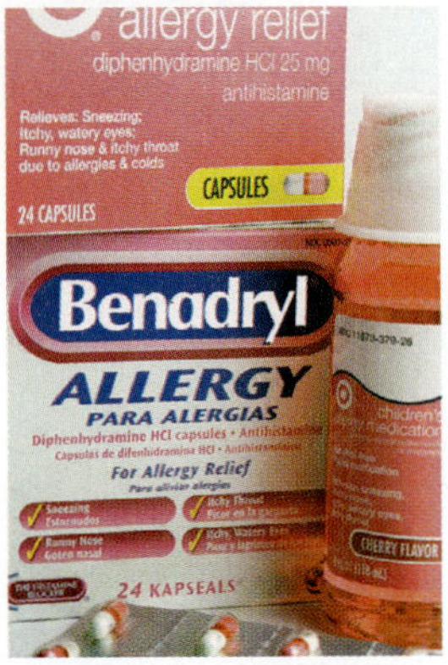

Figure 8-21 OTC antihistamines.

Antihistamines

Antihistamines interfere with the histamine response by blocking the receptors in the upper respiratory tract. Symptoms relieved by antihistamines are sneezing, coughing, watery eyes, and runny nose.

Several OTC antihistamines may cause drowsiness, and patients should be made aware that these agents may interact with other drugs that are sedating, and may impair one's ability to safely operate a vehicle.

Antihistamines associated with drowsiness are brompheniramine, chlorpheniramine, clemastine, diphenhydramine, and triprolidine. Loratadine is an antihistamine that does not cause drowsiness to the extent of agents like diphenhydramine (Figure 8-21).

Antitussives

Antitussives suppress the cough reflex through interacting with the cough center in the central nervous system. These agents are often incorporated into cough syrups and lozenges to decrease the frequency of cough, and as a result, decrease the irritation to the throat. The most common antitussive agents are diphenhydramine and dextromethorphan (DMX).

Decongestants

Decongestants relieve congestion through constricting the blood vessels and shrinking mucus membranes in the nasal passages. This **vasoconstriction** opens airways and facilitates breathing. Patients complaining of a stuffy nose or who indicate that breathing is difficult are likely to request decongestants.

Decongestants are available as systemic agents (tablets and capsules) or as nasal agents (nasal sprays or drops). Because systemic agents are taken by mouth, they have the ability to cause vasoconstriction in any area of the body. In addition, decongestants are sympathomimetic, and will have excitatory effects on the cardiovascular and central nervous systems. For this reason, patients with hypertension, depression, and endocrine disorders should not use the systemic decongestants without first discussing it with a physician. Adverse drug reactions associated with oral decongestants include palpitations, agitation, increased blood pressure, and anxiety. Examples of systemic agents are pseudoephedrine (PSE) and phenylephrine (PE). Table 8-11 identifies conditions for which patients should speak to a physician or pharmacist prior to taking oral decongestants.

Nasal Decongestants

Nasal decongestants directly constrict blood vessels in the nasal passages where they are applied. These agents work rapidly, providing quick relief.

Table 8-11 Restricted Use of Oral Decongestants

Anxiety	Hypertension
Cardiovascular disease	Hyperthyroidism
Coronary artery disease	Insomnia
Depression	Ischemic heart disease
Diabetes mellitus	Parkinson's disease
Glaucoma	Prostatic hypertrophy

vasoconstriction Constriction of blood vessels.

Table 8-12 Examples of Common Respiratory System Agents

Category	Brand Name	Active Ingredient	Dosage Form
Antihistamines	Benadryl	diphenhydramine	Caplet, capsule, liquid
	Claritin	loratadine	Tablet
	Tavist	clemastine	Liquid, tablet
Decongestants	Afrin	oxymetazoline	Nasal spray
	Neo-Synephrine	phenylephrine	Nasal spray
	Sudafed	pseudoephedrine	Liquid, tablet
Expectorants	Robitussin	guaifenesin	Liquid
Combination Products	Actifed	triprolidine, pseudoephedrine	Syrup, tablet
	Drixoral Cold & Flu	acetaminophen, pseudoephedrine, dexbrompheniramine	Tablet
	Motrin IB Sinus	ibuprofen, pseudoephedrine	Tablet
	Robitussin CF	dextromethorphan, guaifenesin, pseudoephedrine	Syrup
	Theraflu Maximum Strength Nighttime	acetaminophen, chlorpheniramine, dextromethorphan, pseudoephedrine	Powder packets
	Tylenol Multi-Symptom Cough	acetaminophen, dextromethorphan	Liquid

They are safer to use in patients with conditions like diabetes and hypertension as they do not exhibit the systemic effects associated with oral decongestants. Rebound nasal congestion is a risk associated with the persistent use of nasal decongestants.

Patients are advised to use these agents for no more than 3 to 4 days. Nasal decongestants are naphazoline, oxymetazoline, phenylephrine, and xylometazoline. Table 8-12 identifies examples of common respiratory system agents.

Caution

Read labels carefully. Patients taking combination cold, cough, and flu products containing acetaminophen should not ingest other products with acetaminophen and should limit their intake of alcohol.

Tech Check

16. What are the categories of cold, cough, and flu active ingredients?(LO 8.5)

17. Which type of agent is available as a nasal spray and as a systemically administered (liquid, tablet) dosage form?(LO 8.6)

Miscellaneous Agents

As there are numerous nonprescription agents that do not fit into any specific category, they are addressed as miscellaneous agents. The agents discussed in this area are agents for dietary supplements, home diagnostic kits, and smoking cessation and weight-loss products. Chapter 9 discusses dietary supplements, including vitamins, minerals, and herbal preparations.

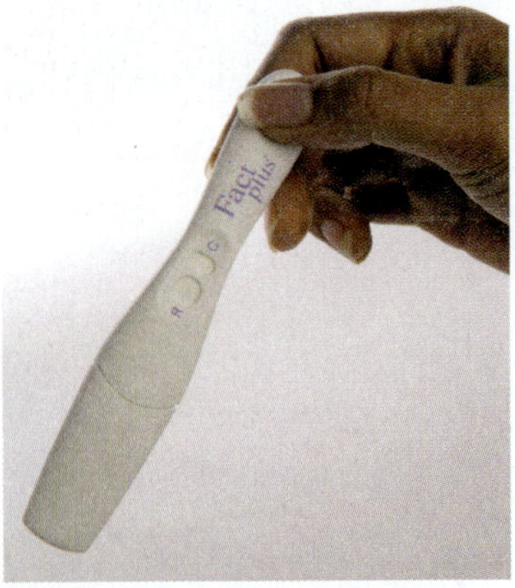

Figure 8-22 Pregnancy test.

Home diagnostic kits are not medications, but are instruments to be used by patients to determine whether or not a particular condition exists. The most common example of a home diagnostic kit is the pregnancy test (Figure 8-22). Available home diagnostic kits in addition to pregnancy tests include cholesterol, menopause, and ovulation. It is important for the pharmacy technician to be aware of these various tests to refer the patient to the appropriate area. The results of these tests are preliminary, and often require confirmation by the patient's physician prior to any action being taken.

Table 8-13 lists common home diagnostic kits with their uses.

Nonprescription smoking cessation agents are designed to provide nicotine to the patient in an effort to wean the individual from cigarettes. Nicotine is provided at a higher dose and is then tapered until the patient no longer needs the OTC product to refrain from smoking. These products contain nicotine incorporated into lozenges, gums, and patches. The individual must stop smoking while using these agents (Figure 8-23).

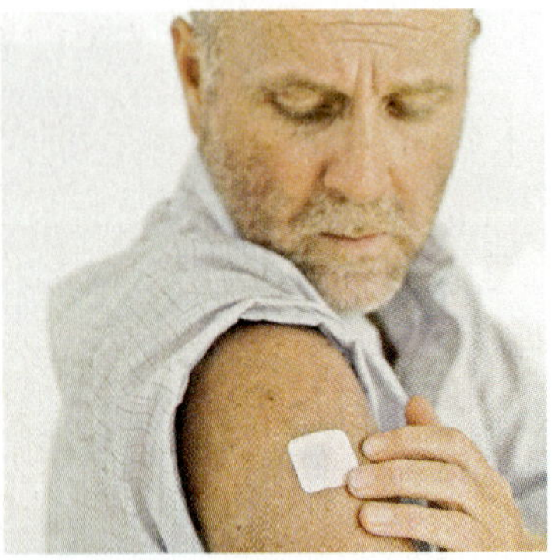

Figure 8-23 Nicotine patch.

Table 8-14 includes examples of smoking cessation agents.

The majority of products available without prescription for weight loss are dietary supplements. Agents are available in multiple forms (solutions, tablets, capsules) and often include multiple agents purported to enhance weight loss (Figure 8-24). Some of these agents are discussed in Chapter 9.

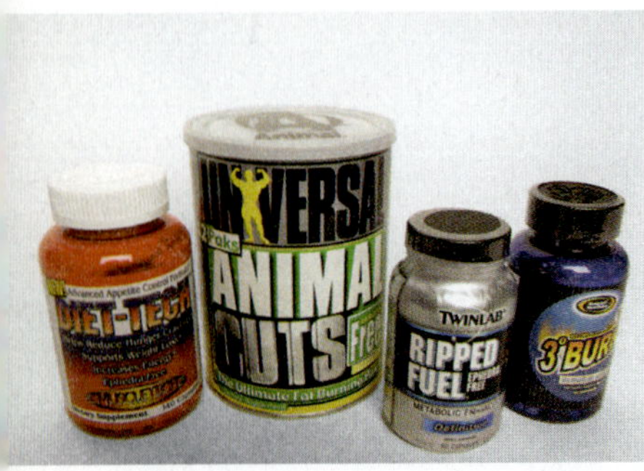

Figure 8-24 Assortment of fat burners and diet pills.

Individuals seeking nonprescription weight-loss agents should be encouraged to adopt a healthier lifestyle, including decreased caloric intake with increased physical exercise. The pharmacy technician should be aware of the potential for abuse of agents. Patients making frequent and/or large purchases of weight-loss agents should be noted and referred to the pharmacist for counseling.

Table 8-13 Types of Home Diagnostic Kits

Blood glucose
Cholesterol
Illicit drugs
Male infertility
Menopause
Ovulation
Pregnancy
Urinary ketones

Table 8-14 Smoking Cessation Agents

Commit lozenge
Nicorette gum
Nicoderm CQ transdermal patch

Chapter Summary

Understanding the basics of OTC agents in the workplace is vital to the pharmacy technician. It is important for the technician to understand the differences between the various categories of OTC medications. Other key points to remember are:

- OTC agents may be acquired without a prescription.
- The FDA governs the use of OTC agents.
- OTC agents undergo more rigorous testing than dietary supplements; however, interactions between the agents may prove harmful.
- Several types of diagnostic kits are available OTC, including tests for illicit drugs, pregnancy tests, ovulation, blood glucose, and cholesterol.

Chapter Review

Case Study Questions

1. What are the contraindications of taking cold medication along with medication for high blood pressure?(LO 8.5, 8.6)
2. How should Peggy handle this situation?(LO 8.2)

At Your Service Questions

1. What type or category of nonprescription medication is Mrs. Quincy requesting?(LO 8.5)
2. Why should she speak to the pharmacist prior to taking anything OTC for her allergies?(LO 8.6)
3. As a pharmacy technician, what do you tell this patient?(LO 8.2)

Multiple Choice

Select the best answer.

1. Which agency is responsible for determining the safety of OTC medications?(LO 8.2)
   a. Drug Enforcement Administration
   b. State Board of Pharmacy
   c. Food and Drug Administration
   d. Centers for Disease Control and Prevention
2. Which of the following patient groups does not need to exercise care when taking OTC preparations?(LO 8.1)
   a. Pediatric
   b. Pregnant
   c. Geriatric
   d. All of the above
3. Which of the following medications is an antifungal medication?(LO 8.6)
   a. Cortaid (hydrocortisone)
   b. Micatin (miconazole)
   c. Benadryl (diphenhydramine)
   d. Caldryl (calamine)
4. Which of the active ingredients is an antitussive agent?(LO 8.6)
   a. Guaifenesin
   b. Naphazoline
   c. Tetrahydrozoline
   d. Dextromethorphan
5. Which of the following has been associated with rebound nasal congestion?(LO 8.6)
   a. Antihistamine tablets
   b. Decongestant nasal sprays
   c. Decongestant nasal tablets
   d. Expectorant syrups
6. Which of the following is indicated for pediculosis?(LO 8.6)
   a. Nix
   b. Caladryl
   c. Cortaid
   d. None of the above

7. Which of the following active ingredients is an expectorant?(LO 8.6)
   a. Guaifenesin
   b. Naphazoline
   c. Tetrahydrozoline
   d. Dextromethorphan
8. Which agent would you take for acid indigestion?(LO 8.5, 8.6)
   a. Bayer (aspirin)
   b. Tylenol (acetaminophen)
   c. Zantac 75 (ranitidine)
   d. Zostrix (capsaicin)
9. OTC oral decongestants should be not be used without the advice of a physician or pharmacist for which conditions?(LO 8.6)
   a. Anxiety
   b. Hypertension
   c. Depression
   d. All of the above
10. Which of the following agents would you least likely use in your eye?(LO 8.5)
    a. Lubricant
    b. Decongestant
    c. Antihistamine
    d. Antibiotic
11. Which of the following is an agent for alopecia?(LO 8.6)
    a. Duofilm
    b. Rogaine
    c. Debrox
    d. Afrin
12. Which of the following agents is used for smoking cessation?(LO 8.6)
    a. Nicorette
    b. Selsun
    c. Tavist
    d. Sensodyne
13. Which of the following agents is an antihistamine?(LO 8.6)
    a. Acetaminophen
    b. Aspirin
    c. Diphenhydramine
    d. Dextromethorphan
14. Which of the following would soften the stool?(LO 8.6)
    a. Colace
    b. Ex-Lax
    c. Imodium
    d. Metamucil
15. Cellufresh is an OTC _____ agent.(LO 8.6)
    a. decongestant
    b. anti-infective
    c. ophthalmic
    d. otic

Critical Thinking Questions

1. Mrs. Taylor is 5 months pregnant and has a cold. She asks you, the pharmacy technician, what agent she could use for her stuffy nose. As the technician, you know the appropriate agents to use for a stuffy nose. What is the best response to Mrs. Taylor.?(LO 8.2, 8.5)
2. Michael is 4 years old and has been taking swimming lessons. His mother tells you he has been experiencing pain in his ears and has a fever. She wants to purchase an earwax removal product. What is your response?(LO 8.2, 8.5)

HIPAA SCENARIO

Sharon Carter and a coworker have been engaging in a mild flirtation at work. Without warning and with no explanation, Bob, Sharon's coworker, begins to avoid her. She asks him if anything is wrong, but he denies it. A few days later Sharon stops by her local pharmacy to refill her medications. She notices Bob leaning on the counter and talking to Joe, a pharmacy technician Sharon has known for a long time. Bob nods at Sharon but does not speak.

At work Sharon continues to ask Bob if something is wrong. Finally he blurts out that his friend Joe told him he saw Sharon purchasing an OTC pregnancy test. Furious, Sharon phones the pharmacy and informs Joe's supervisor of his actions. Joe is later terminated.

Discussion Questions(PTCB II. 73)

1. Should Joe have been terminated for his actions?
2. Is there any justification for Joe's actions?
3. What other courses of action could the supervisor have taken?

Internet Activities

1. Type the name of a common OTC agent into a search engine (MSN, Google, Yahoo). Choose five to seven links to examine in more detail. What type of information is provided about the agent? What are the sources of information? What factors contribute to the validity of the source of information? What factors detract from the credibility of the source? Be prepared to discuss your findings.(LO 8.3, 8.4, 8.5)
2. Go to your state board of pharmacy site. What restrictions exist in your state on the sale of products containing pseudoephedrine? What are the responsibilities of the pharmacy, pharmacist, and pharmacy technician as they relate to this issue?(LO 8.2)

9 Complementary and Alternative Modalities

Key Terms

adulteration
alternative medicine
Ayurvedic medicine
Chinese medicine
complementary medicine
contamination
dietary supplement
Dietary Supplement Health and Education Act (DSHEA) of 1994
integrative medicine
misidentification
proprietary blend
standardization

Learning Outcomes

After completing this chapter, you will be able to:

9.1 Define *complementary* and *alternative medicine*.

9.2 Define *integrative medicine*.

9.3 List and describe types of complementary and alternative medicine.

9.4 List herbs employed in complementary and alternative medicine.

9.5 List other agents employed in complementary and alternative medicine.

9.6 List labeling requirements for dietary supplements.

9.7 Describe the role of the Food and Drug Administration in the safety of dietary supplements.

PTCB

In preparation for the certification examination, you should understand and perform activities associated with the following PTCB Knowledge Statement:

PTCB Knowledge Statement

Domain I. Assisting the Pharmacist in Serving Patients

Knowledge of relative role of drug and nondrug therapy (e.g., herbal remedies, lifestyle modification, smoking cessation) (19)

Case Study

Mr. Johnson approaches the counter at a busy retail pharmacy. He indicates to Sue, the pharmacy technician on duty, that he is looking for herbs to decrease his cholesterol levels and blood pressure. Sue remembers that Mr. Johnson receives prescriptions for those conditions in the pharmacy. Although Sue does not know much about herbal preparations, she is aware that high cholesterol and high blood pressure are serious conditions.

While reading this chapter, keep the following questions in mind:

1. What appropriate action should Sue (as a pharmacy technician) take?(LO 9.1)
2. What constitutes inappropriate action on the part of Sue? What should she not do?(LO 9.1)
3. What should Sue tell Mr. Johnson?(LO 9.1)
4. Do you think Sue should know which dietary supplements Mr. Johnson is most likely looking for?(LO 9.4, 9.5)

Introduction to Complementary and Alternative Modalities(LO 9.1, 9.2, 9.3)

Complementary and alternative modalities encompass all treatment modalities and/or practices of medicine except for traditional Western or conventional medicine.

Complementary and alternative modalities include numerous practices including, but not limited to, **Ayurvedic medicine, Chinese medicine,** massage therapies, and use of **dietary supplements**.

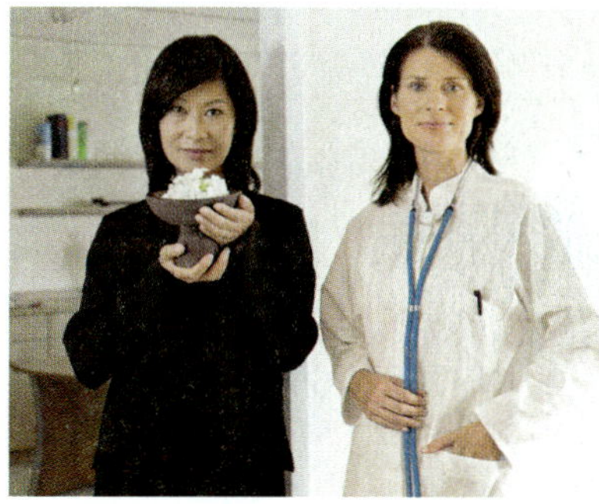

The use of complementary and alternative modalities is on the rise as patients are seeking agents to manage their health problems that are less expensive, have fewer side effects, and are more accessible than traditional medical interventions. **Integrative medicine** is a newer term that is a type of complementary medicine as it employs conventional and alternative methods that are supported by scientific evidence. It is appropriate for a pharmacy technician to ask a customer approaching the counter what other therapies he or she may be using at the time and if the customer would like to ask the pharmacist about the use of those therapies. This chapter highlights the types of complementary and alternative modalities most likely to be encountered by the pharmacy technician, which are primarily dietary supplements. Table 9-1 lists the various examples of complementary and alternative modalities.

Ayurvedic medicine An entire medical system originating in India that utilizes many therapies (yoga, meditation, massage, herbal preparations); also known as Ayurveda.

Table 9-1 Examples of Complementary and Alternative Modalities

Therapy	Description	
Acupressure	Pressure is applied by hand to various areas (channels) in the body to restore balance and health.	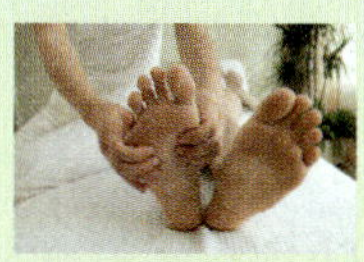
Acupuncture	Needles are inserted into various areas (channels) of the body to restore balance.	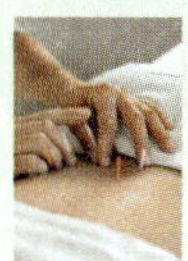

(Continued)

Table 9-1 Examples of Complementary and Alternative Modalities *(Continued)*

Therapy	Description	
Aromatherapy	Essential oils from flowers, herbs, and trees are inhaled to promote health and produce a sense of well-being.	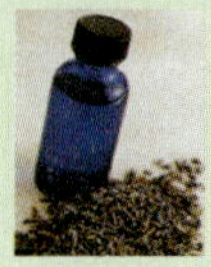
Ayurvedic medicine	Form of medicine originating in India that uses herbal preparations, dietary changes, exercises, and meditation to restore health and promote well-being.	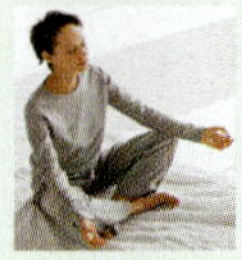
Chinese medicine	Ancient form of medicine originating in China involving herbal and animal source preparations, dietary changes, exercise, and massage as medical components to treat maladies.	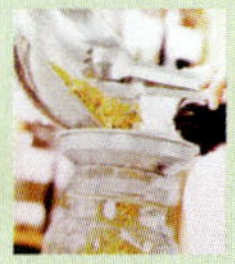
Chiropractic medicine	Adjustments of the spine are made to relieve pressure and/or pain.	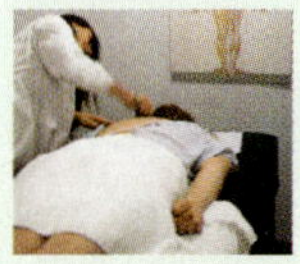
Colonic therapy	Form of therapy that employs the use of cathartics and enemas to cleanse the colon, to promote better health.	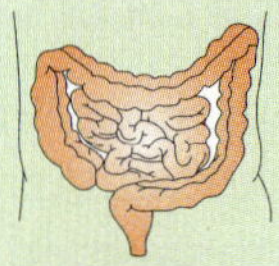
Crystal therapy	Crystals or gems are applied to certain parts of the body to promote healing.	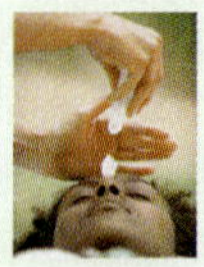
Dietary supplement therapy (herbals, vitamins, minerals)	Over-the-counter preparations are governed by the DSHEA of 1994.	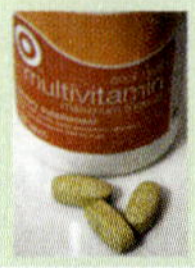
Folk medicine	Remedies based on cultural, ethnic, or racial backgrounds are used to prevent or treat minor illnesses. Usually passed on from generation to generation through word-of-mouth.	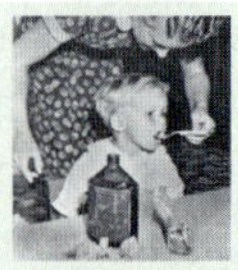
Home remedies (often referred to as folk or ethnic medicine)	May consist of plants, vitamins, or foods to manage a condition.	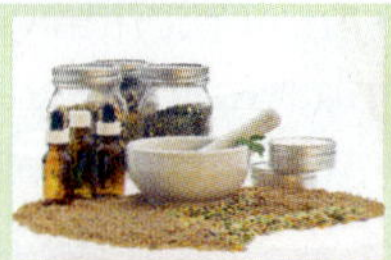
Homeopathy	Based on the principle that the toxin that causes a symptom may relieve that symptom if the toxin is diluted many times.	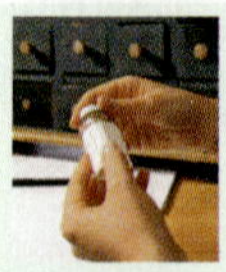
Iridology	Diagnostic tool employed by looking into the iris; the practitioner can determine the deficiencies or conditions responsible for causing illness.	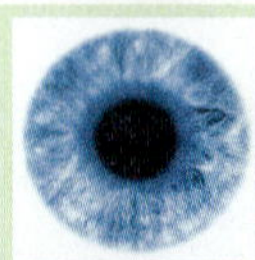
Massage therapy	Movement of parts of the body and human touch are used to alleviate pain, pressure, and promote healing (Rolfing, Shiatsu, Swedish).	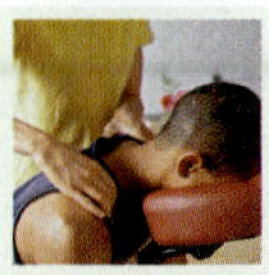

At Your Service

Ms. Kay purchases many over-the-counter (OTC) medications in the pharmacy. Recently, she has added gingko biloba, ginseng, and garlic to her list of frequent purchases. Today, you notice that she is purchasing large quantities of aspirin and ibuprofen with the three herbal products. Prior to ringing up her purchases, you mention to Ms. Kay that you suggest she speak with a pharmacist prior to taking all of these products. Ms. Kay gets upset and says that since herbal products are natural, they are safe.

While reading this chapter, keep the following questions in mind.

1. What potential problem could occur as a result of Ms. Kay taking all of the listed agents?(LO 9.4, 9.5)
2. How might you encourage Ms. Kay to speak with the pharmacist?(LO 9.7)
3. Would you process Ms. Kay's purchases without first having her speak with the pharmacist? Why or why not?(LO 9.2, 9.3)

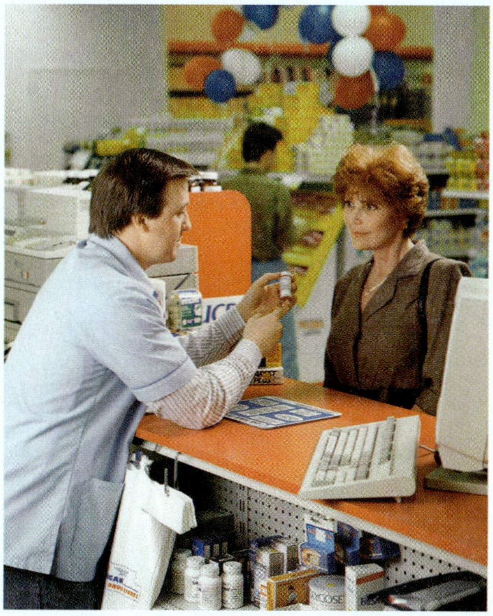

Significance of Complementary and Alternative Modalities(LO 9.1)

While the need for medical care and the cost of that care are consistently increasing, accessibility to care and resources to acquire care have not increased. In addition, many patients have expressed dissatisfaction with medical care as a result of experiencing side effects, prohibitive expense, or decrease in quality of life. As the population in the United States is diverse, it is important to bear in mind that there may be certain cultural beliefs that affect when or if a person seeks conventional medical care. **Complementary medicine** is any nontraditional medical treatment that is used in combination with conventional medicine. **Alternative medicine** is a type of nontraditional medical therapy that is used in place of, or as a substitute for conventional medical treatments. Complementary and alternative modalities may provide relief for some of these patients depending on the modality and the patients' condition. Patients need to know, however, that any treatment, whether traditional or complementary, has the potential to cause harm or risk to them. A natural substance can cause harm.

Complementary and Alternative Modalities(LO 9.1)

Complementary and alternative medicine modalities are not new therapies; for example, Chinese medicine has been used by practitioners for thousands of years. The recent rise in the use of these modalities

Chinese medicine Entire medical system that evolved over thousands of years in China and is based on the concept of balanced "qi" (pronounced "chee") or vital energy. Herbal therapies, diet, and massage are utilized to restore balance in the vital energy.

dietary supplement Any product intended for ingestion that is designed to supplement the diet, and contains at least one of the following agents: vitamin, mineral, herb or other botanical, amino acid, or dietary substance used to increase total daily intake of a constituent, metabolite, or extract.

integrative medicine The combination of components of Western (traditional) medicine with complementary and alternative medicine modalities with scientific evidence of efficacy.

complementary medicine Any nontraditional medical treatment that is used in combination with conventional medicine.

alternative medicine A type of nontraditional medical therapy that is used in place of, or as a substitute for, conventional medicine treatments.

has resulted in the need for pharmacists and pharmacy technicians to be educated regarding the use of these products. Dietary supplements constitute the majority of alternative therapies encountered by pharmacy technicians, including herbal preparations, vitamin and mineral therapies, and animal source products. Many of these products are sold in pharmacies and drug stores, and the pharmacy technician must be knowledgeable about these agents in order to assist the pharmacist in providing efficient and effective pharmaceutical care.

Tech Check

1. What are some reasons for the rise in the use of complementary and alternative medicine modalities?(LO 9.1)
2. List four types of complementary and alternative medicine modalities.(LO 9.1)

Dietary Supplements(LO 9.4, 9.5, 9.6, 9.7)

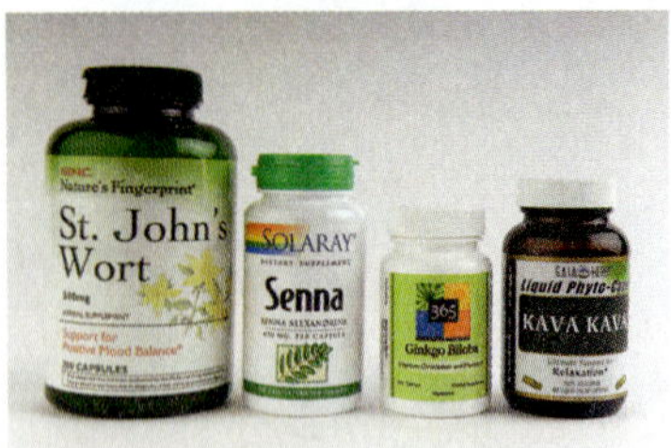

Figure 9-1 Examples of dietary herbal supplements.

A dietary supplement is defined by the Food and Drug Administration (FDA) as any product intended for ingestion and contains at least one of the following agents: vitamin, mineral, herb or other botanical, amino acid, or dietary substance used to increase total daily intake of a constituent, metabolite, or extract (Figure 9-1).

Dietary supplements include herbal preparations, vitamins, minerals, and other miscellaneous agents like shark cartilage and melatonin. The regulation of the dietary supplements is under the auspices of the **Dietary Supplement Health and Education Act (DSHEA) of 1994,** which identifies these agents as dietary supplements and not as drugs. This law also gives the FDA the authority to establish good manufacturing processes for dietary supplements. The FDA also has the responsibility to recall or withdraw a dietary supplement from the market in the event the agent proves to be unsafe. The sale of ephedrine alkaloids was banned by the FDA in 2004, for example. Because dietary supplements are not evaluated through the same process of rigorous clinical trials, as drugs are, no disease-specific claim (e.g., use for intermittent claudication) may be made regarding the product. Dietary supplements can only make structure-function claims (e.g., may enhance circulation) on the package. In addition, the specific labeling requirements of the dietary supplements are outlined below.

- Identification as a dietary supplement, with the word "supplement"
- Statement of identity of product
- Net quantity of contents (number of capsules or tablets)
- Structure-function claim of product with the following statement: "This statement has not been evaluated by the FDA. This product is not intended to diagnose, treat, cure or prevent any disease."
- Directions for use
- Supplement facts panel (including serving size, amount, and active ingredient)
- Other ingredients contained in the product
- Name and place of business of manufacturer, packer, or distributor of the product

Dietary Supplement Health and Education Act (DSHEA) of 1994 Legislation defining dietary supplements and outlining their regulation.

Dietary supplements are best used for chronic conditions that pose no immediate risk or threat to the patient. Supplements should not be used for life-threatening or potentially fatal diseases as their product claims have not been evaluated by the FDA. Patients considering the use of dietary supplements should communicate their intentions to their physicians and pharmacists. Special caution should be used if the patient considering the supplement is attempting to become pregnant, is pregnant, or is nursing. Likewise, the physician should be consulted prior to administration of a supplement to geriatric and pediatric patients. The pharmacy technician can serve as a valuable resource in facilitating open communication between patients and pharmacists. The technician's ability to recognize potential drug interactions and problems is critical in his or her role as a member of the health care team.

Critical Issues of Use

There are several critical issues regarding the use of dietary supplements, particularly herbal preparations. All herbal agents marketed in the United States are considered dietary supplements because they have not undergone the rigorous clinical trials necessary for an agent to be marketed as a drug. Those issues are standardization, adulteration, misidentification, improper preparation, drug interactions, and adverse drug reactions.

Standardization

Standardization means that every unit of a particular dosage form of a dietary supplement has the same content of the purported therapeutic ingredient. Variations in content of the purported therapeutic agent from the same manufacturer have been reported. Standardization is not the same as efficacy (which has to do with the ability of the agent to elicit an effect) or potency (which has to with the relative strength of a substance).

Adulteration

Adulteration refers to the lack of purity, or the lack of contaminants contained in a dietary supplement. Plants in particular may be contaminated with microorganisms, fungi, pesticides, byproducts, or radioactive materials. The FDA has the responsibility to enforce Good Manufacturing Practices (GMPs) to ensure the purity or lack of **contamination** of the product.

Misidentification

Misidentification refers to the discrepancy between the labeling and the contents of a particular preparation. Misidentification is the mislabeling a preparation as containing agents not included in the preparation. An example of misidentification or mislabeling would be to label a product as ginseng, while the contents are actually gingko biloba.

Improper Preparation

Improper preparation refers to the practice of processing plant material in such a manner that inadvertently affects the activity of the therapeutic ingredient. The use of various solvents, exposure to extreme temperatures or light, and age of the plant materials may affect the therapeutic and adverse drug effects of the product. Improper preparation may affect the efficacy, potency, and safety of the dietary supplement.

standardization The consistency of components of the active ingredient from batch to batch and from manufacturer to manufacturer.

adulteration The contamination of a substance with other agents.

contamination The presence of impurities, microorganisms, pesticides, or radioactive substances in a product.

misidentification Mislabeling a preparation as containing agents not included in the preparation.

Table 9-2 Examples of Common Dietary Supplement Drug Interactions

Dietary Supplement	Interacting Agent	Interaction
Garlic, gingko, ginger	Antiplatelet agents, anticoagulants	Increased risk of bleeding
St. John's Wort	Antidepressants	Increased blood pressure
Kava, valerian	Sedatives, benzodiazepines	Increased sedative effects
Ginseng	Decongestants, sympathomimetics	Increased nervousness, insomnia, agitation, palpitations

Drug Interaction

A drug interaction refers to the reaction that occurs as a result of the combination of a dietary supplement with a drug, which may be obtained by prescription or OTC. Use of dietary supplements accompanied with drugs may result in an alteration of drug activity, increased adverse drug reactions, and changes in elimination of the drugs from the body. Likewise, some drugs may affect the action of dietary supplements. The pharmacy technician should be able to recognize potential dietary supplement-drug interactions in order to alert the pharmacist of such a critical situation. The pharmacy technician is often the "front line" of communication in the pharmacy and is often the first member of the pharmacy staff to encounter patients as they approach the counter or make OTC purchases. Refer to Table 9-2 for examples of common dietary supplement drug interactions.

Adverse Effects

An adverse effect refers to a negative, non therapeutic effect associated with the use of a dietary supplement. Consumers often mistakenly believe that natural substances do not cause side effects. Another common misconception is that all natural products are safe to use. Proper patient education is necessary to minimize the incidence of the adverse effects of dietary supplements.

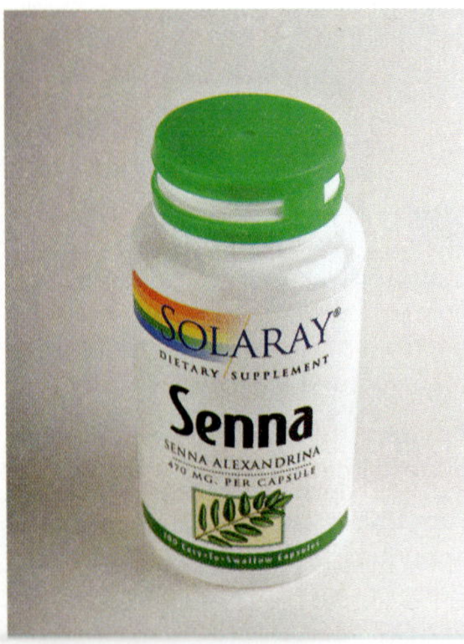

Figure 9-2 Herbal preparation.

Tech Check

3. State the legislation that governs the use of dietary supplements in the United States.(LO 9.7)
4. Define adulteration.(LO 9.7)
5. The reaction that occurs as a result of combining a dietary supplement with a drug is called ________.(LO 9.7)

Herbal Preparations

Herbal preparations are a type of dietary supplement, as are vitamins, minerals, amino acids, and other biologicals. On the OTC market, herbal preparations may be contained in a product as a single agent, or as a component of a **proprietary blend,** or mixture of several agents. Labels must be read carefully to determine the contents of a product. One must also remember that the listed weight or percentage of a particular herbal component does not guarantee the efficacy or safety of the product. Herbal preparations are available in many dosage forms (tinctures, tablets, capsules, creams, gels, elixirs) (Figure 9.2). The dosage form governs the route of administration.

Agents of herbal origin commonly used in the United States are outlined in Table 9-3 include the common name of the agent, the therapeutic claims or uses, adverse effects, and precautions/comments.

Refer to Table 9-3 for the most common herbal preparations and remedies employed in the United States.

proprietary blend Mixture of various herbal, vitamin, and mineral agents to form a component of a specific product.

Caution

Herbal preparations should not be used for acute and/or life-threatening illnesses. Consultation with a physician or pharmacist should precede use of herbal preparations in pregnant or nursing women, children, or elderly people.

Table 9-3 Common Herbal Preparations Used in the United States

Common Name	Use/Claim	Side Effect	Precaution/Comment
Aloe 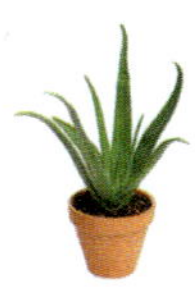	Aids in wound healing for skin infections, burns or psoriasis with topical application	Rash, burning sensation on skin	Ingestion contraindicated in children and pregnant women.
Black cohosh 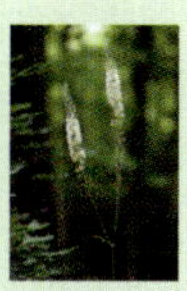	Manages symptoms of menopause, lowers cholesterol	Nausea, dizziness, increased perspiration, reduced pulse, visual disturbances, weight gain	Linked to hepatitis, contraindicated in pregnancy.
Bilberry (*not to be confused with blueberry*) 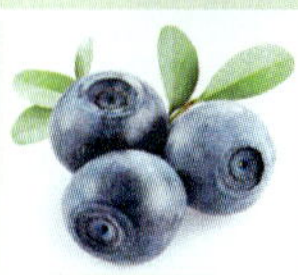	Relieves eye strain and complaints of the gastrointestinal tract	Diarrhea, anemia (high doses of leaves)	Avoid in pregnancy lactation, and children. Avoid in patients with anemia.
Capsicum peppers (Capsaicin)	Acts as irritant (self-defense sprays), exhibits analgesic activity (postsurgical neuralgia or shingles)	Burning sensation upon application to mucus membranes, may cause temporary blindness when sprayed into the eyes, ingestion may cause intense GI burning.	Avoid touching mucus membranes after topical application to avoid burning or stinging.
Chamomile 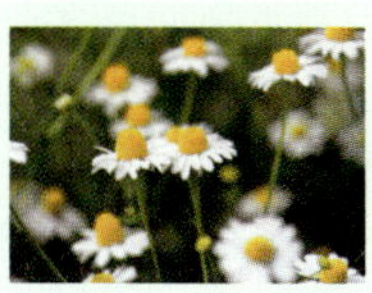	Exhibits anti-inflammatory, gastrointestinal antispasmodic, sedative, anti-allergy activity	Contact dermatitis, anaphylaxis, allergy	Emesis may occur when dried flowering heads are ingested in large quantities.

(Continued)

Table 9-3 Common Herbal Preparations Used in the United States *(Continued)*

Common Name	Use/Claim	Side Effect	Precaution/Comment
Chaste tree 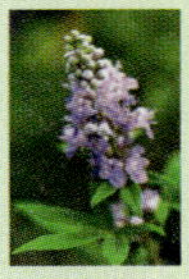	Balances hormones, regulates menstruation, increases lactation, relieves breast pain	Gastrointestinal reactions, itching, rash, headaches, increased menstrual flow	Contraindicated in pregnancy and children.
Echinacea 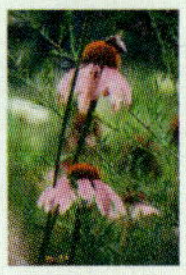	Aids in wound healing, stimulates immune function against viral infections (cold and flu)	Nausea, vomiting, unpleasant taste, abdominal pain, diarrhea, rash	Risk of allergy increased in individuals with allergies to daisy family (ragweed, chrysanthemum, marigold, and daisy).
Garlic 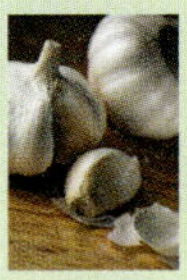	Lowers blood sugar and cholesterol levels, exhibits antiseptic and antibacterial activity	Strong odor, burning of mouth and esophagus, nausea, sweating, lightheadedness	Cautious use for patients taking anticoagulant and/or antiplatelet agents.
Ginger 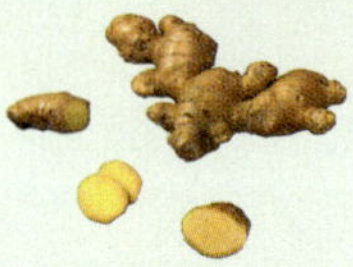	Decreases nausea and vomiting, decreases cholesterol, stimulates circulation, decreases cough, used as flavoring; fungicide, pesticide	High doses may cause drowsiness, and decreased platelet aggregation	Cautious use for patients taking anticoagulant and/or antiplatelet agents.
Gingko 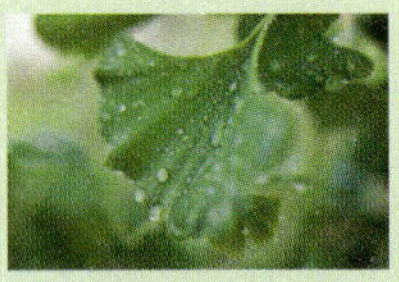	Increases circulation, improves memory, relieves anxiety or stress, alleviates tinnitus, improves symptoms of asthma	Headache, dizziness, palpitations, rash, allergy, nausea, vomiting	Avoid in pregnancy and lactation. May increase bleeding. Seeds contain toxin associated with seizures and death.
Ginseng 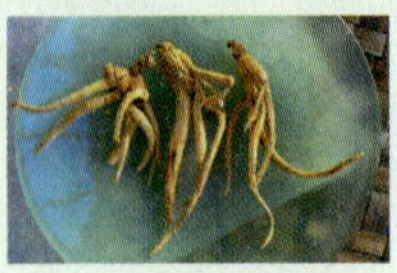	Increases mental and physical capacity for work, relieves fatigue, enhances immune system	Nervousness, agitation, breast nodules, vaginal bleeding, hypoglycemia	Interacts with anticoagulants, loop diuretics, and antipsychotic drugs.
Goldenseal 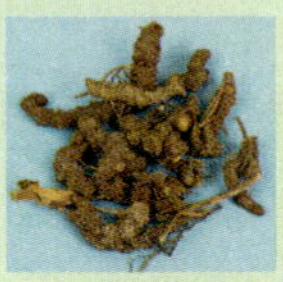	Aids in wound healing, used as an eyewash, improves immune functions against viral infections, such as cold and flu	High doses produce nausea, anxiety, depression, seizures, or paralysis	Contraindicated in pregnancy, lactation, and patients with hypertension.
Green tea 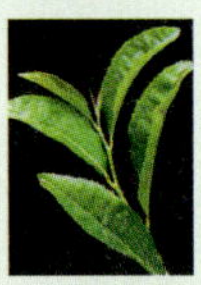	Lowers cholesterol levels, may decrease risk of cancer (antioxidative and antimutagenic effects), prevents cavities	Agitation, nervousness, insomnia, allergic reactions	Use may impair iron metabolism. Avoid use in individuals sensitive to caffeine.
Kava 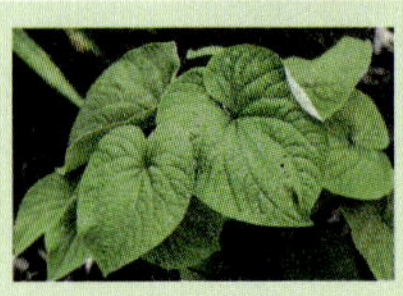	Relieves symptoms associated with stress, exhibits sedative activity	Skin rash, visual disturbances, risk of dependence	Contraindicated in pregnancy, lactation, and patients who have depression. May interact with other sedatives. Not to be used while driving or operating heavy machinery.
Milk thistle 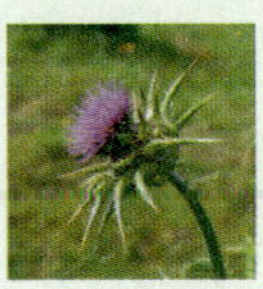	Provides liver protectant effects, manages cirrhosis of the liver, lowers cholesterol	Allergic reactions, stomach upset, nausea, diarrhea	Allergic reactions are more common in individuals who have allergies to plants in the same family (marigold, chrysanthemum, daisy, and ragweed).

(Continued)

Table 9-3 Common Herbal Preparations Used in the United States *(Continued)*

Common Name	Use/Claim	Side Effect	Precaution/Comment
Passion flower	Exhibits sedative activity, reduces symptoms of stress	Drowsiness	May interact with anticoagulants and monoamine oxidase (MAO) inhibitor therapy. Increases the effects of other sedatives; avoid concomitant therapy. Contraindicated in pregnancy as it stimulates uterine contractions.
Saw palmetto 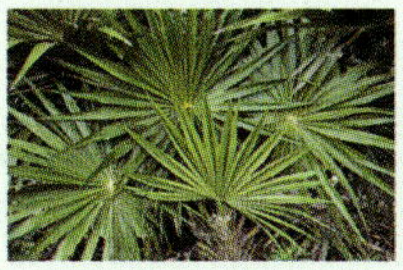	Relieves symptoms of benign prostatic hypertrophy	Nausea	Contraindicated in pregnancy. May interfere with metabolism of hormones.
Senna	Used as a laxative	Cramping, loose stools, electrolyte imbalance, allergic reactions Chronic use has caused discoloration of the colon, reversible finger clubbing, cachexia, laxative dependence	Avoid chronic use.
St. John's wort 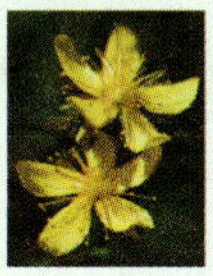	May enhance mood, may have inhibitory effects on viruses	Dry mouth, dizziness, constipation, photosensitivity, confusion, insomnia, nervousness	Products vary in content due to poor standardization of hypericin and hyperforin components. May induce hepatic enzymes. Avoid use with tricyclic antidepressants, selective serotonin reuptake inhibitors (SSRIs), and monoamine oxidase (MAO) inhibitors.
Tea tree oil	May have an inhibitory effect on bacteria	Allergy, eczema, rash	Not for ingestion. Topical application only.
Valerian 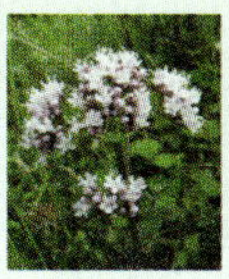 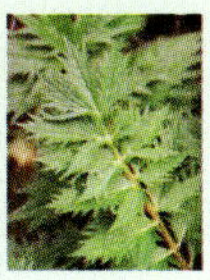	Exhibits sedative activity, used as a flavoring	Drowsiness	Avoid use with other sedative-hypnotics agents.
Wild yam	May help regulate the menstrual cycle, may reduce nausea, may relieve symptoms of urinary tract disorders, rheumatoid arthritis, gas	Nausea, vomiting, diarrhea	No information available.
Witch hazel	Relieves symptoms of hemorrhoids and skin inflammations, may treat damaged veins, stops bleeding from hemorrhoids	Allergy	Avoid internal use, which may cause nausea, vomiting, constipation, impactions, and liver damage.

Source: Guide to Popular Natural Products, 2nd ed. St. Louis, MO: Facts and Comparisons, 2001; **www.rxlist.com** (bilberry); **www.nccam.nih.gov.**

Many herbal preparations may cause risks that outweigh the benefits of their use. Some of these preparations, on the other hand, may exhibit only substantial risk to patients exposed to high doses or long-term use. The National Center for Complementary and Alternative Medicine (**www.nccam.nih.gov**) is a federal agency that provides scientific evidence regarding the use of herbal preparations. Some potentially dangerous herbal preparations when taken alone or in combination with certain medications include:

- Borage
- Chaparral
- Ephedra (Ma huang)
- Licorice root
- St. John's Wort

Keep in mind that herbal supplements may contain other compounds that are also dangerous alone or in combination with medications.

Caution

Natural does not always mean safe.

Tech Check

6. List three herbal dietary supplements that appear to exhibit sedative activity.(LO 9.4)

7. List three agents that may be contained in products used to manage symptoms associated with menopause.(LO 9.4)

8. List three potentially dangerous herbal remedies.(LO 9.4)

Vitamins

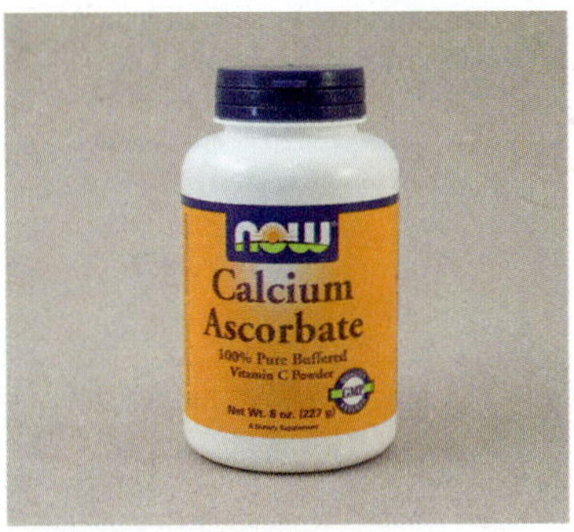

Figure 9-3 Vitamins.

Dietary supplements include vitamins, minerals, and other nonherbal dietary supplements as well as herbal agents previously outlined. The remainder of this chapter focuses on these other types of dietary supplements.

Vitamins are natural substrates found in the body and are essential for proper cellular function (Figure 9-3). The United States Recommended Dietary Allowance (RDA) is the suggested amount of a vitamin to be taken daily in order to meet the nutritional requirements of the body. Vitamins are categorized as dietary supplements, and are generally safe when administered within the limits of the RDA. High doses of vitamins may be dangerous, particularly the fat-soluble vitamins (vitamins A, D, E, and K).

Table 9-4 outlines commonly used vitamins.

Minerals(LO 9.5)

Minerals are elements found in nature, and are generally obtained from food that is consumed. Keeping in mind that the RDA represents the recommended amounts of minerals, there is no evidence to support that

Table 9-4 Vitamins and Their Functions

Agent	Function
Vitamin A	Necessary for maintenance of vision and cellular growth
Vitamin B_1	Necessary for nervous system and muscle function, carbohydrate metabolism
Niacin	Necessary for cholesterol metabolism
Vitamin C	Necessary for collagen formation, aids in absorption of iron
Vitamin B_{12}	Necessary for the maintenance of health nerve cells and red blood cells
Vitamin B_6	Necessary for the formation of neurotransmitters
Vitamin D	Necessary to maintain normal blood vessels, aids in the absorption of calcium
Vitamin E	Necessary for cellular development, antioxidant properties
Folic acid	Necessary for red blood cell development and function, prevents neural tube defects
Vitamin K	Necessary for formation of blood clotting factors

massive doses of minerals will increase one's health. Massive dosages of these mineral agents may actually have negative effects on the health of individuals who consume such large quantities.

Minerals with recommended daily allowances include (Figure 9-4):

- Calcium
- Fluoride
- Iodine
- Iron
- Magnesium
- Phosphorus
- Selenium
- Zinc

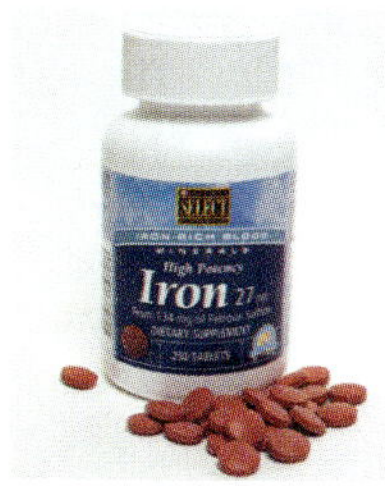

Figure 9-4 Minerals.

Nonherbal Dietary Supplements

Agents previously discussed in this chapter include the following types of dietary supplements, herbal preparations, vitamins, and minerals. There is another type of dietary supplement that does not belong in any of the previously mentioned categories: amino acids, animal or plant source products. For example, although soy is isolated from the soybean plant, it is not considered an herbal preparation. Table 9-5 (p. 262) lists some commonly used nonherbal dietary supplements.

Tech Check

9. Define *vitamin.*(LO 9.5)

10. List three nonherbal dietary supplements.(LO 9.5)

Table 9-5 Common Nonherbal Dietary Supplements

Agent	Claims
Arginine	Stimulates wound healing, reduces risk of heart disease
Beta carotene	Antioxidant, may reduce risk of cancer
Chondroitin sulfate	Improves symptoms of osteoarthritis
Creatine	Enhances physical performance, builds lean body mass
Dehydroepiandrosterone (DHEA)	Slows process of aging, improves immune function
Glucosamine	Relieves pain associated with osteoarthritis
Lactobacillus	Acts as "probiotic" agent
Melatonin	Relieves jet lag, induces sleep
Omega-3 fatty acids	Reduces triglycerides, reduces risk of heart disease
Shark cartilage	Reduces risk of cancer
Soy	Helps manage symptoms of menopause
Spirulina	Antioxidant, source of beta carotene
Ubiquinone (Coenzyme Q10)	Protective effects on the heart

Source: NIH Office of Dietary Supplements, **http://ods.od.nih.gov.**

Chapter Summary

Understanding the complementary and alternative modalities in the workplace is vital to the pharmacy technician. Important points to know are:

- Complementary and alternative medicine modalities include all methods of medical management except traditional or Western medicine.
- Integrative medicine refers to the incorporation of components of traditional and nontraditional treatment modalities tailored to the needs of the patient.
- Types of complementary and alternative medicine modalities include, but are not limited to, acupuncture, acupressure, massage therapy, and dietary supplement therapy.
- Herbal preparations that are employed in complementary/alternative medicine are numerous. Proper use of the herbal preparations depends on understanding that they are not evaluated or categorized as drugs, and therefore cannot be held to the same standards.
- Dietary supplements include vitamins, minerals, amino acids, and herbal preparations. The FDA has outlined specific requirements for the labeling of dietary supplements. Among other things, the label cannot include disease-specific claims.
- The FDA is responsible for ensuring the safety of dietary supplements. The FDA has the responsibility to withdraw or recall a dietary supplement if it is unsafe.

Chapter Review

Case Study Questions

1. What appropriate action should Sue (pharmacy technician) take?(LO 9.1)
2. What constitutes inappropriate action on the part of Sue? What should she *not* do?(LO 9.1)
3. What should Sue tell Mr. Johnson?(LO 9.1)
4. Do you think Sue should know which dietary supplements exhibit some of the effects Mr. Johnson is seeking?(LO 9.4, 9.5)

At Your Service Questions

1. What potential problem could occur as a result of Ms. Kay taking all of the listed agents?(LO 9.4, 9.5)
2. How might you encourage Ms. Kay to speak with the pharmacist?(LO 9.7)
3. Would you process Ms. Kay's purchases without first having her speak with the pharmacist? Why or why not?(LO 9.2, 9.3)

Multiple Choice

Select the best answer.

1. Which legislation is responsible for the regulation of dietary supplements?(LO 9.7)
   a. OBRA
   b. HIPAA
   c. DSHEA
   d. FDA
2. Purity or adulteration is most closely related to ________(LO 9.7)
   a. standardization.
   b. contamination.
   c. integration.
   d. legislation.
3. Which of the following statements regarding complementary and alternative modalities is true?(LO 9.1)
   a. Integrative medicine is the same as complementary and alternative medicine modalities.
   b. Complementary and alternative therapies have just recently come into existence.
   c. Prescription drugs constitute a form of complementary and alternative medicine modalities.
   d. Homeopathy is a form of complementary and alternative modalities.
4. Which of the following is a form of massage therapy?(LO 9.3)
   a. Acupuncture
   b. Rolfing
   c. Iridology
   d. Aroma therapy
5. Which of the following is a component of the labeling requirements for dietary supplements?(LO 9.6)
   a. Statement of purity
   b. Quality of contents
   c. Date of processing
   d. Statement of product identity
6. Which of the following is a critical aspect of dietary supplement use?(LO 9.7)
   a. Integration
   b. Contamination
   c. Classification
   d. Standardization
7. Which of the following dietary supplements is associated with increasing the effects of sedative drugs?(LO 9.4)
   a. Valerian
   b. Gingko
   c. Ginseng
   d. Ephedra
8. Which of the following preparations may be employed to relieve symptoms of benign prostatic hypertrophy?(LO 9.4)
   a. Bilberry
   b. Ginger
   c. Saw palmetto
   d. Rosemary

9. Which of the following agents should be avoided in patients on anticoagulant or antiplatelet therapy?(LO 9.4)
   a. Gingko biloba
   b. Saw palmetto
   c. Ma huang
   d. Black walnut

10. Which of the following vitamins plays a role in blood coagulation?(LO 9.5)
    a. Vitamin A
    b. Vitamin B_6
    c. Vitamin D
    d. Vitamin K

Critical Thinking Questions

1. Why is it necessary for the pharmacy technician to understand the laws, use, and adverse reactions of dietary supplements since the technician does not counsel patients?(LO 9.1, 9.3, 9.6, 9.7)
2. What types of information can the pharmacy technician provide to patients regarding dietary supplements?(LO 9.1, 9.3)
3. Visit a local pharmacy. Choose a product that has been advertised and contains its own proprietary blend. Identify each agent in the proprietary blend and list the potential use for each agent. Also identify situations in which an individual should not take this agent. Present your product and its ingredients in class.(LO 9.4)

HIPAA Scenario

Mr. Kono, a registered pharmacist, compiles a list monthly of patients who are using specific drugs. This list includes complementary and alternative medications such as kava and valerian. Both of these medications are used to relieve symptoms of stress. These alternative medications are contraindicated during pregnancy or when taking other sedatives.

The purpose of the list is to provide the chief of pharmacy with important supply cost data. When Mr. Kono attempted to send the list to his supervisor for editing, he accidentally e-mailed a copy of the March list out to everyone in the pharmacy. A coworker who received the list was angry when he realized his name was on the list for purchasing kava. He demands that Mr. Kono be disciplined.

Discussion Questions(PTCB II. 73)

1. What actions should be taken against Mr. Kono for releasing the medication information data to everyone in the pharmacy?
2. What actions should Mr. Kono and his supervisor take to resolve the situation?

Internet Activities

1. Access **http://dietary-supplements.info.nih.gov/Health_Information/Health_Information.aspx.** Click on Dietary Supplement Fact Sheets. Choose one fact sheet on a dietary supplement. Then go to **www.cfsan.fda.gov/~dms/ds-warn.html.** Scroll down to find information on the dietary supplement you chose from the first Web site. Compare information from the two sites and present your findings to the class.(LO 9.4, 9.5)
2. Go to **www.mayoclinic.com.** Click on Drugs and Supplements. Choose a vitamin or mineral and print out the information sheet. Present your chosen supplement to the class. Indicate whether you would consider taking this supplement. Explain why or why not.(LO 9.4, 9.5)

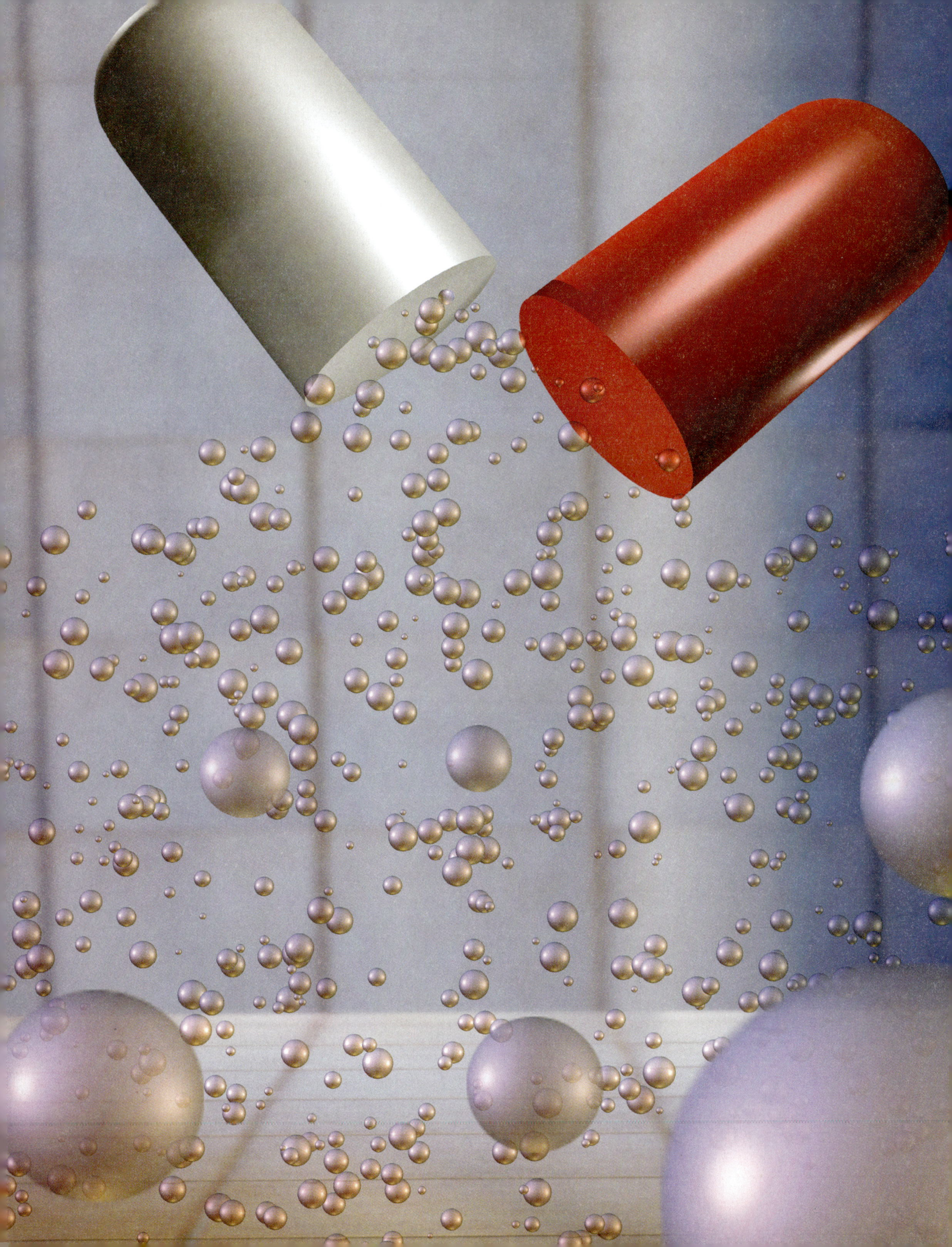

Medication Management and Preparation

Unit 3

Chapter 10 Dosage Forms and Routes of Administration

Chapter 11 Extemporaneous and Sterile Compounding (IV Admixtures)

Chapter 12 Medication Errors

Chapter 13 Referencing

10 Dosage Forms and Routes of Administration

Learning Outcomes

Upon completion of this chapter, you will be able to:

10.1 Differentiate between the various routes of administration used in the practice of pharmacy.

10.2 Compare and contrast the various dosage forms used in pharmacy practice.

10.3 Explain the advantages and disadvantages of a particular dosage form.

10.4 Explain why a particular dosage form of a specific medication would be preferred over a different dosage form of the same medication.

10.5 Identify examples of each dosage form.

10.6 Identify abbreviations associated with the various routes of administration and dosage forms.

PTCB

In preparation for the certification examination, you should understand and perform activities associated with the following PTCB Knowledge Statements:

PTCB Knowledge Statement

Domain I. Assisting the Pharmacist in Serving Patients

Knowledge of pharmaceutical and medical abbreviations and terminology (4)

Knowledge of special directions and precautions for patient/ patient's representative regarding preparation and use of medications (39)

PTCB Knowledge Statement

Domain II. Maintaining Medication and Inventory Control Systems

Knowledge of dosage forms (4)

Key Terms

aerosol
buccal
capsule
cream
douche
dosage forms
emulsion
enema
elixir
excipients
gel
inhalant
intradermal
intramuscular
intravenous
isotonicity
ointment
ophthalmic
oral
otic
parenteral
pastille
pulmonary
pyrogen
rectal
routes of administration
solution
subcutaneous
sublingual
suppository
surfactant

Case Study

A woman asked her husband to stop at the drugstore and bring home some Tylenol. The man became extremely perplexed when looking over the vast selection of Tylenol products at the pharmacy. Did she mean elixir, syrup, suspension, infant drops, tablet, caplet, gel tab, or gel cap? The husband went to the pharmacy counter and asked Andrew, the pharmacy technician, what was the difference between all of these dosage forms.

While reading this chapter, keep the following question in mind:

1. If you were Andrew, what would you tell him? (LO 10.2)

Key Terms

suspension
syrup
tablet
tincture
transdermal
troche
urethral
vaginal

Introduction to Dosage Forms and Routes of Administration (LO 10.1, 10.2)

Pharmacists and pharmacy technicians in the United States process thousands of prescriptions for their customers every day. These prescriptions contain information regarding the dosage form of the medication and its route of administration. A patient's physical and mental condition and the disease state being treated will have an impact on the route of administration and the dosage form selected. This chapter examines the relationship between dosage forms and their route of administration.

At Your Service

A woman and her daughter approach the pharmacy counter with a container of hydrocortisone cream 1% and a container of hydrocortisone ointment 1% for a rash that has appeared on her daughter's arm. The customer knows that both forms of hydrocortisone are the same strength, but she is uncertain which form will work quicker and what the difference is between the two products. The woman informs you that she and her daughter are going to a wedding, and she wants something that will not show on her daughter's skin. You tell the woman that you will inform the pharmacist of her question about the two products.

While reading this chapter think about the following question.

1. Which one of these two products would the pharmacist tell you to recommend? (LO 10.2, 10.3)

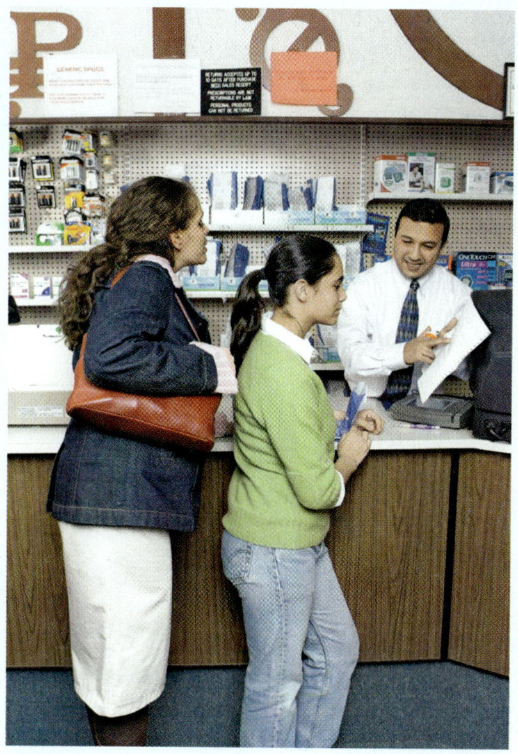

Routes of Administration(LO 10.1)

The route of administration refers to the way a drug is introduced into the body. There are several factors affecting the route of administration of a drug. Is the drug being used for a local or systemic effect? A local effect is one where the drug is applied directly to the site of action; a systemic effect is one where the drug goes through the circulatory system and reaches its site of action. The ease of administration will affect the choice for route of administration (Figure 10-1).

Table 10-1 identifies some of the more common routes of administration and the sites of administration.

A particular medication may be administered using more than one route. The route of administration selected may affect the absorption, distribution, metabolism, and elimination of a drug, as discussed in Chapter 6. It will also affect the onset of action and duration of action.

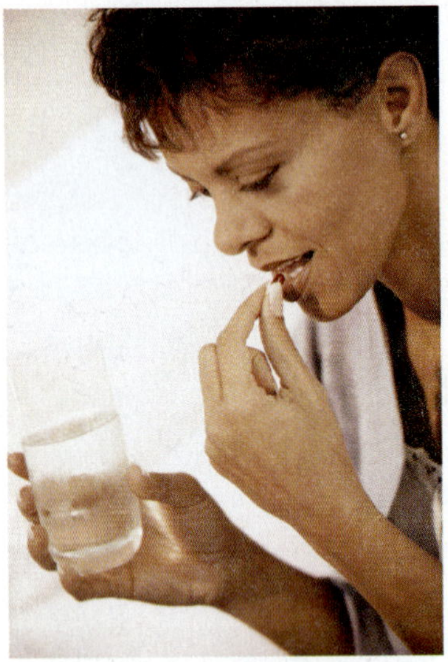

Figure 10-1 **Oral route of administration.**

Oral Administration

The **oral** route of administration is the most convenient route. An oral dosage form is taken by mouth and/or swallowed and the dosage form follows the digestive tract to where it is absorbed in the body. Oral medications do not require any special patient skills.

Table 10-1 Routes of Drug Administration

Route of Administration	Site of Administration
Buccal	Placed between the cheek and gum
Intra-arterial	Injected or infused into an artery
Intradermal	Injected under the skin
Intramuscular	Injected into a muscle
Intraspinal (intrathecal)	Injected or infused into the spine
Intravenous	Injected or infused into a vein
Ophthalmic	Instilled into the eye
Oral	Taken by mouth/swallowed
Otic	Instilled into the ear
Pulmonary	Inhaled into the lungs
Rectal	Inserted into the rectum
Subcutaneous	Injected under the skin
Sublingual	Placed under the tongue
Transdermal	On the skin surface
Urethral	Instilled into the urethra
Vaginal	Inserted into the vagina

oral Most convenient route of medication administration, taken by mouth and /or swallowed.

Examples of oral medications include:

- Tablets
- Capsules
- Solutions
- Syrups
- Elixirs
- Suspensions
- Powders

However, there are disadvantages of oral medications. They have a slower response rate compared to **parenteral** medications, which are medications that are administered by a route that bypasses the digestive system. Examples of parenteral mediations are injections, drops, creams, and patches. Oral medications may have an irregular absorption into the body due to the presence or absence of food in the gastrointestinal tract. The acidic content of the digestive tract may inactivate the medication. In some situations, the oral route may fail to yield a large enough concentration in the body to provide a therapeutic effect. Unfortunately, the oral route of administration cannot be used on patients awaiting anesthesia or in a coma state.

Sublingual Administration

Sublingual tablets are placed under the tongue because of the large blood supply found in the tongue. A medication administered sublingually results in a rapid therapeutic response. A sublingual medication bypasses the digestive system and the first-pass effect. Select medications may be administered sublingually. An example of a sublingual tablet is Nitrostat, which is used for the immediate relief of angina (chest pain) symptoms (Figure 10-2).

Buccal Administration

Buccal medications are placed between the gum and the cheek in the mouth. These medications are rapidly absorbed into the body due to the vascular nature of the mouth. An example of a buccal medication is Mycelex Troche, which is used to treat fungal infections of the mouth and throat (Figure 10-3).

parenteral A drug administered that bypasses the digestive system. Examples of parenteral mediations are injections, drops, creams, and patches.

sublingual Placed under the tongue.

buccal Medication placed between the cheek and gum

Figure 10-2 *(a)* **Nitrostat.** *(b)* **Sublingual tablets should be placed only under the tongue.**

(a) (b)

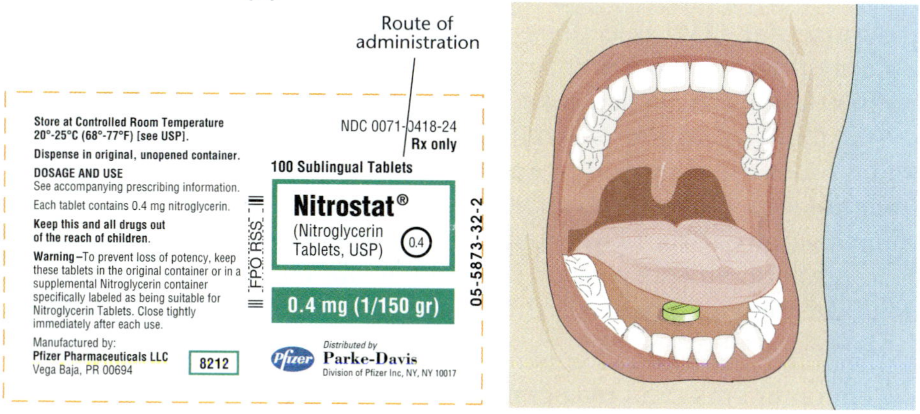

Figure 10-3 **Place a buccal drug between the cheek and gum tissue.**

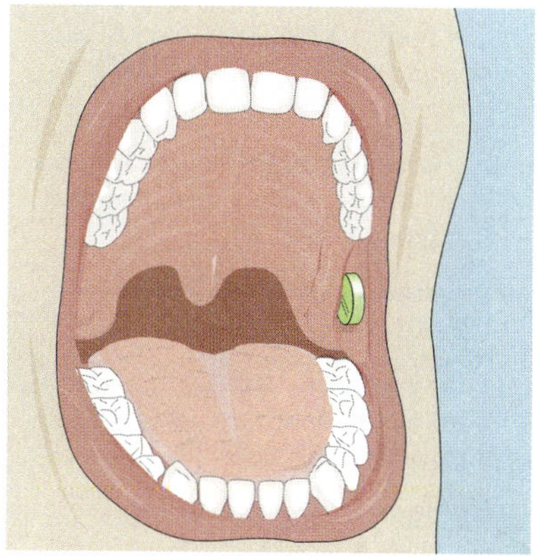

Rectal Administration

Rectal medications are administrated by insertion into the rectum of the body by way of the anus. In many situations, rectal medications are used for their local effect such as in the case of laxatives and the relief of hemorrhoids. However, they may be used for their systemic effect in the treatment of nausea and vomiting in patients who are unable to take oral medications.

Rectal medications include solutions, ointments, and suppositories. Examples of rectal medications include Phenergan suppositories, Cort enemas, and Anusol HC ointment.

Many patients find rectal products inconvenient to use compared to oral medications. Rectal medications have a very irregular and unpredictable rate of absorption into the body. They may be expelled from the rectal cavity.

Injectable Administration

Injectable dosage forms are intended to be injected into the body instead of traveling through the digestive tract like oral medications. This route of administration requires the use of a syringe and needle or an intravenous catheter. Medications may be injected into a blood vessel, different areas of skin tissue, or muscle. Injected medications have a rapid absorption rate compared to oral medications and obtain a therapeutic response sooner.

Some medications have to be injected because they are either destroyed or inactivated in the gastrointestinal tract. This route of administration may be required for patients who are uncooperative, unconscious, or unable to take oral medications. Examples of routes requiring an injection include (Figure 10-4):

- **Intravenous (IV)** injections involve aqueous solutions being injected directly into the patient's vein. These medications include both small- and large-volume injections. Intravenous injections are used in total parenteral nutrition (TPN). Examples of medications available as an IV include Valium and Tenormin.
- **Intradermal (ID)** injections are administered between the upper layers of the skin. The dose is approximately 0.1 mL. Unlike IVs, ID injections are injected into the arm and back. These are usually used for diagnostic purposes, like allergy testing or tuberculin testing. An example is Aplisol.
- **Intramuscular (IM)** injections are injected into the skeletal muscles, primarily the gluteal or lumbar muscles. IM injections may be aqueous or oily solutions or suspensions. A primary concern of IM injections is the possibility of hitting a nerve or a blood vessel. Examples include Bicillin LA and Coly-Mycin M Parenteral.
- **Subcutaneous (sub-Q)** injections are those that are injected into subcutaneous (fatty tissue) layer under the skin. These injections are either aqueous solutions or suspensions. Subcutaneous medications are injected into the abdomen, upper arm, thigh, or buttocks. Insulin is an example.

All injectable medications must meet standards for sterility, particulate matter, contaminants , and **pyrogens**, which are fever-producing substances produced by microorganisms.

rectal Inserted into the rectum of the body by way of the anus.

intravenous (IV) Aqueous solutions injected directly into the patient's vein.

intradermal (ID) Injection administered between the upper layers of the skin.

intramuscular (IM) Injection into the skeletal muscles.

subcutaneous (sub-Q) Injection administered into the fatty tissue layer under the skin.

pyrogen A fever-producing substance produced by microorganisms.

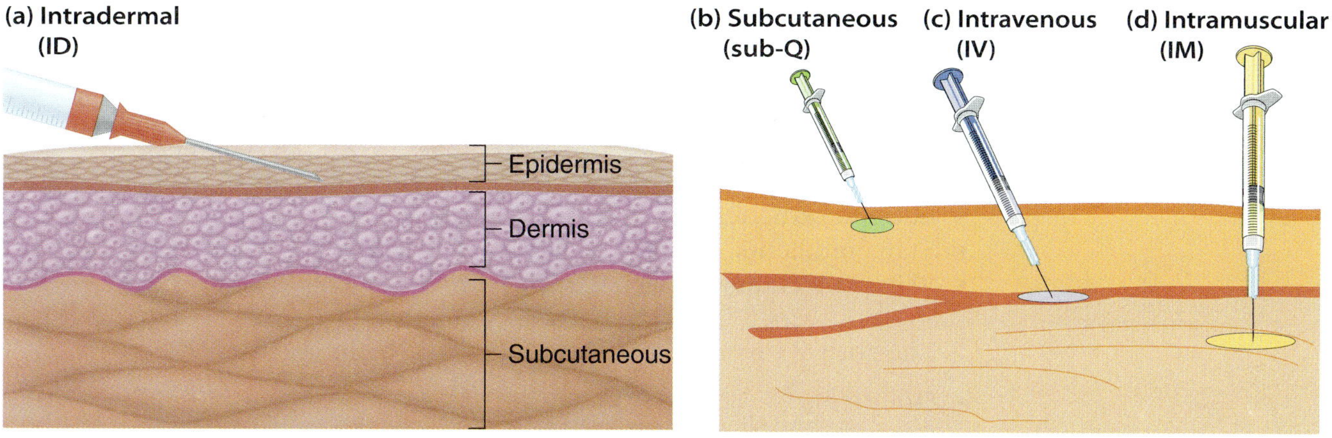

Figure 10-4 Injection needles are placed into separate areas under the skin: (*a*) intradermal: ID, (*b*) subcutaneous: sub-Q, (*c*) intravenous: IV, and (*d*) intramuscular: IM.

The primary disadvantage of parenteral medications is that once it is administered, it is extremely difficult to reverse its action. Injectable medications are more expensive than oral medications due to the costs associated with sterile manufacturing. A parenteral medication may be given by more than one route of administration (Figure 10-5).

Pulmonary Inhalation

Pulmonary agents are inhaled into the lungs (Figure 10-6). The lungs may be used as a route for administration for medications available in the form of a gas or an aerosol. Inhalation products may be administered either orally or by the nose for either their local or systemic effects. Important considerations for inhalation medications include the size of the particle and that consistent penetration occurs within the lungs. General anesthetics are often used in inhalation therapies.

Topical Administration

Topical preparations are used for their local effect because of their prolonged contact with the skin, but they also may be used for their

pulmonary Inhaled into the lungs.

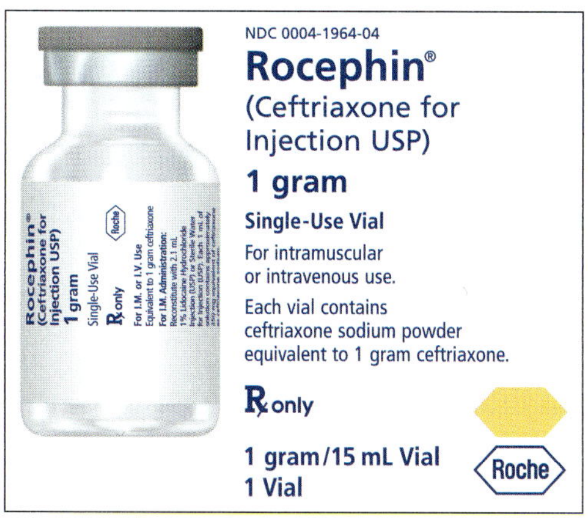

Figure 10-5 Unit dose package of Rocephin for IV or IM administration.

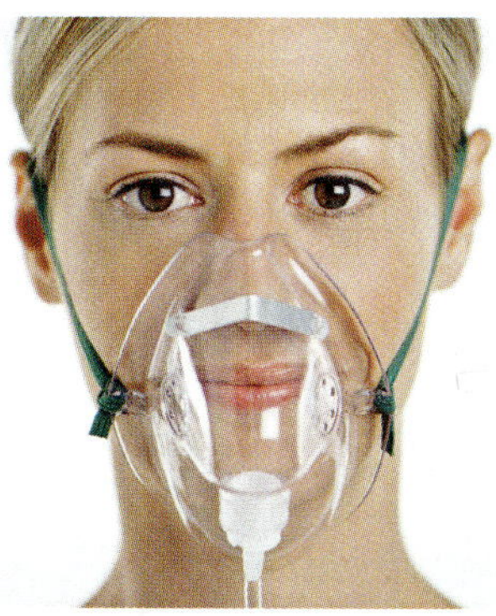

Figure 10-6 Oxygen and other pulmonary agents are inhaled through a mask like this one.

systemic effect. A variety of drug classifications are used for their local effect and include:

- Antiseptics
- Antifungal agents
- Anti-inflammatory products
- Local anesthetics
- Skin emollients
- Skin protectants

The dosage forms administered topically include:

- Ointments
- Creams
- Pastes
- Dry powders
- Aerosol sprays
- Solutions
- Lotions

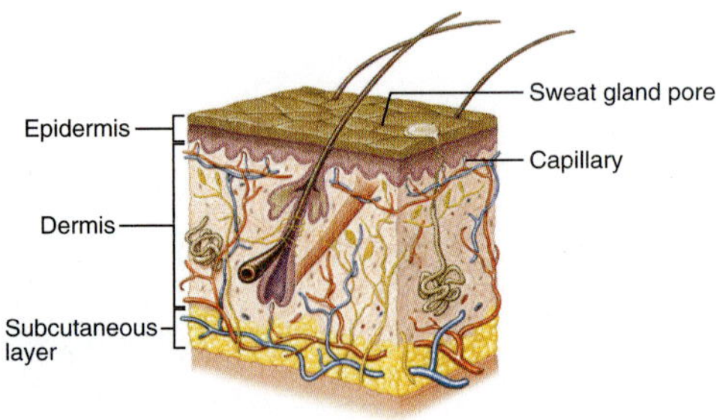

Figure 10-7 Section of skin.

Topical drugs, used systemically, enter the skin through the pores and other structures found in the skin. A medication can enter the capillaries found in the epidermal layer of the skin and find its way into general circulation (Figure 10-7). There are several medications found in transdermal delivery systems (patches) that are used for their systemic effect. For example, nitroglycerin (antianginal), estradiol (hormone), and scopolamine (antinausea and anti-motion sickness) are all medications used for their systemic effect that are administered transdermally.

Nasal Administration

Nasal preparations are used for their local effect involving nasal congestion and allergic rhinitis. Nasal formulations are primarily solutions and suspensions. Other products using the nasal passage include FluMist (flu vaccine) and Stadol NS (migraine treatment).

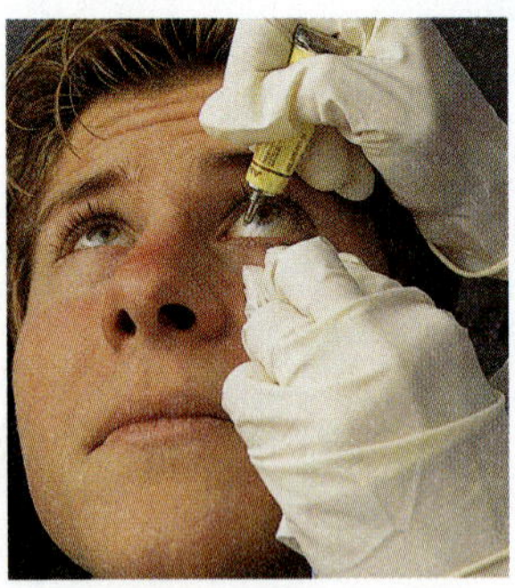

Figure 10-8 Application of eye ointment.

Ophthalmic Administration

Ophthalmic medications use sterile solutions, suspensions, and ointments as dosage forms. Ophthalmic products are used for their local effect with the eye (Figure 10-8). Patient safety and comfort are taken into consideration when selecting a product. Examples of medications include Xalatan and Timoptic.

Otic Administration

Otic administration of medications are used to treat conditions of the ear and are instilled into the ear for a local effect because of their prolonged contact with the affected ear. Pharmaceutical products are used in the ear to soften and remove earwax, combat an earache, or treat an ear infection (Figure 10-9). Examples of otic medications include Cerumenex and Cortisporin otic suspension.

otic Agents used to treat conditions of the ear.

Tech Check

1. What are three routes of drug administration?(LO 10.1)
2. What are two advantages of taking a medication orally?(LO 10.1)
3. What are two disadvantages of the parenteral administration of a medication?(LO 10.1)

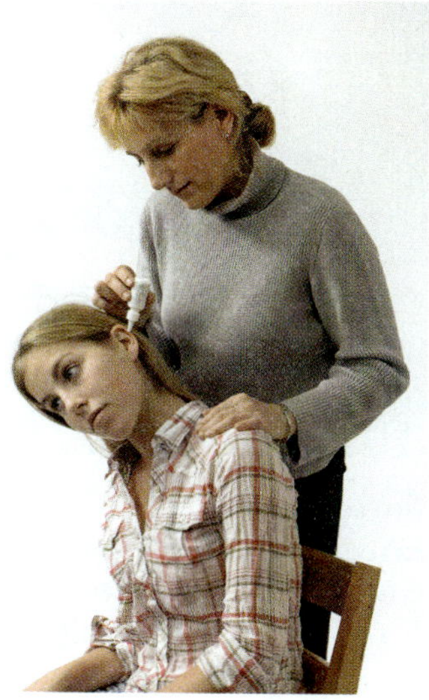

Figure 10-9 Instilling ear drops.

Dosage Forms(LO 10.2, 10.3, 10.4, 10.5)

Tablets

A **tablet** is a solid pharmaceutical dosage form prepared by compression or molding. Some of the advantages of a tablet include:

- Ease of administration
- Readily identifiable
- Accurate dosage

In most situations, tablets should be taken with a full glass of water. Examples of medications available as a tablet include Tylenol, Motrin, Coumadin (Figure 10-11), Synthroid, and Lanoxin.

Tablets come in a variety of shapes, sizes, and weights. Some tablets are scored, which allows one to break them easily to obtain a lower dose of the medication (Figure 10-10).

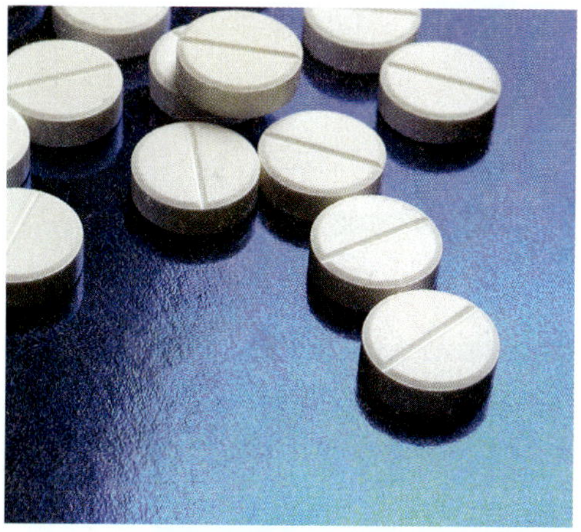

Figure 10-10 Scored tablets.

A tablet may contain diluents, binders, lubricants, glidants, disintegrants, coloring agents, and flavoring agents.

- A diluent is an inert substance used to increase the bulk to make the tablet a functional size for compression. Examples of diluents include lactose, cellulose, mannitol, and dry starch.
- Binders are agents to provide cohesiveness to the powdered material and they include starch, gelatin, and sugars.
- Lubricants aid in the manufacturing process and include talc, magnesium stearate, and polyethylene glycol.
- Glidents are substances that when added to a powder improve its flowability. When a tablet is manufactured, the glidant is added just prior to compression.
- Disintegrants aid in the breakup or disintegration of the tablet after it is administered and their ingredients include corn and potato starch.
- Coloring agents are used to make the tablet more appealing and with unique identification.
- Flavoring agents are used to make the medication more pleasant to the patient.

Types of Tablets

There are many types of tablets used in the practice of pharmacy. Tablets may be prepared either through compression or molding.

- Extended-release (ER) tablets, also known as controlled-release (CR) tablets, are designed to release their medication over a extended period of time following ingestion. There are many advantages of ER tablets over traditional tablets, which include a more constant blood level of the drug, a reduction in the frequency of dosing, improved patient convenience and adherence, a reduction in adverse effects, and a reduction in the

tablet A solid pharmaceutical dosage form prepared by compression or molding.

overall health costs for the patient. An example of an extended-release dosage form is Covera HS.

- Enteric-coated tablets resist solution in the gastric fluid but disintegrate in the intestine. These tablets delay the release of medication until the tablet has passed through the stomach. They are also called delayed-release tablets. E-mycin and Ecotrin are examples of enteric-coated tablets (Figure 10-11).
- Instant disintegrating/dissolving tablets are formulated so they dissolve in the mouth within a minute. Patients having difficulty swallowing find this a convenient dosage form. Claritin RediTab is an example of this type of drug.
- Gelatin-coated tablets are a capsule-shaped compressed tablet that allows the dosage form to be smaller than a capsule filled with an equivalent amount of powder.
- Chewable tablets are formulated so they may be chewed resulting in a pleasant taste left in the mouth, which is easy to swallow. Chewable formulations are used for various antibiotics, children's vitamins, and certain antacids. St. Joseph's Chewable Aspirin, Amoxil, and Tegretol are available in a chewable dosage form (Figure 10-12).
- Effervescent tablets are prepared by compression and may contain either citric or tartaric acid and sodium bicarbonate. Carbon dioxide is released when it is dissolved in water. Effervescent tablets are dissolved in water prior to administration. The tablets should be stored in a tightly closed container that prevents moisture from entering. The patient should be informed that effervescent tablets are not to be swallowed. An example of an effervescent tablet is Alka-Seltzer (Figure 10-13).

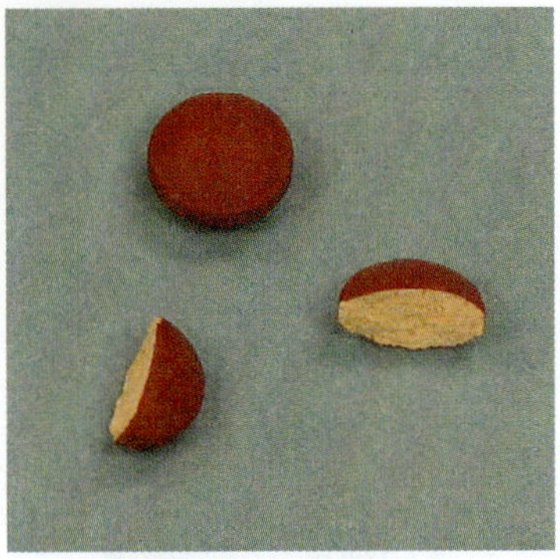

Figure 10-11 **Enteric-coated tablet; one tablet has been split for visualization only.**

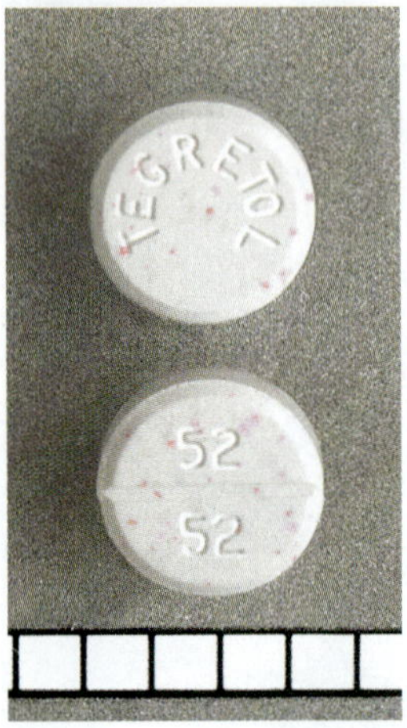

Figure 10-12 **Tegretol.**

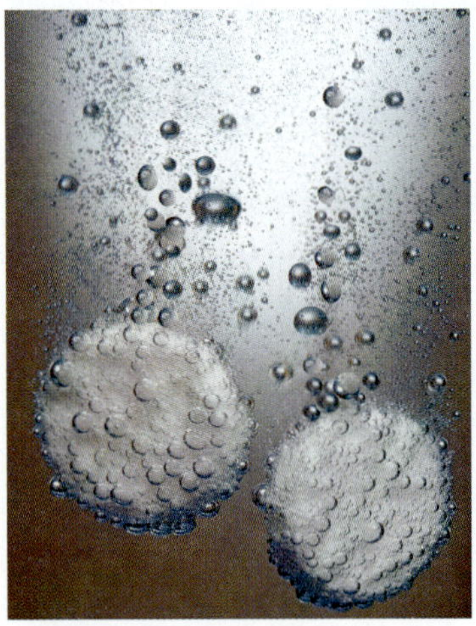

Figure 10-13 **Effervescent tablets.**

Storage

Tablets should be stored in tight containers with low humidity and protected from extreme variations in temperature. Manufacturers pack tablets with a desiccant (drying agent) to absorb moisture. They should be packaged in light-resistant containers to avoid decomposition.

Tech Check

4. What is the difference between controlled-release products and delayed-release tablets?(LO 10.2)
5. Where does an enteric-coated tablet disintegrate?(LO 10.3)
6. Why might an individual wish to take a chewable tablet?(LO 10.3, 10.4)

Capsules

A **capsule** is a solid dosage form in which the drug substance is enclosed in either a hard or soft soluble container or shell of a suitable form of gelatin. Capsules are tasteless and are easily administered. Several examples of products available as capsules include Achromycin, Amoxil, Indocin, and Dalmane (Figure 10-14).

capsule Solid dosage form in which the drug substance is enclosed in either a hard or soft soluble container or shell.

Capsules come in a variety of sizes ranging from 000 to 5. Refer to Table 10-2 for the capacity of each size. Capsules can be manufactured manually using the "punch method" or using manual and automatic machines (Figure 10-15).

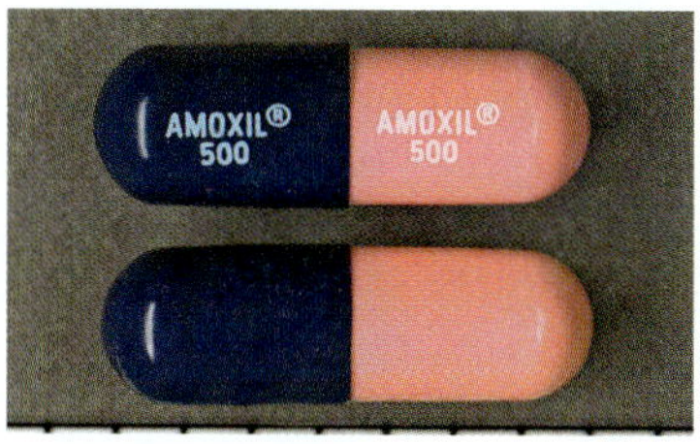

Figure 10-14 Amoxil 500 mg.

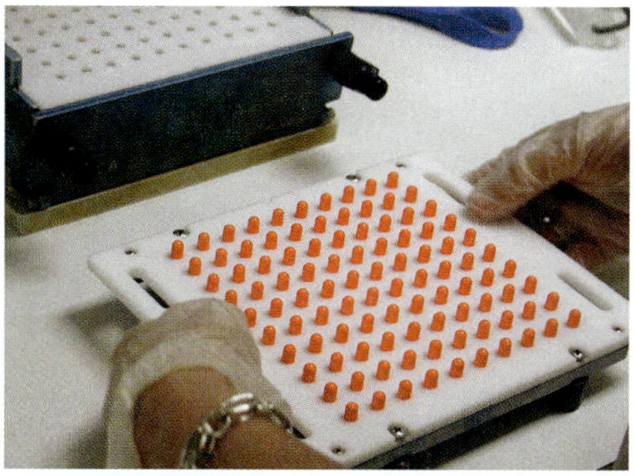

Figure 10-15 Capsules being made by punch method.

Table 10-2 Capsule Size and Capacity

Size	Capacity (weight)	Volume
000	1000 mg	1.37 mL
00	750 mg	0.95 mL
0	500 mg	0.68 mL
1	400 mg	0.5 mL
2	300 mg	0.37 mL
3	200 mg	0.3 mL
4	150 mg	0.2 mL
5	100 mg	0.13 mL

pastille Molded lozenges

troche Compressed lozenges

In addition to the active ingredient contained in the capsule, diluents, or fillers are used to produce the proper capsule volume. Disintegrants assist in the breakup and distribution of the capsule in the stomach, and lubricants such as stearates improve flow properties. Often capsules are used in evaluating new drug products due to the absence of additives.

In most cases, capsules should be swallowed whole. CR capsules, also called sustained-release or ER capsules, release the drug over a long time. If the capsules are not swallowed whole, they may release too much of the drug too quickly for absorption (Figure 10-16).

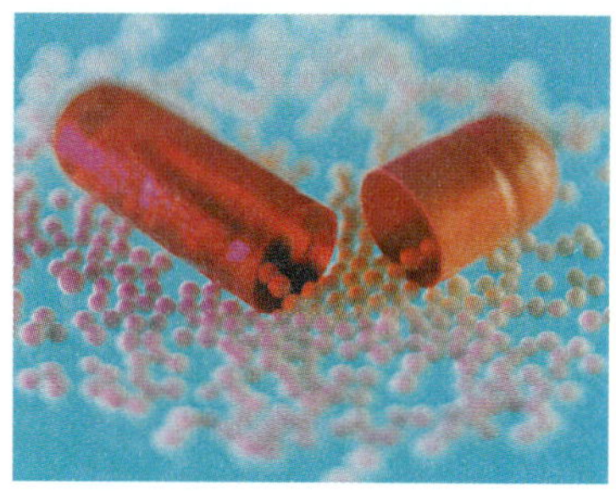

Figure 10-16 Sustained-release capsules.

Pastilles and Troches (Lozenges)

Pastilles, or molded lozenges, and **troches**, or compressed lozenges, are disc-shaped solids containing medicinal agents in a suitable flavored, sweetened base. A pastille or troche is placed in the mouth where it can dissolve slowly and release the active ingredient. Antiseptics, local anesthetics, antibiotics, antihistamines, antitussive, analgesic, or even decongestants have been used in pastilles and troches. An example of a troche is Mycelex Troche (Figure 10-17). An example of a pastille is Sucrets (Figure 10-18).

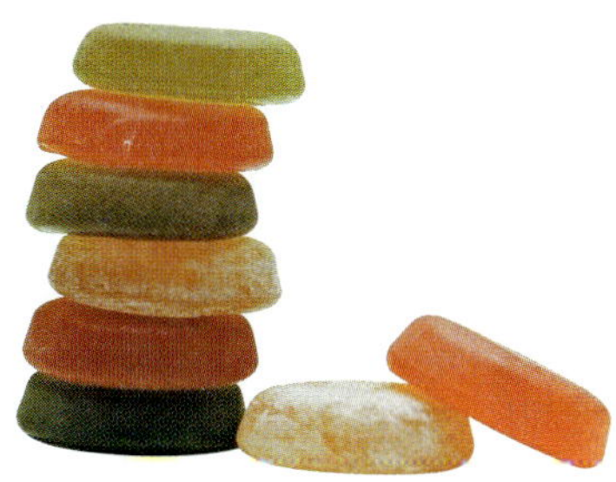

Figure 10-17 Pastille.

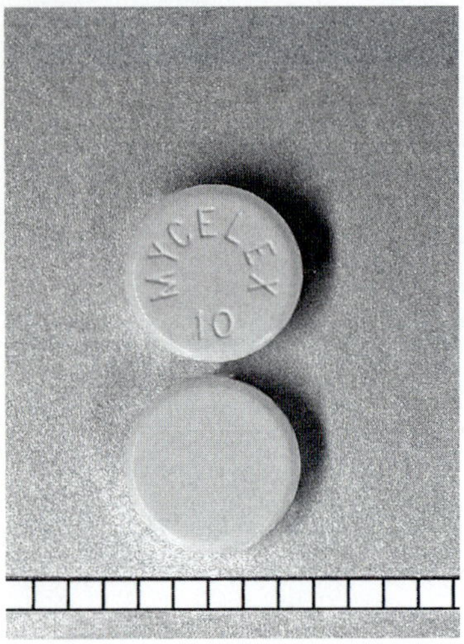

Figure 10-18 Mycelex Troche.

Tech Check

7. Which of the following two sizes of capsules will contain more medication—a size 0 or a size 1?(LO 10.3)

8. What type of ingredients might one find in a capsule besides the active ingredient?(LO 10.2)

Ointments

Ointments are semisolid preparations intended for external application to the skin or mucous membranes. Ointments may be applied to the skin, instilled on the surface of the eyelid, or used nasally, vaginally, or rectally. In most situations, an ointment is used for its local effect (Figure 10-19).

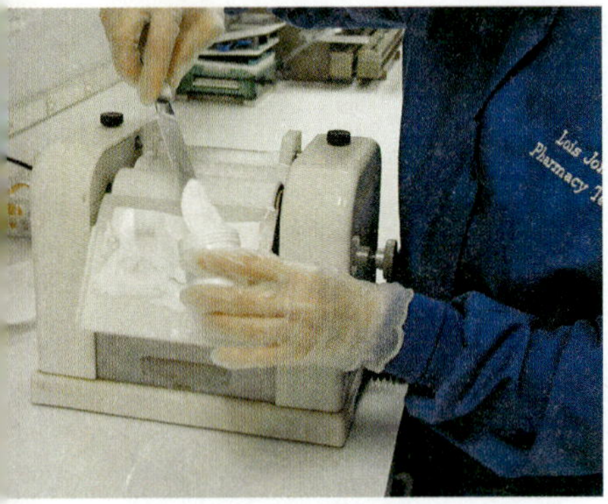

Figure 10-19 Pharmacy technician preparing ointment.

An ointment consists of the ointment base and the active ingredient incorporated into the base. The bases allow a small amount of an aqueous component to be incorporated in them and allow the drug to maintain prolonged contact with the skin. They provide a soothing effect; however, they can be difficult to wash off and they can have a greasy appearance. The bases (oleaginous) include petrolatum (Vaseline), white petrolatum, and white ointment.

Ointments are used in many different therapeutic categories including:

- Antiviral (acyclovir ointment)
- Anesthetics (benzocaine)
- Antibiotic (neomycin and polymyxin B sulfate and bacitracin)
- Antifungal (nystatin)
- Adrenocortical steroids (hydrocortisone)
- Antianginal (nitroglycerin)

Creams

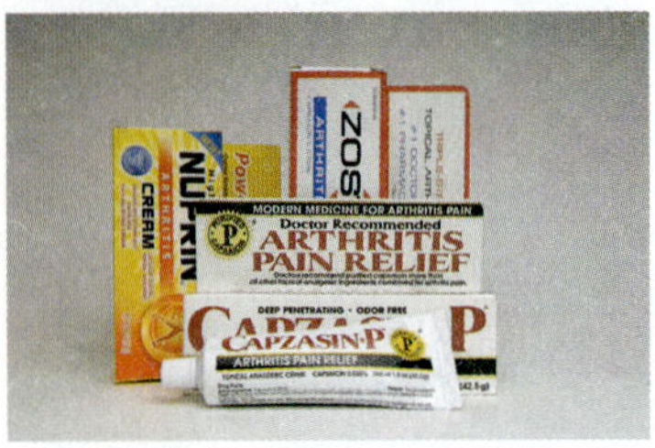

Figure 10-20 Creams.

A **cream** is a semisolid dosage form containing one or more drug substances dissolved in or dispersed in an appropriate base. Creams possess a fluid texture and may be either oil-in-water (O/W) or water-in-oil (W/O). Many of the creams prepared today are O/W emulsions. Advantages of creams over other topical dosage forms include the ease to which they are applied and removed from the skin. Creams may be used vaginally and rectally. Creams are both cosmetically and visually acceptable. After a cream is applied, a thin residue appears on the skin.

Creams are used for many indications including:

- Analgesic (capsaicin)
- Acne (tretinoin)
- Antifungal (clotrimazole)
- Hormone replacement (estradiol)
- Antibiotic (gentamicin)
- Local anesthetic (benzocaine)

ointment A semisolid preparations intended for external application to the skin or mucous membranes.

cream A semisolid dosage form containing one or more drug substances dissolved in or dispersed in an appropriate base.

Gels (Jellies)

Gels, which are also referred to as jellies, are a semisolid dosage form consisting of small particles suspended in a liquid.

One advantage of gels is that they may be used to administer drugs topically or into body cavities. They don't leave a residue like ointments and some creams. Examples of medications available as a gel include:

- Clindamycin (antibiotic)
- Benzoyl peroxide (dermatological)
- Tolnaftate (antifungal)
- Clobetasol(antipruritics)
- Desoximetasone (anti-inflammatory)
- Podofilox (anogenital warts)
- Timolol maleate (glaucoma)
- Acetic acid (maintenance of vaginal acidity)
- Stannous fluoride (dental)

Gels may be used orally, topically, rectally, vaginally, and in the eyes.

Tech Check

9. Provide one example of an ointment base used in preparing ointments.(LO 10.5)
10. Name two locations where ointments may be applied.(LO 10.3)
11. Give an example of a therapeutic category that ointments may be used for.(LO 10.2)

Transdermal Drug Delivery Systems (TDDS)

Transdermal drug delivery systems (TDDS) are also referred to as **transdermal** patches, and assist in the passage of therapeutic quantities of medications through the skin and into systemic circulation (Figure 10-21). TDDS are appropriate for a limited number of medications. The physical and chemical properties of a specific drug will affect its suitability to be considered a candidate for this type of dosage form.

Some of the advantages of TDDS include:

- They can avoid gastrointestinal drug absorption difficulties caused by gastrointestinal factors and any interaction with other substance.
- They can substitute for oral administration, if needed.
- Therapy can be ended quickly if needed.
- They are easily identified in emergency situations.

Despite the advantages of this dosage form, there are several drawbacks:

- Only relatively potent drugs are appropriate for this dosage form.
- Patients may develop contact dermatitis.

Patients should be advised that the rate of absorption would vary with each drug product. TDDS should always be applied to clean, dry skin

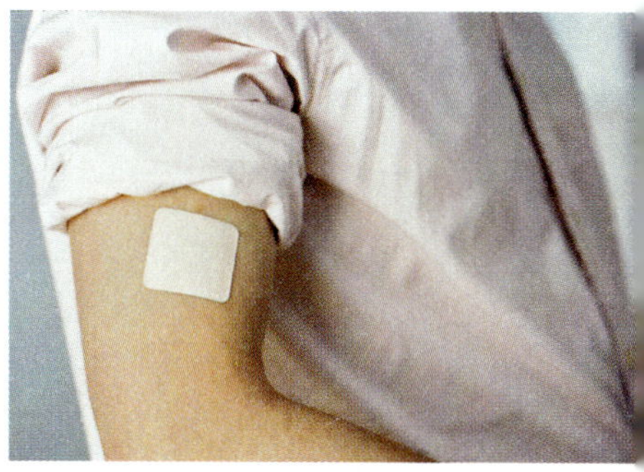

Figure 10-21 Transdermal patch.

gel (jellies) A semisolid dosage form consisting of small particles suspended in a liquid.

transdermal The passage of therapeutic quantities of medications through the skin and into systemic circulation.

areas that are hair free and the application site should be affected either by clothing or body movement. One should be careful not to apply lotions to the body because they alter the rate of absorption of the drug. An individual should not alter the size of product by cutting it down in size. Finally, TDDS should not be reused and should be discarded according to the guidelines established by the drug manufacturer. Examples of TDDS include Transderm Scop, Catapres-TTS, Estraderm, NicoDerm, and Transderm-Nitro.

Suppositories

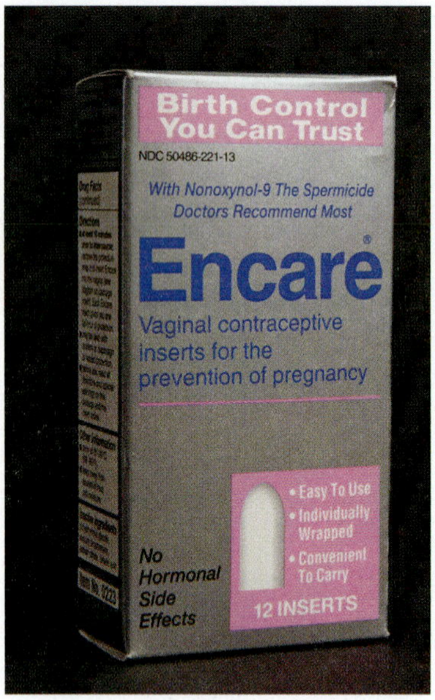

Figure 10-22 Vaginal contraceptive suppository.

A **suppository** is a solid medication dosage formulated to be inserted into the rectum, vagina, or urethra (Figure 10-22). Rectal suppositories are approximately 1 1/2 inches in length. They are cylindrical in shape and may be tapered at one or both ends. Rectal suppositories can be prescribed for infants and small children. **Vaginal** suppositories are generally globular, oval-shaped, or cone-shaped for insertion into the vagina. **Urethral** suppositories (bougies) are slender and pencil-shaped for insertion into the male or female urethra. Male urethral suppositories range from 3 to 6 mm in diameter and measure 140 mm in length; female urethral suppositories are one-half the size of the male suppositories. Suppositories soften, melt, and dissolve at body temperature.

A suppository can provide either local or systemic effects and possess protective or palliative properties. Rectal suppositories being used for their local effect to relieve constipation (bisacodyl) or the pain, irritation, itching, and inflammation associated with hemorrhoids used. Vaginal suppositories are used as contraceptives, antiseptic agents for feminine hygiene, and to combat pathogenic agents (nystatin). Urethral suppositories are used as antibacterial and as local anesthetics.

The rectum can be used for systemic indications because the rectum allows the absorption of many drugs. Examples include acetaminophen (analgesic) and prochlorperazine (nausea and vomiting).

Suppositories using cocoa butter as a base may be made by means of adding the medication into the solid at room temperature. A suppository should melt at body temperature. Cocoa butter may be used to prepare both rectal and vaginal suppositories. Suppositories prepared from cocoa butter substitutes are prepared from fat-type bases such as vegetable oils, coconut, or palm kernel. An advantage of this type of base being used is the ability to have narrow intervals between melting and solidification.

Pellets (Implants)

Pellets or implants are small sterile solid masses consisting of a highly purified medication. They are intended to be implanted in the body, normally by subcutaneous methods, and are expected to provide a continuous release of a medicament over a long period. The primary advantage of this dosage form is that it allows hormones such as testosterone, estradiol, or desoxycorticosterone to be introduced to the body. Examples of pellets or implants include Muse and Norplant.

suppository A solid medication dosage formulated to be inserted into the rectum, vagina, or urethra.

vaginal Inserted into the vagina.

urethral Inserted into the male or female urethra.

Vaginal Inserts

Vaginal inserts are also known as vaginal tablets. They are ovoid in shape and are accompanied by a plastic inserter to be used for inserting the drug into the vagina. An example of a vaginal insert is Semicid.

Solutions

A **solution** is a homogeneous mixture that is prepared by dissolving a solid, liquid, or gas in another liquid. A solution is composed of two distinct parts: a solute and a solvent. The most commonly used solvents include water, ethyl alcohol, and glycerin. In most cases, the solute is the active ingredient but solutes can also be used to provide color, flavor, sweetness, or stability to solution.

Oral Solutions

Oral solutions are liquid preparations intended for oral administration that may contain one or more active ingredients. They may contain flavoring agents, sweetening agents, or coloring agents to improve their appearance and provide a pleasant taste to the patient. Some oral solutions may contain ingredients to prevent the solute from precipitating and crystallizing. Others may contain antimicrobial agents to prevent the growth of bacteria, yeast, and molds. Some solutions may contain sweetening agents such as sorbitol and can be used with diabetic patients. Oral solutions may be made for immediate usage or they may be dispensed in a more concentrated form requiring them to be diluted prior to administration. An example of an oral solution is Potassium Chloride for Oral Solution.

A small sample of drugs available as oral solutions are listed:

- Haldol concentrate—antipsychotic
- Imodium AD—antidiarrheal
- Magnesium citrate—cathartic
- Methadone—narcotic analgesic
- Pediapred—corticosteroid
- Prozac liquid—antidepressant
- Tagamet HCl liquid—H_2 Inhibitor
- Lomotil—antiperistaltic
- Colace syrup—stool softener
- Kaochlor 10% liquid—electrolyte replacement (potassium)

solution A homogeneous mixture that is prepared by dissolving a solid, liquid, or gas in another liquid.

excipient Any more or less of an inert substance added to a drug to give suitable consistency or form to the drug.

Gargles A gargle is an aqueous solution containing antiseptics, antibiotics, and/or anesthetics for treating the pharynx and nasopharynx by forcing air from the lungs through the gargle that is held in the throat and the gargle is later expectorated. In many situations, the gargle is diluted with water prior to use. A gargle is not a mouthwash.

Mouthwashes A mouthwash is an aqueous solution in concentrated form containing one or more active ingredients and **excipients.** which are inert substances added to a drug to give suitable consistency or form to the drug. A mouthwash is used by swishing the liquid in the oral cavity (Figure 10-23). There are two purposes for mouthwashes: therapeutic and cosmetic. A therapeutic mouthwash is used to reduce plaque buildup,

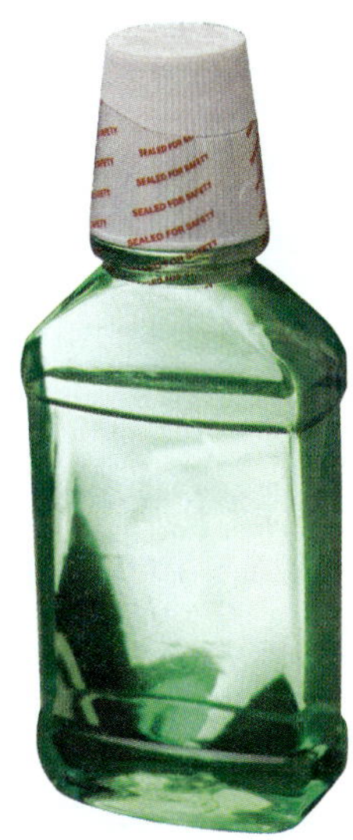

Figure 10-23 Mouthwash.

gingivitis, dental cavities, stomatitis, dry mouth, oral candidiasis, and pain associated with ulcerative oral lesions. Cosmetic mouthwashes are used for bad breath.

There are four classifications of ingredients used in the preparation of mouthwashes:

- Alcohols—used to mask the unpleasant taste of active ingredients, solubilize flavoring agents and as a preservative
- **Surfactants**—used because they aid in the dissolving of flavoring agents and removing the debris caused by the foaming action
- Flavoring—used to mask the unappealing taste of the ingredients (peppermint, spearmint, and wintergreen)
- Coloring agents—used to present an aesthetically appealing appearance

Topical Solutions

A topical solution is normally an aqueous solution but may contain alcohol as the vehicle. Products containing alcohol may cause the area to sting upon application, especially if the skin is broken. Cosolvents may be used to ensure the stability of the product. Topical solutions may be intended to be applied to the skin, but may be applied to mucosal surfaces.

In some instances, a topical solution may appear in the form of a spray. A spray is an aqueous or oleaginous solution in the form of coarse droplets or as finely divided solids to be applied topically. Sprays can be used intranasally to relieve congestion and inflammation and to combat infections. Topical sprays may contain local anesthetics, antiseptics, skin protectants, and analgesics.

Examples of topical solutions include:

- Hibiclens (skin cleanser)
- Lotrimin (antifungal)
- Cleocin T (acne treatment)
- Synalar (topical anti-inflammatory)
- Betadine (anti-infective)
- Efudex (antineoplastic)

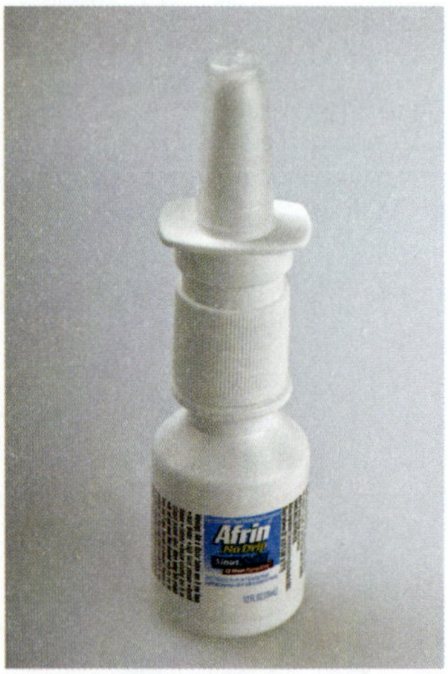

Figure 10-24 Afrin nasal spray.

Nasal Solutions

A nasal solution is normally an aqueous solution administered in the nasal passage in either the form of drops or a spray (Figure 10-24). Nasal solutions are isotonic in nature and may contain antimicrobial preservatives. These solutions may be in the form of an emulsion or suspension. Nasal solutions are packaged in either a plastic dropper or spray bottles holding 15 to 30 mL of the solution and should be tightly closed during non-use. The patient should discard the nasal solution if the solution changes color or if a precipitate develops.

Examples of nasal solutions include:

- NasalCrom nasal solution (allergic rhinitis)
- Oxytocin nasal solution (synthetic hormone replacement)
- Stadol NS (migraine)
- Afrin nasal spray (decongestant)
- Ocean Mist (nasal moisturizer)

surfactant An emulsifying agent that stabilizes an emulsion from preventing small droplets from becoming large droplets.

Otic Solutions

An otic solution is prepared under sterile conditions. Otic solutions are also known as eardrops. The patient should be informed to warm the bottle by rubbing between the hands prior to using the product. When administering eardrops, it is best to have someone other than the patient instill them. The patient should be informed to stay stationary on the side for a brief period after application. Eardrops should be stored out of the reach of small children.

Otic or ear solutions may contain:

- Analgesics (benzocaine)
- Antibiotics (neomycin)
- Earwax removal (carbamide peroxide)
- Anti-inflammatory agents (cortisone)

Examples of otic solutions include:

- Cortisporin otic solution
- Auralgan otic solution
- Cerumenex ear drops

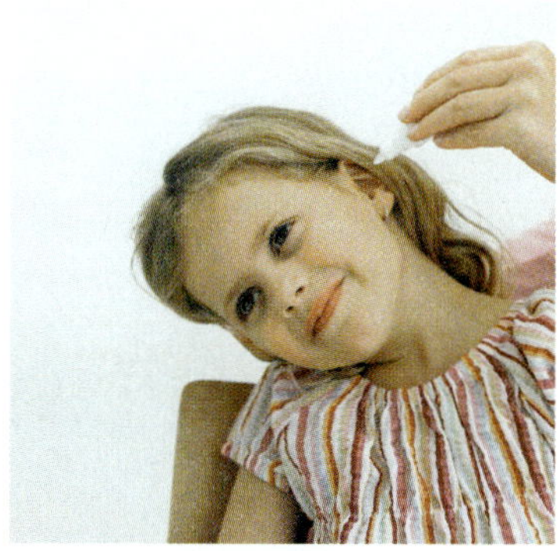

Figure 10-25 Ear drops.

Douches

A **douche** is an aqueous solution directed against a part or into a body cavity. A douche serves either as a cleansing agent or as an antiseptic agent. An eye douche is used to remove a particle from the eye, pharyngeal douches are used to prepare the throat for an operation, and vaginal douches are use to cleanse the vagina and for hygienic purposes. Ingredients used in douches include benzalkonium chloride, sodium borate solution, and sodium bicarbonate. A vaginal douche may contain antimicrobial agents, anesthetics, antipruritics, astringents, or surfactants. An example of a vaginal douche is Summer's Eve.

Enemas

An **enema** is a rectal dosage form used to evacuate the bowel or to affect a local disease. Enemas are of one of two types: evacuant and retention. An enema may possess nutritive, sedative, stimulating properties or contain radiopaque agents for diagnostic purposes of the lower bowel. Evacuant enemas may contain sodium chloride, sodium bicarbonate, or sodium monohydrate to evacuate the bowel. Evacuant enemas may occupy a volume up to 2 pints. Retention enemas are retained in the small intestine and occupy a much smaller volume (150 mL) compared to evacuant enemas. The retention enema may use vehicles such as ethanol and propylene glycol to carry the medication. Examples of enemas include Cort-Dome enema, Rowasa enema, and Fleet's enema.

Tech Check

12. What routes may be used in the administration of a solution?(LO 10.1)

13. What are the two components of a solution?(LO 10.2)

14. What is the route of administration for an enema?(LO 10.1)

douche Aqueous solution directed against a part or into a body cavity.

enema Rectal dosage form used to evacuate the bowel or to affect a local disease.

Syrups

A **syrup** is a concentrated solution of sugar in water or other aqueous solutions with or without flavoring agents and medicinal substances. In some situations, syrup may contain either sorbitol or glycerin to prevent crystallization of the sucrose. Alcohol may be used in a syrup as a preservative or as a solvent for the active ingredient. Antimicrobial preservatives (i.e., benzoic acid, sodium benzoate, and methyl-, propyl-, and butylaparabens) are used to prevent microbial growth from developing. Flavors are used to enhance the taste of the syrup and colors are used to make the syrup more eye appealing to the patient. One advantage of syrups over other oral dosage forms is their ability to mask the bitter taste of the active ingredient.

Syrups can be made by the following methods:

- Solution of the ingredients with the aid of heat
- Solution of the ingredients by agitation without the use of heat
- Addition of sucrose to a prepared medicated liquid or to a flavored liquid

Medicated syrups are used to contain many different drug classifications for both children and adults. Examples include:

- Proventil syrup (bronchodilator)
- Robitussin syrup (expectorant)
- Phenergan syrup (anti-emetic)
- Symmetrel syrup (antiviral)
- Colace syrup (stool softener)
- Demerol syrup (analgesic)
- Depakene syrup (anticonvulsant)
- Benylin (antitussive)
- Lactulose (cathartic)
- Reglan (gastrointestinal stimulant)

Nonmedicinal syrups provide a vehicle for active ingredients during compounding. Examples of nonmedicated syrups include:

- Simple syrup (85% solution of sucrose and water)
- Cherry syrup
- Cocoa syrup
- Ora-Sweet

Tech Check

15. What is an advantage of using a syrup?(LO 10.3)

16. What are two functions of alcohol in a syrup?(LO 10.3)

17. What are two basic categories of syrups?(LO 10.3)

syrup A concentrated solution of sugar in water or other aqueous solutions with or without flavoring agents and medicinal substances.

elixir Clear, pleasantly flavored, sweetened hydro-alcoholic liquid for oral use.

Elixirs

Elixirs are clear, pleasantly flavored, sweetened hydro-alcoholic liquids for oral use. They may be either medicated or nonmedicated (Figure 10-26). Elixirs contain ethanol (alcohol) and water, but may contain glycerin, sorbitol, propylene glycol, flavoring agents, preservatives, and syrups. Elixirs are more fluid than syrups due to the use of less-thick substances, such as alcohol, and they are not as sweet. The alcohol content found in elixirs can range from 3% to 23%.

Examples of elixirs include:

- Benadryl elixir (antihistamine)
- Tylenol elixir (OTC analgesic and antipyretic)
- Dexamethasone elixir (corticosteroid)
- Lanoxin pediatric elixir (cardiotonic agent)

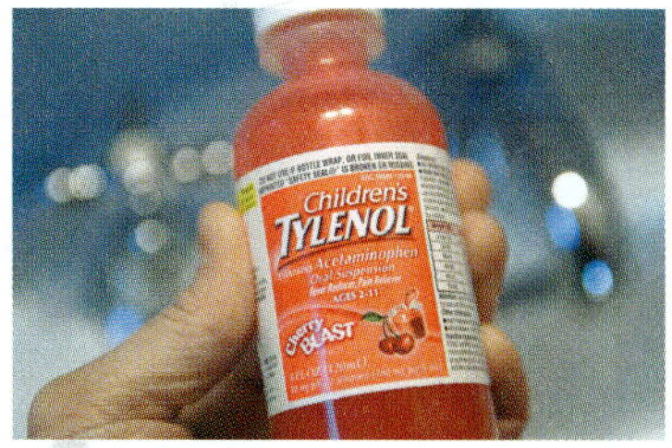

Figure 10-26 Children's Tylenol.

Tech Check

18. What type of patient should be extremely careful of syrups?(LO 10.3)

19. What is a disadvantage of a syrup?(LO 10.3)

20. Which is more fluid: elixir or syrup?(LO 10.3)

21. Name an elixir that treats pain and fever.(LO 10.3)

Tinctures

Tinctures are either alcoholic or hydro-alcoholic solutions prepared from either vegetable or chemical substances. Tinctures may be taken orally or applied topically. Tinctures vary in their preparation, the strength of the active ingredient, their alcohol content, and their function. The concentration of tinctures ranges from 10% to 80%. The alcohol content of a tincture eliminates microbial growth and keeps the active ingredient in solution. Tinctures must be tightly closed, protected from extreme temperatures, and stored in light-resistant containers.

Examples of tinctures include:

- Belladonna tincture
- Tincture of benzoin
- Tincture of iodine
- Tincture of opium

Disperse Systems

A disperse system is one that contains an undissolved ingredient in a vehicle. The dispersed ingredient (usually a solid) in the vehicle is referred to as the dispersed phase and the vehicle (usually a liquid) is referred to as the dispersing phase or dispersing medium. Dispersions may consist of a solid dispersed in a liquid, liquid dispersed in another liquid, or a liquid dispersed in a gas. The particle size of the dispersed phase may vary in size. The larger the particle size will result in a greater likelihood that it will separate in a dispersing medium. Examples of disperse systems include emulsions, suspensions, magmas, gels, and aerosols.

Emulsions

According to the *United States Pharmacopeia (USP)*, an **emulsion** is a two-phase system in which one liquid is dispersed throughout another liquid in the form of small droplets. When oil is the dispersed phase and an aqueous solution is the continuous phase, the system is known as an O/W emulsion. Conversely, when water or an aqueous solution is the dispersed phase and oil or oleaginous material is the continuous phase, the system is

tincture Alcoholic or hydro-alcoholic solutions prepared from vegetable or chemical substances.

emulsion A two phase system in which one liquid is dispersed throughout another liquid in the form of small droplets.

designated as a W/O emulsion. Emulsions are stabilized through the usage of emulsifying agents, which prevent small droplets from becoming larger droplets. An emulsifying agent is a surfactant that provides a barrier. An emulsion may be used orally, topically, or parenterally.

Emulsification is the process that allows a pharmacist or pharmacy technician to compound relatively constant and uniform mixtures of two immiscible liquids. Emulsification is necessary for O/W emulsions to be taken orally by using a flavored aqueous solution. Topical emulsions may either be O/W or W/O depending on the therapeutic agents being used, the desire of having a softening effect, and the physical conditions of the skin.

Emulsifying agents must be well suited with the other ingredients in the emulsion. These agents cannot interfere with the stability or affect the effectiveness of the active ingredient. Emulsifying agents should not cause injury to the patient taking or applying the medication. They should be odorless, tasteless, and colorless.

Emulsions can be compounded using several different methods depending upon the nature of the ingredients and the equipment used. Emulsions should be protected from extreme heat and cold during either shipping or storage. An emulsion can be affected by light, air, and other microorganisms; therefore, the storage of an emulsion is extremely important. Two examples of emulsions are castor oil and Mylicon drops.

Suspensions

Suspensions are liquid preparations consisting of solid particles dispersed throughout a liquid phase in which the particles are not soluble. Suspensions may be available for immediate use or may be required to be reconstituted prior to use. If it is required to be reconstituted the label will read "for Oral Suspension."

Oral suspensions are liquid preparations containing solid particles dispersed in a liquid vehicle with appropriate flavoring agents for oral use. Oral suspensions need to shaken well before taking.

Examples of oral suspensions include:

- Amoxicillin suspension
- Zithromax suspension
- Tylenol suspension

Tech Check

22. What type of agent is required in the preparation of an emulsion?(LO 10.2)

23. What are the two types of emulsion?(LO 10.3)

24. Give an example of a suspension.(LO 10.5)

Injectable Parenteral Preparations

There are five general types of preparations that may be used for parenteral administration. These preparations may contain buffers and preservatives and include:

- Drug injection—liquid preparations that are drug substances or solutions
- Drug for injection—dry solids that upon the addition of suitable vehicles yield solutions conforming to all respects to the requirements for injections

suspension A liquid preparation consisting of solid particles dispersed throughout a liquid phase in which the particles are not soluble.

- Drug injectable emulsion—liquid preparation of drug substances dissolved or dispersed in suitable emulsion mixture
- Drug injectable suspension—liquid preparations of solids suspended in a suitable liquid medium.
- Drug for injectable suspension—dry solids that upon the addition of suitable vehicles yield preparations conforming in all respects to the requirements for injectable suspensions.

Injectable parenteral solutions and suspensions differ from other types of solutions and suspensions due to the following:

- Solvents or vehicles used must meet special purity standards based on the *United States Pharmacopeia–National Formulary* (*USP–NF*) criteria, which ensure their safety.
- The usage of buffers, stabilizers, and antimicrobial preservatives may be restricted in select parenteral products. The use of coloring agents is prohibited.
- Product must meet sterility standards and be pyrogen-free.
- Parenteral products must meet *USP–NF* standards regarding particulate matter.
- They must be prepared in an environmentally controlled area to ensure sanitation and that the individuals preparing them possess specific skills obtained through training.
- Parenteral products must be packaged in hermetic containers.
- Parenteral containers are filled in a slight excess to the amount to be withdrawn.
- Restrictions apply to the number of injections permitted on multiple-dose containers.
- Specific labeling requirements must be followed.

Table 10-3 (p. 288) lists solutions and usage of intravenous solutions.

There are two different types of containers that may be used in the preparation of injectable parenteral medications: single-dose and multiple-dose containers.

A single-dose container is a tightly sealed container holding a quantity of sterile drug for injection intended for parenteral administration as a single dose, and when opened it cannot be resealed. A single-dose container does not contain a preservative. Single-dose containers include vials and ampoules.

A multiple-dose container is a tightly sealed container that permits withdrawal of successive portions of the contents without changing the strength, quality, or purity of the remaining solution (suspension). Unlike a single-dose container, it does contain a preservative.

Large-volume parenterals (LVPs) are those that have a volume greater than 100 mL. They are used to replenish body fluids (water) and provide electrolytes and nutrition. They are injected into the body by slow intravenous infusion with or without a controlled-rate infusion system (Figure 10-27).

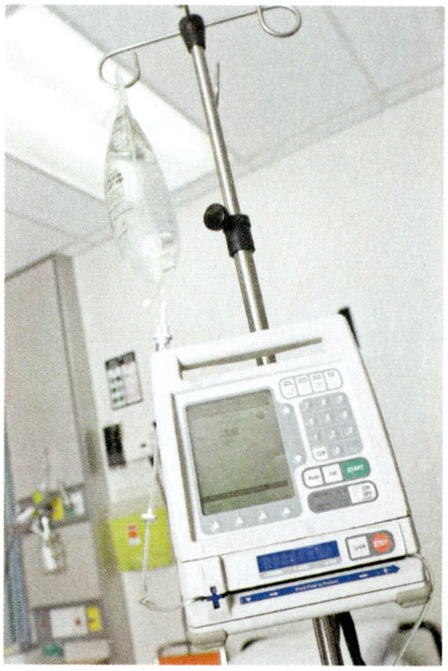

Figure 10-27 IV drip, controlled rate.

Examples of large-volume parenterals include:

- Dextrose injection (fluid and nutrient replenisher)
- Sodium chloride injection (fluid and electrolyte replenisher)
- Lactated Ringer's injection (system alkalinizer; fluid and electrolyte replenisher)

Table 10-3 Vehicles Used as Intravenous Solutions

Solution	Usage
Water for injection	Used in the preparation of injectable products, which will be sterilized after their preparation.
Purified water	Used in the preparation of injectable products, which will be sterilized after their preparation.
Sterile water for injection	Used as a solvent, vehicle, or diluent for already sterilized and packaged injectable medications.
Bacteriostatic water for injection	Used as a sterile vehicle in the preparation of small volumes of injectable preparations. Comes in vials containing 30 mL or less.
Sodium chloride injection	Used as a sterile vehicle in the preparation of solutions or suspensions of drugs for parenteral administration. Sodium chloride injection is used to flush catheter lines.
Bacteriostatic sodium chloride injection	Not suitable for mixing with all medications. May be used to flush catheters. Bacteriostatic sodium chloride injection is available in vials containing 30 mL or less. Cannot be used in newborns.
Ringer's injection	Employed as a vehicle for other drugs or as a replacement for lost electrolytes.

Tech Check

25. What are two differences between parenteral solutions and other types of solutions?(LO 10.2, 10.3, 10.4)

26. Name a large-volume parenteral.(LO 10.5)

27. Name a use for a large-volume parenteral.(LO 10.3)

28. What are two vehicles used as intravenous solutions?(LO 10.2, 10.3, 10.4)

Inhalants

According to the *USP*, an **inhalant** is an inhalation product that consists of drugs or combinations of drugs that, due to its high vapor pressure, can be carried by an air current into the respiratory system where it exerts its effect. An inhalation preparation is intended to deliver a drug into the respiratory system of an individual. It is used to relieve symptoms of bronchial and nasal congestion.

inhalant Drugs or combinations of drugs that, due to its high vapor pressure, can be carried by an air current into the respiratory system.

Inhalants maybe delivered with a nebulizer if the droplets are extremely fine and uniform in size. The solution may be inhaled directly from the nebulizer or with intermittent positive pressure breathing machine. Another method of introducing an inhalant into the respiratory tract is with a metered-dose inhaler (MDI). An MDI is a propellant-driven drug suspension or solution in a liquefied-gas propellant. Most MDIs contain more than 100 doses in the container (Figure 10-28). Examples of medications available as inhalations include Flonase, Atrovent, and NasalCrom.

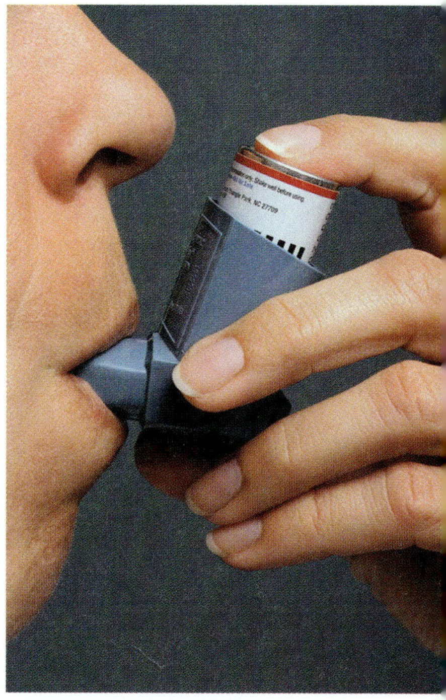

Figure 10-28 Metered-dose inhaler (MDI).

Aerosols

Aerosols are products that are packaged under pressure and contain therapeutically active ingredients that are released upon activation of an appropriate valve. Aerosols are used for topical application to the skin and for local application into the nose, mouth, or lungs. They may deliver the active ingredient either in a continuous or in a metered-dose inhaler method.

Examples of aerosols include Proventil inhalation aerosol, Atrovent inhalation aerosol, and Intal inhaler.

Tech Check

29. What body organ system is utilized by inhalation products?(LO 10.1)

30. What is the meaning of "MDI"?(LO 10.2)

Ophthalmic Preparations

Ophthalmic agents are used to treat surface or intraocular conditions to include infections of the eyes or eyelids due to bacteria, fungi, or virus. Ophthalmic preparations are used to treat allergic or infectious conjunctivitis, inflammation of the eye, elevated intraocular pressure, glaucoma, and symptoms of dry eye.

Ophthalmic agents may be used either topically or systemically. These agents may contain:

- Anesthetics (tetracaine)
- Antibiotics (sulfacetamide and polymyxin B-bacitracin)
- Antifungal agents (Amphotericin B)
- Anti-inflammatory agents (prednisolone)
- Antiviral agents (vidarabine)
- Astringents (zinc sulfate)
- Beta-adrenergic blocking agents (timolol)
- Miotics (pilocarpine)
- Mydriatics/cycloplegics (atropine)
- Protectants/artificial tears (carboxymethyl cellulose)
- Vasoconstrictors/decongestants (naphazoline)

Ophthalmic Solutions

Ophthalmic solutions are sterile solutions that are free from foreign particles and compounded and packaged especially for the instillation into the eye. Ophthalmic solutions must take into consideration the toxicity of the drug, buffers, preservatives, and **isotonicity,** which means relating to or exhibit equal osmotic pressure. Lacrimal fluid is isotonic with blood and therefore ophthalmic solutions should be isotonic. Buffering agents prevent an increase in the pH, which can affect both the stability and

aerosol Product that is packaged under pressure and contains therapeutically active ingredients that are released upon activation of an appropriate valve.

ophthalmic Agents used to treat surface or intraocular conditions of the eyes or eyelids.

isotonicity Relating to or exhibiting equal osmotic pressure.

solubility of the medication. A buffering system should be selected that will not cause precipitation of the drug or cause deterioration of the drug.

Ophthalmic solutions may be packaged in multiple-dose containers when intended for use by one patient. All ophthalmic containers must be sealed and tamper-proof to ensure the sterility of the substance is present upon opening the container. Each container of ophthalmic solution contains ingredients to prevent the growth of or to destroy microorganisms accidentally introduced upon opening of the container. Examples of ophthalmic solutions include Betoptic (glaucoma agent) and Decadron Ophthalmic Solution (anti-inflammatory).

Ophthalmic Suspensions

Ophthalmic suspensions are sterile liquid preparations containing solid particles dispersed in a liquid vehicle intended for application into the eye. Ophthalmic suspensions must be sterilized and often contain preservatives to prevent microbes from developing. Other considerations include particles found in ophthalmic suspensions are micronized to prevent any irritation and/or scratching to the cornea. Ophthalmic suspensions should never be dispensed if it appears that a precipitate has formed. Timoptic and Tobrex are examples of an ophthalmic suspension.

Ophthalmic Ointments

Ophthalmic ointments are intended to be applied to the eye. The formulation allows the drug to stay in contact with the eye longer than either suspensions or solutions, but can also result in blurred vision. These are usually administered at night when possible to reduce discomfort from effect on vision.

Examples of ophthalmic ointments include:

- Bacitracin ophthalmic ointment
- Garamycin ophthalmic ointment
- Vira-A ophthalmic ointment
- Neosporin ophthalmic ointment

Tech Check

31. What is a primary concern for all ophthalmic products?(LO 10.3)

32. What is a usage of ophthalmic products?(LO 10.3)

Dosage Form Abbreviations(LO 10.6)

Medical prescribers utilize various pharmacy abbreviations when writing prescriptions and medication orders. Both pharmacists and pharmacy technicians must be able to correctly identify the abbreviations used by prescribers in prescriptions or the medication orders will result in prescription (medication) errors.

The pharmacy technician should never guess at an abbreviation used in a prescription but rather should verify it with the pharmacist or the prescriber. A listing of some of the more commonly used dosage abbreviations is found in Table 10-4.

Table 10-4 Dosage Forms and Abbreviations

Abbreviation	Dosage Form
cap	capsule
cr	cream
elix	elixir
emul	emulsion
liq	liquid
oint	ointment
pulv	powder
soln	solution
supp	suppository
susp	suspension
syr	syrup
tinct	tincture
tab	tablet
ung	ointment

Chapter Summary

Understanding dosage forms, abbreviations, and routes of administration is vital to the pharmacy technician. Important points to know are:

- There are many different routes by which a drug may be administered to a patient; however, not all medications can be administered by every route.
- There are many different dosage forms, but not all medications are available in every dosage form.
- Specific characteristics of each drug will determine its route of administration and the dosage form to be used.
- A particular disease or condition may have an effect on the dosage form and route of administration.

Table 10-5 provides a summary of the routes of administration for each dosage form.

Table 10-5 Dosage Forms Available for Administration by Various Routes of Administration

	Nasal	Oral	Injection	Sublingual	Pulmonary	Topical	Ophthalmic	Otic	Rectal	Vaginal
Aerosol					X	X				
Capsule		X								
Cream						X			X	X
Elixir		X								
Emulsion						X				
Gel		X				X				
Lotion						X				
Ointment	X					X	X		X	
Pastes						X				
Powder		X			X	X				
Spray	X				X					
Solution	X	X	X		X	X	X	X	X	X
Suppository									X	X
Suspension		X	X				X	X		
Syrup		X								
Tablet		X		X						
Troche/Pastille/ Lozenge		X								

Chapter Review

Case Study Question

1. If you were Andrew, what would you tell the customer?(LO 10.2)

At Your Service Question

1. Which one of these two products would the pharmacist recommend?(LO 10.2, 10.3)

Multiple Choice

Select the best answer.

1. Which oral dosage form has a special coating that prevents it from disintegrating until it reaches the intestine?(LO 10.2, 10.3, 10.4)
   a. Enteric-coated tablet
   b. Sustained-release capsule
   c. Time-release capsule
   d. All of the above
2. Which oral dosage form is a clear, sweetened, usually hydro-alcoholic liquid containing flavoring substances and sometimes medicinal agents for oral use?(LO 10.2)
   a. Aromatic water
   b. Elixir
   c. Syrup
   d. Tincture
3. What term refers to the type of ingredient that, when added to a substance, reduces the strength of the substance?(LO 10.2)
   a. Binder
   b. Buffer
   c. Diluent
   d. Excipient
4. Which of the following is an advantage of an oral dosage form?(LO 10.3)
   a. Easy to administer
   b. Easy to reverse effects if ingested accidentally
   c. Relatively inexpensive
   d. All of the above
5. Which of the following is *not* a capsule size?(LO 10.4)
   a. 000
   b. 00
   c. 6
   d. 1
   e. 2
6. Which of the following is a parenteral route of administration?(LO 10.1)
   a. Inhalation
   b. Sublingual
   c. Topically
   d. All of the above
7. Into which of the following body orifices may a suppository be inserted?(LO 10.1, 10.3)
   a. Rectum
   b. Urethra
   c. Vagina
   d. All of the above
8. Which of the following is least likely to be an elixir?(LO 10.3)
   a. Bendryl
   b. Tylenol
   c. Colace
   d. Lanoxin
9. Which of the following dosage forms would be administered orally?(LO 10.3.)
   a. Suspension
   b. Troche
   c. Injection
   d. Inhalant
10. Which of the following is a method for injecting a parenteral dosage form (may select more than one)?(LO 10.1)
    a. Intramuscular
    b. Intravenous
    c. Subcutaneous
    d. All of the above
11. Which of the following dosage forms has an irregular absorption rate?(LO 10.3)
    a. Capsule
    b. Solution
    c. Suppository
    d. Tablet
12. Which of the following routes of administration would yield the quickest response for the patient?(LO 10.1)
    a. Intramuscular
    b. Intravenous
    c. Oral
    d. Topical
13. What type of tablet leaves a pleasant taste in the mouth?(LO 10.3)
    a. Delayed release
    b. Enteric coated
    c. Chewable
    d. Gelatin coated

14. What type of tablet dissolves under the tongue?(LO 10.2)
    a. Buccal
    b. Chewable
    c. Instant disintegrating
    d. Sublingual
15. What is another term for a pastille or troche?(LO 10.2)
    a. Film-coated tablet
    b. Lozenge
    c. Placebo
    d. Sugar-coated tablet
16. Which of the following is an advantage of a transdermal drug delivery system (may select more than one)?(LO 10.3)
    a. Avoidance of first-pass effect
    b. Easily identifiable during emergency situations
    c. Prompt termination of therapy
    d. All of the above
17. Which of the following types of solutions may be used in preparing intravenous solutions?(LO 10.4)
    a. Bacteriostatic water for injection
    b. Purified water
    c. Sodium chloride injection
    d. All of the above
18. Which of the following may be a site of application for an aerosol?(LO 10.1)
    a. Mouth
    b. Nose
    c. Skin
    d. All of the above
19. Which of the following may be used as a base for a suppository?(LO 10.2)
    a. Cocoa butter
    b. Glycerin
    c. PEG
    d. All of the above
20. How many phases are found in an emulsion?(LO 10.3)
    a. One
    b. Two
    c. Three
    d. Four

True/False

Print *T* for True or *F* for False for each statement. If a statement is false, correct it to make it true.

_______ 1. Ophthalmic medications are sterile preparations.(LO 10.2)

_______ 2. An MDI is used with IVs.(LO 10.3)

_______ 3. Parenteral products must be pyrogen-free.(LO 10.2)

_______ 4. CR capsules are also called ER capsules.(LO 10.2)

_______ 5. Enteric-coated and extended-release dosage forms are the same.(LO 10.2)

_______ 6. Elixirs are clear in appearance.(LO 10.2)

_______ 7. All elixirs contain a medication.(LO 10.2)

_______ 8. Film-coated tablets are the same as sugar-coated tablets.(LO 10.2)

_______ 9. A large-volume parenteral contains a volume of 50 mL or more.(LO 10.2)

_______ 10. A sublingual tablet is placed between the gum and the cheek.(LO 10.2)

Abbreviations

Print the word or phrase for the following dosage abbreviations.

cap ____________________
emul ____________________
MDI ____________________
pulv ____________________
sol ____________________
supp ____________________
susp ____________________
syr ____________________
tab ____________________
ung ____________________

Critical Thinking Questions

1. A patient brings in the following prescription:

   Phenergan 25 mg tab #12

   i tab po q4-6 h prn nausea and vomiting

   a. What might you question about this prescription?(LO 10.1)

   b. How might this situation be resolved?(LO 10.2)

2. A mother brings in the following prescription for her 4-year-old son. What concern do you have about this prescription?(LO 10.3)

   Amoxil 250 mg #30

   i tab po tid

3. A patient brings in a prescription for Antabuse. While waiting for the prescription, the patient asks you if he or she can purchase a bottle of elixir of terpin hydrate with codeine. What is the potential problem with this situation?(LO 10.3)

4. What auxiliary label should be affixed to a bottle containing a suspension?(LO 10.3)

HIPAA Scenario

Joannie's roommate, Karen, is a pharmacy technician at the pharmacy where Joannie routinely fills her prescriptions. One day Karen sees that Joannie's doctor has phoned in a prescription for birth control pills for her. Karen fills the prescription and takes it home. Over dinner she mentions what she has done, thinking she has done Joannie a favor by saving her a trip to the pharmacy. Joannie becomes livid, telling Karen that she has no right to violate her privacy. Stunned, Karen leaves the table and vows never to do a favor for Joannie again.

Discussion Questions(PTCB II. 73)

1. Is Joannie right to be angry with Karen for filling her prescription?)
2. Would Joannie have a case if she were to report Karen to her supervisor for invasion of privacy and violation of HIPAA law?
3. Should Karen have filled Joannie's prescription?

Internet Activities

1. Use the Internet to find out what requirements the Center for Biologics Evaluation and Research has established for biological products.(LO 10.2)
2. Search the FDA Office of Biotechnology's Web site for any recently approved or pending biotechnology products. What are they and what is their indication?(LO 10.1)

Extemporaneous and Sterile Compounding (IV Admixture)

11

Learning Outcomes

Upon completion of this chapter, you will be able to:

11.1 Define *extemporaneous compounding.*

11.2 Define *sterile compounding.*

11.3 Identify types of products produced by sterile compounding.

11.4 Identify pharmacy settings where nonsterile compounding occurs.

11.5 Identify common pharmacy equipment or supplies used in extemporaneous compounding.

11.6 Articulate which types of preparations must be prepared using aseptic technique and which do not require aseptic technique.

11.7 Identify pharmacy settings where sterile compounding occurs.

11.8 Define *aseptic technique.*

11.9 Describe how aseptic technique relates to infection control.

11.10 Explain and describe cleaning and use of the laminar flow hood.

11.11 Describe the use of personal protective equipment in sterile compounding.

11.12 Identify the regulations associated with sterile compounding.

Key Terms

alligation
aseptic technique
extemporaneous compounding
infection control
IV
IV piggyback
laminar flow hood
levigation
reconstitution
sepsis
sterile compounding
TPN
triturate
USP<797>

PTCB

In preparation for the certification examination, you should understand and perform activities associated with the following PTCB Knowledge Statements:

PTCB Knowledge Statement

Domain I. Assisting the Pharmacist in Serving Patients

Knowledge of practice site policies and procedures regarding prescriptions or medication orders (20)

Knowledge of procedures to prepare IV admixtures (55)

Knowledge of procedures to prepare total parenteral nutrition (57)

Knowledge of procedures to prepare reconstituted injectable medications (58)

Knowledge of aseptic technique (65)

Knowledge of infection control procedures (66)

Case Study

Marcos, CPhT, has been the senior pharmacy technician at ABC Infusion Services for the past 5 years. ABC Infusion Services provides intravenous medications and TPNs for patients who receive the medications at home. Nurses assist patients at home with medication administration. As the senior technician, Marcos oversees four other pharmacy technicians and works closely with the pharmacists and drivers. Marcos is responsible for checking the laminar flow hoods and doing microbiologic studies in the sterile compounding area, as well as IV admixture. Yesterday, during a busy period, Marcos noticed that the newest technician, Jack, placed the labels to be adhered to the IV bags in the hood to speed processing. Jack also likes to keep a pen in the hood so he can easily initial his work.

While reading this chapter, keep the following questions in mind:

1. Is Jack using proper aseptic technique?(LO 11.2, 11.8)
2. What are the potential risks that can occur?(LO 11.9, 11.10)
3. What is Marcos's responsibility as the senior technician?(LO 11.9, 11.12)
4. What should Marcos do?(LO 11.9)

Introduction to Compounding(LO 11.1, 11.2)

Compounding is the manufacture of medicinal agents by the pharmacy technician or pharmacist. Although the majority of medications today arrive from the manufacturer in a form for direct administration to patients, compounding has again become a significant portion of modern pharmacy practice. Compounding allows for dosage and dosage form administration to be tailored to the patient, resulting in individualized therapy. Compounding may also be necessary when a particular pharmaceutical agent is not stable in its final form and must be compounded for administration immediately prior to dispensing for administration. Compounding may be described as either extemporaneous (nonsterile) or sterile compounding. **Aseptic technique** is the process used in sterile compounding that reduces the risk of contamination and helps ensure the sterility of a product.

Extemporaneous compounding or nonsterile compounding is the manufacture of a medication for administration that does not require aseptic technique. An example of a dosage form or medication that is compounded in this manner is a cream for topical application. The pharmacy technician and pharmacist should still wear gloves and follow techniques to limit the contamination of the product.

In recent years, there has been an increase in extemporaneous compounding as prescribers in specialty areas (such as dermatology) are requiring more individualized pharmacologic therapy for their patients.

Sterile compounding is the manufacture of pharmaceutical products in a sterile environment requiring the use of aseptic technique to help ensure the absence of pathogens and contaminates. These products are not available in the form for patient administration or are unstable and must be prepared immediately prior to administration to the patient. Proper aseptic technique allows for the maintenance of product sterility. As sterile compounds are free of pathogens and contaminants,

aseptic technique Process that reduces the risk of contamination and helps ensure the sterility of a product.

extemporaneous compounding The manufacture of pharmaceutical products in a nonsterile environment.

sterile compounding The manufacture of pharmaceutical products in an sterile environment.

At Your Service

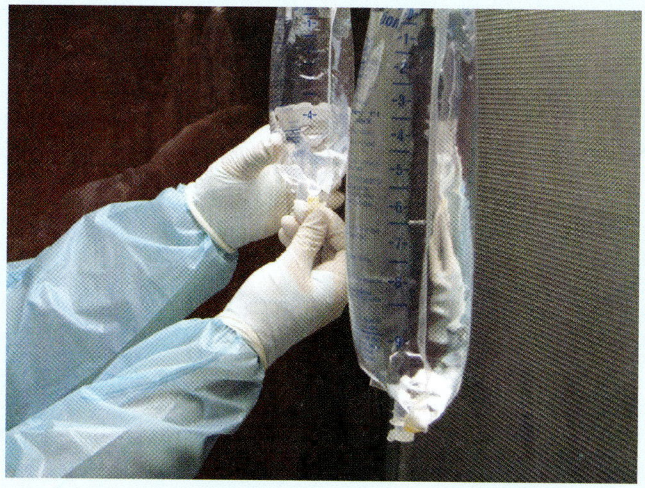

Pat is a pharmacy technician at Community Medical Center. She often prepares intravenous admixture products, including total parenteral nutrition (TPN) and chemotherapy. Pat recently received a written order from the nurses' station for IV hydration fluids for a patient. It does not take Pat much time to prepare the IV. A nurse comes from the nurses' station asking if the IV is ready for the patient. The nurse says the patient needs it right away and does not understand why Pat will not hand her the prepared IV until after the pharmacist checks it. After all, Pat is a very experienced technician. The nurse says she will check the IV before she gives it to the patient anyway.

While reading this chapter, keep the following questions in mind.

1. Is the nurse right or wrong? Explain.(LO 11.3)
2. How should Pat respond to the nurse?(LO 11.12)
3. What should Pat do?(LO 11.12)

special care must be taken to preserve the sterility of these compounds for administration to patients. This chapter will discuss major aspects of sterile compounding as they pertain to the responsibilities and duties of the pharmacy technician.

Exemporaneous Compounding(LO 11.1, 11.4, 11.5, 11.6)

Extemporaneous compounding is the manufacture of pharmaceutical products in a nonsterile environment. Nonsterile compounding often involves the preparation of tablets, capsules, lotions, or ointments when sterile preparation is not necessary because the medication is not being administered via a route where sterile compounding is required (Figure 11-1).

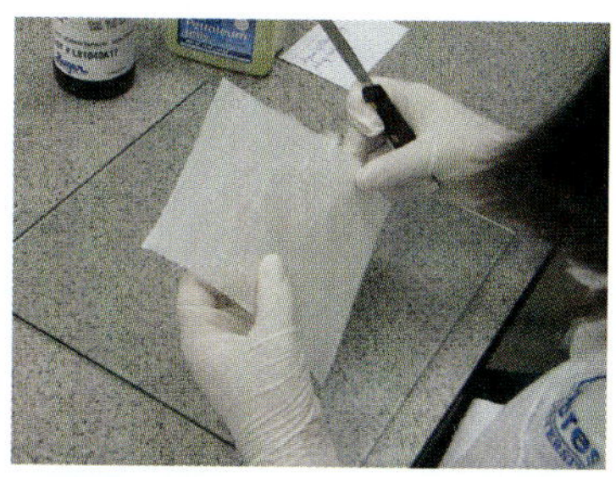

Figure 11-1 Compounding equipment and supplies.

Dosage forms that may be compounded using the extemporaneous method include:

- Capsules
- Creams
- Gels
- Lotions
- Ointments
- Pastes
- Soaps
- Solutions

- Suppositories
- Tablets
- Wet dressings

Pharmacy technicians may perform extemporaneous compounding in either outpatient or inpatient settings, with an increasing number working in pharmacies that specialize in compounding. It is important for the pharmacy technician to remember that although an aseptic environment may not be required for extemporaneous compounding, it is still desirable. The pharmacy technician must make every effort to prepare a product that is free from contaminants of any kind.

> **Caution**
>
> The pharmacy technician should always wear gloves while compounding a medication to limit the risk of contamination of the product prior to dispensing.

Equipment and Tools

In order for pharmacy technicians to be proficient in extemporaneous compounding, they must be familiar with the equipment and supplies commonly used in compounding. The proper use, care, and cleaning of the equipment is also a responsibility of pharmacy technicians, and is critical for the proper preparation of the compounded product to avoid adulteration and contamination. Examples of compounding equipment include the mortar and pestle and the Class A balance (Figure 11-2). Supplies are items that are used in compounding, but are disposable and are usually used only once. Gelatin capsules and waxed paper are examples of supplies employed in extemporaneous compounding. Table 11-1 (p. 299) lists common types of equipment and supplies used in extemporaneous compounding.

Extemporaneous Compounding Techniques

Although the pharmacy technician will be required to compound various types of preparations, two common techniques are outlined below as examples of methods for extemporaneous compounding. The following technique will provide guidance for the pharmacy technician in compounding.

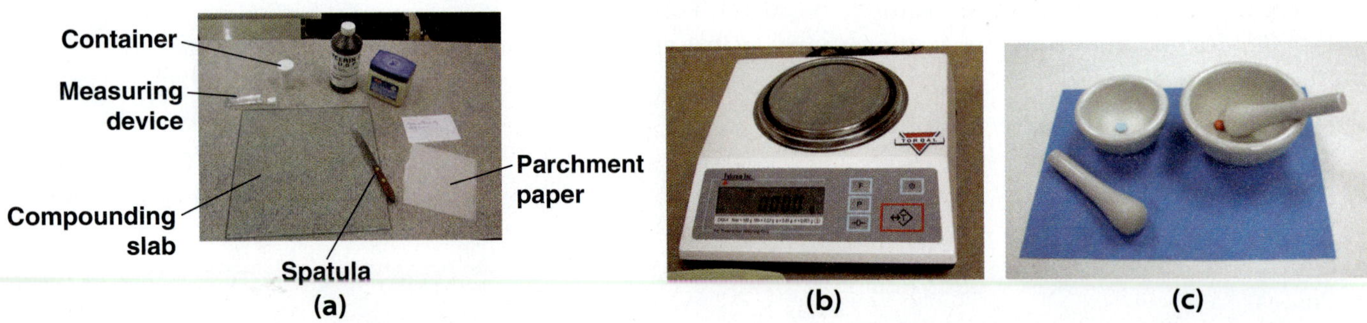

Figure 11-2 (*a*) Compounding slab, spatula, parchment paper, container, and measuring device. (*b*) Balance. (*c*) Mortar and pestle.

Table 11-1 Common Equipment and Supplies Used for Extemporaneous Compounding

Equipment	Supplies
Class A balance	Suppository molds
Pipette	Filters
Mortar and pestle	Parchment paper
Spatula	Gelatin capsules
Graduated cylinders	Containers
Beakers	Labels
Bunsen burner	Syringes
Compounding slab	Weighing papers
Thermometers	Flasks

Preparation of an Ointment (Figure 11-3)

1. Read the prescription.
2. Consult the pharmacist if you are unsure of any part of the prescription, especially the quantities of the various components.
3. Perform any necessary calculations and recheck while reviewing the prescription.
4. Gather all of the necessary active and inactive ingredients.
5. Gather all necessary equipment, including a mortar and pestle, balance, ointment slab, parchment paper, spatula, and container.
6. Weigh the appropriate amount of solid powder on the Class A balance. Set aside.
7. Weigh the appropriate amount of ointment base on balance. Set aside.(See Figure a)
8. Using the mortar and pestle, **triturate** the solid particles until they exhibit a fine, powdery consistency. This will aid in the incorporation into the ointment.(See Figure b)
9. Using a spatula and ointment slab, slowly incorporate small amounts of the powder into the ointment base to ensure even and complete incorporation (**levigation**).(See Figure c)

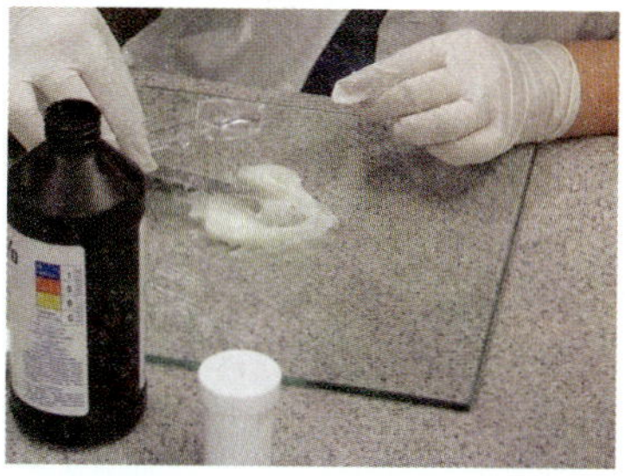

Figure 11-3 Extemporaneous (nonsterile) compounding of an ointment.

triturate To crush or grind solid particles using a mortar and pestle to decrease particle size for ease of incorporation into a compounded preparation.

levigation The gradual circular motion used to incorporate solid particles into a diluent.

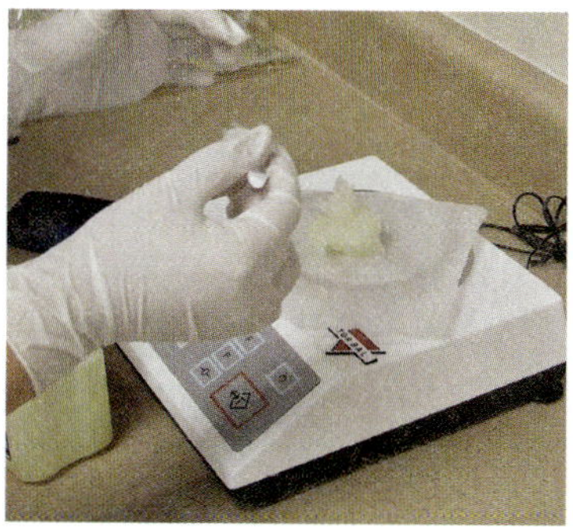

(a)

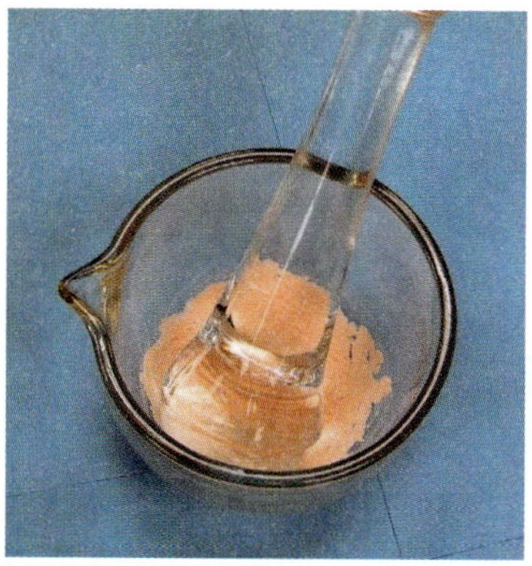

(b)

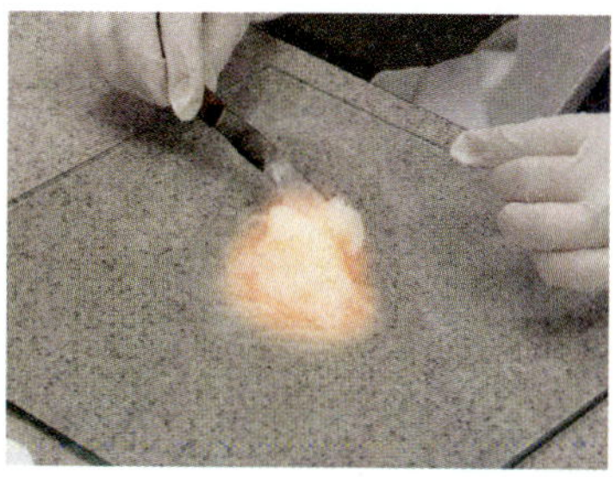

(c)

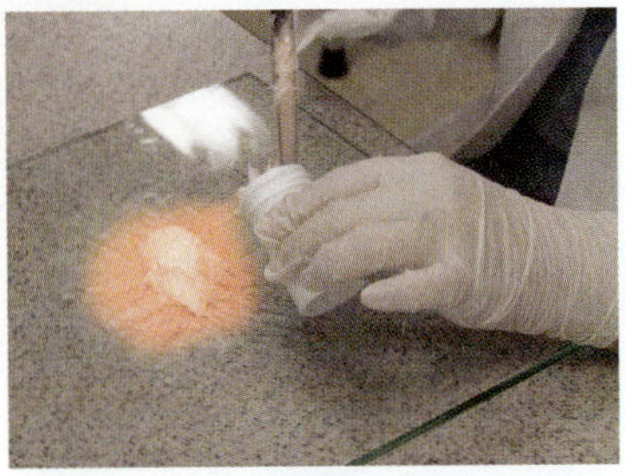
(d)

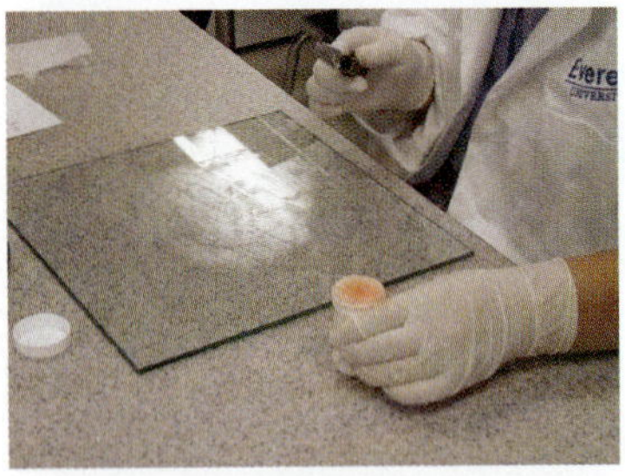
(e)

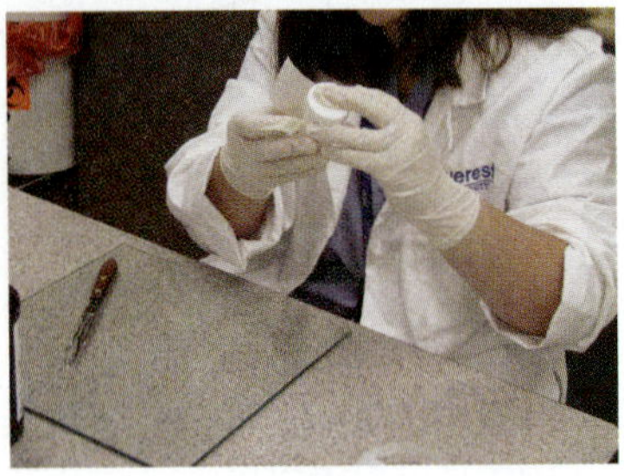
(f)

10. Using a spatula, take the container for dispensing and insert the ointment, first lining the walls of the container with the ointment, and then filling in the middle.(See Figure d)
11. Tap the filled container gently to remove air pockets. Gently "finish" by incorporating ointment high on the insides of the container into the center of the container, providing a cleaner appearance.(See Figure e)
12. Move the spatula in a circular motion gently over the top of the ointment to enhance appearance.
13. Close the container, affix the label, and affix appropriate auxiliary labels. For example: "For external use only."(See Figure f)
14. Keep all source containers and calculations handy for the pharmacist to check.
15. Thoroughly clean and store equipment.

Preparation of Suppositories

1. Read the prescription.
2. Consult the pharmacist if you are unsure of any part of the prescription, especially the quantities of the various components.
3. Perform any necessary calculations and recheck while reviewing the prescription.
4. Gather all of the necessary active and inactive ingredients.
5. Gather all necessary equipment, including a mortar and pestle, balance, beaker, magnetic stirrer, electric hot plate, parchment paper, spatula, and disposable suppository strip molds.
6. If the prescription indicates that a solid substance is to be incorporated into the dosage form, weigh the appropriate amount of solid powder on the Class A balance. Set aside.
7. Decrease the particle size of the solid by triturating to a fine powder using a mortar and pestle.
8. Carefully melt the suppository base using a beaker and hot plate.
9. Slowly incorporate the solid particles into the melted base to ensure even distribution.
10. Allow the mixture to cool slightly (but not to the point of solidification) and slowly pour into the suppository molds.
11. Allow to cool completely. Refrigeration may be required.
12. Affix a label to the container for the suppositories.
13. Affix the appropriate auxiliary labels. For example: "For rectal use only" or "Refrigerate."
14. Leave calculations and all materials available to the pharmacist for checking.
15. Thoroughly clean and store equipment.

Caution

When compounding, it is advisable to double-check your calculations and the process with the pharmacist prior to completing the compounded product to avoid errors and waste.

Tech Check

1. List three pieces of equipment that may be used in compounding.(LO 11.5)
2. List three types of supplies that may be used in compounding.(LO 11.5)
3. Which item is always used while compounding, regardless of the product?(LO 11.11)
4. Compounding should always begin with ______.(LO 11.1, 11.2)

Sterile Compounding(LO 11.2, 11.3, 11.6, 11.7, 11.8, 11.9, 11.10, 11.12)

Sterile compounding is the manufacture of pharmaceutical products using aseptic technique. Products prepared using sterile compounding include intravenous admixture (TPN, **IV piggybacks, IV** infusions, prefilled syringes for IV push), irrigation solutions, and ophthalmic preparations (Figure 11-3).

Sterile compounding results in a product that is free from microorganisms (like bacteria), pyrogens (fever-producing agents), and other contaminants (like particulate matter).

ASHP (American Society of Health-System Pharmacists) guidelines indicate that the pharmacy is responsible for making sure all products prepared using sterile compounding are:

- Therapeutically and pharmaceutically appropriate
- Free from microbial and pyrogenic contaminants
- Free from particulate and toxic contaminants
- Made up of the correct amounts of the prescribed agents
- Properly labeled, distributed, and stored

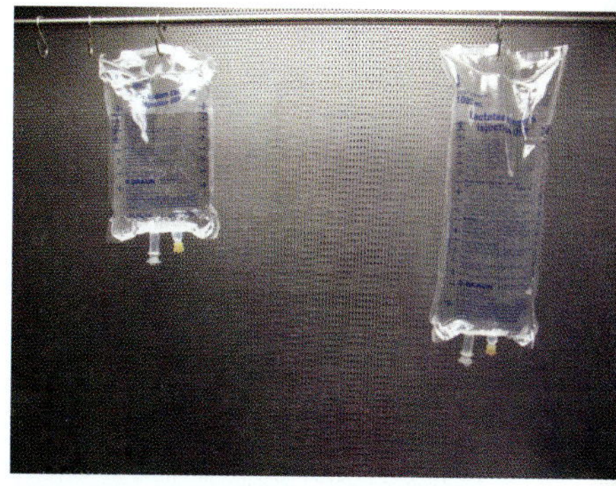

Figure 11-4 IV solutions.

The stability of the preparation must be considered in the compounding. Some items need to be protected from light, and are therefore delivered to the floor in a light-resistant bag with an auxiliary label indicating that the preparation needs to be protected from light. Some items may require refrigeration or freezing prior to and/or after compounding. In the preparation of sterile products, it is also important to consider that certain combinations of products are incompatible and may result in a precipitate. After compounding clear IV solutions, the technician must check for a precipitate by holding the bag up to a light source and by using a black and white panel for visual inspection.

Sterile compounding is no longer limited to the hospital or inpatient setting. Compounding pharmacies are often equipped to provide both nonsterile and sterile compounded products. Home infusion service pharmacies and long-term care pharmacies also have facilities to do sterile compounding. Pharmacy technicians are responsible for every aspect of sterile compounding except for the final check of the product. Although the pharmacist has responsibility of the final check, the technician should check his or her own work prior to having the pharmacist review it.

Medication routes requiring sterile compounding are:

- Intra-arterial
- Intracardiac

IV piggyback Small-volume intravenous medication (usually containing an antibiotic) that is added on to an existing catheter site through the tubing.

IV Intravenous, intravenously; medication administration into the vein.

- Intradermal
- Intramuscular
- Intrathecal
- Intravenous (may be administered IV piggyback, IV infusion, or IV push)
- Ophthalmic
- Subcutaneous

Role of the Pharmacy Technician

The pharmacy technician is responsible for preparing and sorting labels; filling the medication order; checking the generated label against the prescription; performing necessary calculations (including **alligation** when needed); retrieving the needed drugs, diluents, equipment, and supplies from stock; employing aseptic technique in the preparation of the medication; checking for particulate matter; and affixing the label to the packaging. After the pharmacist provides the final check, the technician may deliver the compounded products to the nurses' station. The pharmacy technician is also responsible for maintaining stock and supplies, dispensing records, and for ensuring proper storage of medications, as well as cleaning and maintenance of the **laminar flow hood** and other pharmacy equipment and documentation of such.

Tech Check

5. According to the ASHP, the pharmacy is responsible to ensure that sterile compounded products are ________.(LO 11.12)

6. List three routes of administration requiring sterile compounding.(LO 11.6)

Equipment used in Sterile Compounding

There are many types of equipment the pharmacy technician will need to use to perform sterile compounding using aseptic technique. Types of equipment can be divided into disposable items (such as personal protective equipment, needles, and syringes, tubing) and nondisposable items (such as laminar flow hoods and automated IV compounding equipment). Tables 11-2 and 11-3 identify equipment and solutions commonly used in sterile compounding.

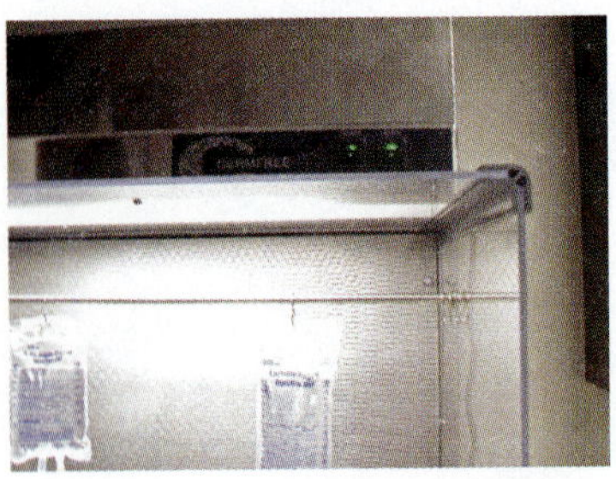

Figure 11-5 Laminar flow hood.

The laminar flow hood uses a HEPA filter through which jets of airflow keep contamination from settling onto and into the products being combined for the final compounded product (Figure 11-5).

The airflow in laminar flow hoods is either horizontal or vertical. Horizontal laminar flow is effective for sterile compounding using nonhazardous drugs or substances. The horizontal flow of air comes outward from the back of the cabinet out toward the pharmacy technician preparing items in the hood. The horizontal flow of air limits the contact of pathogens that may have been introduced into the hood by the pharmacy technician to the products in the hood. The pharmacy technician must still use proper aseptic technique while working in the hood to ensure that the final product is sterile.

Vertical flow hoods have air jets flowing down from the top of the hood. They are used to decrease contamination that may be introduced by the

alligation Mathematical method to determine the respective percentages of a compounded product.

laminar flow hood Apparatus used in sterile compounding that employs air jets to assist in providing a sterile environment.

Table 11-2 Equipment and Supplies Used in Sterile Compounding

Nondisposable Item	Disposable Item
Automated pumps	70% isopropyl alcohol
Laminar flow hood	Alcohol pads
TPN admixture machine	Evacuation containers
	Filtered needles
	IV bags
	Low-lint disposable towels
	Mini-spike
	Needles
	Personal protective equipment (gloves, gowns, masks, hair covers, shoe covers)
	Syringe caps
	Syringes
	Transfer needles
	Tubing

Table 11-3 Common Intravenous Solutions

1/2NS	Half Normal Saline (0.45% NaCl)
D10NS	10% dextrose in normal saline
D10W	10% dextrose in water
D5/1/2NS	5% dextrose in 0.45% NaCl
D5/NS	5% dextrose in normal saline
D5W	5% dextrose in water
LR	Lactated Ringer's Solution
NS	Normal saline (0.9% NaCl)

pharmacy technician and also to protect the technician from particles from the substances used in compounding. Vertical flow hoods also have a protective glass shield that descends from the top of the cabinet to provide further protection to the pharmacy technician. As with the horizontal flow hood, proper aseptic technique must be employed to ensure sterility of the final product. The technician handling hazardous substances must be aware of proper storage, handling, and disposal of hazardous substances. In instances where a technician is handling a hazardous substance in compounding, he or she should wear two pairs of gloves, with the inner pair placed with the cuffs under the gown, and the outer pair with cuffs over the outside of the cuff of the gown. Any spills are to be cleaned up immediately, with disposal of contaminated towels, gowns, or gloves in the properly marked hazardous disposal bags, which are placed in marked, closed containers. Vertical laminar flow hoods are used in the compounding of chemotherapeutic agents. Refer to Chapter 2 for information on the handling, storage, and disposal of hazardous substances.

The pharmacy technician is responsible for the care and cleaning of the laminar flow hood.

- The laminar flow hood must be turned on for at least 30 minutes prior to sterile compounding.
- The hood is to be cleaned thoroughly, including the side Plexiglas panels and the horizontal surface with 70% isopropyl alcohol and low-lint disposable towels.
- It is important that the surface is completely dry prior to compounding, as it is in the drying of the alcohol that pathogens are eliminated.

Other nondisposable equipment includes compounding machines for TPN compounding and other IV additive machines. Proper care and maintenance of the machines are important to ensure the accuracy and sterility of the product. These machines are placed within the laminar flow hood and must be cleaned prior to placement into the hood.

Disposable equipment includes equipment used in the preparation of the product and equipment used to decrease contamination of the product or the pharmacy technician. Disposable equipment, like syringes and needles, are used only once to reduce contamination. The re-using of needles may cause contamination and coring (pieces of the rubber seal on the vial being introduced into the product). The pharmacy technician may want to use a mini-spike if medication needs to be removed from a vial multiple times.

Figure 11-6 Gauges of needles.

Several types of needles are used in sterile compounding. There are regular needles, vented needles that allow for the transfer of air, and filtered needles that allow for filtration of particles. The gauge of the needle refers to the size of the bore (diameter, or the opening through which drug is initially drawn). Note that the lower the gauge number, the larger the size of the bore (Figure 11-6).

Techniques Used in Sterile Compounding (LO 11.7, 11.8, 11.9, 11.10, 11.11)

Aseptic Technique

As mentioned previously, proper aseptic technique is required to produce sterile compounded products. The primary way the pathogen contamination is reduced is through proper handwashing technique, although gloves will be worn during compounding. The reason hands are washed is that every article that is touched is at risk for contamination, including personal protective equipment (Figure 11-7a, b).

Proper technique for sterile compounding begins with cleaning the laminar flow hood, while wearing a closed front gown, gloves, mask, and hair cover. All surfaces to be punctured are to be wiped with 70% isopropyl alcohol wipes. If wipes are not available, 70% isopropyl alcohol spray can be applied to the rubber seals or ampule necks and allowed to dry (Figure 11-8).

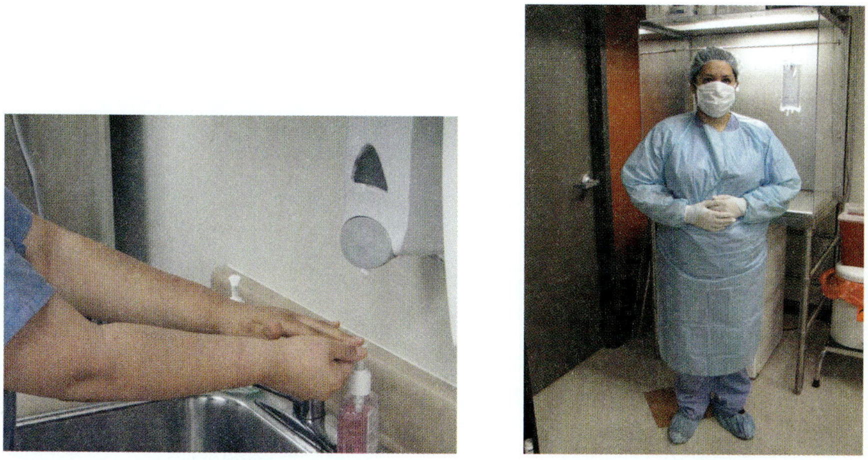

(a) (b)

Figure 11-7 (*a*) Hand washing. (*b*) Personal protective equipment.

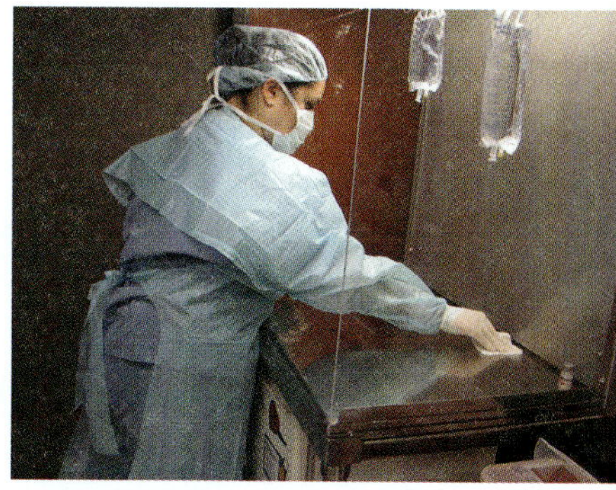

Figure 11-8 Cleaning the hood.

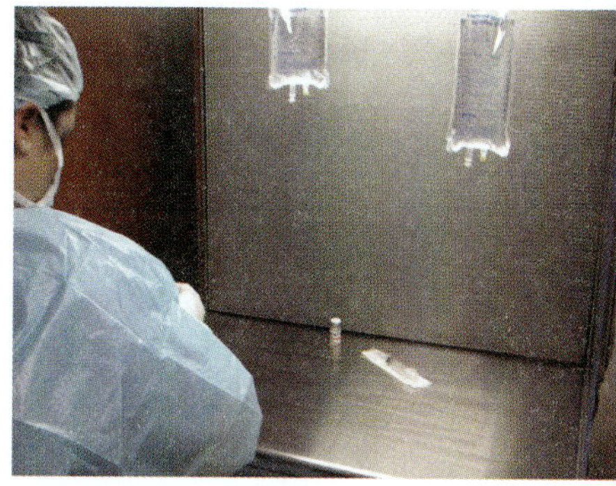

Figure 11-9 Placement of items inside hood.

When working in the laminar flow hood, make sure you are working at least 6 inches into the hood.

It is important to remember to preserve an unobstructed flow of air in the laminar flow hood. This means larger items should not be placed directly behind shorter items because this will interfere with airflow contact. Do not arrange vials in such a way that they are touching each other. This will interfere with the proper flow of the air jets, and increase the risk of contamination (Figure 11-9).

IV Additive Solutions

Intravenous additive solutions involve an agent being injected into a high-volume IV bag for administration to a patient. In a clean hood, with all puncture ports cleaned with alcohol (Figure 11-10) and supplies ready, the technician will draw up an amount of air equal to the amount of additive to be injected into the solution. The air is injected into the additive. The vial containing the additive is inverted and the specified volume is removed by pulling back the plunger (Figure 11-11). The needle is removed and the agent is added to the IV bag (Figure 11-12). A seal is placed over the injection port, and the technician checks for particles and precipitates by holding the bag up toward the light and in front of a white and black panel. The label is then placed on the bag.

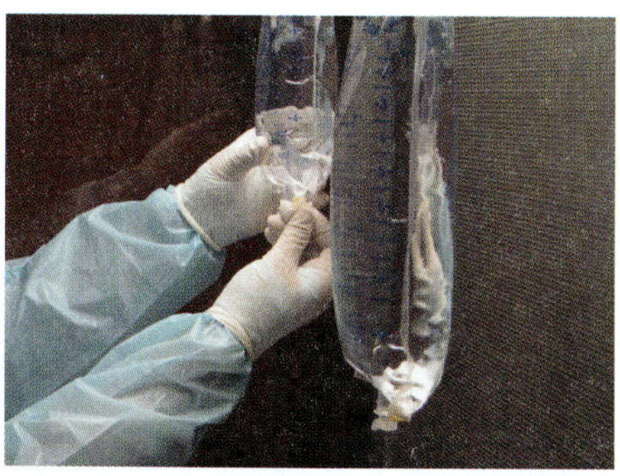

Figure 11-10 Puncture port cleaned with alcohol.

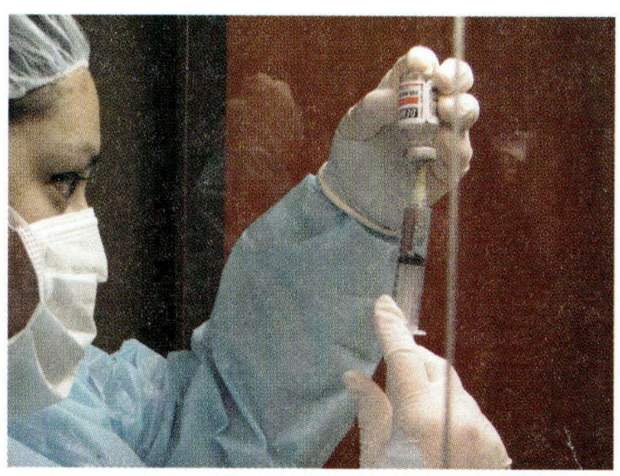

Figure 11-11 Liquid agent is removed from vial.

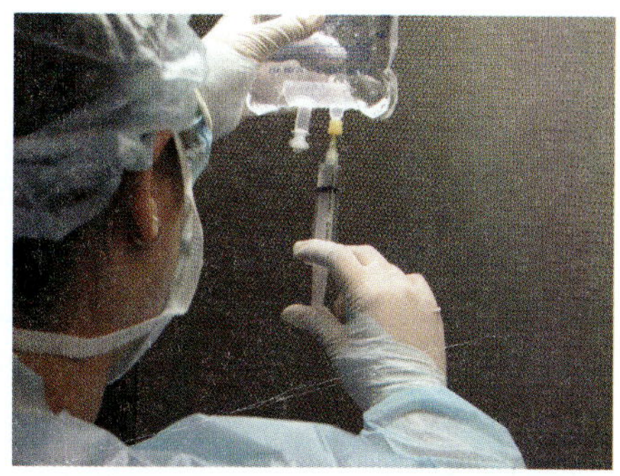

Figure 11-12 Agent is added to IV bag.

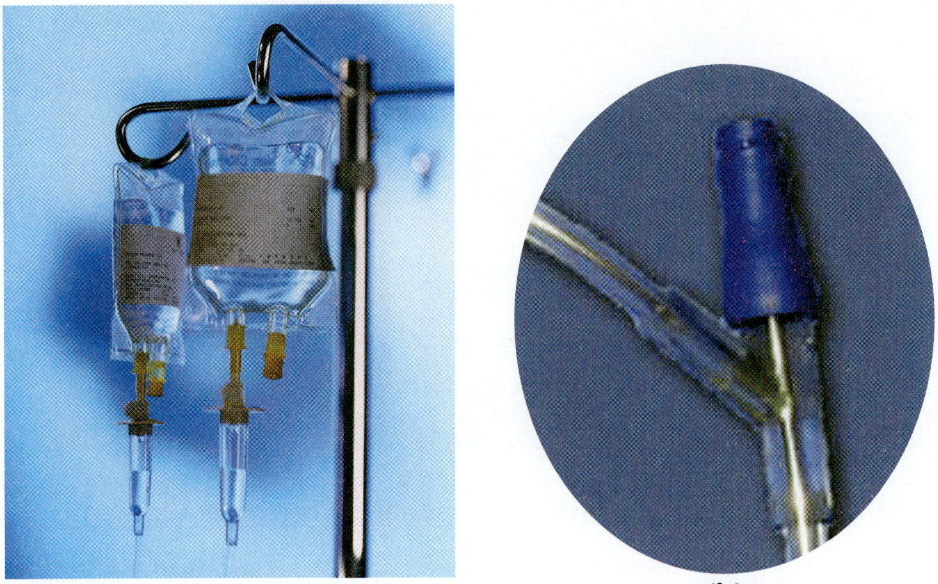

(a) (b)

Figure 11-13 *(a)* **IV piggyback solutions.** *(b)* **Y-site in tubing.**

IV piggyback solutions involve addition of agents, usually antibiotics, to small-volume solutions, ranging from 50 to 100 mL. IV piggyback solutions are introduced into an existing catheter site at a fork (y-site) in the tubing (Figure 11-13a, b).

When transferring liquid from an ampule to an IV bag, a filtered needle must be used to avoid the inclusion of glass particles. Coring (rubber particle introduction into the vial) may be limited by placing the needle, beveled side up at a 45° angle to touch the target entry point and then raised to a 90° angle to puncture the rubber seal. When transferring any solutions, do not touch the shaft of the plunger, as pathogens can be introduced into the solution.

See Tables 11-4 and 11-5 for a list of aseptic technique "do's and don'ts."

Caution

Remember to check the medication order and label carefully before you begin compounding. Double-check calculations to verify that the appropriate amount of agent is added. As with nonsterile compounding, review calculations and procedures prior to compounding to save materials and time.

Infection Control

All members of the health care team must be engaged in **infection control.** Awareness of infection control is critical when medications are being compounded for entry directly into a patient's vein. **Sepsis,** an infection in the bloodstream, can result if infection control guidelines are not followed. Universal precautions apply to any person who may come into contact with blood and other body fluids. The primary means of infection control is proper hand-washing technique. Hands must be washed before donning

infection control Methods to decrease contamination and disease due to pathogens.

sepsis Bacterial infection disseminated in the bloodstream.

Table 11-4 List of Aseptic Technique "Do's"

Do . . .
Clean the laminar flow hood at the beginning of each shift and document its cleaning.
Wash hands thoroughly often even though you are wearing gloves.
Change gloves often.
Gather all needed pharmaceuticals, syringes, diluents, and other equipment prior to beginning the compound.
Compound one order at a time to avoid errors.
Spray gloves with 70% isopropyl alcohol and let them dry in the hood prior to compounding. Repeat periodically throughout your shift.
Wear a hair cover and keep hair away from compounding area.
Dispose of syringes and needles in a covered sharps container.
Check for particulate matter prior to labeling clear solutions using black and white panels.
Wear a gown with a closed front.
Clean all articles placed in laminar flow hood with 70% isopropyl alcohol.
Remove torn gloves and soiled personal protective equipment immediately.

Table 11-5 List of Aseptic Technique "Don'ts"

Do Not . . .
Do not wear excessive jewelry or cosmetics while performing sterile compounding.
Do not speak, cough, or sneeze into the hood.
Do not attempt to remove or clean the HEPA filter in the laminar flow hood.
Do not wear artificial nails or chipped nail polish.
Do not place pens, labels, or other papers in the hood.
Do not eat or drink or bring food into the compounding area.
Do not re-cap, crush, or break needles.
Do not block the flow of air from the laminar flow hood.
Do not re-use needles or syringes.
Do not work in the laminar flow hood without wearing gloves.
Do not break ampules using bare hands.
Do not continue to wear soiled personal protective equipment (gowns) after spills.

gloves and after their removal. Gloves must be worn to protect against contamination. In the event of a tear in the gloves, they must be removed immediately. The hands are then washed again, and a new pair of gloves is donned. It is important to remember that universal precautions are designed to guard against the spread of infection, whether from patient to

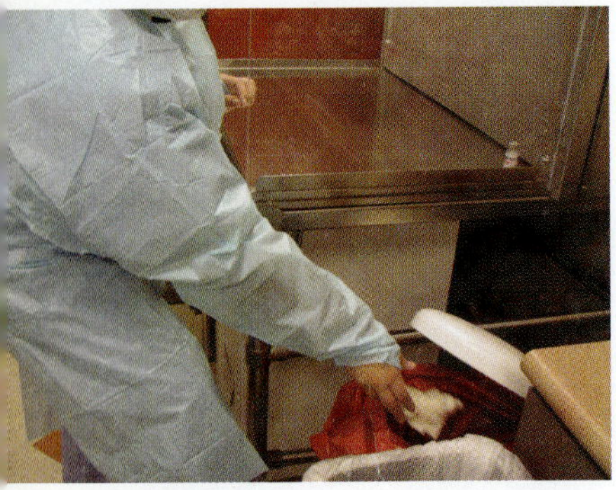

Figure 11-14 Disposing of gloves in biohazardous waste bag.

health care professional, or the other way around. If a pharmacy technician accidently sticks himself with a needle while working in the laminar flow hood and begins to bleed, it presents a risk to any patient who receives medications compounded in that contaminated environment. Any gloves, gowns, or other equipment soiled with blood or body fluids should be disposed of in a biohazardous waste bag (Figure 11-14).

Reconstitution

Reconstitution is the dissolving of a powder in a diluent. In sterile compounding, reconstitution requires the use of sterile water for injection to be introduced into the vial of powder to be dissolved. The plunger of the syringe is pulled back to the volume of diluent needed for the reconstitution. This volume of air is injected into the sterile water for injection, allowing for easy withdrawal of an equal amount of diluent. The diluent is then injected into the powder to be reconstituted. An equal amount of air is withdrawn from the vial to equalize the pressure. The vial is shaken (depending on the directions) and the resulting solution is ready to be added to a higher volume IV solution.

Total Parenteral Nutrition (TPN)

Total parenteral nutrition (**TPN**) is synonymous with IV feeding. TPN is used when a patient cannot obtain adequate nutrition via oral feeding consisting primarily of dextrose, amino acids, and lipids (fat). TPN is highly individualized, and is based upon a patient's caloric requirements, extent of disease, existing conditions, and catheter site. Following the aseptic technique for all sterile compounding, additives to the TPN are introduced to the dextrose, as it is clear and can be checked for particles and precipitates. Other agents are often added to the TPN, like multiple vitamins and minerals. Amino acids are added to the dextrose mixture. The lipids are the final large volume added. It is critical that the pharmacy technician know the protocol in his or her institution.

Chemotherapy

All of the same sterile compounding with aseptic techniques are employed while preparing chemotherapy. There are a few differences, however.

- The vertical laminar flow hood is used.
- The pharmacy technician should wear two pairs of gloves. In the event that the outer pair becomes contaminated, the gloves can be removed without allowing contact between the chemotherapeutic agents and the skin.
- The technician lays a sterile gauze pad on the floor of the hood to set items on as it facilitates cleaning up any spills.
- The sharps container is located inside the hood to contain any dispersal of hazardous particles.
- Personal protective equipment (masks, gloves, gowns) that becomes soiled while compounding chemotherapeutic agents should be removed immediately and disposed of in hazardous waste bags.

reconstitution The addition of a diluent (usually sterile water) to dissolve or suspend a powder in a liquid.

TPN Total parenteral nutrition, also known as hyperalimentation; nutritional support (calories, protein, multivitamins) administered intravenously.

Seals are placed on the IV bags that are then placed into marked chemotherapy bags along with auxiliary labels indicating chemotherapeutic contents. Chemotherapeutic agents require special handling, and are delivered to the floor separate from other IV products.

Tech Check

7. When cleaning the laminar flow hood, it is important to clean the _________.(LO 11.10)
8. The use of black and white panels or screens after IV admixture is to _________.(LO 11.12)
9. List the major components of TPN.(LO 11.3, 11.6)
10. List three "Do's" for pharmacy technicians when performing sterile compounding.(LO 11.9, 11.10, 11.11)
11. List three "Don'ts" for pharmacy technicians when performing sterile compounding.(LO 11.9, 11.10, 11.11)

Agencies/Regulations Governing Sterile Compounding

On January 1, 2004, the *United States Pharmacopeia* published **USP<797>,** a set of official and enforceable regulations governing sterile compounding. As adherence to USP <797> is a requirement, it is enforced by boards of pharmacy (BOP), The Joint Commission (TJC), formerly Joint Commission on Accreditation of Healthcare Organizations (JCAHO), the Food and Drug Administration (FDA), and other regulatory agencies. USP <797> applies to any facility that performs sterile compounding. It also applies to any health care professional involved in handling sterile compounded products, including doctors, nurses, pharmacists, and pharmacy technicians. USP <797> is concerned with the following areas:

- Risk-level assessment
- Environmental quality control
- Process and preparation quality control
- Personnel training, competence, and performance

Source: ES Kastango: *The ASHP Discussion Guide for Compounding Sterile Preparations: Summary and Implementation of USP<797>*. Bethesda, MD: ASHP, 2005.

The pharmacy technician has many responsibilities with respect to sterile compounding. The use of universal precautions and aseptic technique are essential in the compounding of sterile products. Knowledge of USP <797> regulations is also important for the proper compounding of sterile products. The pharmacy technician must also be aware of the various types of products produced by sterile compounding and the specific issues that pertain to each product type.

Tech Check

12. _________ is an official and enforceable set of regulations pertaining specifically to sterile compounded products.(LO 11.12)

USP<797> First set of official and enforceable regulations involving sterile compounding.

Chapter Summary

Understanding the uses and procedures of sterile and nonsterile compounding is vital to the pharmacy technician. Important points to remember are:

- Compounding is the manufacture of pharmaceutical preparations and may involve both sterile and nonsterile methods.
- Dosage forms produced by nonsterile compounding are those used in situations where the risk of infection is low, and include agents for topical or external use, such as ointments or creams.
- Products produced by sterile compounding include intravenous and ophthalmic preparations, where the risk of infection to the patient is high.
- Pharmacy settings where sterile compounding occurs are not limited to institutions, but also include outpatient pharmacies that are properly equipped to prepare parenterally administered agents.
- Aseptic technique is utilized by health professionals to minimize the transfer of pathogens to the patient.
- As proper cleaning of the laminar flow hood is a critical element of infection control, its cleaning and maintenance must be documented and kept on file as part of the pharmacy's records.
- The proper use of personal protective equipment in sterile compounding is important to limit transfer of pathogens from the pharmacy technician into the product being compounded.
- USP <797> is a set of enforceable regulations that govern sterile compounding and the environments in which such activity can occur.

Chapter Review

Case Study Questions

1. Is Jack using proper aseptic technique?(LO 11.2, 11.8)
2. What are the potential risks that can occur?(LO 11.9, 11.10)
3. What is Marcos's responsibility as the senior technician?(LO 11.9, 11.12)
4. What should Marcos do?(LO 11.9)

At Your Service Questions

1. Is the nurse right or wrong? Explain.(LO 11.3)
2. How should Pat respond to the nurse?(LO 11.12)
3. What should Pat do?(LO 11.12)

Multiple Choice

1. Topical creams requiring compounding usually do *not* require ______(LO 11.6)
   a. laminar flow hood.
   b. accurate calculations.
   c. wearing gloves.
   d. cleaning equipment after use.
2. Levigation refers to ______(LO 11.5)
   a. increasing solid particle size.
   b. decreasing solid particle size.
   c. filtering solids from a liquid mixture.
   d. incorporating a solid into a diluent.
3. The pharmacy technician should always wear ______ while doing any type of compounding.(LO 11.5, 11.11)
   a. shoe covers
   b. gloves
   c. goggles
   d. none of the above

4. Which of the following is a type of supply for use in nonsterile compounding?(LO 11.5)
   a. Class A balance
   b. Beakers
   c. Flasks
   d. Syringes

5. Which of the following preparations requires sterile compounding?(LO 11.6)
   a. Capsules
   b. Creams
   c. Total parenteral nutrition
   d. Suppositories

6. The laminar flow hood must be on for at least ______ minutes prior to beginning sterile compounding.(LO 11.10)
   a. 15
   b. 30
   c. 45
   d. 60

7. The pharmacy technician must work at least ______ inches into the laminar flow hood.(LO 11.10)
   a. 6
   b. 12
   c. 18
   d. none of the above

8. ______ is used to clean the laminar flow hood and puncture points.(LO 11.9, 11.10)
   a. 0.9% NaCl
   b. 5% dextrose in water
   c. 70% isopropyl alcohol
   d. 0.45% NaCl

9. Which of the following would you least likely perform during proper aseptic technique?(LO 11.8)
   a. Use personal protective equipment
   b. Clean the hood
   c. Clean the filter of the hood
   d. Wash hands

10. Which of the following involves small volumes of IV fluids?(LO 11.3, 11.6)
    a. TPN
    b. Large-volume IV solutions
    c. IV piggyback solutions
    d. None of the above

11. Which of the following staff or personnel must meet USP <797> standards?(LO 11.12)
    a. Pharmacists
    b. Nurses
    c. Pharmacy technicians
    d. All of the above

12. Which of the following is *not* a route of administration requiring sterile compounding?(LO 11.3, 11.6)
    a. Intravenous
    b. Intramuscular
    c. Ophthalmic
    d. Intranasal

13. Which of the following is the same as intravenous feeding?(LO 11.3, 11.6)
    a. Chemotherapy
    b. IV piggyback
    c. Total parenteral nutrition
    d. Prefilled syringes

14. Which of the following agencies can enforce USP <797> regulations?(LO 11.12)
    a. Boards of pharmacy
    b. FDA
    c. TJC (formerly JCAHO)
    d. All of the above

15. Pharmacy technicians should wash hands______ (LO 11.9)
    a. before putting on gloves.
    b. after removing gloves.
    c. throughout the day while at work.
    d. all of the above.

16. Compounding always begins with______ (LO 11.1, 11.2)
    a. calculations.
    b. gathering all materials.
    c. weighing powders.
    d. reading the prescription.

17. Compounding always ends with______ (LO 11.5, 11.10)
    a. gathering all materials.
    b. doing calculations.
    c. typing the label.
    d. cleaning all equipment.

18. Pharmacy technicians contribute to infection control by ______ (LO 11.9)
    a. using aseptic technique.
    b. wearing gloves.
    c. properly cleaning the laminar flow hood.
    d. all of the above.

19. Which of the following best indicates intravenous feedings?(LO 11.3)
    a. Oral nutrition
    b. Total parenteral nutrition
    c. Enteral nutrition
    d. None of the above

20. Which of the following is compounded in a vertical laminar flow hood?(LO 11.3, 11.6)
    a. TPN
    b. IV piggyback
    c. Ointments
    d. Chemotherapeutic agents

Matching

Match the term with its appropriate definition.

_______ 1. Triturate

_______ 2. Levigate

_______ 3. Reconstitute

_______ 4. Compound

_______ 5. Aseptic

a. Incorporating a solid with a liquid

b. Decreasing particle size through grinding

c. Manufacturing a dosage form in a pharmacy setting

d. Absence of pathogens

e. Slow and even incorporation of solid particles into a base using circular motions

Critical Thinking Questions

1. If you observed someone using inappropriate aseptic technique, what would you do or say?(LO 11.8) What risks are presented if you do or say nothing?(LO 11.9, 11.12)
2. Why is it important that all health professionals know aseptic technique and adhere to USP <797> regulations?(LO 11.12)
3. Would you be afraid to compound chemotherapeutic agents?(LO 11.3) Why or why not?(LO 11.11, 11.12)

HIPAA Scenario

After a patient, Larry Newsome, picked up his compounded nicotine lollipops for smoking cessation, the pharmacist realized that the caution label "Keep out of the reach of children" was not included on the packaging, and that he had failed to counsel Mr. Newsome on this topic. The pharmacist asked technician Fred to contact the patient so that he could counsel the patient over the phone.

Discussion Questions(PTCB II. 73)

1. In what manner is consistent with the HIPAA law for Fred to contact the patient?
2. What concerns should the technician and the pharmacist have in addition to the labeling?

Internet Activities

1. Access **www.ashp.org.** Locate information on USP<797>. Choose one article on the Web site. Read the article and identify how the issues discussed impact the practice of pharmacy technicians. Be prepared to discuss your article and comments in class.(LO 11.12)
2. Access **www.usp.org.** Click on the "About Us" link. Write a brief paragraph on the role of the *United States Pharmacopeia* listing at least three services it provides.(LO 11.12)

12

Medication Errors

Learning Outcomes

Upon completion of this chapter, you will be able to:

12.1 Define *error* according to the Institute of Medicine (IOM).

12.2 Identify types of medication errors.

12.3 Identify causes of medication errors.

12.4 Identify common prescribing errors observed by pharmacists.

12.5 Recognize costs associated with medication errors.

12.6 List methods to reduce medication errors.

12.7 Explain the NCC MERP index for categorizing medication errors.

12.8 Explain the problems identified by ISMP and solutions to these problems.

12.9 State the IOM's recommendations to improve patient safety.

12.10 Identify ways the patient can assist in reducing prescription errors.

12.11 Differentiate between the types of dispensing errors.

12.12 Explain why there is not a valid defense for a prescription error.

12.13 Identify a "high-alert medication."

12.14 Explain National Patient Goals that have been established by The Joint Commission (TJC).

12.15 Discuss e-prescribing.

12.16 Identify the various agencies that oversee the reporting of medication errors and the processes that have been established to do so.

Key Terms

error

Institute for Safe Medication Practices (ISMP)

medication error

MEDMARX

MedWatch

negligence

U.S. Pharmacopeia (USP)

Vaccine Adverse Event Reporting System (VAERS)

PTCB

In preparation for the certification examination, you should understand and perform activities associated with the following PTCB Knowledge Statements:

PTCB Knowledge Statement

Domain I. Assisting the Pharmacist in Serving Patients

Knowledge of pharmaceutical, medical, and legal developments which impact on the practice of pharmacy (2)
Knowledge of techniques for detecting prescription errors (25)
Knowledge of quality improvement methods (49)

PTCB Knowledge Statement

Domain III. Participating in the Administration and Management of Pharmacy

Knowledge of quality improvement standards and guidelines (10)

Case Study

In November 1994, a single catastrophic death and a second permanent, debilitating injury at the Dana-Farber Cancer Institute sent the staff and public reeling. Betsy Lehman, a 39-year-old *Boston Globe* health reporter and mother of two, succumbed to a chemotherapeutic overdose. She was undergoing an advanced breast cancer drug protocol as part of a Harvard research study. Another patient, 52-year-old Maureen Bateman, was seriously injured because of the same unintentional mis-treatment. What is perhaps the most chilling aspect of the story is that the error was detected 8 weeks later by a data manager. If it had not been a research protocol, it is possible that no one would have noticed the four fold larger dosage of cyclo-phosphamide administered for 4 days straight to each patient instead of quartered across the days. Lehman died from heart failure the day before she was due to be discharged, 3 weeks after she received the fatal high doses. Bateman also suffered from cardiac toxicities, but she died in 1997 from her cancer.

While reading this chapter, keep the following questions in mind:

1. Who could have prevented the overdose from occurring? (LO 12.3)
2. What should the pharmacy team have done when filling the prescription? (LO 12.3)

Source: Organizational Change in the Face of Highly Public Errors, **http://webmm.ahrq.gov/index.aspx**.

Introduction to Medication Errors(LO 12.3)

In 2000, the Institute of Medicine (IOM) released its critical report on the American health care system titled *To Err Is Human*. The exact number of dispensing errors and of miss-filled prescriptions is unknown. Medication errors can be caused by physicians, nurses, pharmacists, pharmacy technicians, and other medical personnel. *Nobody is exempt from making an error!*

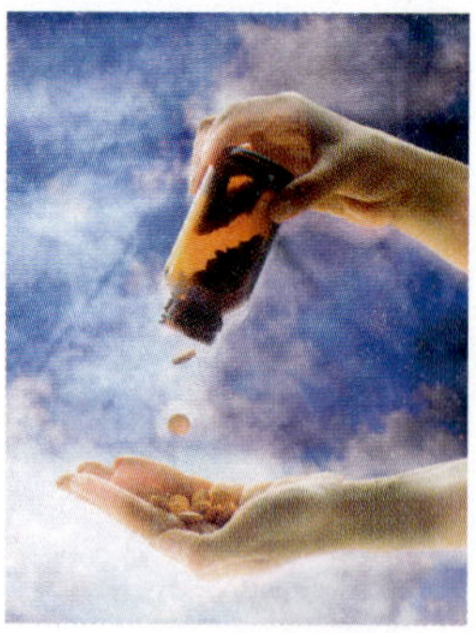

Figure 12-1 Medication errors can be fatal.

error Failure of a planned action to be completed as intended or the use of a wrong plan to achieve an aim.

Medication Errors(LO 12.1,12.7)

The IOM defines an **error** as a "failure of a planned action to be completed as intended or the use of a wrong plan to achieve an aim." A medical error can occur in many different forms, such as diagnostic, technical, or even wound infection. Unfortunately, the largest cause of medical errors involves medication (Figure 12-1). According to the National Coordinating Council for Medication Error Reporting and Prevention (NCC MERP), a **medication error** is "any preventable event that may cause or lead to inappropriate medication use or patient harm, while the medication is in the control of [a] health care professional, health care product, procedures, and systems, including prescribing; order communication; product

At Your Service

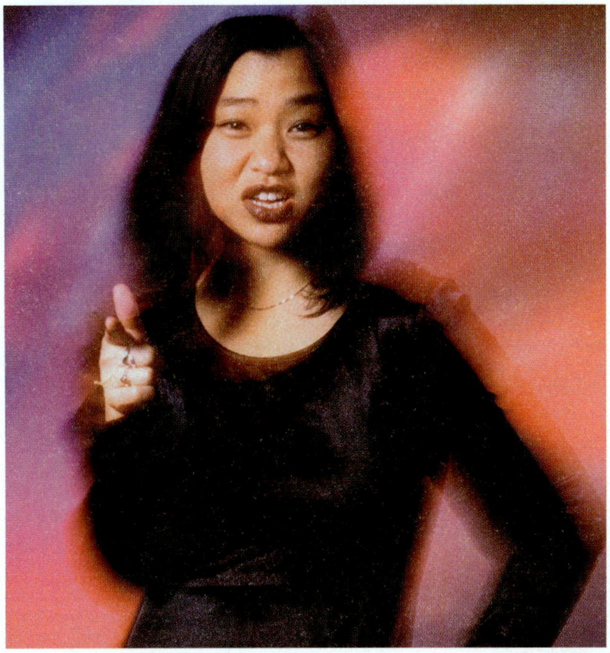

Mary Smith, a customer of Your Friendly Pharmacy, brings in a prescription from her doctor's office on Friday at 8 pm and hands it to the pharmacy technician. The technician notices the physician failed to write Mary's name on the prescription. The technician informs Mary that her name is not on the prescription, and that the pharmacy must verify the prescription with her physician. Mary becomes irritated with the technician and says, "The physician handed the prescription to me, so therefore it must be my prescription! Check my profile!"

The pharmacy technician checks Mary's profile and finds out that Mary has never received this medication from Your Friendly Pharmacy.

While reading this chapter, keep the following questions in mind.

1. What should the pharmacy technician do?(LO 12.4)
2. What could happen if the pharmacy fills the prescription without verifying the prescription with the physician?(LO 12.1)
3. Could the pharmacy use as an excuse that it filled the prescription because the patient demanded it?(LO 12.3)

labeling, packaging, nomenclature; compounding; dispensing; distribution; administration; education; monitoring; and *use*."

The NCC MERP has organized medications into nine categories based on four major error groupings:

- No Error
- Error, No Harm
- Error, Harm
- Error, Death

These four error groupings are affected by the amount of harm, monitoring, intervention, and intervention to sustain life. Harm is an impairment of the physical, emotional, or psychological function or structure of the body and or pain resulting from the error. Monitoring involves observing and recording the relevant physiological or psychological signs. Intervention includes the change in therapy or active medical/surgical treatment. Intervention necessary to sustain life includes cardiovascular and respiratory support. These nine categories are described in Table 12-1.

The nine different categories of medication errors will have different impacts on patients and their families, as shown in Table 12-2.

medication error "Any preventable event that may cause or lead to inappropriate medication use or patient harm, while the medication is in the control of [a] health care professional, health care product, procedures, and systems, including prescribing; order communication; product labeling, packaging, nomenclature; compounding; dispensing; distribution; administration; education; monitoring; and use."

Table 12-1 Categories of Medication Errors

Category	Example
Category A: No error has occurred or circumstances or events that have the capacity to commit error are present.	An example of this would be the similar packaging or labeling of a drug product, such as AcipHex and Aricept. Both of these drugs' packaging has a blue band going across the front of the package and the tablets' color is yellow.
Category B: An error has occurred but the error did not reach the patient. In this situation, errors are discovered and intercepted before they reach the patient. An error of "omission" is not considered a Category B. In addition, these errors are not "potential" (something that can develop or become actual) errors.	Examples of a Category B include when the wrong product is sent to the floor or unit but detected before being administered to the patient; a wrong dose is prepared but detected before being dispensed or administered; a wrong dose or directions is prescribed but is detected before being dispensed or administered.
Category C: An error has occurred that reached the patient but did not cause the patient harm.	An example of a Category C medication error would include routine blood work for phenytoin revealing a sudden decrease of phenytoin level. The patient has been taking the wrong dose of medication, or a patient with no known allergies is administered one dose of acetaminophen 325 mg when none was ordered.
Category D: An error has occurred that reached the patient and required monitoring to confirm that it resulted in no harm to the patient and/or required intervention to preclude harm.	An example would be an improper dose of insulin administered to a patient with diabetes. Because of this error, the patient's blood glucose is being monitored every hour. Another example is when a patient with a diagnosed penicillin allergy is ordered and administered cephalexin and, upon notification of a potential cross-sensitivity, the practitioner orders diphenhydramine to preclude a reaction.
Category E: In this situation, an actual error occurred, reached the patient, and may have contributed to or resulted in temporary harm to the patient and the patient required intervention. Types of intervention may include a change in therapy or active medical/surgical treatment.	An example of a Category E would find a patient being administered an extra dose of a non steroidal anti-inflammatory drug. The patient complains of abdominal discomfort, and requires an antacid.
Category F: An actual error occurred that reached the patient. The patient required an initial hospitalization due to the error. This error may have contributed to or resulted in temporary harm to the patient. The patient's length of stay may increase or he or she may require a higher level of medical care.	An example of a Category F would be an improper dose of insulin administered to a patient with diabetes. The patient experiences CNS disturbances resulting in a prolonged hospital stay for additional treatment and monitoring.
Category G: A Category G results when an actual error occurs and reaches the patient. This error may have contributed to or resulted in permanent patient harm. Permanent harm may include a loss of physical or emotional functions, which may include neurological impairment or loss of limb.	An example of Category G results if an improper dose of insulin is administered to a patient with diabetes. The patient becomes hypoglycemic, experiences seizures, and suffers from permanent neurological impairment.
Category H: This category results when an error occurs, reaches the patient, and the patient requires intervention needed to sustain life. Without intervention, the patient would most likely die.	An example of Category H would be if an improper dose is administered to a patient with diabetes. The patient becomes unresponsive and requires cardiopulmonary resuscitation. The patient fully recovers after receiving CPR and hospitalization is not extended.
Category I: In this situation, an error occurs, reaches the patient, and may have contributed to the patient's death.	An example of Category I is if a terminally ill hospice patient is ordered "concentrated morphine 0.1 mL (2 mg) every 2 hours as needed," but instead is given two 1-mL doses (20 mg). The patient dies after the second dose. Death was imminent, but it is uncertain if death was a result of the overdose. The patient's outcome may have been a result of the medication error, but the error may have contributed to the patient's death.

Table 12-2 Prescription Error Facts

- 1.5 million Americans are sickened, injured, or killed each year due to prescription errors.
- A hospitalized patient will experience at least one prescription error for each day he or she is hospitalized.
- A prescription error can add more than $8,750 to the hospital bill of a patient.
- $3.5 billion are spent each year to treat prescription-related errors occurring in hospitals.
- Deaths due to preventable adverse effects exceed the number of deaths attributed to vehicle accidents, breast cancer, or AIDS.
- Prescription errors cause 400,000 preventable injuries and deaths in hospitals each year.
- Medication errors cause 800,000 preventable injuries and deaths to elderly people in nursing homes each year.
- Drug errors cause 530,000 preventable injuries and deaths in Medicare recipients in outpatient facilities each year.

Source: BD Franklin, C Vincent, M Schachtner, N Barber: The incidence of prescribing errors in hospital inpatients. *Drug Saf.* 2005;28:891–900.

Tech Check

1. What are the four major error groupings established by the NCC MERP?(LO 12.7)

Types of Errors(LO 12.2, 12.4, 12.11)

Prescribing Errors

The most common types of prescription errors committed by physicians include prescribing an inappropriate dose, prescribing the wrong medication for a particular condition, and failing to monitor for side effects (Figure 12-2). The Joint Commission (TJC), formerly JCAHO, conducted a survey with community pharmacists and released these findings in the September 2004 edition of the *Joint Commission Journal on Quality and Safety*. These findings identified the following types of prescribing errors:

- Route of administration not specified
- Patient allergies
- Incorrect strength of medication
- Incomplete medication name
- Quantity and refills omitted
- Early refills for narcotics
- Prescriber failure to provide dates on prescription for controlled substances
- Additional directions required

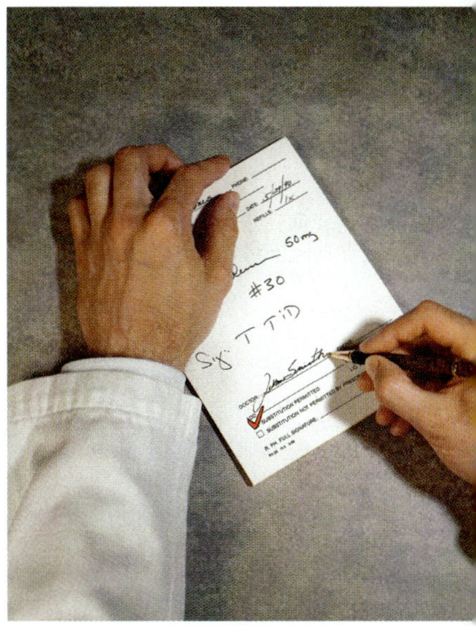

Figure 12-2 Prescription errors can be a result of incomplete or incorrect information.

Every one of these findings required additional clarification by the pharmacy staff before filling the prescription.

In this same survey, TJC demonstrated that the format of many of the prescription pads analyzed is not adequate to reduce prescription errors. All states specify similar requirements for a prescription, which include:

- Patient's name and address
- Prescriber's name and address
- Prescriber's DEA number for controlled substances
- Date the prescription is written
- Name, strength, dosage form, and quantity of medication
- Route of administration,
- Number of authorized refills
- Directions for use (to include dose and frequency)

Prescription forms A, B, and C represent a variety of prescription pad formats. According to TJC survey, which of the prescription pad formats do you think resulted in fewer omissions by a physician?

If you selected prescription form C, you have identified the prescription pad format that most physicians preferred in this study. This prescription pad reduced the greatest number of prescribing problems and omission errors by physicians.

Form A

Andrew J Prescriber MD
Prescriber's address; Prescriber's telephone number

Patient Name Date

Address DOB
Rx

DEA BP5555555 M.D.
Substitution is mandatory unless presriber writes "brand necessary" or "no substitution"

(a)

Form B

Andrew J Prescriber
Prescriber's address; Prescriber's phone number

Patient Name Date

Address DOB

Medication Name Form

Strength MILLIgrams MICROgrams

Dose One Tab or Cap Two Tabs or Caps Puffs Units

	Route		Frequency		Refills
Oral	eAr	Left	Daily	QAM	None
Topical	Nasal	Right	BID	Nightly	1 2 3
Rectal	eYe	Both	TID	Weekly	4 5 6
Inhaled	Subcutaneous		QID	PRN	1 Year
Other:			Other:		Other:

Quantity (#) Thirty Sixty Ninety One-Hundred-Eighty

Indication
Additional Directions
DEA #BP5555555 MD
Substitution is mandatory unless prescriber writes, "brand necessary" or "no substitution."

(b)

Form C

Andrew J Prescriber
Prescriber's address
Prescriber's phone and fax numbers
DEA BP5555555

Patient Name **Date**
Address **DOB**

Medication Name and Strength (digits and words) MILLIgrams MILLIgrams per ml Percent
Form Tab or Cap Inhaler Cream Chewable Tablet Liquid Nebulizer
Dose(digits & wds)

Tab or Cap **Route** **Frequency**
One Units Oral Topical eAr Left Daily TID QAM
Two Puffs Rectal Inhaled Nasal Right BID QID Nightly
Half TEAspoon Subcutaneous eYe Both prn Weekly

Quantity or Duration One Five Seven Fourteen Thirty Sixty Days Months Doses
Refills Zero One Two Three Six One Year

Indication
Additional Directions
M.D.
Substitution is mandatory unless the prescriber writes "brand necessary" or "no substitution"

(c)

Figure 12-3 Examples of prescription formats.

Types of Dispensing Errors

There are two types of dispensing errors committed by pharmacists: mechanical errors and judgmental errors. A mechanical error occurs in the preparation and the processing of a prescription (Figure 12-4). An example of a mechanical error would be if the pharmacist read the prescription properly, but dispensed the wrong medication to the patient. A judgment error may occur in the screening of a patient, performing a drug utilization review, or during the counseling of a patient. If a pharmacy technician commits a dispensing error, it will be a mechanical error because pharmacy technicians are not permitted to perform judgmental duties in the pharmacy. A mechanical error is the most common type of error.

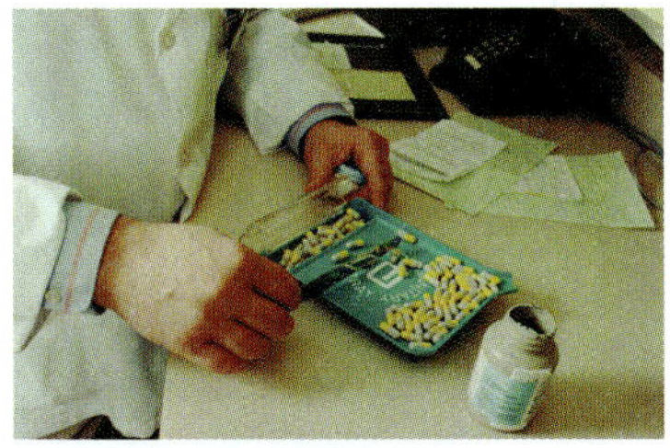

Figure 12-4 A mechanical error is a type of dispensing error.

Errors must be tracked and recorded in order to prevent further errors. In 2001, **MEDMARX**, a national, Internet-accessible database that hospitals and health care systems use to track and trend adverse drug reactions and medication errors, reported the types of medication errors committed by pharmacies as seen in Table 12-3 (MEDMARX will be discussed in detail later in this chapter).

MEDMARX A national, Internet-accessible database that hospitals and health care systems use to track and trend adverse drug reactions and medication errors. Hospitals and health care systems participate in MEDMARX voluntarily and subscribe to it on an annual basis.

Administration Errors

Prescription errors can take many forms regardless of the age or experience of the practitioner. In a hospital setting, there has been documentation according to the Massachusetts Coalition for the Prevention of Medical Errors of the following occurring:

- Enteral formulas given parenterally
- Oral medications given intravenously
- Intravenous medications administered intrathecally
- Intramuscular preparations administered intravenously
- Epidural and intravenous lines mixed up
- Intravenous syringes used to measure doses of oral medications
- Intravenous medications used orally

Table 12-3 Medication Errors Committed by Pharmacies

Error	Number of Cases	Percentage Reported
Omission errors	27,714	29%
Improper dose/quantity	20,024	21%
Prescribing errors	13,634	14%
Wrong drug	12,689	13%
Wrong time	6,899	7%
Extra dose	6,387	7%
Wrong patient	5,054	5%
Wrong drug preparation	4,275	4%
Wrong dosage form	1,885	2%
Wrong route	1,743	2%
Wrong administration technique	1,315	1%

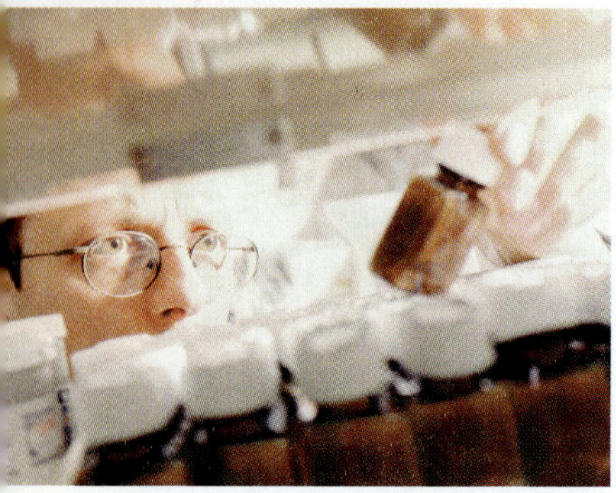

Figure 12-5 Interruptions in the prescription process can create medication errors.

Tech Check

2. What are three examples of prescribing errors?(LO 12.4)

3. What are three examples of dispensing errors?(LO 12.11)

4. What are three examples of administration errors?(LO 12.11)

5. Why do you think administration errors occur?(LO 12.3)

6. What can be done to prevent administration errors?(LO 12.6)

Causes of Errors(LO 12.3)

Many studies have been conducted by various researchers throughout the United States to identify the factors leading to the causes of prescription errors. MEDMARX conducted a study and released its findings in 2001 of the causes of prescription errors.

- Performance deficit—35,690 cases (38%)
- Procedure/protocol not followed—18,981 cases (20%)
- Transcription inaccurate/omitted—13,860 cases (15%)
- Documentation—11,622 cases (12%)
- Computer entry—10,353 (11%)
- Knowledge deficit—9,356 cases (10%)
- Communication—9,342 (10%)
- Written order—5,363 (6%)
- Drug distribution center—3,868 (4%)
- Handwriting illegible or unclear—3,258 (3%)

The perception among pharmacists is that prescription errors are increasing in both community and institutional pharmacy practice. Pharmacists believe the leading causes of prescription errors are based upon the workload of the pharmacists and the working conditions in pharmacies. Pharmacists believe that as the number of prescriptions per hour increases, the likelihood of errors increases also. It is believed that an increase in errors will occur if a pharmacist is tired or is under extreme pressure to fill prescriptions quicker.

According to the National Association of Chain Drug Stores, between 2004 and 2010 the supply of community pharmacists is expected to increase only 7.8% versus an estimated 27% increase in number of prescriptions dispensed, going from 3.27 billion in 2003 to over 4.1 billion in 2010. If this prediction comes true, one may assume that there will be an increase in prescription errors in the years to come.

Many pharmacists state that interruptions in the prescription process create errors (Figure 12-5). Interruptions such as the phone ringing and excessive noise in the pharmacy area cause lapses in the pharmacist's concentration. Pharmacists have cited similar medication names, packaging, and labeling as a source of prescription errors.

U.S. Pharmacopeia (USP) The United States Pharmacopeia (USP) is an official public standards–setting authority for all prescription and over-the-counter medicines and other health care products manufactured or sold in the United States.

Organizational Causes of Errors

The **U.S. Pharmacopeia (USP)** is an official standards setting authority for all prescription and over-the-counter medicines and other health care products manufactures or sold in the United States, which has identified three categories of organizational causes of medication errors: technical, organizational, and human factors. A technical error is latent in nature and may be caused by either external, design, material, label, or form factors. External failures are beyond the control of the organization; a design failure results from poor design; a material failure is to a product defect beyond the control of the organization; labeling failures occur due to the label, such as the size, adhesive used, appearance, print or format; and a form failure occurs due to confusing or incomplete information being provided.

An organizational factor is a hidden error and may be the result of external forces, policies and procedures, knowledge lapses, management priorities, or the culture of the organization. External errors are beyond the control of the organization, policies and procedures are implemented due to a failure of the quality of the procedure, knowledge failures result from inadequate knowledge, and management priorities failures result from management decisions creating conflicting demands.

Unlike technical or organizational factors, human factors are active errors and take the form of external forces, knowledge-based lapses, rule-based lapses, qualifications, coordination, verification, intervention, monitoring, or skill-based lapses. A knowledge-based error occurs due to the inability of individuals to apply their existing knowledge. Rule-based errors involve the application of existing rules. Qualification factors occur due to an incorrect fit between an individual's qualification, training, education, or the task. Coordination factors lack task coordination within the organization. Verification factors occur because of failing to make a complete assessment of the situation before starting an intervention. Intervention factors occur because of poor task planning and execution. Inappropriate monitoring of a patient is considered a human factor. Skill-based factors are those that rely on "automatic" tasks, which require little or no conscious attending during the execution of the task. Patient factors are not taken into consideration because they occur outside the organization.

negligence A tort related to defective products where the defendant has breached a duty of due care and caused harm to the plaintiff. The failure of a corporate director or officer to exercise the duty of care while conducting the corporation's business.

Tech Check

7. What are three factors that contribute to prescription errors?(LO 12.3)

8. What are the three categories of organizational causes or errors? Provide an example of each.(LO 12.3)

Consequences of Errors(LO 12.5, 12.12)

There are no words that a pharmacist can say to a patient or the patient's family to express sorrow for committing a prescription error. A prescription error may result in a patient's injury and/or death, and may lead to legal consequences for the pharmacist or the pharmacy. Consider the examples in Table 12-4.

If pharmacists commit a prescription error, they are held liable for their actions under the theory of negligence. Pharmacists cannot make errors, whether mechanical or judgmental. They have a legal duty to provide patients with the best possible care, and any deviation from this duty would result in their **negligence**, which is punishable under tort law. (refer to chapter 4 to review laws; Figure 12-6). Originally, pharmacists had a legal responsibility in the dispensing of medication. It has now evolved to include counseling patients.

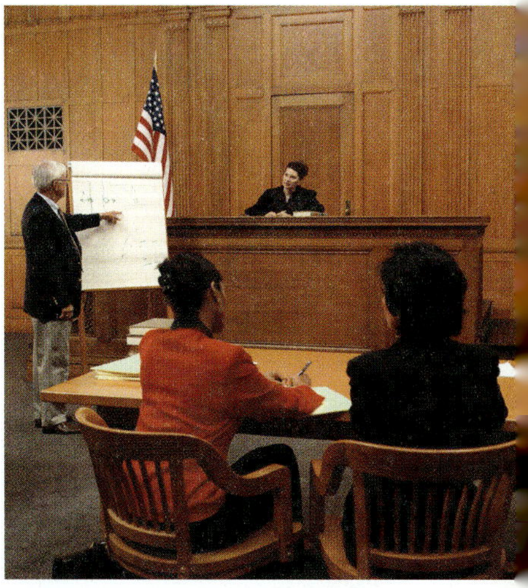

Figure 12-6 Negligence is punishable under tort law.

Table 12-4 Results of Prescription Errors

Error	Result
A pharmacist sold zinc sulfate to a pregnant woman instead of Epsom salts.	Both the woman and the child died.
A patient was poisoned after pharmacist dispensed corrosive sublimate instead of the antiseptic chlorodyne.	The patient died.
A patient received another person's prescription bottle in a bag labeled with the patient's name.	Pharmacy was found negligent.
A pharmacist refilled a prescription for Dymelor with Aldomet.	Patient developed uncontrolled diabetes and suffered stroke. Pharmacy received a $1.4 million judgment against it.
A man received Cycrin instead of Coumadin, suffered a heart attack, then a stroke, and finally went into a coma.	Pharmacy received a $6 million judgment to compensate the man and all costs associated for the patient in a special care facility.
A pharmacist mistranscribed telephoned prescription for Calcitrol resulting in the patient receiving twice the intended dose.	Pharmacy received an $8 million judgment against it.
A patient with diabetes requested semi-lente insulin from the pharmacy clerk. The clerk asked for "some lente." The patient used it for several days before suffering injury.	Pharmacy received a $350,000 judgment against it.

Sources: P Knudsen, H Herborg, et al. Preventing medication errors in community pharmacy, frequency and seriousness of medication errors. *Qual Saf Health Care.* 2007;21:291–296; Pharmacists Mutual Insurance Company. The pharmacists mutual claim study, **www.phmic.com/web.nsf/17e8baa11ffecbc586256d0200661c2b/3641346e2tbbf4a48625714f0078c029?Open Document**.

As a result of numerous court findings, pharmacists must be skillful in dealing with medications, but also cautious in their actions. They must use care in their dispensing of medications. The courts have ruled that even though the actions of pharmacists are not intentional, they are guilty of negligence nonetheless.

- A pharmacist cannot offer any valid defense for committing a prescription error.
- Increasing prescription volume is not a defense.
- Physicians' poor handwriting is not a defense.
- Numerous interruptions, such as the phone ringing excessively and noise occurring in the prescription area, are not a defense.
- Working long hours as a result of no relief help is not a defense.
- A pharmacy technician giving a patient the wrong prescription bag with another person's medication is not a defense.

There are *no* legal defenses if a prescription error occurs.

Tech Check

9. What excuse may be used in the case of a prescription error?(LO 12.12)

Methods to Reduce Prescription Errors (LO 12.4, 12.6, 12.8, 12.9, 12.13, 12.14)

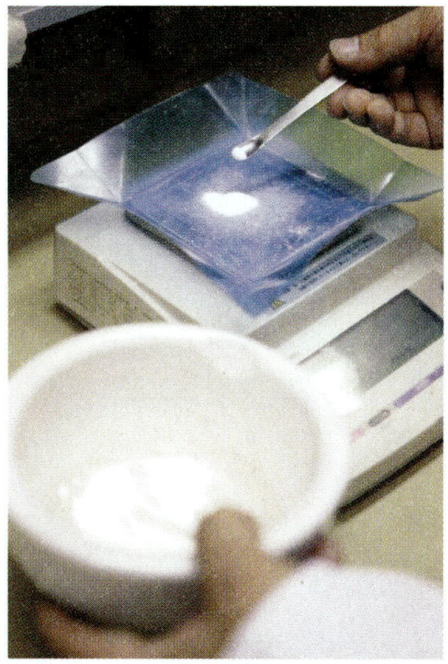

Figure 12-7 A detailed process is used to identify medication errors.

The reduction of prescription errors must begin with a detailed process to identify medication errors (Figure 12-7). There are multiple tools available to an organization to identify medication errors, which include the Failure Mode and Effect Analysis (FMEA), TJC Patient Safety Goals and Medication Management Standards, reports issued by MEDMARX, the National Quality Forum, and the IOM.

FMEA has released an index titled Highest Ranking Criticality Indexes. This index identifies

- Lethal drugs available as floor stock
- Mistakes in calculating doses
- Incorrectly calculating flow rates and doses for IVs
- Failure of properly checking patient arm bands prior to medication administration
- Excessive medications in nursing floor stock rooms/areas

In 2004, TJC released a statement titled "National Patient Safety Goals for 2004." TJC established several goals to improve patient safety. Refer to Table 12-5.

Identifying Medication Errors

Numerous organizations are actively conducting research on medication errors and analyzing the data. These organizations include TJC, USP, and the **Institute for Safe Medication Practices (ISMP)**, which is a nonprofit organization that educates the health community and consumers about safe medication practices. The data analysis examines trends on a monthly, quarterly, and yearly basis. Trends are cross-referenced by the error category, type of error, and cause of error.

These trends may compare other periods and indicate when specific initiatives have been implemented by an institution. Other forms of analysis may include:

- Harmful versus nonharmful errors
- Occurrence of the error, such as prescribing, transcribing, dispensing, administering, or monitoring

Table 12-5 TJC Goals to Improve Patient Safety

Goal	Focus
Improve the accuracy of patient identification	Focuses on preventing the wrong patient from receiving incorrect medication
Improve the effectiveness of communication among caregivers	Encompasses "verbal orders," "pharmacy abbreviations," and "brand/generic names that sound or look alike" as issues in communication among health care providers
Improve the safety of using high-alert medications	Examines both generic names and therapeutic classes
Improve the safety of using infusion pumps	Examines pump failures, pump malfunction, and improper doses received because of the pump

Institute for Safe Medication Practices (ISMP) A nonprofit organization educating the health care community and consumers about safe medication practices.

- Identification of who committed the error, whether it is a registered nurse, pharmacy technician, respiratory therapist, unit secretary/clerk, pharmacist, physician, licensed practical/vocational nurse, or other ancillary personnel
- Location of the initial error, such as a nursing (patient care) unit, pharmacy, emergency department, pediatrics, intensive care unit, radiology, outpatient surgery department, or other location

As a result of this analysis, the USP has identified the Top 10 Products in Categories A-I. These include:

- Insulin—12.93%
- Morphine—8.62%
- Potassium chloride—8.62%
- Albuterol—7.76%
- Heparin—6.90%
- Cefazolin—6.03%
- Levofloxacin—5.17%
- Warfarin—5.17%
- Vancomycin—5.17%
- Furosemide—5.17%

Another analysis of the Top 10 Products in Category E-I found the following results:

- Insulin—22.73%
- Morphine—18.18%
- Heparin—9.09%
- Fentanyl—9.09%
- Hydromorphone—9.09%
- Potassium chloride—4.55%
- Warfarin—4.55%
- Meperidine—4.55%
- Vancomycin—4.55%
- Furosemide—4.55%
- Metoprolol—4.55%

Both pharmacists and pharmacy technicians must be extremely careful when dispensing medications.

Assessment of Errors

After a pharmacy has identified a medication error, an action should be made to prevent the error from occurring again. In 2001, MEDMARX reported that the following actions were taken by organizations upon discovery of a medication error.

- Informed staff member who made the initial error (66%)
- Informed staff member who was also involved in the error (19%)
- Provided education/training (15%)
- Took no action (14%)
- Enhanced communication process (12%)
- Informed patient/caregiver of medication error (3%)
- Changed policy or procedure

Unfortunately, weaker actions are most often employed instead of stronger actions.

Preventing Errors

Both TJC and ISMP have identified abbreviations and symbols that may result in medication errors due to problems in communication. Initially, TJC issued the "Do Not Use" list of abbreviations and symbols. ISMP expanded the list, which is found in Table 12-6. ISMP is hoping that all health care organizations and practitioners will adopt this list.

Table 12-6 ISMP List of Error-Prone Abbreviations, Symbols, and Dose Designations

Abbreviation	Meaning	Possible Error	Solution
Ug	Microgram	Mistaken as "mg"	Use "mcg"
AD, AS, AU	Right ear, left ear, each ear	Mistaken as OD, OS, OU (right eye, left eye, each eye)	Use "right ear," "left ear," or "each ear"
OD, OS, OU	Right eye, left eye, each eye	Mistaken as AD, AS, AU (right ear, left ear, each ear)	Use "right eye," "left eye," or "each eye"
BT	Bedtime	Mistaken as "BID" (twice daily)	Use "bedtime"
cc	Cubic centimeter	Mistaken as "u" (units)	Use "mL"
D/C	Discharge or discontinue	Premature discontinuation of medications if D/C (intended to mean discharge) has been misinterpreted as "discontinued" when followed by a list of discharge medications	Use "discharge" and "discontinue"
IJ	Injection	Mistaken as "IV" or "intrajugular"	Use "injection"
IN	Intranasal	Mistaken as "IM" or "IV"	Use "intranasal" or "NAS"
HS	Half-strength	Mistaken as bedtime	Use "half-strength"
hs	At bedtime, hour of sleep	Mistaken as half-strength	Use "bedtime"
IU*	International Unit	Mistaken as IV (intravenous) or 10 (ten)	Use "units"
o.d. or OD	Once daily	Mistaken as "right eye" (OD—oculus dexter) leading to oral liquid medications administered in the eye	Use "daily"
OJ	Orange juice	Mistaken as OD or OS (right or left eye); drugs meant to be diluted in orange juice may be given in the eye	Use "orange juice"
Per os	By mouth; orally	The "os" can be mistaken as "left eye" (OS—oculus sinister)	Use "PO," "by mouth," or "orally"
q.d. or QD*	Every day	Mistaken as q.i.d., especially if the period after the "q" or the tail of the "q" is misunderstood as an "i"	Use "daily"
qhs	Nightly at bedtime	Mistaken as "qhr" or every hour	Use "nightly"
qn	Nightly or at bedtime	Mistaken as "qh" (every hour)	Use "nightly" or "at bedtime"

(Continued)

Table 12-6 ISMP List of Error-Prone Abbreviations, Symbols, and Dose Designations *(Continued)*

q.o.d. or QOD*	Every other day	Mistaken as "q.d." (daily) or "q.i.d. (four times daily if the "o" is poorly written	Use "every other day"
q1d	Daily	Mistaken as q.i.d. (four times daily)	Use "daily"
q6PM	Every evening at 6 pm	Mistaken as every 6 hours	Use "6 pm nightly" or "6 pm daily"
SC, SQ, sub q	Subcutaneous	SC mistaken as SL (sublingual); SQ mistaken as "5 every;" the "q" in "sub q" has been mistaken as "every" (e.g., a heparin dose ordered "sub q 2 hours before surgery" misunderstood as every 2 hours before surgery)	Use "subcut" or "subcutaneously"
ss	Sliding scale (insulin) or ½ (apothecary)	Mistaken as "55"	Spell out "sliding scale;" use "one-half" or "1/2"
SSRI	Sliding scale regular insulin	Mistaken as selective-serotonin reuptake inhibitor	Spell out "sliding scale (insulin)"
SSI	Sliding scale insulin	Mistaken as strong solution of iodine (Lugol's)	Spell out "sliding scale (insulin)"
i/d	Once daily	Mistaken as "tid"	Use "1 daily"
TIW or tiw	3 times a week	Mistaken as "3 times a day" or "twice in a week"	Use "3 times weekly"
U or u*	Unit	Mistaken as the number 0 or 4, causing a 10-fold overdose or greater (e.g., 4U seen as "40" or 4u seen as "44"); mistaken as "cc" so dose given in volume instead of units (e.g., 4u seen as 4 cc)	Use "unit"
Dose Designation and Other Information	**Intended Meaning**	**Misinterpretation**	**Correction**
Trailing zero after decimal point (e.g.,1.0 mg)*	1 mg	Mistaken as 10 mg if the decimal point is not seen.	Do not use trailing zeros for doses expressed in whole numbers.
Naked decimal point (e.g., 5 mg)*	0.5 mg	Mistaken as 5 mg if the decimal point is not seen.	Use zero before a decimal point when the dose is less than a whole unit.
Drug name and dose run together (especially problematic for drug names that end in l such as Inderal 40 mg or Tegretol 300 mg)	Inderal 40 mg Tegretol 300 mg	Mistaken as Inderal 140 mg Mistaken as Tegretol 1300 mg.	Place adequate space between the drug name, dose, and unit of measure.
Numerical dose and unit of measure together (e.g., 10 mg, 100 mL)	10 mg 100 mL	The "m" is sometimes mistaken as a zero or two zeros, risking a 10- or 100-fold overdose.	Place adequate space between the dose and the unit of measure.
Abbreviations such as mg or mL with a period following the abbreviation	mg mL	The period is unnecessary and could be mistaken as the number 1 if written poorly.	Use mg, mL, etc. without a terminal period.

(Continued)

Table 12-6 ISMP List of Error-Prone Abbreviations, Symbols, and Dose Designations *(Continued)*

Large doses without properly placed commas (e.g., 100000 units or 1000000 units)	100,000 units 1,000,000 units	100000 has been mistaken as 10,000 or 1,000,000; 1000000 has been mistaken as 100,000.	Use commas for dosing units at or above 1,000, or use words such as 100 "thousand" or 1 "million" to improve readability.
Drug Name Abbreviation	**Intended Meaning**	**Misinterpretation**	**Correction**
ARA A	vidarabine	Mistaken as cytarabine (ARA C)	Use complete drug name
AZT	zidovudine (Retrovir)	Mistaken as azathioprine or aztreonam	Use complete drug name
CPZ	Compazine (prochlorperazine)	Mistaken as chlorpromazine	Use complete drug name
DPT	Demerol-Phenergan-Thorazine	Mistaken as diphtheria-pertussis-tetanus (vaccine)	Use complete drug name
DTO	Diluted tincture of opium, or deodorized tincture of opium (Paregoric)	Mistaken as tincture of opium	Use complete drug name
HCl	hydrochloric acid or hydrochloride	Mistaken as potassium chloride (The H is misinterpreted as K)	Use complete drug name unless expressed as a salt of a drug
HCT	hydrocortisone	Mistaken as hydrochlorothiazide	Use complete drug name
HCTZ	hydrochlorothiazide	Mistaken as hydrocortisone (seen as HCT250 mg)	Use complete drug name
MgSO4*	Magnesium sulfate	Mistaken as morphine sulfate	Use complete drug name
MS, MSO4*	Morphine sulfate	Mistaken as magnesium sulfate	Use complete drug name
MTX	Methotrexate	Mistaken as mitoxantrone	Use complete drug name
PCA	Procainamide	Mistaken as patient-controlled analgesia	Use complete drug name
PTU	Propylthiouracil	Mistaken as mercaptopurine	Use complete drug name
T3	Tylenol with Codeine No. 3	Mistaken as liothyronine	Use complete drug name
TAC	Triamcinolone	Mistaken as tetracaine, adrenalin, cocaine	Use complete drug name
TNK	TNKase	Mistaken as "TPA"	Use complete drug name
ZnSo4	Zinc sulfate	Mistaken as morphine sulfate	Use complete drug name
Stemmed drug names	Intended meaning	Misinterpretation	Correction
"Nitro" drip	Nitroglycerin infusion	Mistaken as sodium nitroprusside infusion	Use complete drug name
"Norflex"	Norfloxacin	Mistaken as Norflex	Use complete drug name
"IV Vanc"	Intravenous vancomycin	Mistaken as Invanz	Use complete drug name

*These abbreviations are included on TJC's "minimum list" of dangerous abbreviations, acronyms, and symbols that must be included on an organization's "Do Not Use" list, effective January 1, 2004. Visit **www.jointcommission.org** for more information about this TJC requirement.

An omission error is "the failure to carry out some of the actions necessary to achieve a desired goal." An omission error in a prescription involves missing or incomplete information required to appropriately or legally dispense a prescription.

Another area of concern for both pharmacists and pharmacy technicians is the numerous drugs that either are spelled or sound similar. ISMP has identified these medications and issued a comprehensive list, which is found in Appendix B of this text.

High-Alert Medications

According to the ISMP, a high-alert medication is defined as "those medications that are involved in a high percentage of errors and/or sentinel events and/or carry a higher risk for abuse, errors or other adverse outcomes. It is a medication that, if misused, could cause serious harmful consequences to the patient."

The Institute for Safe Medication Practices (ISMP) has issued a list of both specific categories of medications, which if taken incorrectly may cause significant harm to the patient. They include:

- Adrenergic agonists, IV (e.g., epinephrine)
- Adrenergic antagonists, IV (e.g., propranolol)
- Anesthetic agents, inhaled and IV (e.g. propofol)
- Cardioplegic solutions
- Chemotherapeutic agents, parenteral and oral
- Dextrose, hypertonic, 20% or greater
- Dialysis solutions, peritoneal and hemodialysis
- Epidural or intrathecal medications
- Glycoprotein IIb/IIIa inhibitors (e.g., eptifibatide)
- Hypoglycemic agents
- Inotropic medications, IV (e.g., digoxin)
- Liposomal forms of medications (e.g., liposomal amphotericin B)
- Moderate sedation agents, IV (e.g., midazolam)
- Moderate sedation agents, oral, for children (e.g., chloral hydrate)
- Narcotic/opiates, IV and oral (including liquid concentrates, immediate- and sustained-release formulations)
- Neuromuscular blocking agents (e.g., succinylcholine)
- Radiocontrast agents, IV
- Thrombolytic/fibrinolytics, IV (e.g., tenecteplase)
- Total parenteral solutions

The ISMP identified the following medications as having the possibility to cause harm to a patient if they are not used correctly:

- amiodarone, IV
- colchicine injection
- heparin, low molecular weight, injection
- heparin, unfractionated, IV
- insulin, subcutaneous and IV
- lidocaine, IV
- magnesium sulfate injection
- methotrexate, oral, nononcologic use
- nesiritide
- nitroprusside sodium for injection
- potassium chloride for injection concentrate

- potassium phosphate injection
- sodium chloride injection, hypertonic (more than 0.9% concentration)
- warfarin

Tech Check

10. What are two goals outlined by TJC in its National Patient Safety Goals of 2004?(LO 12.14)

11. What three medications that have contributed to the largest number of medication errors?(LO 12.13)

12. What are three examples of action taken by an organization after a medication error has occurred?(LO 12.6)

Prevention of Prescribing Errors(LO 12.6, 12.15)

Prescription Writing

All prescription documents should be legible (Figure 12-8). The information on the prescription should contain a brief notation of the usage of the medication unless the prescriber considers it inappropriate. All prescriptions should be written in metric units; in other words, the apothecary and avoirdupois systems should not be used. A prescriber should indicate the age and weight of the patient; this practice can eliminate numerous errors in pediatric and geriatric populations. All medication orders should include the drug name, the exact metric weight, or concentration. The pharmacist should check with the prescriber for any information that is missing or questionable. A leading zero always precedes a decimal expression of less than one; terminal zeros should never be used after a decimal (10-fold error in drug strengths have occurred with the inappropriate use of zeros). Prescribers should avoid using abbreviations for both drug names and Latin terms.

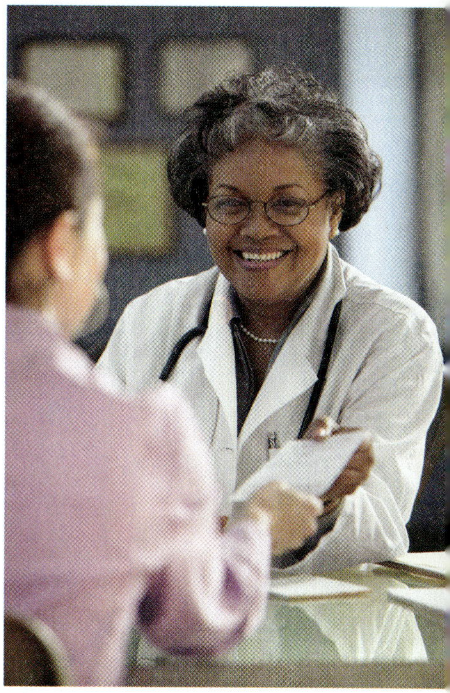

Figure 12-8 All prescription documents should be legible and written in metric units of measurement.

Verbal Prescriptions

Verbal prescription orders should be limited to emergency situations where written or electronic prescriptions are not possible. Any questions with a verbal order should be clarified before it is filled by the pharmacist.

Health care organizations should establish policies and procedures for the usage of verbal prescriptions/medication orders. These policies should address the limitations and prohibitions on the usage of verbal orders, and guidelines should be established for clear and effective communication to include who may send and receive a verbal order. The NCC MERP recommends that verbal orders for antineoplastic agents should not be permitted due to their narrow margin of safety.

Verbal orders should indicate the name of patient; the age and weight of the patient, the drug name; the dosage form; the exact strength or concentration; dose, frequency, and route; quantity and/or duration of therapy; purpose or indication; specific instructions for use; the name of the prescriber and telephone number; and the name of the individual transmitting the order. During the communication of the verbal order, the name of the drug should be confirmed by any of the following: spelling the drug name, providing both the brand and generic names of the medication, and providing the indication of the use. To avoid any confusion with drug name modifiers, such as prefixes and suffixes, additional spelling-assistance methods should be used. Instructions for uses should be provided without abbreviations. The pharmacist receiving the verbal order should write down the complete order to enter it into the computer, then read it back to the prescriber and receive confirmation.

Electronic Prescribing

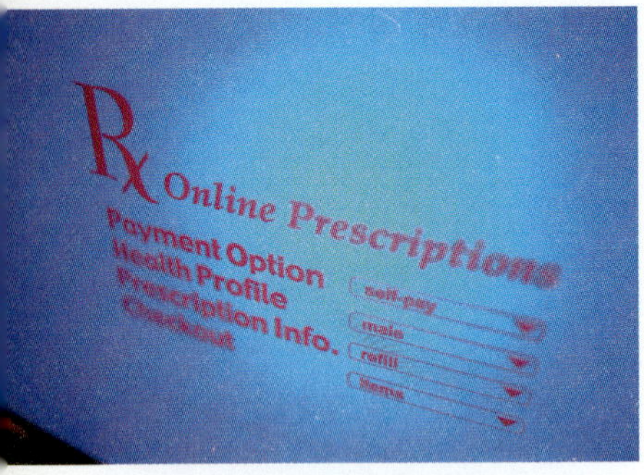

Figure 12-9 Electronic prescriptions can reduce the potential for medication errors.

Electronic prescribing, or e-prescribing, is a complete electronic transmission of prescription information from a prescriber's software application to the pharmacy site. Electronic prescribing is not the usage of faxes, scanned images of the prescription, or an e-mailed prescription. The prescription is formatted and encrypted during transmission using the "NCPDP Script" standard, which was developed by the National Council for Prescription Drug Programs (NCPDP). Electronic prescribing flows in both directions—from the physician's office to the pharmacy and vice versa. Now there is a heavy emphasis for e-prescribing to be implemented in the United States by 2010.

The core benefits of electronic prescribing include:

- Eliminating illegible prescriptions
- Using clinical decision support to reduce preventable errors, such as drug-drug interactions, drug allergy reactions, dosing errors, and therapeutic duplication
- Enhancing communication between clinician and patient
- Enhancing communication through all parts of the prescribing chain
- Increasing access to important reference and patient information
- Providing clinicians with cost information
- Improving work efficiency

E-prescribing saves time for both physicians and their staffs. It reduces the number of faxes and telephone calls for authorization during office hours. Electronic prescribing also reduces requests from the pharmacist for clarification on new prescriptions. E-prescribing is convenient for the patient and improves patient safety by reducing the potential for medication errors due to illegible and misread prescriptions and sound-alike and look-alike drugs (Figure 12-9).

Consider the following estimates:

- The Leapfrog Group has estimated that a computerized system could reduce prescribing errors by up to 86%, the length of hospital stays by 1 day, and hospital charges.
- E-Health Initiative suggests that e-prescribing technology could prevent more than 2.1 million drug events and 190,000 hospitalizations, thereby saving $29 billion annually.
- Topics in Health Information Management found that two e-prescribing devices cut prescription average refill from 15 minutes (time spent on hold before orders were taken) to an average 69 seconds.

E-prescribing will primarily benefit patients, pharmacists, and prescribers. The observed benefits include increased patient safety, increased quality of care, increased efficiency, and increased convenience. Increased patient safety results from a reduction in misread or misunderstood handwritten prescriptions or medications with similar-sounding names.

The quality of patient care is improved because more information can be collected about the patient for both the pharmacist and the prescriber. Types of information that would be more readily available include age, height, weight, race, and gender of the patient; this information will permit the pharmacist to assess a particular medication prescribed for a patient. Other information collected could include drug allergies, diagnosis codes, and lab values.

An increase in the efficiency of processing prescriptions could occur because the pharmacy may receive the prescription prior to the patient leaving the physician's office. The time spent on calling in prescriptions and faxing prescriptions from the physician's office to the pharmacy or obtaining a refill authorization from a physician's office is reduced. This saving in time will allow shorter waiting times in a pharmacy for a patient and will result in an improvement in customer service.

Many state boards of pharmacy allow for e-prescribing of noncontrolled substances. The DEA is evaluating e-prescribing for controlled substances, where the largest obstacle is with Schedule II medications. The pharmacist must have the original prescription prior to dispensing, except in situations for emergency prescribing and long-term care facilities. E-prescribing will continue to benefit patients, pharmacists, and physicians in the future.

Dispensing Medications

All prescriptions/orders should be reviewed by a pharmacist prior to dispensing. Any order that is incomplete, illegible, or of concern should be clarified using an established process for resolving questions. Patient profiles should be current and contain adequate information that allows the pharmacist to assess the appropriateness of a prescription/order.

The dispensing area should be properly designed to prevent errors. The design of the pharmacy should address fatigue-reducing environmental conditions (e.g., adequate lighting, air conditioning, noise-level abatement, and ergonomic fixtures), minimize distractions (e.g., telephone and personnel interruptions, clutter, unrelated tasks), and provide sufficient staffing and other resources for workload.

The pharmacy's inventory should be arranged to help differentiate medications from one another. This may be accomplished with visual discriminators such as signs or markers. This is extremely important where confusion may exist between or among strengths, similar-looking labels, and names that sound or appear similar.

The prescription department should utilize a series of checks and balances to assess the accuracy of the dispensing process prior to the medication being provided to the patient. Other methods of checking may include automation (e.g., bar coding systems), computer systems, and patient profiles. Prescription labels should be read a minimum of three times: when selecting the medication, during the packaging of the medication, and when returning the medication to the shelf.

The pharmacy department staff should triple-check the replenishment of the regular medication stock or automated dispensing machines, such as Pyxis, to ensure accuracy of product and precision of placement (e.g., when selecting the product, before the product leaves the pharmacy, and prior to placing the product in the automated dispensing machine/cabinet).

As a result of OBRA-90 (Omnibus Budget Reconciliation Act of 1990), pharmacists are required to counsel patients at the time of dispensing. Counseling the patient should be viewed as an opportunity to verify the accuracy of dispensing and that the patient understands proper medication use. Counseling should include the indications for the use of the medication as well as the precautions and warnings. The patient also should be informed of the expected outcomes from the medication and any possible adverse reactions and interactions with food or other medications. In addition, the patient should be informed of what to do when adverse reactions or interactions do occur, and how to store the medication.

All pharmacy staff, pharmacists, and pharmacy technicians should receive ongoing training on accepted standards relating to the dispensing process with the goal of prescription error reduction. Policies and procedures should be established by the pharmacy for the dispensing process.

Bar Coding

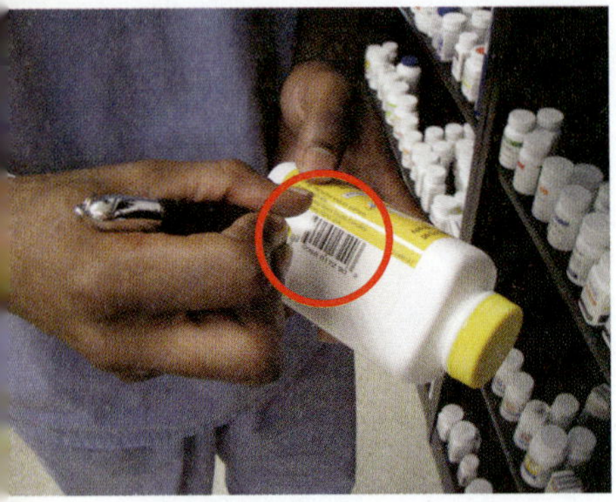

Figure 12-10 Bar coding can improve patient safety.

Patient safety can be improved with machine-readable bar codes, which can be standardized and found on medication packages and containers (Figure 12-10). Using scannable bar codes can guarantee that the correct drug and dosage form are being administered to the correct patient.

To eliminate dispensing errors with the usage of bar codes, each bar code will be required to contain the NDC number, the lot (control/batch) number, and the expiration date of the medication. To be properly implemented the NDC number, lot number, and expiration date must appear uniform on all packaging. In addition, the density of the bar code will need to be consistent to ensure that an accurate scan each time.

The bar code should be included on all immediate container labels of all commercially available prescription and nonprescription medications, regardless of the dosage form. The standardized bar code should appear on every unit-of-use packaging, to include single-unit, single-dose, unit-dose, unit-of-use, multiple-unit, and multiple-dose containers. The use of bar codes will enhance patient safety through the reduction of medication errors.

Labeling and Packaging Preventions

There are several ways health care organizations are able to reduce medication errors due to labeling and packaging of drug products. Health care organizations can utilize machine-readable coding, such as bar coding, in the management of the medication use process.

A second key area in error reduction involves the storage of medications from bulk delivery to point of use. In selecting the storage and location of these products, special consideration should be given to distinguishing similar products. Specific medications appearing in concentrated forms or that have a high potential for risk should be stored in specific locations. Another consideration is the access and accountability of floor stock medications. A health care organization needs to consider the safety and accountability of access to pharmaceuticals when a pharmacist is not present, such as the access to floor stock and access to the pharmacy when the pharmacy is closed.

Prescription Scanning

Today, pharmacies scan prescriptions upon their receipt. This process entails entering the prescription information into the pharmacy's computer system. Next, the medication is selected and the bar code is scanned. If the medication's bar code matches the information in the computer system, one is able to continue with the prescription processing. If the information does not match, one must determine the problem and correct it before proceeding further. At no time should the process be bypassed by either the pharmacy technician or the pharmacist. Prescription scanning eliminates errors in prescription processing.

Pharmaceutical Industry Assistance

The pharmaceutical industry can assist both the FDA and USP to establish and implement uniform bar code standards for all medications. Second, the pharmaceutical industry can assist in the development of technology to read bar codes properly. A third area is selecting trade names that are not similar to current brand or generic names. The pharmaceutical industry can modify their packaging to differentiate them from other strengths of a particular medication, such as using different colors for different strengths.

Continuous Quality Improvement (CQI)

For pharmacy organizations using a continuous quality improvement (CQI) process, quality is improved when the probability of desired outcomes has increased and undesired outcomes have decreased. CQI is more prominent in institutional pharmacy than community pharmacy practice. It is extremely important to discover the factual basis of a problem instead of the cause or nature of the problem. Promptly recording any related information will help the pharmacy team discover why the mistake occurred. The creation of a database of useful information is paramount within a health care organization. The following information is beneficial:

- Was the prescription telephoned to the pharmacy or was it transmitted in writing (paper, fax, or computer)?
- Was the prescription new or a refill?
- Was the prescription prepared for a person who chose to wait for it, or was it prepared for the "will call" or delivery area?
- How many hours did the pharmacist who made the error work on the date of the dispensing error?
- Take the number of prescriptions filled on the day of error by the pharmacist who made the error and divide it by the number of hours worked by that pharmacist to calculate an average of prescriptions filled per hour on that day by the pharmacist.
- How many other pharmacists were working at the time the dispensing error occurred?
- How many support staff members were working at the time the dispensing error occurred?

- Was the pharmacist involved with the dispensing error a regular staff member at the pharmacy, or was the pharmacist an occasional staff member (such as a floater or relief pharmacist)?
- During the shift on which the dispensing error occurred, was the pharmacist involved with the error performing several different dispensing functions throughout the shift, or did the pharmacist focus on a single dispensing function for all or most of the shift?
- Was the prescription dispensed to the patient or to another patient acting for the patient?
- Is it documented in writing that the person who received the medication was counseled by the pharmacist?
- Did the patient ingest the erroneously dispensed medication, and if so, what was the consequence for the patient?

Workload has long been attributed to a major cause of prescription errors. A pharmacist who is asked to fill more prescriptions per unit of time may not fill all of the prescriptions accurately. Due to managed-care restrictions on pharmacy reimbursement, a pharmacy will be required to fill more prescriptions to maintain a steady level of income. An increase in the number of prescriptions filled results in less time per prescription and may result in more errors.

Another area examined is the determination of a "safe rate" of prescriptions processed; this has been unsuccessful for many reasons. First, some prescriptions require more time to process, such as compounds or medications requiring reconstitution. Second, some pharmacists work more efficiently than other pharmacists do. Third, a pharmacy may employ more clerical help or technological support than another pharmacy.

All activities performed within a pharmacy should be done purposefully, according to the system, in which each specific action is understood to cause a specific result and changes can be performed on the system. A well-designed system will produce positive outcomes and a poorly designed system will yield poor results. The pharmacy system should allow a competent and caring pharmacist to produce good results. If a pharmacist is alleged to have made a mistake, it is extremely important that the pharmacist is able to describe the system used. There should be sufficient checks and balances in place to reduce errors.

Tech Check

13. What are three benefits of e-prescribing?(LO 12.15)

14. What are three things prescribers can do when writing prescriptions to reduce errors?(LO 12.4, 12..6)

15. What are three things that can be done when dispensing medications to reduce medication errors?(LO 12.6)

Regulatory Oversight(LO 12.10, 12.16)

A state board of pharmacy is responsible for the practice of pharmacy within the state (Figure 12-11). It possesses permissive authority, not mandatory authority. The state board of pharmacy has the authority to admonish a pharmacist, assess a fine to the pharmacist who errs, or even suspend the license to practice pharmacy within the state.

Overall, the use of punishment has been shown not to be an effective means of reducing prescription errors. Once an error has occurred, it cannot be reversed. Errors occur because of multiple factors and placing blame on a particular individual will not solve the problem. In the majority of situations, the system has failed!

The IOM recommends that a health care regulator, which includes the state board of pharmacy, regulate to implement "meaningful patient safety programs with defined executive responsibility." In other words, state boards of pharmacy wish to ensure that systems are developed to enable pharmacists and pharmacy technicians to do their best. It is the responsibility of the institution to design its system and to improve safety of the system to improve the system's outcomes.

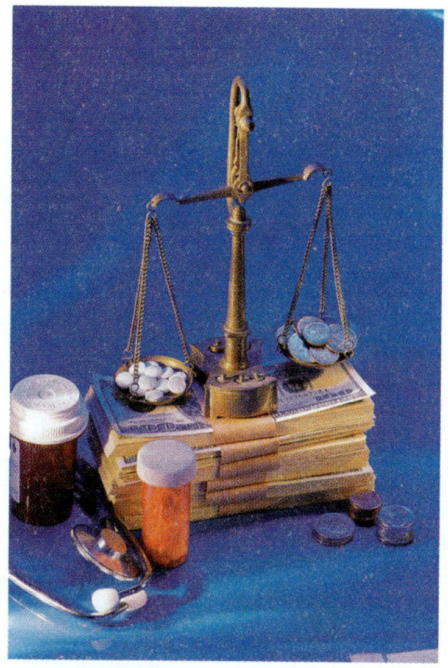

Figure 12-11 A state board of pharmacy is responsible for the practice of pharmacy within the state.

MedWatch

The FDA has the responsibility for ensuring the safety and efficacy of all regulated marketed medical products. **MedWatch,** the FDA Safety Information and Adverse Event Reporting Program (**www.accessdata.fda.gov/scripts/medwatch/**), serves both health care professionals and the medical product–using public. Practitioners can report medication issues by using FDA Form 3500 or FDA Form 3500A (Figures 12-12 and 12-13). MedWatch provides important and timely clinical information about safety issues involving medical products, including prescription and over-the-counter (OTC) drugs, biologics, medical and radiation-emitting devices, and special nutritional products (e.g., medical foods, dietary supplements, and infant formulas). Medical product safety alerts, recalls, withdrawals, and important labeling changes that may affect the health of all Americans are quickly disseminated to the medical community and the public via the MedWatch Web site and the MedWatch E-list.

Vaccine Adverse Event Reporting System (VAERS)

The **Vaccine Adverse Event Reporting System (VAERS)** is a valuable tool for postmarketing safety surveillance (monitoring after a product has been approved and is on the market). Although extensive studies are required for licensure of new vaccines, postmarketing research and surveillance are necessary to identify safety issues that may only be detected following vaccination of a much larger and more diverse population. Rare events may not become known before licensure. Sometimes an event is noted, but the evidence may not be adequate to conclude that a noted event is due to the vaccine.

VAERS is a program created as an outgrowth of the National Childhood Vaccine Injury Act of 1986 (NCVIA) and is administered by the Food and Drug Administration (FDA) and the Centers for Disease Control and Prevention (CDC). VAERS accepts reports of adverse events that may be associated with U.S.-licensed vaccines from health care providers, manufacturers, and the public (Figure 12-14). The FDA continually monitors VAERS reports for any unexpected patterns or changes in rates of adverse events.

MedWatch The FDA Safety Information and Adverse Event Reporting Program that serves both health care professionals and the medical product–using public.

Vaccine Adverse Event Reporting System (VAERS) A cooperative program for vaccine safety of the Centers for Disease Control and Prevention (CDC) and the Food and Drug Administration (FDA). VAERS is a postmarketing safety surveillance program, collecting information about adverse events (possible side effects) that occur after the administration of U.S.-licensed vaccines.

Figure 12-12 Form 3500 for FDA Voluntary Reporting.

Next Page | Reset Form

U.S. Department of Health and Human Services

MEDWATCH

The FDA Safety Information and Adverse Event Reporting Program General Instructions

For VOLUNTARY reporting of adverse events, product problems and product use errors

Page 1 of 12

Form Approved: OMB No. 0910-0291, Expires: 12/31/2011
See OMB statement on reverse.

FDA USE ONLY
Triage unit sequence #

PLEASE TYPE OR USE BLACK INK

A. PATIENT INFORMATION Section A - Help

1. **Patient Identifier** — In confidence
2. **Age at Time of Event or Date of Birth:**
3. **Sex** ☐ Female ☐ Male
4. **Weight** ______ lb or ______ kg

B. ADVERSE EVENT, PRODUCT PROBLEM OR ERROR

Check all that apply: Section B - Help

1. ☐ **Adverse Event** ☐ **Product Problem** *(e.g., defects/malfunctions)*
☐ **Product Use Error** ☐ **Problem with Different Manufacturer of Same Medicine**

2. **Outcomes Attributed to Adverse Event** *(Check all that apply)*
☐ Death: ______ *(mm/dd/yyyy)* ☐ Disability or Permanent Damage
☐ Life-threatening ☐ Congenital Anomaly/Birth Defect
☐ Hospitalization - initial or prolonged ☐ Other Serious (Important Medical Events)
☐ Required Intervention to Prevent Permanent Impairment/Damage (Devices)

3. **Date of Event** *(mm/dd/yyyy)*
4. **Date of this Report** *(mm/dd/yyyy)*
5. **Describe Event, Problem or Product Use Error**

(Continue on page 3)

6. **Relevant Tests/Laboratory Data, Including Dates**

(Continue on page 3)

7. **Other Relevant History, Including Preexisting Medical Conditions** *(e.g., allergies, race, pregnancy, smoking and alcohol use, liver/kidney problems, etc.)*

C. PRODUCT AVAILABILITY Section C - Help

Product Available for Evaluation? *(Do not send product to FDA)*
☐ Yes ☐ No ☐ Returned to Manufacturer on: ______ *(mm/dd/yyyy)*

D. SUSPECT PRODUCT(S) Section D - Help

1. **Name, Strength, Manufacturer** *(from product label)*
#1 Name:
Strength:
Manufacturer:
#2 Name:
Strength:
Manufacturer:

2. **Dose or Amount** | **Frequency** | **Route**
#1
#2

3. **Dates of Use** *(If unknown, give duration) from/to (or best estimate)*
#1
#2

4. **Diagnosis or Reason for Use** *(Indication)*
#1
#2

5. **Event Abated After Use Stopped or Dose Reduced?**
#1 ☐ Yes ☐ No ☐ Doesn't Apply
#2 ☐ Yes ☐ No ☐ Doesn't Apply

6. **Lot #**
#1
#2

7. **Expiration Date**
#1
#2

8. **Event Reappeared After Reintroduction?**
#1 ☐ Yes ☐ No ☐ Doesn't Apply
#2 ☐ Yes ☐ No ☐ Doesn't Apply

9. **NDC # or Unique ID**

E. SUSPECT MEDICAL DEVICE Section E - Help

1. **Brand Name**
2. **Common Device Name**
3. **Manufacturer Name, City and State**
4. **Model #** | **Lot #**
Catalog # | **Expiration Date** *(mm/dd/yyyy)*
Serial # | **Other #**
5. **Operator of Device**
☐ Health Professional
☐ Lay User/Patient
☐ Other:
6. **If Implanted, Give Date** *(mm/dd/yyyy)*
7. **If Explanted, Give Date** *(mm/dd/yyyy)*
8. **Is this a Single-use Device that was Reprocessed and Reused on a Patient?**
☐ Yes ☐ No
9. **If Yes to Item No. 8, Enter Name and Address of Reprocessor**

F. OTHER (CONCOMITANT) MEDICAL PRODUCTS

Product names and therapy dates *(exclude treatment of event)* Section F - Help

(Continue on page 3)

G. REPORTER ***(See confidentiality section on back)*** Section G - Help

1. **Name and Address**
Name:
Address:
City: State: ZIP:

Phone # | **E-mail**

2. **Health Professional?** ☐ Yes ☐ No
3. **Occupation**
4. **Also Reported to:**
☐ Manufacturer
☐ User Facility
☐ Distributor/Importer
5. **If you do NOT want your identity disclosed to the manufacturer, place an "X" in this box:** ☐

FORM FDA 3500 (1/09) Submission of a report does not constitute an admission that medical personnel or the product caused or contributed to the event.

Figure 12-13 Form 3500A for FDA Mandatory Reporting.

Print | Next Page | Reset Form

Form Approved: OMB No. 09 10-029 1, Expires 12/31/11
See OMB statement on reverse.

U.S. Department of Health and Human Services
Food and Drug Administration

MEDWATCH

FORM FDA 3500A (1/09)

General Instructions

For use by user-facilities, importers, distributors and manufacturers for MANDATORY reporting

Page 1 of 15

Mfr Report #

UF/Importer Report #

FDA Use Only

PLEASE TYPE OR USE BLACK INK

A. PATIENT INFORMATION Section A - Help

1. **Patient Identifier** — In confidence
2. **Age at Time of Event:** or **Date of Birth:**
3. **Sex** — ☐ Female ☐ Male
4. **Weight** — lbs or kgs

B. ADVERSE EVENT OR PRODUCT PROBLEM Section B - Help

1. ☐ **Adverse Event** and/or ☐ **Product Problem** *(e.g., defects/malfunctions)*
2. **Outcomes Attributed to Adverse Event** *(Check all that apply)*
   - ☐ Death: *(mm/dd/yyyy)*
   - ☐ Disability or Permanent Damage
   - ☐ Life-threatening
   - ☐ Congenital Anomaly/Birth Defect
   - ☐ Hospitalization - initial or prolonged
   - ☐ Other Serious (Important Medical Events)
   - ☐ Required Intervention to Prevent Permanent Impairment/Damage (Devices)
3. **Date of Event** *(mm/dd/yyyy)*
4. **Date of This Report** *(mm/dd/yyyy)*
5. **Describe Event or Problem**
6. **Relevant Tests/Laboratory Data, Including Dates**
7. **Other Relevant History, Including Preexisting Medical Conditions** *(e.g., allergies, race, pregnancy, smoking and alcohol use, hepatic/renal dysfunction, etc.)*

Submission of a report does not constitute an admission that medical personnel, user facility, importer, distributor, manufacturer or product caused or contributed to the event.

C. SUSPECT PRODUCT(S) Section C - Help

1. **Name** *(Give labeled strength & mfr/labeler)* #1 #2
2. **Dose, Frequency & Route Used** #1 #2
3. **Therapy Dates** *(If unknown, give duration) from/to (or best estimate)* #1 #2
4. **Diagnosis for Use** *(Indication)* #1 #2
5. **Event Abated After Use Stopped or Dose Reduced?** #1 ☐ Yes ☐ No ☐ Doesn't Apply; #2 ☐ Yes ☐ No ☐ Doesn't Apply
6. **Lot #** #1 #2
7. **Exp. Date** #1 #2
8. **Event Reappeared After Reintroduction?** #1 ☐ Yes ☐ No ☐ Doesn't Apply; #2 ☐ Yes ☐ No ☐ Doesn't Apply
9. **NDC# or Unique ID**
10. **Concomitant Medical Products and Therapy Dates** *(Exclude treatment of event)*

D. SUSPECT MEDICAL DEVICE Section D - Help

1. **Brand Name**
2. **Common Device Name**
3. **Manufacturer Name, City and State**
4. **Model #** — **Lot #** — **Catalog #** — **Expiration Date** *(mm/dd/yyyy)* — **Serial #** — **Other #**
5. **Operator of Device** — ☐ Health Professional ☐ Lay User/Patient ☐ Other:
6. **If Implanted, Give Date** *(mm/dd/yyyy)*
7. **If Explanted, Give Date** *(mm/dd/yyyy)*
8. **Is this a Single-use Device that was Reprocessed and Reused on a Patient?** ☐ Yes ☐ No
9. **If Yes to Item No. 8, Enter Name and Address of Reprocessor**
10. **Device Available for Evaluation?** *(Do not send to FDA)* ☐ Yes ☐ No ☐ Returned to Manufacturer on: *(mm/dd/yyyy)*
11. **Concomitant Medical Products and Therapy Dates** *(Exclude treatment of event)*

E. INITIAL REPORTER Section E - Help

1. **Name and Address** — **Phone #**
2. **Health Professional?** ☐ Yes ☐ No
3. **Occupation**
4. **Initial Reporter Also Sent Report to FDA** ☐ Yes ☐ No ☐ Unk.

Figure 12-14 VAERS Reporting Form.

WEBSITE: www.vaers.hhs.gov E-MAIL: info@vaers.org FAX: 1-877-721-0366

VAERS

VACCINE ADVERSE EVENT REPORTING SYSTEM
24 Hour Toll-Free Information 1-800-822-7967
P.O. Box 1100, Rockville, MD 20849-1100
PATIENT IDENTITY KEPT CONFIDENTIAL

For CDC/FDA Use Only
VAERS Number ____________
Date Received ____________

Patient Name:	Vaccine administered by (Name):	Form completed by (Name):
Last First M.I.	Responsible Physician ____________	Relation to Patient ☐ Vaccine Provider ☐ Patient/Parent ☐ Manufacturer ☐ Other
Address	Facility Name/Address	Address *(if different from patient or provider)*
City State Zip	City State Zip	City State Zip
Telephone no. (____) ____________	Telephone no. (____) ____________	Telephone no. (____) ____________

1. State	2. County where administered	3. Date of birth __/__/__ mm dd yy	4. Patient age	5. Sex ☐ M ☐ F	6. Date form completed __/__/__ mm dd yy

7. Describe adverse events(s) (symptoms, signs, time course) and treatment, if any

8. Check all appropriate:
☐ Patient died (date __/__/__ mm dd yy)
☐ Life threatening illness
☐ Required emergency room/doctor visit
☐ Required hospitalization (________days)
☐ Resulted in prolongation of hospitalization
☐ Resulted in permanent disability
☐ None of the above

9. Patient recovered ☐ YES ☐ NO ☐ UNKNOWN

10. Date of vaccination __/__/__ mm dd yy Time ________ AM PM

11. Adverse event onset __/__/__ mm dd yy Time ________ AM PM

12. Relevant diagnostic tests/laboratory data

13. Enter all vaccines given on date listed in no. 10

	Vaccine (type)	Manufacturer	Lot number	Route/Site	No. Previous Doses
a.					
b.					
c.					
d.					

14. Any other vaccinations within 4 weeks prior to the date listed in no. 10

	Vaccine (type)	Manufacturer	Lot number	Route/Site	No. Previous doses	Date given
a.						
b.						

15. Vaccinated at:
☐ Private doctor's office/hospital ☐ Military clinic/hospital
☐ Public health clinic/hospital ☐ Other/unknown

16. Vaccine purchased with:
☐ Private funds ☐ Military funds
☐ Public funds ☐ Other/unknown

17. Other medications

18. Illness at time of vaccination (specify)

19. Pre-existing physician-diagnosed allergies, birth defects, medical conditions (specify)

20. Have you reported this adverse event previously? ☐ No ☐ To health department ☐ To doctor ☐ To manufacturer

Only for children 5 and under

22. Birth weight ________ lb. ________ oz.

23. No. of brothers and sisters

21. Adverse event following prior vaccination (check all applicable, specify)

	Adverse Event	Onset Age	Type Vaccine	Dose no. in series
☐ In patient				
☐ In brother or sister				

Only for reports submitted by manufacturer/immunization project

24. Mfr./imm. proj. report no.

25. Date received by mfr./imm.proj.

26. 15 day report? ☐ Yes ☐ No

27. Report type ☐ Initial ☐ Follow-Up

Health care providers and manufacturers are required by law (42 USC 300aa-25) to report reactions to vaccines listed in the Table of Reportable Events Following Immunization. Reports for reactions to other vaccines are voluntary except when required as a condition of immunization grant awards.

Form VAERS-1(FDA)

MEDMARX

MEDMARX is a national, Internet-accessible database that hospitals and health care systems use to track and trend adverse reactions and medication errors. The program is voluntary and one subscribes to it on a yearly basis. MEDMARX is a quality improvement tool that facilitates productive and efficient documentation, reporting, analysis, tracking, trending, and prevention of drug events.

Features of MEDMARX include:

- Allows anonymous reporting of adverse drug events
- Captures information on actions taken and makes recommendations to avoid future adverse drug events
- Provides automatic completion of TJC root cause analysis template and FDA's MedWatch forms

MEDMARX allows both hospitals and health care systems to:

- Improve patient safety and standard of care within an institution
- Prevent medication errors and adverse drug reactions through proactive measures to identify potential problems
- Eliminate the high costs and risks associated with medication errors and adverse drug reactions
- Provide insight into trends and best practices from a comprehensive national database

USP-ISMP Medication Errors Reporting Program (MERP)

All health care practitioners who encounter actual or potential medication errors are encouraged to report them confidentially and anonymously to the USP-ISMP Medication Errors Reporting Program (MERP). This program analyzes and disseminates recommendations for prevention of errors. Both regulatory agencies and pharmaceutical manufacturers are notified of needed changes in products. The failure to report such incidents would allow these safety issues to go unchecked in the future.

Types of errors to be reported include misinterpretations, miscalculations, misadministrations, difficulty in interpreting handwritten orders, and misunderstanding of verbal orders. Other concerns include confusion over look-alike/sound-alike drugs, incorrect route of administration, and misuse of medical equipment.

When reporting an error the following information should be included:

- Describe the error or preventable adverse drug reaction. What went wrong?
- Was this an actual medication error (reached the patient) or are you expressing concern about a potential error or writing about an error that was discovered before it reached the patient?
- What was the patient outcome?
- In what type of practice site (hospital, private office, retail pharmacy, drug company, long-term care facility) did the error occur?
- What are the generic names (INNs or official names) of all products involved?
- What are the brand names of all products involved?

- What was the dosage form, concentration, or strength?
- How was the error discovered/intercepted?
- What are your recommendations for error prevention?

It is through the reporting of errors that future errors may be prevented.

Patient Role in Medication Error Reduction

The American Pharmacists Association (APhA) believes that the patient can play an integral role in reducing medication errors. Based on a study conducted by the APhA, only 55% of the patients surveyed could identify the active ingredient in their prescription medications but more than 55% could identify the main ingredients in their nonprescription medications, vitamins, mineral supplements, and herbal or natural products.

The APhA recommends that the pharmacy patient do the following:

- Use one pharmacy. If the pharmacy patient uses the same pharmacy, the pharmacy staff will be able to perform a more accurate drug utilization review of your prescription, OTC, vitamins, mineral supplements, or natural products.
- Know your medicine. Patients should know the names of the medications you are taking, why you are taking them, and how they make you feel. You should inform your pharmacist if the medication looks different or it makes you feel different.
- Know your pharmacist. If you know your pharmacist, you will be more likely to discuss medication issues with him or her.
- Keep a list of all of your medications. This list should include prescription medications, nonprescription drugs, herbal, and other dietary supplements.

Tech Check

16. What form is used by practitioners to report medication issues?(LO 12.16)

17. Who uses MEDMARX?(LO 12.16)

18. Who uses MERP?(LO 12.16)

19. What is one thing patients can do to assist in reducing prescription errors?(LO 12.10)

Chapter Summary

Understanding the cause and prevention of medication errors is vital to the pharmacy technician. Important points to know are:

- Errors may occur during the prescribing, dispensing, counseling, and administration processes.
- Errors can never be completely eliminated from the practice of pharmacy; however, both the pharmacist and pharmacy technician can work to reduce these errors.
- Upon discovery of a medication error, it is important to identify the cause of the error and find solutions to prevent the error from occurring again.
- Reporting medication errors through the MedWatch, VAERS, MEDMARX, and the USP-ISMP systems will play a major role in the reduction and prevention of medication errors.
- In the future, electronic prescribing will play a major role in the reduction of medication errors.

Chapter Review

Case Study Questions

1. Who could have prevented the overdose from occurring?(LO 12.3)
2. What should the pharmacy team have done when filling the prescription?(LO 12.3)

At Your Service Questions

1. What should the pharmacy technician do?(LO 12.4)
2. What could happen if the pharmacy fills the prescription without verifying the prescription with the physician?(LO 12.1)
3. Could the pharmacy team use as an excuse that they filled the prescription because the patient demanded it?(LO 12.3)

Multiple Choice

Select the best answer.

1. Which of the following is a cause for medication errors?(LO 12.3)
   a. Failed communication
   b. Dose miscalculations
   c. Lack of patient education
   d. All of the above
2. According to most research, the perceived dispensing error rate among pharmacists is(LO 12.4)
   a. increasing.
   b. decreasing.
   c. remaining constant.
   d. undetermined.
3. Which of the following is an explanation of a failed communication?(LO 12.2)
   a. Perfect handwriting
   b. Lack of patient education
   c. A miscalculated drug dose
   d. Similar route
4. What explanation does a pharmacist most often use for a dispensing error?(LO 12.3)
   a. Overwork and fatigue
   b. Having to counsel patients
   c. Improperly trained pharmacy technicians
   d. Improperly supervised pharmacy technicians
5. Which of the following would be considered incorrect drug administration?(LO 12.2)
   a. Incorrect patient
   b. Incorrect route
   c. Incorrect time
   d. All of the above
6. Which of the following is a true statement regarding similar drug names?(LO 12.13
   a. Are encouraged by the FDA
   b. Rarely cause confusion among pharmacists
   c. Are responsible for about 15% of reported errors
   d. All of the above
7. Which of the following is a type of medical error?(LO 12.2)
   a. Diagnostic
   b. Technical
   c. Wound infection
   d. All are examples of medical errors
8. At what rate is there a greater likelihood that a prescription error may occur?(LO 12.3)
   a. Filling 10 prescriptions per hour
   b. Filling 12 prescriptions per hour
   c. Filling 15 prescriptions per hour
   d. Filling 17 prescriptions per hour
9. Which of the following is likely to cause an interruption or distraction in a pharmacy?(LO 12.3)
   a. Automatic dispensing machines
   b. Faxes
   c. Interruptions such as the telephone ringing
   d. Automatic telephone refill systems

10. How many times should a pharmacist or pharmacy technician read a prescription?(LO 12.6)
    a. 1 time
    b. 2 times
    c. 3 times
    d. Varies based upon the expertise of the individual

11. Which of the following statements most correctly describes the attitude of courts toward dispensing errors of pharmacists?(LO 12.12)
    a. Courts will punish a pharmacist if they can show that the pharmacist intentionally made an error.
    b. Courts will punish a pharmacist if there is a loss of human life.
    c. Courts will punish the pharmacist if it is shown that there is a continuous pattern of errors.
    d. Courts will ordinarily find a pharmacist legally liable for any dispensing error.

12. Which of the following is least likely to reduce the number of prescription errors by a pharmacist?(LO 12.6)
    a. Frequent checking of prescriptions
    b. Increased use of adequately trained support personnel
    c. Working faster so there is no backlog of prescriptions
    d. Providing patients with comfortable waiting areas

13. What is the purpose of quality assurance programs?(LO 12.6)
    a. Document the causes of errors and implement programs to reduce them
    b. Provide evidence for state disciplinary actions
    c. Reduce the use of technicians in dispensing activities
    d. All of the above

14. Which of the following is being done to reduce the number of prescription errors?(LO 12.6)
    a. Limit the number of hours a pharmacist may work in a pay period
    b. Limit the number of pharmacy technicians a pharmacist may supervise
    c. Set limits for the number of prescriptions that a pharmacist may process on a shift
    d. All of the above

15. What effect does patient counseling have on dispensing errors?(LO 12.6)
    a. Increases the number of errors
    b. Increases the detection of errors before they reach the patient
    c. Increases time in filling a prescription
    d. Has no effect on errors being committed

16. Which of the following is true about the reporting of prescription errors?(LO 12.16)
    a. Reporting is required by all boards of pharmacy.
    b. All errors must be reported to the FDA.
    c. State reporting systems increase the number of penalties awarded.
    d. There is a growing trend for a state reporting system in conjunction with quality assurance programs.

17. Which of the following contributes to the largest percentage of medication errors according to MEDMARX?(LO 12.3)
    a. Communication
    b. Computer entry
    c. Documentation
    d. Performance deficit

18. According to MEDMARX, which of the following constitutes the largest percentage of types of prescription errors?(LO 12.2)
    a. Improper dose/quantity
    b. Omission errors
    c. Prescribing errors
    d. Wrong drug

19. Which of the following organizations is responsible for the postmarketing surveillance of vaccines?(LO 12.16)
    a. TJC
    b. MEDMARX
    c. MedWatch
    d. VAERS

20. Which of the following medications result in the greatest percentage of medication errors?(LO 12.13)
    a. Insulin
    b. Morphine
    c. Potassium chloride
    d. Warfarin

Identify the omission or error in the following prescriptions:

Rx. 1

Andrew J. Prescriber
1000 Buzz Aldrin Dr., Suite 103
Reston, VA 20194
703-435-1111

Mary E. Shed — March 10, 2012
1000 Wilson Blvd. — Arlington, VA 22209

Inderal 5 mg — #30
1 tab po every day
Refill × 3

Dr. Andrew J. Prescriber

Rx. 2

Andrew J. Prescriber
1000 Buzz Aldrin Dr., Suite 103
Reston, VA 20194
703-435-1111
FP5555555

Hector Belt — March 8, 2012
1000 Armstrong Ave. — Reston, VA 20194

Robitussin AC — 240 g
1 teaspoonful po q 6-8 hrs prn cough

Dr. Andrew J. Prescriber

Rx. 3

Andrew J. Prescriber
1000 Buzz Aldrin Dr., Suite 103
Reston, VA 20194
703-435-1111

Matthew Shult — March 9, 2012
200 Thomas Jefferson Way — Reston, VA 20194

Cortisorin Otic Soln — 8 mL
Instill one drop in right eye for conjunctivitis

Dr. Andrew J. Prescriber

Rx. 4

Andrew J. Prescriber
1000 Buzz Aldrin Dr., Suite 103
Reston, VA 20194
703-435-1111

Patrick Amano — March 1, 2012
100 Brown Belt TKD Way — Great Falls, VA 11111
Amoxicillin 250 mg/5 mL Suspension — 150 mL
Inject 5 mL IV every 8 hours

Dr. Andrew J. Prescriber

Rx. 5

Andrew J. Prescriber
1000 Buzz Aldrin Dr., Suite 103
Reston, VA 20194
703-435-1111

Matt Jones — March 6, 2012
2222 Subunit Rd. — Reston, VA 20190
Tessalon Perles #30
Chew one perle q 8 hours
Refill × 1

Dr. Andrew J. Prescriber

Critical Thinking Questions

1. Assume you are a patient and the pharmacist informs you that you received the incorrect strength of a medication. How would you react?(LO 12.3)
2. If you were a pharmacist, would you admit that you made a prescription error to a patient? Why?(LO 12.9)
3. Should a health care organization punish individuals for reporting prescription errors that they made or commend them for their honesty? Why?(LO 12.9)

HIPAA Scenario

Elena Rodriquez, CPhT, a retail pharmacy technician, is filling a prescription for 30 0.125 mg generic digoxin tablets for patient Carol Mason. Upon opening the stock bottle to count out 30 tablets, Elena notices that the stock bottle contains both white and yellow tablets of the same size. The color of the generic digoxin 0.125 mg tablets from the manufacturer is yellow. Elena believes that what most likely happened is that either a pharmacy technician or a pharmacist had previously removed both the 0.125 mg generic digoxin and 0.25 mg generic digoxin stock bottles from the shelf at the same time, opened the stock bottle of 0.25-mg generic digoxin (white) tablets, and after counting out the number of tables needed to fill the prescription, accidentally put the extra 0.25 mg generic digoxin (white) tablets into the *wrong* bottle of 0.125 mg generic digoxin (yellow) tablets.

Drug Name
Digoxin
Strength(s)
0.125 mg
Drug Name, Imprint(s), Manufacturer/Distributor
Duramed

Drug Name
Digoxin
Strength(s)
0.125 mg
Imprint(s)
LANOXIN Y3B
Manufacturer/Distributor
Vangard Labs Inc

Drug Name
Digoxin
Strength(s)
0.25 mg
Imprint(s), Manufacturer/Distributor
Duramed

Discussion Questions(PTCB II. 73)

1. What should the technician do?
2. Should Elena separate out the two colors of tablets and place the white tablets into the bottle of 0.25-mg digoxin?
3. What impact, if any, on previous patients does this scenario present?
4. What questions should the technician and pharmacist have?
5. How does this scenario relate to HIPAA?

Internet Activities

1. What safeguards to reduce prescription errors have been implemented by your state board of pharmacy?(LO 12.16)
2. Visit **www.jointcommission.org** and identify recommendations to reduce medication errors proposed by TJC.(LO 12.16)
3. Explore **www.fda.org** and identify the programs associated with the FDA to reduce prescription errors.(LO 12.16)

13 Referencing

Key Terms

biologicals
biotechnology
brand name
carcinogenesis
cosmeceuticals
etiology
formulary
monoclonal antibodies
monograph
mutagenesis
nutraceuticals
personal digital assistant (PDA)

Learning Outcomes

Upon completion of this chapter, you will be able to:

13.1 Differentiate between primary, secondary, and tertiary literature.

13.2 Explain the importance of maintaining a library in a pharmacy.

13.3 Compare and contrast the components of various reference books.

13.4 Define the meaning of the terms found in a drug monograph.

13.5 Identify the appropriate reference books for a particular setting.

13.6 Discover the use of the Internet in obtaining information affecting pharmacy practice.

13.7 Identify various pharmacy Internet sites and the information they contain.

13.8 Understand the application of technology in obtaining pharmacy information.

PTCB

In preparation for the certification examination, you should understand and perform activities associated with the following PTCB Knowledge Statement:

PTCB Knowledge Statement

Domain I. Assisting the Pharmacist in Serving Patients

Knowledge of drug information sources including printed and electronic reference materials (15)

Case Study

Dr. Andrew J. Shedlock called Your Neighborhood Pharmacy to obtain information on drug interactions with a newly approved medication, Duetact. The pharmacy technician answered the phone promptly and relayed the question to the pharmacist on duty. The pharmacist instructed the technician to look up the medication in the pharmacy's library. The technician looked at the vast collection of reference books maintained at the pharmacy, which included the *USP–NF*, the *PDR*, *Remington's Pharmaceutical Sciences: The Science and Practice of Pharmacy*, and *Drug Facts and Comparisons*. The pharmacy technician chose *Drug Facts and Comparisons* and looked up the drug in the reference book.

While reading this chapter, keep the following question in mind:

1. Did the pharmacy technician choose the correct reference book? Why or why not?(LO 13.5)

Introduction to Referencing(LO 13.2)

The *Millis Report* published in the mid-1970s stated that the practice of pharmacy includes the dispensing of both medication and information. Since a pharmacist may be providing (dispensing) information to a patient or health care provider, it is extremely important that a pharmacy possesses an up-to-date library. The pharmacist may ask the pharmacy technician to look up a specific piece of information regarding a medication. It is important for the technician to be able to access the information correctly and promptly.

All pharmacies are required to maintain a current copy of the *United States Pharmacopoeia–National Formulary (USP–NF)* and the federal Controlled Substance Act. Each state board of pharmacy may have regulations outlining required references to be maintained by a pharmacy. The pharmacy selects references appropriate for the practice. This library may consist of bound books or digital resources.

Types of Reference Sources(LO 13.1)

There are three types of sources—primary, secondary, and tertiary—that are used in the practice of pharmacy.

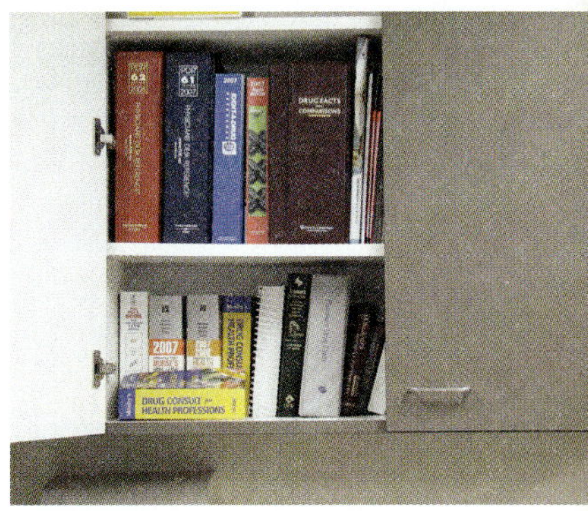

Figure 13-1 Reference books.

- Primary literature for pharmacies is found in various scientific and professional journals. Primary sources include the original studies, and reports found in journals, monographs, and published conference proceedings. Examples of journals include *JAMA: Journal of the American Medical Association, American Journal of Health-System Pharmacy,* and *New England Journal of Medicine.*
- Secondary sources consist of literature to identify primary and other sources, to include bibliographies, abstracting, and indexing services. Secondary sources can be accessed via the Internet. A secondary resource includes review articles. The main disadvantage of secondary sources is that they are expensive and may not be used by pharmacists and pharmacy technicians. Secondary sources must be selected on the scope of the topic.

At Your Service

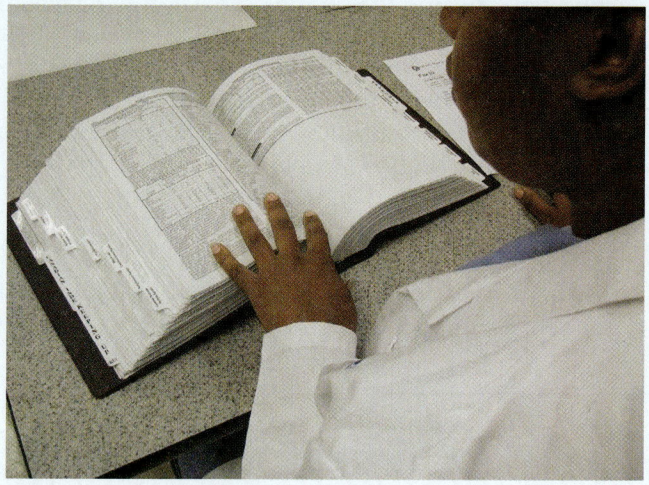

Recently, there have been numerous medication errors occurring at AEGIS Community Hospital regarding the anticoagulant, Coumadin. The pharmacy director is extremely disturbed about this situation due to its life-threatening implications. He assigns his lead pharmacy technician, AJ, to research the problem and to find out if the problem is unique for AEGIS Community Hospital or if it is occurring at other hospitals.

Several hours later, AJ presents his findings to the pharmacy director. According to his research, the Institute for Safe Medication Practices (ISMP) includes Coumadin among its list of drugs that have a heightened risk of causing significant patient harm when used in error. The Joint Commission (TJC), formerly Joint Commission on Accreditation of Healthcare Organizations (JCAHO), recommends that patients receiving anticoagulants receive individualized care through a defined process that includes standardized ordering, dispensing, administration, monitoring, and education.

According to MEDMARX, Coumadin was involved in 1.4% of reported hospital medication errors in 2006. The pharmacy director is extremely impressed with AJ's work and the source of his information.

After a lengthy discussion with members of the Pharmacy and Therapeutic Committee, new guidelines were established for the use of Coumadin within AEGIS Community Hospital. Within 30 days, the number of medication errors involving Coumadin had decreased by 99%.

While reading this chapter, keep the following questions in mind:

1. Where did AJ find this information?(LO 13.5)
2. Why is the need for information important?(LO 13.2)
3. Do all reference materials provide the same information?(LO 13.3)
4. Would you know where to find specific information if a similar situation occurred?(LO 13.5)

- Tertiary sources include general reference books and textbooks (Figure 13-1). Tertiary sources can be used to provide general information for the pharmacist or pharmacy technician. Two outstanding textbooks include *Remington: The Science and Practice of Pharmacy* and *Goodman and Gilman's The Pharmacologic Basis of Therapeutics,* which will be discussed in detail later in the chapter.

Pharmacists provide information to both health care providers and their patients. Being able to inform a physician about the indications, contraindications, and adverse effects of a specific medication may have a profound effect on a patient's treatment and response to that treatment. OBRA-90 required that an offer be made to all pharmacy patients for counseling by the pharmacist. The information provided during counseling may include how to take the medication, possible adverse effects, and what to do if a dose is missed. The information provided should be explained to the patient in terms that the patient will understand. Depending on the pharmacy, setting will determine which reference books are maintained by a pharmacy.

A database is a primary reference source. There are two primary advantages of databases over print sources. Databases are more current than print media and they are easy to use when seeking information.

MEDLINE is produced by the U.S. National Library of Medicine, **www.nlm.nih.gov,** and provides coverage of over 4,000 medical journals. It is subsidized by the U.S. government and can be accessed by using one of two free search engines: PubMed and Internet Grateful Med. MEDLINE is available through other vendors via the Internet, CD-ROMs, or on tape. MEDLINE's strength is in its clinical and therapeutic information (Figure 13-2).

EMBASE is another medical database, but of slightly smaller magnitude than MEDLINE. The primary difference between MEDLINE and EMBASE is that EMBASE is based upon European drug literature instead of U.S. drug literature. EMBASE is made available by two online vendors, Dialog and Ovid, and can be purchased as CD-ROMs.

MEDMARX (**www.medmarx.com**) is an Internet-accessible medication errors database that enables hospitals to report medication errors anonymously to a centralized program and can be used as part of a hospital's internal quality improvement (Figure 13-3). This database provides guidelines for collecting medication error data as well as standardized criteria and methods for reporting, tracking, preventing, and comparing medication error data. MEDMARX allows an institution to view errors and prevention strategies of other participating institutions.

BIOSIS Previews is a scientific database that is an online version of *Biological Abstracts* and *Bioresearch*. BIOSIS focuses on the life sciences, especially the preclinical toxicity and carcinogenicity studies. In addition to these three major databases, there are many specialized databases, which are listed in Table 13-1.

Tech Check

1. What are the differences between primary, secondary, and tertiary pharmacy sources?(LO 13.1)
2. Give an example of a primary, secondary, and tertiary pharmacy reference.(LO 13.1)

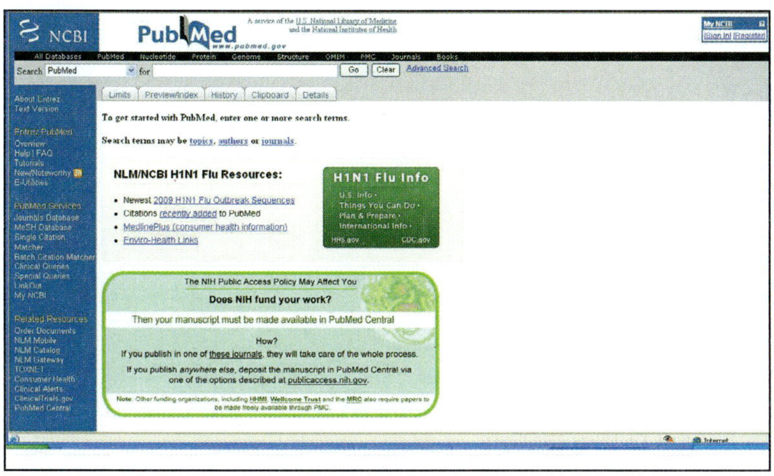

Figure 13-2 PubMed.

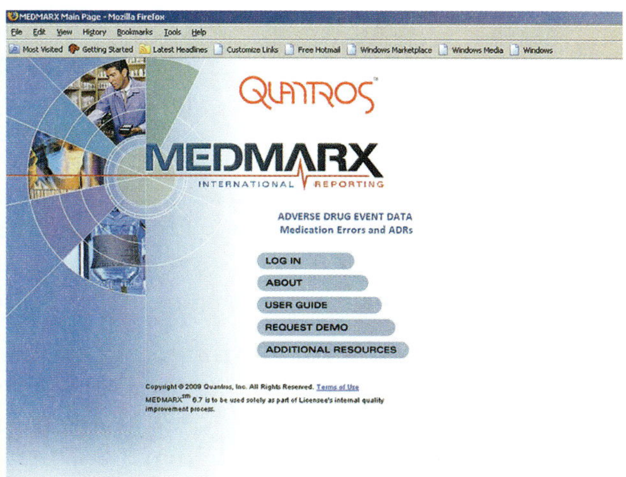

Figure 13-3 MEDMARX.

Table 13-1 Specialized Databases

Database	Specialty
ADIS LMS Drug Alerts	Clinical trials
Derwent Drug File	Drug development and manufacture
Diogenes FDA Regulatory Updates	News stories and unpublished documents relating to U.S. regulation
F-D-C Reports	F-D-C text newsletters to include *Prescription Pharmaceuticals & Biotechnology* and *Nonprescription Pharmaceuticals and Nutritionals*
Iowa Drug Information Service	Indexes of journals by disease and drug therapy
MSDS Database	An online index of Material Safety Data Sheets for USP's entire catalog of more than 2,000 Reference Standards. The database is updated daily.
NDA Pipeline: New Drugs	Tracks drugs through discovery, clinical trials, new drug application, and approval/disapproval by the FDA
Pharmaceutical News Index	Indexes pharmaceutical industry newsletters
Pharmaprojects	Worldwide progress on pharmaceutical products
SEDBASE	Analysis of side effects of drugs in literature
TOXLIT	Toxicity information
Unlisted Drugs	Drug products in active development that are not listed in standard reference work

Commonly Used Pharmacy Reference Books(LO 13.3,13.4,13.5)

There are many different types of reference books available for use in a pharmacy. Pharmacopeias, formularies, and compendia are all examples of various reference books. A pharmacopoeia discusses the therapeutic uses of a drug but also provides official information on the purity, strength, and quality of a specific product. A **formulary** is a listing of approved drugs for an institution or third-party provider. A compendia provides concise information on the therapeutic uses of a medication and may include the pharmacology, pharmacokinetics, contraindication, adverse effects, and specific warnings in the form of a monograph.

United States Pharmacopoeia–National Formulary (USP–NF)

The *USP–NF* is the official compendia for drugs marketed in the United States (Figure 13-4). It contains pharmacopeial standards for medicines, dosage forms, drug substances, excipients, medical devices, and dietary supplements. *USP–NF* in English is available in print, online, and CD formats; *USP–NF* in Spanish is available in print format only.

formulary An approved list of medications to be used in an institution or to be reimbursed by an insurance company.

The *USP–NF* is a single-volume combination of two official compendia, the *United States Pharmacopeia (USP)* and the *National Formulary (NF)*. A **monograph** includes the name of the ingredient or preparation; the definition; packaging, storage, and labeling requirements; and the specification. The specification consists of a series of tests, procedures for the tests, and acceptance criteria. These tests and procedures require the use of official USP Reference Standards. Medicinal ingredients and products will have the stipulated strength, quality, and purity if they conform to the requirements of the monograph. Tests and procedures referred to in multiple monographs are described in detail in the *USP–NF* general chapters. Monographs for drug substances and preparations are featured in the *USP*. Monographs for dietary supplements and ingredients appear in a separate section of the *USP*. Excipient monographs are included in the *NF*.

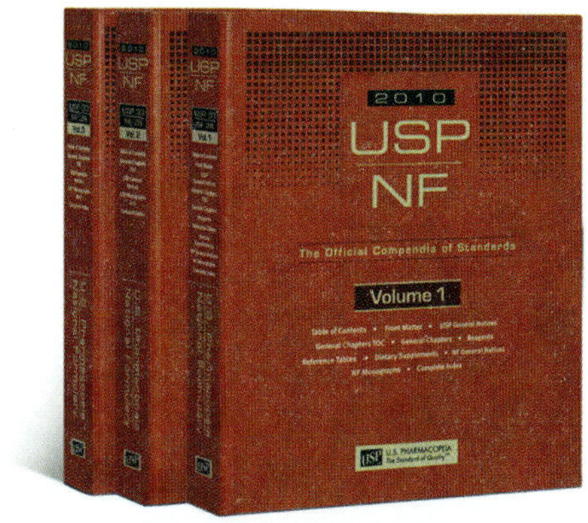

Figure 13-4 ***United States Pharmacopeia (USP)* and the *National Formulary (NF)*.**

The U.S. Federal Food, Drug and Cosmetics Act designates the *USP–NF* as the official compendia for drugs marketed in the United States. A drug product in the U.S. market must conform to the standards in *USP–NF* to avoid possible charges of adulteration and misbranding. The *USP–NF* is also widely used by scientists in industries producing prescription and nonprescription medications, biological and **biotechnology** products. Biotechnology is the field of study that combines the science of biology, chemistry, and immunology to produce synthetic, unique drugs with specific therapeutic effects, blood and blood products, cosmetics, dietary supplements, medical devices, gases, and veterinary medicine. The *USP–NF* is used in quality control and quality assurance programs, regulatory affairs, and research and development and is an important reference for pharmacies and medical and pharmacy schools. Meeting *USP–NF* standards is accepted globally as assurance of high quality. USP creates and continuously revises *USP–NF* standards through a unique public-private collaborative process, which involves the pharmaceutical industry as well as government and other interested parties from anywhere in the world.

monograph A written document that includes the name of the ingredient or preparation; the definition; packaging, storage, and labeling requirements; and the specification.

biotechnology The field of study that combines the science of biology, chemistry, and immunology to produce synthetic, unique drugs with specific therapeutic effects.

Approved Drug Products with Therapeutic Equivalence Evaluations (Orange Book)

The *Approved Drug Products with Therapeutic Equivalence Evaluations* (referred to as the *Orange Book*) is an example of a formulary established by the FDA. It is published yearly and is updated monthly with new drugs (Figure 13-5). The *Orange Book* identifies drug products approved on the basis of safety and effectiveness by the FDA under the Federal Food, Drug and Cosmetic Act. The monthly supplements provide information on newly approved drugs, changes and revisions to current data including therapeutic equivalence evaluations, and updated patent and exclusivity data. It does not include information on medications marketed prior to 1938. The *Orange Book* is used by state governments, hospitals, and third-party insurance plans to develop formularies. It is available in both print and electronic format. The electronic format allows one to search the approved drug list by active ingredient, proprietary name, the applicant holder, or applicant number.

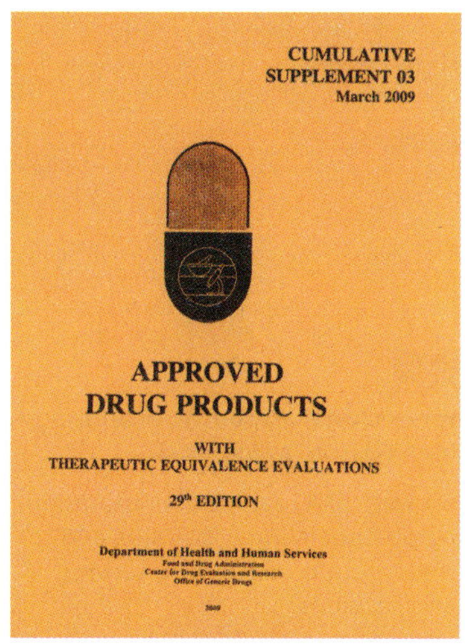

Figure 13.5 ***Approved Drug Products with Therapeutic Equivalence Evaluations* (referred to as the Orange Book).**

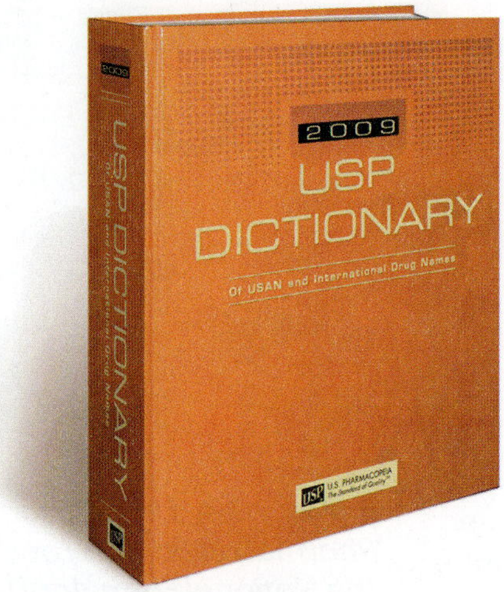

Figure 13-6 **The *USP Dictionary of USAN and International Drug Names.***

The *USP Dictionary of USAN and International Drug Names*

The *USP Dictionary of USAN and International Drug Names* is used by pharmacists, nurses, and other health care providers for regulatory/compendial affairs, quality assurance, research and development, quality control, patent and trademark law, technical documentation, and drug information and safety (Figure 13-6).

Some of the advantages of resource include:

- Ensuring official compliance to product labeling in order to obtain new drug approval and to avoid "misbranded" products
- Determining established generic drug names to use in advertising and brochures as required by U.S. federal law
- Preserving trademark rights to drug brand names by using proper generic names
- Avoiding errors in reports, correspondence, articles, and package inserts
- Grouping drug products into families
- Avoiding serious verbal medication errors

The *USP Dictionary of USAN and International Drug Names* contains the following information:

- Generic or U.S. adopted names
- Brand names
- Chemical names
- International Nonproprietary Names (INNs)
- British Approved Names (BANs)
- Japanese Accepted Names (JANs)
- Official USP–NF names
- FDA-established names
- Drug manufacturers' names
- Graphical chemical structures
- Molecular weights and formulas
- Pharmacologic and/or therapeutic categories
- Code designations
- VA classification system for medications
- USAN submission forms
- Drug pronunciation guide

The resource is available in both print and online formats.

The Merck Index

The Merck Index contains over 10,000 monographs on various drug products (Figure 13-7). These compounds include human and veterinary drugs; biotech drugs and **monoclonal antibodies**, which are antibodies derived from a single cell; substances used for medical imaging; natural and **biologicals** products, which are medicinal preparations made from living organisms and their products, including serums and vaccines; **nutraceuticals**, which are foodstuffs (as a fortified food or dietary supplement) that is held to provide health or medical benefits in addition to its basic nutritional value, and **cosmeceuticals**, which are preparations that contain both pharmaceutical and cosmetic properties; laboratory reagents and catalysts; dyes, colors, and indicators; food additives and nutritional supplements; flavors and fragrances; agricultural chemicals, pesticides, and herbicides; and industrial and specialty chemicals.

monoclonal antibody An antibody derived from a single cell.

biological A medicinal preparation made from living organisms and their products, including serums and vaccines.

nutraceutical A foodstuff (as a fortified food or dietary supplement) that is held to provide health or medical benefits in addition to its basic nutritional value.

cosmeceutical A preparation that contains both pharmaceutical and cosmetic properties.

The Merck Index provides the chemical, common, and generic names; trademarks and associated companies; chemical structures; molecular formulae, weights, and percentage composition; capsule statements identifying compound classes and scientific significance; scientific and patent literature references; physical and toxicity data; therapeutic and commercial uses; and caution and hazard information. *The Merck Index* is available in print and comes with a companion CD.

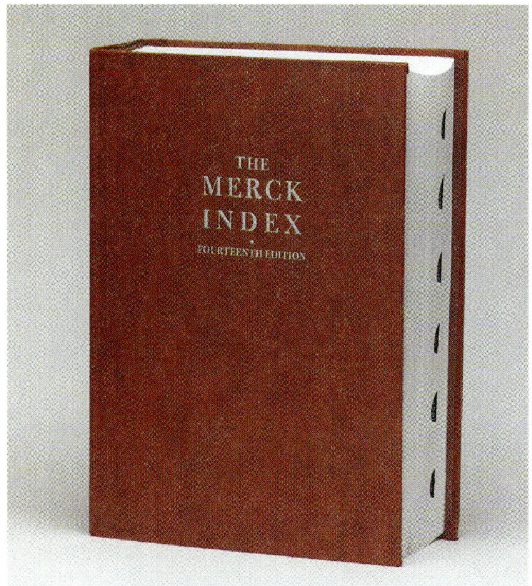

Figure 13-7 ***The Merck Index.***

Drug Facts and Comparisons (F & C)

Drug Facts and Comparisons (F & C) is a comprehensive drug information reference featuring more than 22,000 products. It is available in print media, online, or using a PDA. *Drug Facts and Comparisons* contains prescription and OTC drug product information, drug-herb-food interactions, natural products, and patient information. Specifically, the resource includes:

- Drug interaction facts
- Reviews of natural products
- Nonprescription drug therapies
- Med Facts
- Drug Interaction Facts: herbal supplements and food
- Drug Identification Tool
- A to Z drug facts
- Pregnancy and lactation warnings
- Black box warnings

The print version is updated on a monthly basis.

There are many advantages of the electronic version of *Drug Facts and Comparisons* over the print version:

- Allows user to conduct simple and advanced searches across numerous publications in real time.
- Drug news is updated on a daily basis.
- Reviews comparative tables of therapeutic groups.
- Provides a comprehensive drug identification tool.
- Allows the user print sections of monographs or tables.
- Provides patient education in the form of a Med Guide.
- Allows user search by NDC number using the drug identifier tool.

The PDA version contains A2z Drugs and iFacts, Antibiogram, Antidotes, and Herballx. The advantage of the PDA form is its portability.

Physicians' Desk Reference (PDR)

The *Physicians' Desk Reference* (*PDR*) is a commercially published compilation of manufacturers' prescribing information (package insert) on prescription drugs, updated annually (Figure 13-8). While designed to provide physicians with the full legally mandated information relevant to writing prescriptions (just as its name suggests), it is widely used by other medical specialists.

The PDR is organized into five categories: the manufacturers' index, brand and generic index, product category index, product identification guide, and product information. The product information is organized alphabetically by the drug manufacturer and drug product.

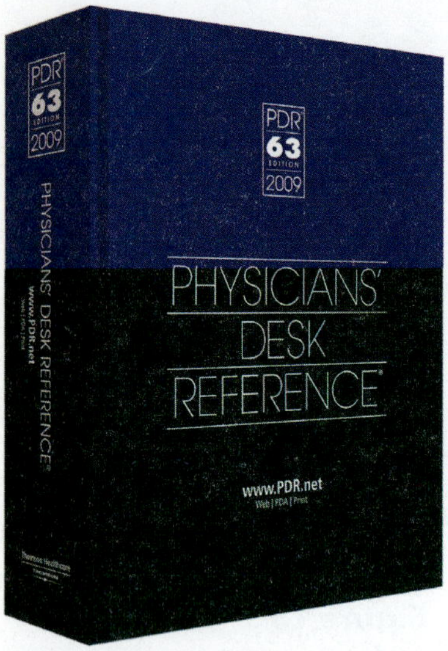

Figure 13-8
The *Physicians' Desk Reference (PDR)*.

carcinogenesis Production of a cancer.

mutagenesis The induction of a genetic mutation.

Each drug monograph contains the following information:

- Brand name.
- Generic name.
- Description.
- Clinical pharmacology: Contains pharmacokinetic information, which includes the absorption, distribution, metabolism, and excretion of the drug entity, as well as mechanism of action and pharmacodynamics of the medication.
- Indications and usage: Defines the condition and population for whom the drug is intended. Indications are specific in nature.
- Contraindications: States when the medication is not to be used in patients, when the risks outweigh the benefits of the medication. All information on contraindication is based on evidence, not theoretical beliefs.
- Warnings: Includes adverse reactions, potential safety hazards, limitation in use imposed by them, and any particular steps to be taken if a situation occurs.
- Precautions: The precaution section contains the following subdivisions:
    - General: Any special care to be provided by prescriber not included in the labeling.
    - Information for patient: Any information that the patient should be aware of for the safe use of the product. If a Patient Product Insert (PPI) is to be provided, it is mentioned in this section.
    - Laboratory tests: Any laboratory tests needed to monitor the use of the product. This may include liver function tests and appropriate blood work to be performed.
    - Drug interactions and drug-laboratory interactions: Any significant interactions that the drug may have with other drugs or with routine lab tests.
    - **Carcinogenesis, mutagenesis,** impairment of fertility: Any data from animal carcinogenicity and fertility studies are presented.
    - Pregnancy: Provides information on the use of the medication on the unborn fetus.
    - Labor and delivery: If the drug has a recognized use during labor and delivery, the effects of the drug on the mother and fetus are included.
    - Nursing mothers: Information about the excretion of the drug in human milk is included.
    - Pediatric use: If the medication has a pediatric indication but must be supported by well-controlled studies.
- Adverse reactions: A listing of the reported side effects associated with the medication. The list may be subcategorized by the system or the percent of cases reported.
- Drug abuse and dependence: Any potential psychological and/or physiological dependence.
- Overdosage: Any potential situations involving overdosage, which may include clinical or laboratory findings. Possible treatments to counteract overdosage are included.
- Dosage and administration: Detailed information regarding proper dosing schedules.
- How supplied: Strength, form, and descriptions of available dosage forms and units in which they are packaged.

PDR for Nonprescription Drugs, Dietary Supplements, and Herbs

PDR for Nonprescription Drugs, Dietary Supplements, and Herbs provides detailed information for OTC drugs, dietary supplements, and herbs (Figure 13-9).

There are nine sections in this reference book:

- Section 1—Manufacturer's Index: Shows all participating manufacturers, including addresses, phone numbers, and emergency contacts. It identifies each manufacturer's products.
- Section 2—Product Name Index: Products are listed alphabetically by brand name.
- Section 3—Product Category Index: Lists all fully described products by prescribing category.
- Section 4—Active Ingredients Index: Cross-references generic ingredients of all product descriptions.
- Section 5—Companion Drug Index: Lists symptoms occurring during prescription drug therapy and presents over-the-counter products that may be recommended for relief.
- Section 6—Product Identification Guide: Shows full-color, actual-sized photos of tablets and capsules. Arranged alphabetically by manufacturer.
- Section 7—Nonprescription Drug Information: Products are arranged alphabetically by brand name within each therapeutic category.
- Section 8—Dietary Supplement and Herbal Information: Provides a variety of natural remedies and nutritional supplements marketed under DSHEA 1994.
- Section 9—Product Comparison Tables: Lists over 20 tables comparing ingredient and dosing information, organized by therapeutic category. Includes antifungals, cough-cold-flu products, psoriasis products, weight management products, and more.

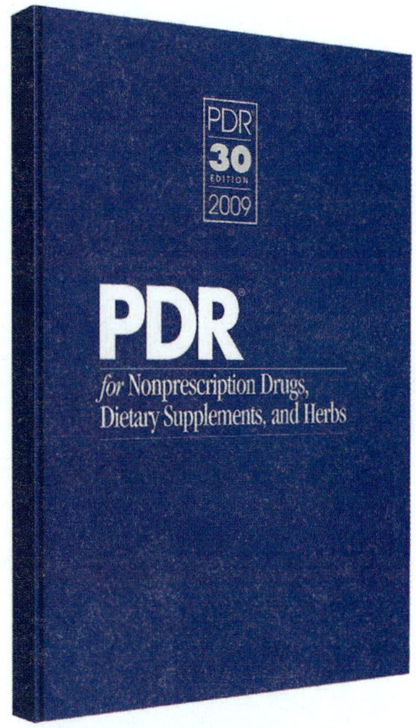

Figure 13-9 ***PDR for Nonprescription Drugs, Dietary Supplements, and Herbs.***

Other PDR Products

Other PDR products include:

- *PDR Pharmacopoeia Pocket Guide* provides important dispensing information and is arranged in a tabular format. It supplies FDA-approved dosing information and black box warning summaries of over 1,500 drugs.
- *PDR for Nutritional Supplements* provides a comprehensive, unbiased source of evidence-based information of nutritional supplements.
- *PDR for Herbal Medications* consists of updated monographs to include the efficacy, safety, potential interactions, clinical trials, case reports, and meta-analysis results of herbal medications. Each monograph discusses the effects, contraindications, precautions, adverse reactions, and dosage sections for each herbal medication.
- *PDR for Ophthalmic Medicines* provides the practitioner with information on the drugs and equipment used in the practice of ophthalmology and optometry.
- *PDR Drug Guide for Mental Health Professionals* provides detailed information on 75 common psychotropic medications.

Red Book

Red Book provides extensive pricing information for both prescription and OTC products available in the United States (Figure 13-10).

Red Book is 10 chapters in length with the following content:

- Emergency Information, which includes the FDA MedWatch Form, the Vaccine Adverse Event Reporting Form, poison antidote chart, poison control centers, and drug information centers.
- Clinical Reference Guide presents a listing of drugs that should not be crushed, sugar-free products, alcohol-free products, sulfite-containing products, drugs that cause photosensitivity, lactose- and galactose-free drugs, vitamin comparison table, drug-food interactions, drug-alcohol interactions, drug-tobacco interactions, use in pregnancy ratings, drugs excreted in breast milk, and common laboratory values.
- Herbal Medicine guide offers information on the more popular herbs, herbal terminology, herbs requiring supervision, herbal contraindications, herb-drug interactions, a glossary of scientific and common names, and a list of verified herbal indications.
- Practice Management and Professional Development provides information on disease management programs, disease management credentialing, nontraditional PharmD programs, handheld prescription systems, and dosing instructions in Spanish.
- Pharmacy and health care organizations contain information on national pharmacy organizations, state pharmacy associations, state boards of pharmacy, state Drug Utilization Review Offices, federal government offices, state Medicaid program offices, DEA office directory, state controlled substances scheduling authorities, and valuable Web sites.
- Drug Reimbursement Information supplies information on state AIDS drug assistance programs, patient assistance programs, Medicaid upper-limit prices, Medicaid reimbursement for drugs by state, pharmacy benefit managers (PBMs), and NCPDP standard billing units.
- Manufacturer/Wholesaler Information contains a manufacturer directory, pharmaceutical wholesaler directory, and OBRA participating manufacturers.
- Product Identification Guide contains 300 full-color photographs of prescription and over-the-counter medications and a listing of look-alike, sound-alike drug names.
- Rx Product Listings provides a key to prescription product listings to include standard dosage form descriptions, route of administration, abbreviations, and ingredient abbreviations, a Top 200 brand-name drug list, a Top-200 generic prescription drug list, new FDA-approved entities for the year, generics approved during the year, and prescription drug listings.
- OTC/Non-Drug Product Listings is very similar the Rx product listings, but contains information for OTC and nondrug products.

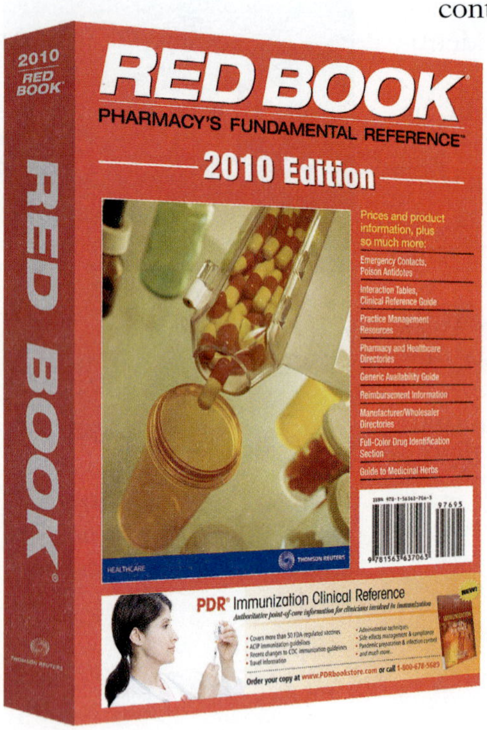

Figure 13-10 ***Red Book.***

This reference book provides average wholesale prices (AWPs), direct prices (DPs), and maximum allowable costs (MACs) for prescription drugs. *Red Book* provides suggested retail prices and the correct NDC numbers for all FDA-approved drugs. This reference book is published yearly.

USP <797> Guidebook to Proposed Revision Guidelines

USP <797> Guidebook to Proposed Revision Guidelines provides the practice standards to help ensure that compounded sterile preparations are of high quality. *USP Chapter <797>, Pharmaceutical Compounding: Sterile Preparations* is the first set of enforceable sterile compounding standards issued by the United States Pharmacopeia (USP). *USP Chapter <797>* describes the procedures and requirements for compounding sterile preparations and sets the standards that apply to all settings in which sterile preparations are compounded. The book is intended to assist hospitals, pharmacists, and pharmacy technicians with the interpretation of the proposed revisions. The resource contains the following information:

- Proposed Revisions to General Chapter<797>
- Current official full text of *USP <797> Pharmaceutical Compounding-Sterile Preparations*
- Introduction: General Chapter <797> and the USP revision process
- Enforceability and recognition of General Chapter <797>
- Rationale for Major Changes Proposed for the In-Process Revision of *USP General Chapter <797> Pharmaceutical Compounding-Sterile Preparations*
- Frequently Asked Questions regarding General Chapter <797>

Remington's Pharmaceutical Sciences: The Science and Practice of Pharmacy

Remington's Pharmaceutical Sciences: The Science and Practice of Pharmacy is a comprehensive reference book providing essential information on the practice of pharmacy. The content is divided into 8 parts or 10 sections:

- Part 1: Orientation
- Part 2: Pharmaceutics
- Part 3: Pharmaceutical Chemistry
- Part 4: Pharmaceutical Testing: Analysis and Control
- Part 5: Pharmaceutical Manufacturing
- Part 6: Pharmacodynamics
- Part 7: Pharmaceutical and Medicinal Agents
- Part 8: Pharmacy Practice, which is subdivided into three sections: Pharmacy, Administration, and Fundamentals of Pharmacy Practice and Patient Care

Remington's provides detailed information on ophthalmic products, medicated topicals, oral solid dosage forms, coatings of oral pharmaceutical dosage forms, controlled-released drug delivery systems, quality assurance and control, stability of pharmaceutical products, bioavailability and bioequivalence testing, pharmaceutical necessities, nutrition in pharmacy practice, self-care/diagnostic products, complementary and alternative medical health care, vitamins and other nutrients, ambulatory patient care, institutional patient care, long-term care facilities, patient communication and compliance, pharmacoepidemiology, integrated health care delivery services, and home health patient care. The resource is published every 5 years.

AAP Red Book: Report of the Committee on Infectious Diseases

AAP *Red Book: Report of the Committee on Infectious Diseases* (American Academy of Pediatrics) contains recommendations on the clinical manifestations, **etiology** (the science dealing with the cause of disease), epidemiology, diagnosis, and treatment of over 200 diseases (Figure 13-11).

The AAP *Red Book* provides information on active and passive immunization, school health, blood safety, STDs, drug therapy, and antimicrobial prophylaxis. It addresses combination vaccines, standards for child and adult immunization, West Nile virus, and the American Heart Association's recommendations for the prevention of bacterial endocarditis.

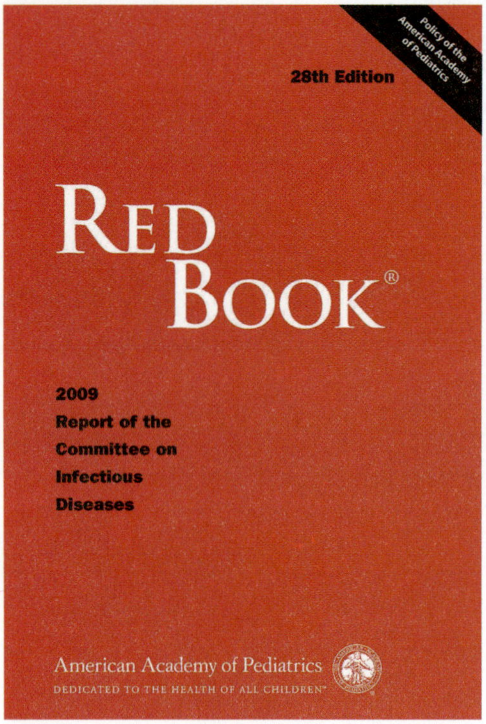

Figure 13-11 AAP *Red Book, Report of the Committee of Infectious Disease.*

Handbook on Injectable Drugs

Handbook on Injectable Drugs is a comprehensive source of drug compatibility and stability. This reference provides essential information on over 350 medications. It is cross-referenced with *AHFS Drug Information.* The *Handbook on Injectable Drugs* provides information regarding the preparation, storage, and administration of injectable medications.

AHFS Drug Information

AHFS Drug Information is an unbiased source of information on over 40,000 represented medicines and 100,000 represented drug products. It contains both off-labeled and labeled uses of medications, drug interactions, cautions and toxicity, dosage and methods of administration, chemistry and stability, referenced laboratory and test inferences, and pharmacology and pharmacokinetics.

Ident-A-Drug

Ident-A-Drug provides an accurate identification of oral tablets and capsules available in the United States by the identification code imprinted on the medication, their color, and the shape of the product. Ident-A-Drug provides the National Drug Code (NDC number) of the medication, its drug classification, and its schedule if it is a controlled substance.

Goodman & Gilman's The Pharmacological Basis of Therapeutics

Goodman & Gilman's The Pharmacological Basis of Therapeutics is a comprehensive drug reference for physicians and pharmacists. This book provides comprehensive disease coverage and accurate therapeutic solutions; you can identify all aspects of drug interaction, toxic effects, and chemical properties that may affect different body systems. *Goodman & Gilman's* is a valuable reference to improve patient safety. One is able to find complete drug dosage information.

Professional's Handbook of Complementary and Alternative Medicines

Professional's Handbook of Complementary and Alternative Medicines provides research on herbal agents in common use today. Monographs are

etiology The science dealing with the causes of disease.

based on the results of clinical studies, examining the existing evidence and comparing it with the manufacturers' claims. The monographs contain the most common generic names, synonyms, common trade names, common forms, sources, chemical components, actions, reported uses, dosages, and adverse reactions broken down by body system, interactions, contraindications, and precautions.

Neofax

Neofax provides a comprehensive selection of useful drug and infant nutritional data. It includes the newest approved medications for neonates, updates on existing neonatal drugs, drug monographs indexed alphabetically by drug class, human milk and infant formula comparison tables, recommended concentrations for administrations to neonates, and newborn metric conversion tables.

Trissel's Stability of Compounded Formulations

Trissel's Stability of Compounded Formulations summarizes specific formulation and stability studies. The book helps the pharmacy team determine whether formulated compounds and repackaged formulations will be stable for the anticipated duration of use, as well as properly stored. It explains how to formulate in accordance with documented standards, and counsel patients on the use and storage of compounded medications. The text contains monographs on over 355 products arranged alphabetically by nonproprietary name. The monograph contains information on the properties of medication, general stability considerations, and stability reports of compounded preparations and compatibility with other drug products. This reference book also contains an index of nonproprietary and brand names.

American Drug Index

American Drug Index contains over 22,000 prescription and OTC medications with cross-indexing of trade names, generics, and drug classes. This reference book provides information on the manufacturer, pronunciation, active ingredients, dose forms, strengths, packaging, and uses. It contains a comprehensive index indicating which drugs should not be chewed or crushed, drug names that look alike or sound alike, storage requirements for USP drugs, trademark glossary, and normal laboratory values. It is available in print format or on a CD-ROM. The book may be used in all types of pharmacies.

Tech Check

3. What is the official compendium in the United States?(LO 13.5)
4. What is a formulary?(LO 13.5)
5. What is a drug monograph?(LO 13.4)
6. Give five examples of information found in a drug monograph.(LO 13.4)
7. In which pharmacy setting might one find Neofax?(LO 13.5)
8. What is the importance of Ident-A-Drug?(LO 13.5)

Internet References(LO 13.6, 13.7)

Many pharmacies today have access to the Internet and therefore are able to access the most up-to-date information regarding diseases and appropriate protocol of treatment. Many of the reference sources previously cited can be found on the Internet. It is extremely important that a pharmacy technician develop appropriate computer skills to be able to navigate around the Internet. Internet references include the following:

- American Pharmacists Association (**www.aphanet.org**) was founded in 1852 as the American Pharmaceutical Association. The APhA represents pharmacists, pharmaceutical scientists, pharmacy students, and pharmacy technicians whose goal is to assist pharmacists improve medication use and advance patient care. The APhA provides professional information and education for both pharmacists and pharmacy technicians. Members of the APhA are eligible to participate in continuing education. The APhA publishes *Pharmacy Today, JAPhA,* and *JPharmSci.*
- *Drug Topics* (**www.drugtopics.com**) is an online newsmagazine that is published twice a month on all phases of the practice of pharmacy. Practitioners in community pharmacy, health-system pharmacy, HMOs, and consultant and mail-order pharmacies find this resource beneficial. *Drug Topics* focuses on managed-care trends; professional issues; national and state government activities; new prescription drugs, OTCs, and health and beauty care products; retail management and store operations; and new merchandising and marketing techniques. This newsmagazine provides continuing education for both pharmacists and pharmacy technicians.
- The Food and Drug Administration's Web site (**www.fda.gov**) provides a wealth of information for all health care providers, including pharmacists and pharmacy technicians and for the public. This site provides information on food, drugs, medical devices, biologics, animal feed and drugs, cosmetics, radiation-emitting products, and combination products. Information is available on both food and drug recalls within the past 60 days and new drug product approvals and controversial topics affecting medication in the United States. Through this Web site, one can report adverse reactions, product quality problems, and product use errors. FDA safety data can be accessed through the Adverse Event Reporting System (AERS) and Vaccine Adverse Event Reporting System (VAERS). Both health care professionals and the medical product–using public are able to access MedWatch, which provides clinical information about safety issues involving medical products, including prescription and OTC drugs.
- Center for Biologics Evaluation and Research (CBER) is found via the FDA Web site or at **www.fda.gov/cber.** This site provides information on allergenics, blood, cellular and gene therapy, tissues, vaccines, and xenotransplantation. The information is helpful for both the health care professional and the consumer. The site identifies shortages in biologicals, which may be helpful for those working in hospitals. Another component of the FDA Web site is the Center for Drug Evaluation and Research (CDER) at **www.fda.gov/cder**. CDER provides assistance in obtaining both regular and emergency investigational drugs. Fact Sheets about specific drugs for patients are available in both English and Spanish.

- HealthSTAR contains citations to the published literature from 1975 to the present on health services, technology, administration, and research. HealthSTAR provides information on both the clinical and nonclinical aspects of health care delivery. This database contains both citations and abstracts when available to journal articles, monographs, technical reports, meeting abstracts, and papers and government documents. HealthSTAR is produced with the assistance of the National Library of Medicine and the American Hospital Association.
- Medline Plus (**www.nlm.nih.gov/medlineplus**) is a service of the U.S. National Library of Medicine and the National Institutes of Health and uses information from other government agencies and health-related organizations. This Web site provides access to medical journal articles; 740 topics on conditions, diseases, and wellness; extensive information on drugs (prescription, OTC, herbs, and supplements); an illustrated encyclopedia and a medical dictionary; interactive patient tutorials; studies for new drugs and treatments; health information for older adults; directories on physicians, dentists, and hospitals; and the latest in health news. This Web site is also available in Spanish.
- *Pharmacy Times* was established as a medium for practical pharmacy information in 1897 and is available in both print format and on the Internet at **www.pharmacytimes.com**. *Pharmacy Times*'s goal is to provide practical and reliable information on improving patient care in the pharmacy practice. The clinical information in *Pharmacy Times* assists the pharmacy staff during the counseling of patients and with interactions with physicians. Recently, *Pharmacy Times* has expanded its content to include pharmacy technology and health systems pharmacy. The publication provides Accreditation Council for Pharmacy Education (ACPE) endorsed continuing education, which includes topics such as prescription errors, drug interactions, pharmacy technology, disease state management, patient counseling, and pharmacy law.
- *Rx Times* (**www.rxtimes.com**) features news, columns, and information for the pharmaceutical industry. The Web site provides extensive national content, continuing education, classifieds, employment listings, and a Web directory.
- *U.S. Pharmacist* is available in print format and on the Internet at **www.uspharmacist.com.** *U.S. Pharmacist* is a monthly journal that provides both pharmacists and pharmacy technicians with up-to-date, peer-reviewed clinical articles pertinent to contemporary pharmacy in a variety of settings, including community pharmacy, hospitals, managed-care systems, ambulatory care clinics, home health care organizations, long-term care facilities, and the pharmacy industry. Both pharmacists and pharmacy technicians are able to obtain continuing education credits approved by the ACPE. Each monthly edition focuses on a specific issue as follows:

January	General Pharmacy
February	Cardiovascular
March	New Drugs
April	Dermatologic Disorders
May	Pain Management
June	General Pharmacy
July	Respiratory Diseases

August	Men's Health
September	Women's Health
October	New Drugs
November	Psychotropic
December	General Pharmacy

In addition to these topics, oncology supplements are issued in January, April, July, and October; a generic supplement is released in June; a senior care supplement is distributed in October; and a diabetes supplement is provided in November. Refer to Table 13-2 for a list of valuable Internet Web sites.

Table 13-2 Pharmacy Internet Web Sites

Web Site	Type of Information Found on Site
www.acpe-accredit.org	Provides national accreditation for professional pharmacy degrees and continuing education
www.amcp.org	Home page for the Academy of Managed Care Pharmacy
www.aphanet.org	Provides association and pharmacy news, health information, continuing education, and pharmacy training programs
www.ashp.org	Home page for the American Society of Health-System Pharmacists
www.cdc.gov	Centers for Disease Control and Prevention; features current public health issues, as well as a listing of disease and health topics
www.clinicaltrials.gov	A search engine for information on clinical trials and medical research
www.cms.gov	Site for the Centers for Medicare and Medicaid Services; provides reimbursement information at the federal and state levels
www.dea.gov	Home page of the Drug Enforcement Administration
www.drugs.com	Searchable database of drugs, medical conditions, drug interactions; it provides a pill identifier
www.fda.gov	Home page of the Food and Drug Administration; offers information on drugs, cosmetics, and food safety
www.fda.gov/cder/index/html	Site of the FDA's Center for Drug Evaluation and Research; offers drug information and regulatory guidance with links to *Drug Approvals, Orange Book, National Drug Code Directory, MedWatch,* and *Drug Shortages*
www.health.nih.gov	Provides health reports and studies from the National Institutes of Health database
www.intelihealth.com	Sponsored by Aetna U.S. Healthcare; provides health information from Harvard Medical School, as well as listings of health resources and links to medical search engines
www.libuiowa.edu.hardin.md	Sponsored by the University of Iowa's Hardin Library for the Health Sciences; provides a listing of Web sites by medical specialty
www.mayoclinic.com	Offers health and drug information, including a Drug Watch Index that monitors recent approvals and recalls
www.medconnect.com	Provides news and resources for health care professionals, including continuing education for pharmacists
www.medlineplus.gov	Part of the National Library of Medicine database; provides health and drug information, medical dictionaries and encyclopedias, directories for locating health care organizations, and providers

Table 13-2 Pharmacy Internet Web Sites *(Continued)*

Web Site	Type of Information Found on Site
www.medscape.com	Provides peer-reviewed, practice-oriented information on diseases, pharmacotherapy, managed care, and links to medical journals for health care professionals and consumers; contains continuing education courses
www.ncpanet.org	Home of the National Community Pharmacists Association; represents the political interests of independent pharmacists at the federal and state level; contains professional news and continuing education
www.nlm.nih.gov	Site of the National Library of Medicine; PubMed and Medline Plus allow users to search the NLM database
www.pdrhealth.com	Consumer site for the *Physicians' Desk Reference;* provides practitioners and patients with drug information on prescription and OTC products as well as herbal and dietary supplements
www.pharmacist.com	Features professional resources such as licensing information, monthly updates on drug therapy developments, and online continuing education
www.pharmscope.com	Reports on current practices and trends affecting managed-care pharmacy
www.rxfactstat.com	Offers continuing education and a biweekly newsletter of new drug information
www.rxlist.com	Provides searchable database of prescription and OTC drug information and interactions
www.tnp.com	Site of *The Natural Pharmacist* and provides information on alternative and complementary medicine
www.webmd.com	Provides news and health information for consumers and health care professionals
www.ptcb.org	Web site for the Pharmacy Technician Certification Board that provides information regarding pharmacy technician certification
www.rxtec.net	Home page for pharmacy technician organization
www.pharmacytechnician.com	American Association of Pharmacy Technicians
www.pharmacytechnician.org	National Pharmacy Technician Association is the world's largest organization established specifically for pharmacy technicians
www.drugtopics.com	Offers the latest pharmacy and medical news as well as continuing education
www.pharmacytimes.com	Site of *Pharmacy Times* and continuing education
www.rxtimes.com	Site of *Rx Times* and continuing education
www.uspharmacist.com	Site of *U.S. Pharmacist* and continuing education
www.powerpak.com	Site for continuing education for both pharmacists and pharmacy technicians

Tech Check

9. Which pharmacy-related Web site is associated with the National Institutes of Health?(LO 13.7)

10. What Web site would you use to find information on the PTCB exam?(LO 13.7)

11. What is the name of a Web site where you may obtain continuing education to satisfy your requirements for recertification?(LO 13.7)

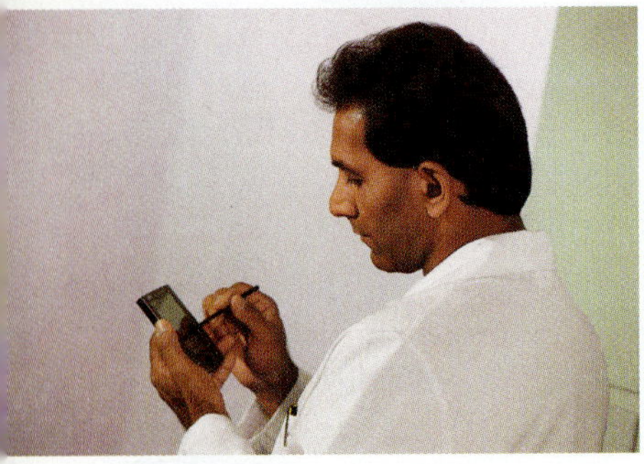

Figure 13-12 PDA.

personal digital assistant (PDA) A handheld device that runs on its own battery power so that it may be used anywhere.

Personal Digital Assistants (PDAs) and Pharmacy Software(LO 13.8)

A **personal digital assistant (PDA)** is a small mobile handheld device that provides computing and information storage and retrieval capabilities for personal and business use (Figure 13-12). The term *handheld* is another name for a PDA. PDAs are being used more in the practice of pharmacy as reference tools for both pharmacists and pharmacy technicians.

Epocrates is a type of pharmaceutical software that can be downloaded to a mobile PDA. Epocrates provides up-to-date information for the health care professional. One is able to download some of the software free, while other data may require a subscription for 1 to 2 years. A comparison of the various Epocrates products and their features are contained in Table 13-3.

Table 13-3 Epocrates PDA

	Epocrates Rx	Epocrates Rx Pro	Epocrates Medical Dictionary	Epocrates Coder	Epocrates Essentials	Epocrates Essentials Deluxe
Drug monograph, health plan formularies	X	X			X	X
Drug interaction checker, calculators	X	X			X	X
Infectious disease treatment guide		X			X	X
Alternative (herbal) medicines		X			X	X
IV compatibility checker		X			X	X
Disease monographs, symptom assessment						X
Diagnostic and laboratory tests					X	X
ICD-9 and CPT codes				X		X
Medical dictionary			X			X
Free content updates/medical news	X	X	X	X	X	X
Mobile CME	X	X	X	X	X	X
Med Tools Applications	X	X	X	X	X	X
International drug name indexes	X	X	X	X	X	X

Chapter Summary

Understanding the cause and prevention of medication errors is vital to the pharmacy technician. Important points to know are:

- Pharmacy information may be primary, secondary, or tertiary.
- Pharmacy information may be found in databases, journals, formularies, and reference books.
- All pharmacies must contain a library that is reflective of the pharmacy's practice.
- A pharmacy technician needs to be able to select the correct reference source and locate

the material being requested promptly for the pharmacist.

- The Internet contains valuable pharmacy information for the pharmacy team. It also can be a source of continuing education for both pharmacists and pharmacy technicians.
- Pharmacy software has become available to be used on PDAs.

Chapter Review

Case Study Question

1. Did the pharmacy technician choose the correct reference book? Why or why not?[LO 13.5]

At Your Service Questions

1. Where did AJ find this information?[LO 13.5]
2. Why is the need for information important?[LO 13.2]
3. Do all reference materials provide the same information?[LO 13.3]
4. Would you know where to find specific information if a similar situation occurred?[LO 13.5]

Multiple Choice

Select the best answer.

1. Which reference book would be beneficial to a retail pharmacy if it were seeking pricing information?[LO 13.5]
   a. *Blue Book*
   b. *Orange Book*
   c. *Red Book*
   d. All of the above
2. Which reference book consists of patient product inserts from drug manufacturers and is marketed to physicians?[LO 13.5]
   a. *Drug Facts and Comparisons*
   b. *PDR*
   c. *USP DI*
   d. *USP–NF*
3. Which reference book is updated monthly?[LO 13.5]
   a. *Drug Facts and Comparisons*
   b. *Orange Book*
   c. *PDR*
   d. *USP DI*
4. Which pharmacy reference book contains pharmacy standards?[LO 13.5]
   a. *F & C*
   b. *USP–NF*
   c. *USP DI*
   d. All of the above
5. Which pharmacy reference book is published every 5 years?[LO 13.x5]
   a. *Martindale's Pharmaceutical Sciences*
   b. *PDR*
   c. *Remington's Pharmaceutical Sciences*
   d. *USP DI*
6. Which of the following pharmacy reference books is required in a pharmacy's library?[LO 13.5]
   a. *Drug Facts and Comparisons*
   b. *PDR*
   c. *Remington's Pharmaceutical Sciences*
   d. *USP–NF*

7. Which pharmacy reference book provides valuable information regarding bioequivalence?(LO 13.5)
   a. *Blue Book*
   b. *Green Book*
   c. *Orange Book*
   d. *Red Book*

8. What is another name for *Approved Drug Products with Therapeutic Equivalence Evaluations?*(LO 13.5)
   a. *Blue Book*
   b. *Green Book*
   c. *Orange Book*
   d. *Red Book*

9. Which of the following pieces of information would be contained in a drug monograph?(LO 13.4)
   a. Contraindications
   b. Description
   c. Indications
   d. All of the above

10. Which of the following is *not* a primary source of information?(LO 13.1)
    a. EMBASE
    b. MEDLINE
    c. *New England Journal of Medicine*
    d. *PDR*

11. If one was seeking information on side effects of a medication, which of the following databases would provide this information?(LO 13.1)
    a. ADIS LMS Drug Alerts
    b. Diogenes FDA Regulatory Updates
    c. F-D-C Reports
    d. SEDBASE

12. Which of the following sources of drug literature is most common in pharmacies?(LO 13.1)
    a. Primary
    b. Secondary
    c. Tertiary
    d. Quandinary

13. Which of the following is an example of a tertiary reference source?(LO 13.1)
    a. *Approved Drug Products with Therapeutic Equivalence Evaluations*
    b. *Drug Facts and Comparison*
    c. *United States Pharmacopoeia—National Formulary*
    d. All of the above

14. Which reference book is cross-referenced with the *Handbook on Injectable Drugs?*(LO 13.5)
    a. AAP *Red Book*
    b. *AHFS Drug Information*
    c. *PDR*
    d. *USP–NF*

15. Which pharmacy magazine dedicates a specific topic to be presented on a monthly basis?(LO 13.7)
    a. *Chain Drug Review*
    b. *Pharmacy Times*
    c. *Rx Times*
    d. *U.S. Pharmacist*

16. What is a formulary?(LO 13.1)
    a. An approved listing of medications to be used within an organization
    b. A listing of drugs made by a particular drug manufacturer
    c. A listing of drugs recalled by a drug manufacturer
    d. A listing of drugs with the same indication

17. Which organization accredits continuing education for pharmacy technicians?(LO 13.6)
    a. ACPE
    b. DEA
    c. FDA
    d. USP

18. Which of the following references provides only information related to infants?(LO 13.5,)
    a. *Trissel's*
    b. *Goodman and Gilman's*
    c. *Neofax*
    d. *AHFS*

19. Which month of the year would one find information focused on cardiovascular issues in *U.S. Pharmacist?*(LO 13.6, 13.7)
    a. January
    b. February
    c. March
    d. December

20. If one was looking for specific information involving the practice of pharmacy, which reference book would one select?(LO 13.5)
    a. *Facts and Comparisons*
    b. *The Merck Manual*
    c. *Remington's Pharmaceutical Sciences: The Science and Practice of Pharmacy*
    d. *USP DI*

21. Which legislation designates the *USP–NF* as the official compendia for drugs marketed in the United States?(LO 13.1)
    a. Dietary Supplement Heath Education Act
    b. Federal Food, Drug and Cosmetics Act
    c. OBRA-90
    d. Pure Food and Drug Act

22. Which pharmacy reference provides information on drug compatibility and stability?(LO 13.5)
    a. AAP *Red Book*
    b. *AHFS Drug Information*
    c. *Approved Drug Products with Therapeutic Equivalence*
    d. *Handbook on Injectable Drugs*

Matching

Match the abbreviation or acronym with its full name.

_______ 1. AERS
_______ 2. *F & C*
_______ 3. FDA
_______ 4. OTC
_______ 5. PDA
_______ 6. *PDR*
_______ 7. USAN
_______ 8. *PBM*
_______ 9. *USP–NF*
_______ 10. VAERS

a. Food and Drug Administration
b. *Physicians' Desk Reference*
c. *United States Pharmacopoeia–National Formulary*
d. Adverse Event Reporting System
e. *Pharmacy Benefit Manager*
f. Vaccine Adverse Event Reporting System
g. Over-the-counter
h. United States adopted names
i. *Facts and Comparisons*
j. Personal digital assistant

Critical Thinking Questions

1. A patient enters the pharmacy and asks you to explain the difference between a proprietary drug and a nonproprietary drug. What would you tell them?(LO 13.3)
2. A patient has purchased a copy of *The Pill Book*. She is seeking additional information on her medications. She panics when she sees the list of adverse affects of the medications. How would you explain adverse effects to the patient?(LO 13.4)
3. Which pharmacy reference book do you find most appropriate for your pharmacy setting? Why?(LO 13.5)
4. You have processed a prescription for a patient and the prescription is rejected because the drug is not part of the prescription plan's formulary. The patient asks you what a formulary is. How would you explain it?(LO 13.5)

HIPAA Scenario

Patient Dora Lavince broke her leg while slipping on a wet surface at her workplace at Save-Alot Grocery Store. She was placed on two prescription medications:

Ansaid 800 mg tid × 14 days
Vicodin q8 h prn severe pain × 7 days

Pharmacy technician Janet received a call from a workers' compensation agent, Della Barter, who asked for a faxed copy of the patient's complete prescription history. Upon receiving the patient's history, Della called Janet and asked several questions regarding the medication.

Discussion Questions(PTCB II. 73)

1. Della asked Janet if generic forms of both medications are available. Where could Janet find this information?
2. Are pharmacy technicians permitted to look up information for an individual?

Internet Activities

1. Visit one of the following pharmacy Web sites: **www.pharmacytimes.com**, **www.uspharamacist.com**, or **www.powerpak.com**. Select a continuing education article; read it and then answer the questions at the end of the article. Submit it for continuing education credit.(LO 13.6, 13.7)

2. Visit **www.usp.org** and select one of the following topics found under Chapter <797> and report your findings to the class.(LO 13.7)
    - Single-Dose versus Multiple-Dose Containers
    - Additional Personnel Requirements
    - Personnel Cleansing and Garbing
    - Disinfectant and Cleaning

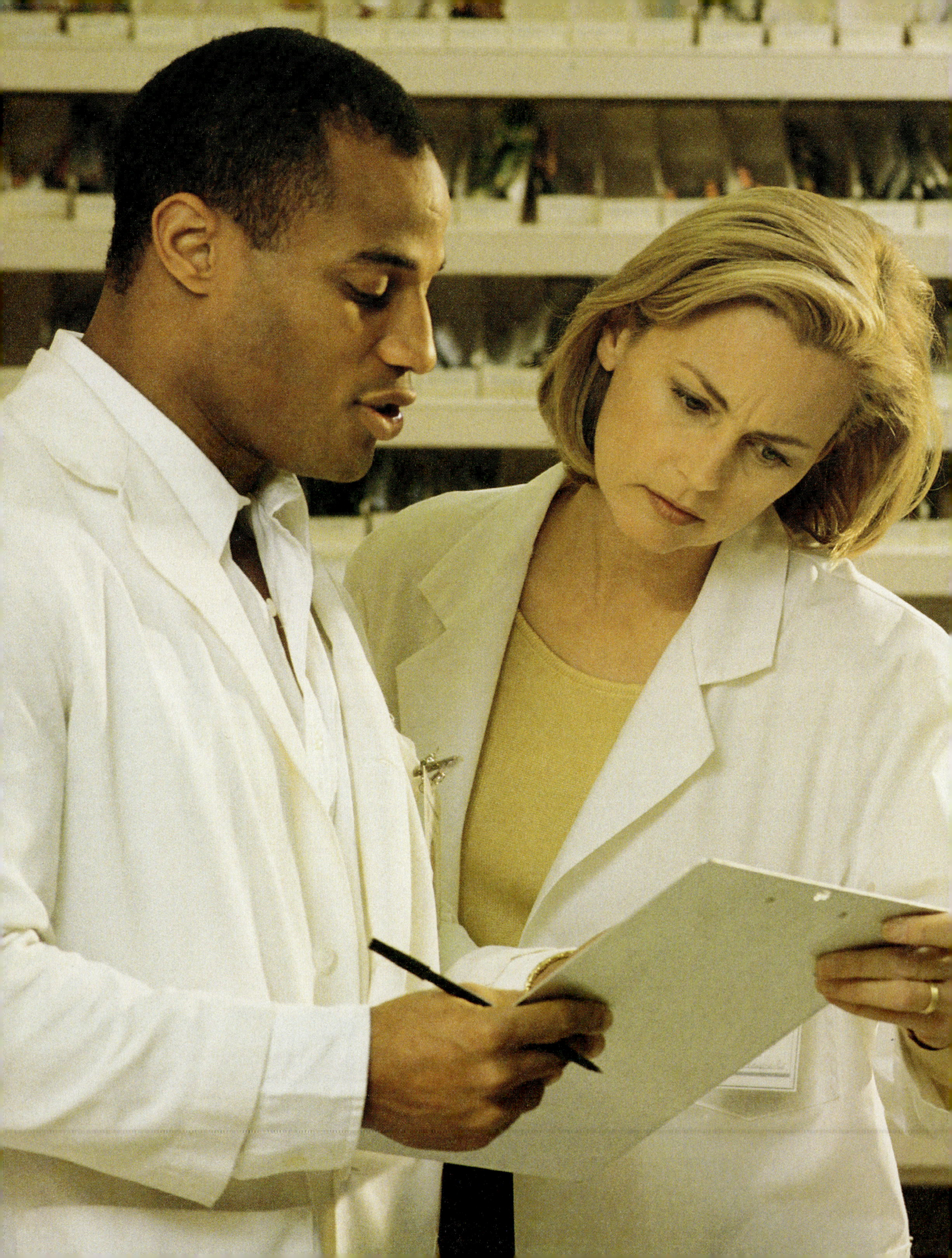

Unit 4

Practice Settings

Chapter 14 Retail Setting

Chapter 15 Hospital/Inpatient Setting

Chapter 16 Other Environments

Chapter 17 Inventory Management

14 Retail Setting

Learning Outcomes

Upon completion of this chapter, you will be able to:

14.1 Describe the layout of a retail pharmacy.
14.2 List the different types of retail pharmacies.
14.3 List the components of a prescription.
14.4 List information needed to fill a prescription.
14.5 Describe how to process a prescription.
14.6 Understand the connection between retail pharmacy and customer service.
14.7 Explain the various reasons why a prescription may be rejected by a third-party payer.
14.8 Understand how to find insurance information from the insurance card.
14.9 Describe the importance of the "flow of service."
14.10 Identify the various categories of OTC medications found in a retail pharmacy.
14.11 Define the role of the pharmacy technician and the duties assigned to him or her in a retail pharmacy.
14.12 Explain the importance of the pharmacy's computer system.

Key Terms

adjudication
drug utilization evaluation (DUE)
health maintenance organization (HMO)
independent practice association (IPA)
preferred provider organization (PPO)

PTCB

In preparation for the certification examination, you should understand and perform activities associated with the following PTCB Knowledge Statements:

PTCB Knowledge Statement

Domain I. Assisting the Pharmacist in Serving Patients

Knowledge of pharmaceutical and medical abbreviations and terminology (4)
Knowledge of generic and brand names of pharmaceuticals (5)
Knowledge of information to be obtained from patient/patient's representative (21)
Knowledge of non-prescription (over-the-counter) formulations (28)
Knowledge of packaging requirements (33)
Knowledge of NDC number components (34)
Knowledge of information for prescription or medication order labels (36)
Knowledge of requirements regarding auxiliary labels (37)
Knowledge of requirements regarding patient package inserts (38)

Knowledge of quality improvement methods. (49)

Knowledge of pharmacy-related computer software for documenting the dispensing of prescriptions or prescriptions or medication orders (69)

Knowledge of reimbursement policies and plans (75)

Knowledge of legal requirements for pharmacist counseling of patient/patient's representative (76)

PTCB Knowledge Statement

Domain II. Maintaining Medication and Inventory Control Systems

Knowledge of formulary or approved stock list (5)

Knowledge of products used in packaging and repackaging (12)

PTCB Knowledge Statement

Domain III. Participation in the Administration and Management of Pharmacy Practice

Knowledge of roles and responsibilities of pharmacists, pharmacy technicians, and other pharmacy employees (7)

Knowledge of legal and regulatory requirements for personnel, facilities, equipment, and supplies (8)

Knowledge of state board of pharmacy regulations (11)

Knowledge of sanitation requirements (19)

Knowledge of manual and computer-based systems for storing, receiving, and using pharmacy-related information (26)

Case Study

Tina Williams, a pharmacy technician, works for MacArthur's chain pharmacy. She comes in and takes over the prescription drop-off window. While accepting prescriptions from patients, Mrs. Jones enters and presents Tina with a new prescription and a new insurance card. Mrs. Jones tells her that the medication is one she has never taken and she needs to start taking it immediately, so she will wait for the prescription to be filled.

Tina shows her where she can wait and starts to process the prescription. Before Mrs. Jones walks away, she asks Tina if she can tell her where to find the dishwashing liquid. Tina informs Mrs. Jones where to find the dishwashing liquid. Mrs. Jones thanks her and walks away.

Tina continues to process her prescription. The telephone rings and she answers it while continuing to type. Mr. Smith, the customer on the phone, asks for a price on 30 Prozac 20 mg capsules. Tina switches screens and gives him a price of $119.99. When Tina switches screens back to Mrs. Jones, she finds that there is an insurance rejection code.

The rejection code states "patient is not covered." Tina pages Mrs. Jones to the pharmacy. She tells her about the problem and that it will require her to contact the PBM (prescription benefits manager). Tina calls the PBM to find out why the patient is not covered. The operator tells Tina that the person is not found in their system and Mrs. Jones should contact her human resources office.

Tina pages Mrs. Jones to the pharmacy and tells her what she needs to do. Mrs. Jones asks how much the medication would cost without her insurance. Tina looks up the price for Avonex injection and tells her that it will cost $423.67. Tina also notices that the computer system says that they are out of the medication. Tina checks the refrigerator to verify this. She tells Mrs. Jones that they are temporarily out of the medication but will be able to have it for her tomorrow afternoon. Mrs. Jones agrees to this because it would enable her to fix her insurance problem.

While reading this chapter, keep the following questions in mind:

1. Why is multitasking important?(LO 14.9)
2. Why is it important to know your computer system?(LO 14.7, 14.8)
3. What are some examples of customer service being observed in this retail pharmacy by Tina?(LO 14.6)

Introduction to the Retail Setting(LO 14.6)

Retail pharmacy is a challenging and rewarding environment for many people. Successful pharmacy technicians are detail-oriented and enjoy working with a diverse group of people. This setting requires an individual to be able to multitask, which means being able to perform multiple tasks simultaneously. Retail pharmacy requires an individual to possess superb customer service skills because of the personal contact with people who are dropping off and picking up their prescriptions.

There are many different types of retail pharmacies and each is designed to meet the specific needs of a particular customer. Depending on the pharmacy, technicians may be assigned a variety of duties but each of these duties places the welfare of the patient first. Some of their duties may include data entry, prescription processing, prescription compounding, inventory management, and handling of insurance problems; however, the most important duty of any pharmacy technician is that of a customer service specialist. Pharmacy technicians may be assigned a title such as senior technician, lead (head) technician, inventory specialist, or compounding technician.

At Your Service

Monday is the busiest day of the week in the pharmacy. Karen, the pharmacy technician, is at the in-window with six people waiting to give her their prescriptions.

Meanwhile, Chris, another pharmacy technician, is busy pulling and counting out medications. He looks up and notices the line of customers at the in-window. He stops what he is doing to help Karen.

Rose is scheduled to come in early on Monday, because the warehouse shipment is being delivered and she wants to get it put away promptly. She notices how busy the pharmacy is and assists with the waiting customers at the out-window.

By the time Karen, Chris, and Rose have assisted all of the waiting customers, the warehouse order arrives. Rose and Chris start to put away the order.

Chris asks Rose, "Would you teach me how to place the order?"

Rose says, "Sure, and I would like you to explain how to handle insurance problems."

Tim, the pharmacy manager, overhears the conversation and tells them, "It's a great idea to learn everything you can in the pharmacy, so if one person is sick someone else can pick up where the sick person left off. It also helps the pharmacy to run smoother when everyone is able and willing to help each other."

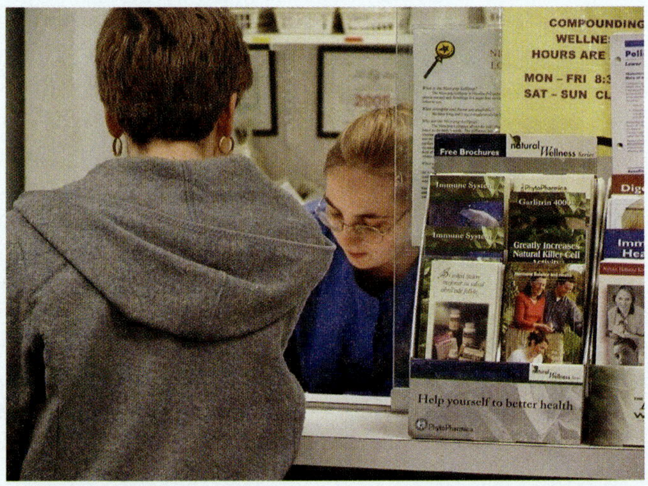

While reading this chapter, keep the following questions in mind:

1. What is the role of the pharmacy technician in a retail pharmacy?(LO 14.11)
2. What are some of the duties a pharmacy technician may be responsible for performing while working in a retail pharmacy?(LO 14.11)
3. Why is teamwork important in a retail pharmacy?(LO 14.11)

Retail Pharmacy(LO 14.1, 14.2)

A retail pharmacy can be divided into two major areas—the pharmacy and the front end.

The pharmacy consists of the pharmacy department, where an individual is able to obtain a filled prescription that has been prescribed from a medical doctor or other individual with prescribing authority. The front-end merchandise includes OTCs, health and beauty items, cosmetics, stationary and school supplies, snacks, sundry items, and even seasonal merchandise; not all of these categories may be found in all pharmacies (Figure 14-1). It is important that a pharmacy technician know where products are located within the store.

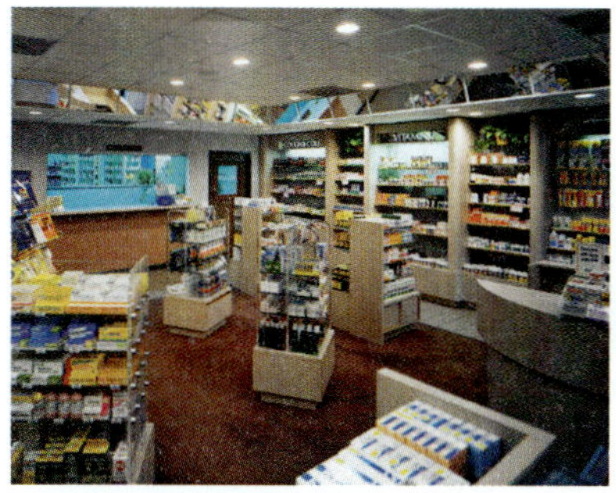

Figure 14-1 **Front-end merchandise.**

Types of Retail Pharmacies

Retail pharmacies may be designed and merchandised differently, but they have many common elements. Some pharmacies may have a drive-through window and others are strictly walk-up.

Medications are arranged on the shelf in alphabetical order, by either generic or brand name (Figure 14-2). Drugs may be arranged by dosage form, such as topical agents, inhalers, ophthalmic and otic agents, suppositories, small and large liquids, and reconstituted liquids. The assortment and quantity of drugs may vary by pharmacy depending on its prescription volume.

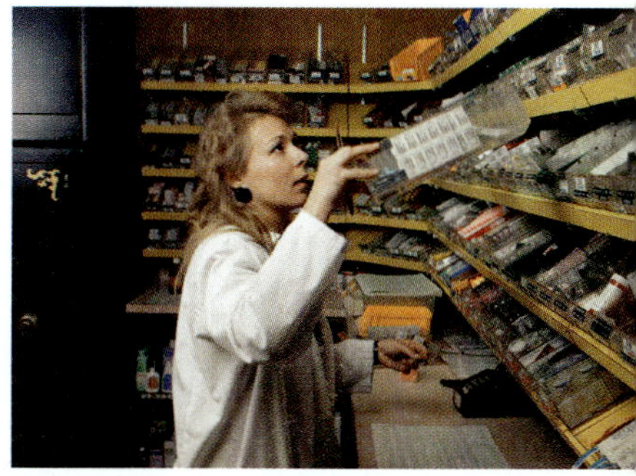

Figure 14-2 **Medications are arranged in alphabetical order.**

The state board of pharmacy oversees the practice of pharmacy within the state. The state board of pharmacy conducts an inspection prior to the issuance of a pharmacy permit to ensure pharmacy regulations are being followed. These regulations specify a minimum amount of counter space and specific equipment required in the operation of the pharmacy. Some of the equipment required in a pharmacy includes:

- Sink with both hot and cold running water
- Adequate refrigeration facilities with a monitoring thermometer
- Current dispensing information references consistent with the scope of the pharmacy practice
- Prescription balance sensitive to 15 mg or an electronic scale
- Metric weights
- An accepted burglar alarm consistent with industry standards
- Other equipment consistent with the pharmacy's scope of practice, which may include mortars and pestles (glass, wedge wood, or porcelain), graduate cylinders, stirring rods, spatulas, weighing papers, ointment slabs, reconstitution tubes, pill counting trays, and suppository molds
- Supplies consistent with the scope of the practice such as prescription bags, prescription pads, vials, bottles, ointment jars, labels, auxiliary labels, and printer paper

Chain Pharmacies

These are stores with the same name and owned by a corporation. A corporation has a board of directors who oversee the operation of the company and ensure that the interests of the stockholders of the company are met. In addition to carrying prescription medications, a chain pharmacy may carry a variety of products, such as OTC medications, health and beauty aids, and school and stationary supplies. CVS and Walgreen's are examples

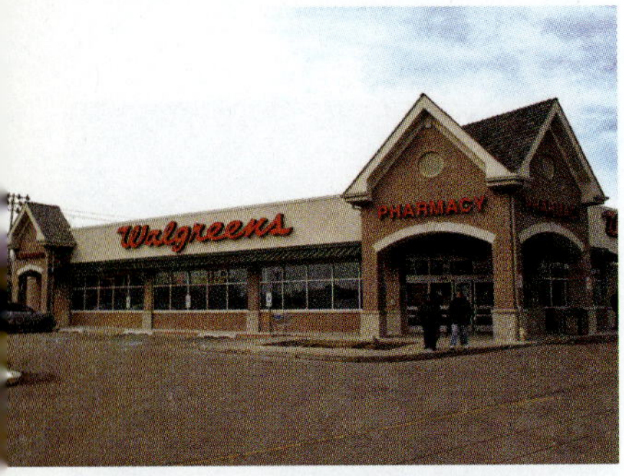

Figure 14-3 Chain pharmacy Walgreens.

of a traditional chain pharmacy, where their primary focus is medication (Figure 14-3). Other mass merchandiser types of chains may contain a pharmacy such as Target, a discounter such as Walmart, a membership club such as Costco, or a grocery store such as Safeway. Chain pharmacies occupy more space than either a franchise or independent pharmacy.

Some of the design elements of chain pharmacies include:

- In-windows—The in-window is where customers drop off prescriptions to be filled.
- Out-windows—The out-window is where customers pick up prescriptions and may purchase other items at that time.
- Patient consultation area—This is a private area where the pharmacist may answer questions that customers might have in private. This is a requirement of both OBRA-90 and HIPAA.

Franchise Pharmacies

A franchise pharmacy has characteristics of both independent and chain pharmacies. A franchiser allows for the exclusive use of the company's name to an owner of a drugstore. However, the owner has flexibility in setting up and running the store. Medicine Shoppe is an example of a franchise pharmacy.

Outpatient Pharmacies (Ambulatory Pharmacies)

An outpatient pharmacy is a pharmacy within the hospital where discharged patients are able to obtain their medication before they go home. If the hospital has outpatient services (e.g., outpatient surgery), those patients may also have their prescriptions filled in this pharmacy. Other outpatient health care facilities, such as urgent care centers, also have outpatient pharmacies. However, not all hospitals or other outpatient facilties have an outpatient pharmacy.

Independent Pharmacies

Independent pharmacies are owned by a single person or partners. The owners make all decisions affecting the business. The number of independent pharmacies is decreasing due to increased competition of the chain pharmacies and requirements established by managed care.

Pharmacy technicians must possess skills to be able to work in any of these retail pharmacy organizations. Regardless of their size or the merchandise they carry, they all process prescriptions.

Both pharmacists and pharmacy technicians at all pharmacies must observe federal, state, and local laws. Some of the federal laws are:

- Food, Drug and Cosmetic Act of 1938
- Durham-Humphrey Amendment
- Kefauver-Harris Amendment
- Poison Control Act
- Comprehensive Drug Abuse Prevention and Control Act
- Omnibus Budget Reconciliation Act (OBRA-90)
- Health Insurance Portability and Accountability Act (HIPAA)
- Medicare Modernization Act (MMA)

These laws are discussed in greater detail in Chapter 4.

Tech Check

1. Name the different types of retail stores.(LO 14.2)
2. What is a common component of all retail pharmacies?(LO 14.6)

Flow of Service(LO 14.3, 14.4, 14.5, 14.6, 14.9)

Flow of service refers to the critical path by which a prescription is processed when it arrives in the pharmacy. The flow of service is affected by the type of pharmacy and the volume of prescriptions being processed. Each work area in a pharmacy may be considered a separate workstation (Figure 14-4).

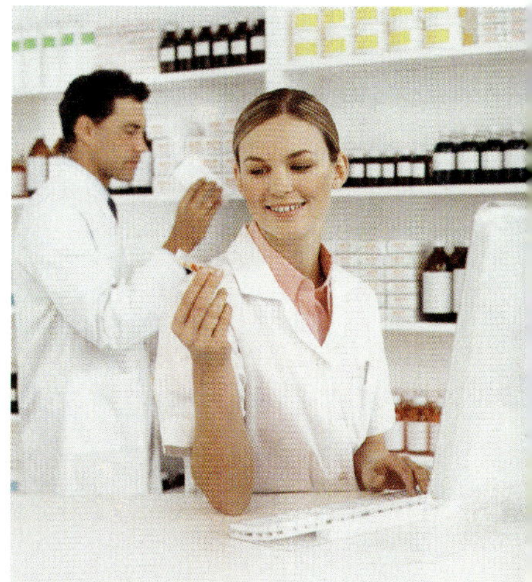

Figure 14-4 There are different work areas in the pharmacy.

In a low-volume pharmacy, there may be one pharmacist, one technician, and one cashier working at a time. In this scenario, the technician might be working at the in-window taking new prescriptions, accepting refills, and inputting them (via data entry) into the computer. If the pharmacy technician is not working with a customer, he or she may pull the medications, count them out, and place the label on the vial with the medication inside it. The technician may place the filled medication vial, drug monograph, original medication bottle, and prescription to the side for the pharmacist to perform the final check. It is the responsibility of the pharmacist to sign off on each completed prescription.

In a high-volume pharmacy, there may be a technician at the in-window, and a technician pulling and counting out medications. A technician may be assigned to work at the drive-through window or handle insurance problems. In some extremely busy stores, there may be a pharmacy technician assigned specifically to perform inventory duties. This person may assist other technicians during busy times, but working with inventory is his or her main job. The number of technicians that a pharmacist may supervise at one time may be determined by state pharmacy regulations.

Prescription Processing

Pharmacy technicians must be able to read and interpret a patient's prescription (Figure 14-5). There are specific parts of a prescription that must be present before it can be filled.

The components of a prescription are:

- Prescriber information—Name, address, telephone number, and other information identifying the prescriber.
- Date—The date that the prescription was written.
- Patient information—Name, address, birth date, and other information to identify the patient.
- Inscription—Medication prescribed, including generic or brand name, strength, and quantity.
- Subscription—Instructions to the pharmacist dispensing the medication. This may include generic substitution and refill authorization.
- Signa—Instructions to the patient.
- Signature—Prescriber's signature for handwritten prescriptions. The prescriber's signature must be in ink but it cannot be a stamped signature.
- DEA number—Required for prescriptions of Schedules II, III, IV, and V medications only.

Table 14-1 Common Prescription Abbreviations

Abbreviation	Meaning
aa	Of each
ac	Before meals
ad	Up to
ad lib	Freely, at pleasure
am	Morning
aq	Water
bid	Twice a day
BM	Bowel movement
BP	Blood pressure
BS	Blood sugar
c̄	With
caps	Capsule
cc	Cubic centimeter
CHF	Congestive heart failure
COPD	Chronic obstructive pulmonary disease
disp	Dispense
dtd	Give of such doses
elix	Elixir
gm (g)	Gram
GERD	Gastroesophageal reflux disease reflux disease
gr	Grain
gtt(s)	Drop(s)
HA	Headache
kg	Kilogram
L	Liter
m	Mix
mcg	Microgram
mEq	Milliequivalent
mg	Milligram
mL	Milliliter
MOM	Milk of magnesia
MS	Morphine sulfate
MVI	Multivitamin
N&V	Nausea and vomiting
non rep /NR	Do not repeat
OJ	Orange juice
pc	After meals
po	By mouth
pr	By rectum
prn	As needed
pulv	A powder
q	Each or every
ISMP	Every other day
q4h	Every 4 hours
q6h	Every 6 hours
q12h	Every 12 hours
qs	Sufficient quantity
qs ad	Sufficient quantity to make up to
s̄	Without
ss	One-half
Sig	Write on label
SL	Sublingual
SOB	Shortness of breath
sol	Solution
stat	Immediately
supp	Suppository
Susp	Suspension
syr	Syrup
T	Temperature
tab	Tablet
TB	Tuberculosis
tbsp	Tablespoon
tid	Three times daily
top	Topical
tsp	Teaspoon
ud, ut dict	As directed
UTI	Urinary tract infection
URI	Upper respiratory infection
wk	Week

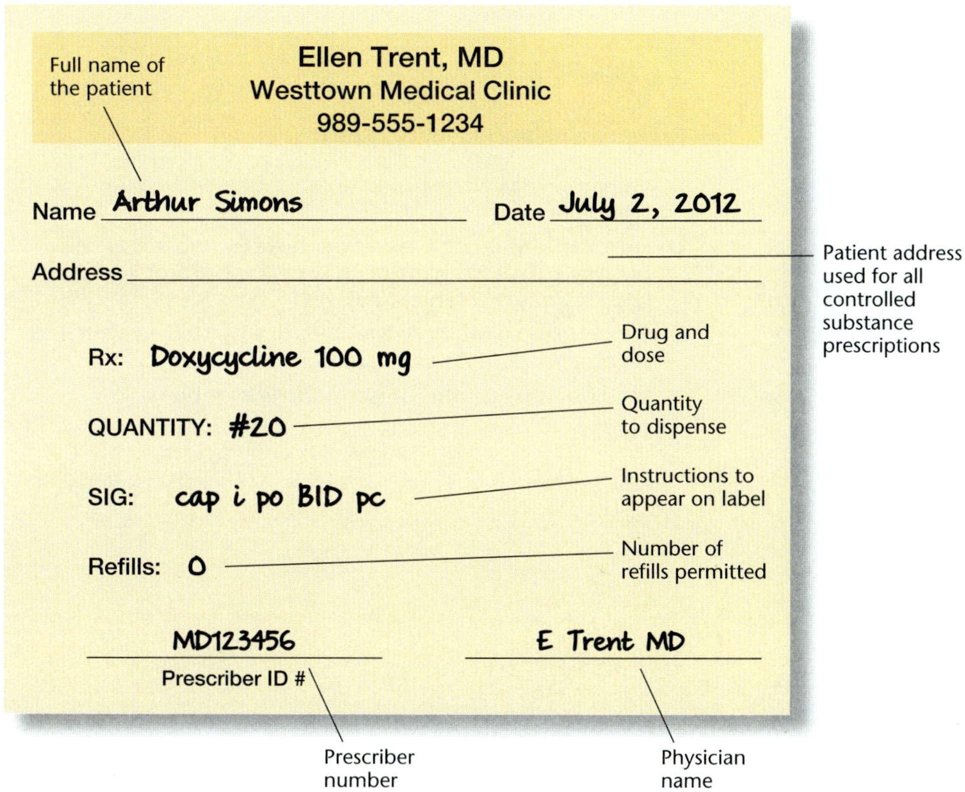

Figure 14-5 A typical outpatient prescription.

The directions on a prescription may be written in Latin, and as a pharmacy technician you will have to learn these common abbreviations (Table 14-1). When processing a prescription it is also important to know how to calculate a day's supply and quantity. Day's supply can be calculated by the following formula:

$$\text{Day's supply} = \frac{\text{Total quantity dispensed}}{\text{Total quantity taken per day}}$$

The physician may not indicate the quantity to be dispensed on a prescription; rather he or she may provide the pharmacy with how many days the patient should take the medicine. In pharmacy practice, a month is 30 days in length. See Table 14-2.

Receiving the Prescription

When you receive a new prescription from the patient or patient representative, it is important to look at the prescription to ensure that it has been completely filled out properly. Before allowing the patient to leave, you should ask if the person has had a prescription processed at your pharmacy before. If not, you will need to obtain information necessary to process the prescription. At this point, you may give the customer a patient profile, a form that will allow the customer to write down all personal information in privacy. Figure 14-6 is a sample patient profile. Patient profiles help reduce prescription errors and may prevent the patient from experiencing unnecessary reactions. If your pharmacy does not provide use a patient profile form, you should obtain the following information:

- The correct spelling of the name
- Home address

Table 14-2 Interpreting a Prescription

Information on Prescription	What It Means
Dr. Joseph Johnson 123 Main St. Anytown, USA 33358 265-555-4379 Name: Amy Smith Date: 7/28 Address: 895 Croissant Drive Anytown, USA 33358 Rx: Augmentin 500 mg i tab po bid × 10 days ______ Voluntary Formulary Permitted ______ Brand Name Medically Necessary Label ______________ DEA ______________ Signature: Joseph Johnson	To Determine the Quantity to Be Dispensed 1. We know that Amy should take 1 tablet twice a day for 10 days. 2. First step—Multiply 1 tablet per dose by two doses per day equals 2 tablets per day or (1 tab/dose)(2 doses/day) = 2 tablets/day. 3. Second step—Multiply 2 tablets/day by 10 days which is equal to 20 tablets or (2 tablets/day)(10 days). 4. Your quantity for this prescription is 20 tablets.
Dr. Joseph Johnson 123 Main St. Anytown, USA 33358 265-555-4379 Name: Amy Smith Date: 7/28 Address: 895 Croissant Drive Anytown, USA 33358 Rx: Tussi Organidin ii tsp po tid Qty 240 mL _______ Voluntary Formulary Permitted _______ Brand Name Medically Necessary Label ______________ DEA ______________ Signature: Joseph Johnson	To Calculate Day's Supply 1. Amy is taking 2 teaspoons (10 mL) per dose and is taking three doses per day. 2. First step—(10 mL/dose)(3 doses/day) = 30 mL/day 3. Second step—Days supply is equal to quantity dispensed divided by quantity taken per day. $\frac{240\text{ mL}}{30\text{ mL/day}}$ = 8 days supply. 4. Therefore, the medication will last the patient 8 days.

- Home and work telephone numbers
- Date of birth
- Allergies (drug and food)
- Insurance information

Once you have this information, you should review the prescription to make sure that all of the information required for a prescription is present. It should include:

Patient Information

First name: ____________________ Middle initial Last name: ________________
Address: ____________________________________
City: ______________________________________
State: _____________________________ Zip: _______________________
Phone: ___________________ E-z off caps ___ Yes ____ No
Allergies: ________________________
Male _________ Female _________
Date of birth: ______________________
Insurance company name: ____
Insurance ID number: _______________________________
Insurance group number: ____________________________

Figure 14-6 Patient profile.

- Date
- Physician's address
- Physician's telephone and fax number
- DEA number (if applicable)
- Name of drug
- Strength of drug (not all medications have a strength)
- Quantity
- Signa
- Refills (if any)
- Doctor's signature

The date on the prescription is extremely important. If the prescription is a noncontrolled drug the prescription is valid for 1 year from the date it was written (please check state regulations). If the date was not written on the prescription and the medication is for a noncontrolled drug then you list the date the prescription was brought to you.

In the practice of pharmacy, state laws over rule Federal law. Federal law states that prescriptions for Schedule II medications are valid for 60 days. However, many states laws rule that prescriptions for Schedule II medications are only valid for 7 days from the date it is written. It is necessary for the pharmacy technician to know the state law regarding prescriptions for Schedule II medications. Prescriptions for Schedules III to V drug are valid for only 6 months from the date written. If the date is missing on Schedules III to V medication they are, you will need to contact the physician to verify the date it was written. In addition, you may need to verify that the DEA number is listed on the prescription if it is a controlled substance.

Once you have made sure that everything you need is on the prescription, you should look on the shelf to make sure that the drug is available for you to fill. Refer to the following sample prescriptions on page 382.

Review the prescriptions. Would you be able to fill them? If not, list why and how you would explain it to the patient.

In addition to a prescription being brought in to the pharmacy by the patient or patient representative, a prescription may be telephoned in to the pharmacy by the physician. In most states, pharmacy technicians are not permitted to accept telephoned prescriptions from physicians; they

Sam Gooding
9461 Chum Ave.
Any town, USA. 44456
Phone: 123-555-4466 Fax: 123-555-4467
Name: _Susan Moore________ Date: __7/6____
Address: __995 Apple St.__Anytown, USA 44456____________

Rx
Naprosyn 500 mg
i tab po q 8 h prn pain
#25

Label: ___ Refills: _____
DEA: __AG1234563__

Signature: __Sam Gooding______

Dr. Sharon Watson
456 Somewhere Lane
Anytown, USA 44458
123-555-4698

Name:_____Joe Smith___________________Date:_7/5____________
Address:____875 Palm St.____ Anytown, USA 44458

Rx:

Prozac
i po qd

Label:_________
Refills: 2

DEA:______________

Signature:_____Sharon Watson _______

must notify the pharmacist that a doctor's office is attempting to call in a new prescription. A physician's office may fax a new prescription in to the pharmacy and the pharmacy technician is permitted to remove it from the fax machine. Some states may allow a patient to fax in a prescription but the person must present the original prescription before it is picked up.

Processing the Prescription

Processing a prescription begins when you enter the information into the computer and is completed when the patient receives the filled prescription.

Entering Patient Information

For a new prescription, the first thing you do is type in the patient's name. If the patient has not been to the pharmacy before you will need to enter all of the patient's personal information. The computer will prompt you for specific patient and prescription information (Figure 14-7).

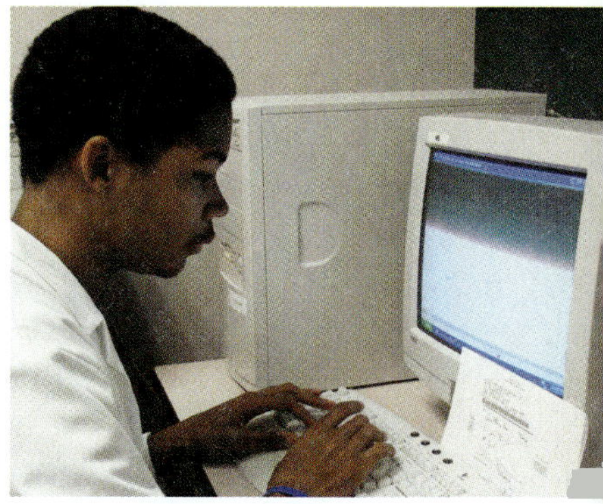

Figure 14-7 Entering prescription into the computer.

Computer Systems Computer systems vary from employer to employer, but all require the same information to enter. Many pharmacies have developed their own sig codes (abbreviations that are used to allow the pharmacy personnel from having to type out every word). There are many universal pharmacy abbreviations with which a pharmacy technician must be familiar. The Joint Commission (TJC), formerly Joint Commission of Accreditation of Healthcare Organizations (JCAHO), has issued its "Do Not Use List" that was discussed in Chapter 12 because of prescription errors due to abbreviations. However, many physicians may continue to use these abbreviations.

Entering the Doctor's Information

A pharmacy technician may be required to enter the doctor's information into the computer system (Figure 14-8). If a physician's information is not on file at your pharmacy, the computer entry screen will come up automatically. If you find yourself in this situation, you will be prompted by the computer system to enter the physician's specific information in a manner very similar to that of entering a new patient.

All the information that you need for the physician should be found on the prescription and will include:

- Physician's name
- Physician's office address
- Physician's office telephone number
- Fax number
- DEA number
- State license number (may be a legal requirement for specific states)

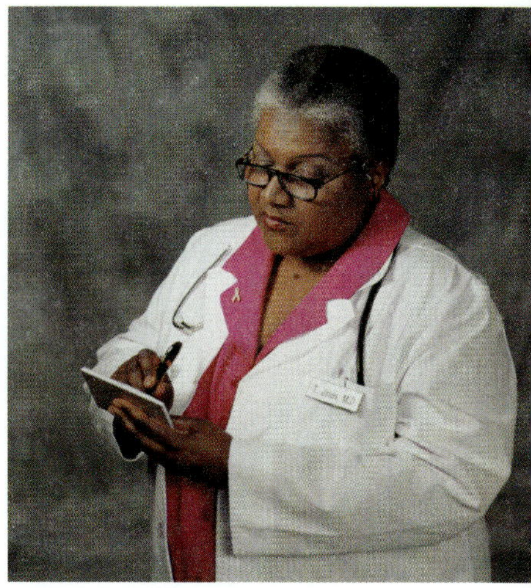

Figure 14-8 Physician's information may need to be entered into the computer system.

Brand Name Versus Generic When doctors request brand name medications, they must hand write either "medically necessary" or "dispense as written" on the prescription form for it to be valid. The abbreviation for "dispense as written" is DAW, and specific DAW codes are used in pharmacy practice for reimbursement. A pharmacy technician must be aware of the state regulations regarding generic substitution of medications. If a patient requests that he or she wants the brand name drug when a generic drug is available and has been approved by the physician, the pharmacist may dispense it. However, if a patient wishes to receive a generic drug when the physician has not initially approved it, the pharmacist must contact the physician for approval before dispensing it. If the physician approves the use of the generic, it must be documented on the hard copy of the prescription.

Reimbursement and DAW Codes It is extremely important that a pharmacy be properly reimbursed for its services rendered by third-party payers. The pharmacy technician must be able to read the prescription properly and select the correct DAW code for proper reimbursement. The failure to select the correct code may result in the pharmacy losing money at that moment or in the future if the pharmacy is audited by a third-party provider.

DAW codes used in the practice of pharmacy are the following:

0 – Generic or no generic available
1 – Name brand product "Medically Necessary"
2 – Patient selected the brand product
3 – Pharmacist selected the brand product
4 – No generic available—not in stock
5 – "Branded generic" brand dispensed as pharmacy's generic
6 – Override DAW code
7 – Brand mandated by state law
8 – Brand product not available in the market place

A third-party provider may schedule a prescription audit at any time and visit the pharmacy to examine specific prescriptions filled for clients. During an audit inspectors verify that a valid prescription exists, the pharmacy entered the correct DAW code based upon the physician's wishes, and that patient signature logs are being maintained. The signature logs indicate the prescriptions were picked up by the patients. If an auditor finds something wrong or missing, he or she may deny payment to the pharmacy or request that the pharmacy reimburse the insurance provider for overpayment.

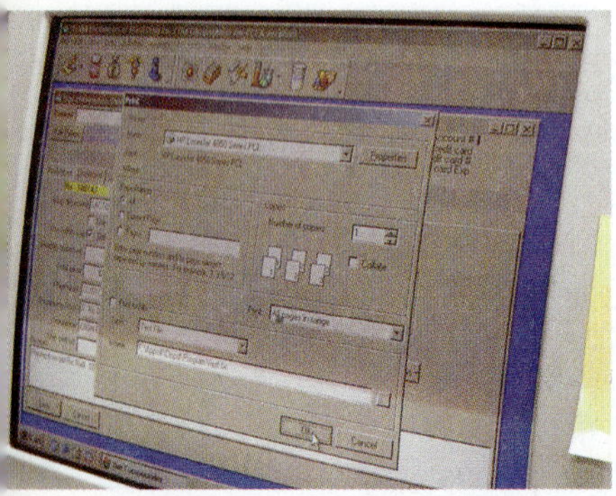

Figure 14-9 Prescriptions are submitted for payment to a third party provider on line.

adjudication An electronic online billing of prescriptions, that ensures prompt payment to the pharmacy and reduces the number of rejected prescriptions.

drug utilization evaluation (DUE) The process that examines whether prescription drugs are being used efficiently and appropriately within a prescription drug benefit.

Adjudication

After you have entered all of the necessary information, the system should take you back to the prescription screen, where you will be prompted to provide the name of the medication.

Many times by entering only the first few letters of the medication's name, you will be taken to a screen that allows you to select the correct medication. It is possible to enter the drug by using a medication's NDC number. You will be asked the quantity of the medication and number of refills approved by the physician. You also will be asked to enter the signa of the prescription where you may be able to use "sig codes." It is at this point that a prescription is submitted for payment to a third-party provider (Figure 14-9). This process is known as online **adjudication,** which is an electronic online billing of prescriptions, that ensures prompt payment to the pharmacy and reduces the number of rejected prescriptions, and is discussed in greater detail later in the chapter.

Drug Utilization Evaluation

The next step in processing the prescription is **drug utilization evaluation (DUE),** formerly referred to as drug utilization review (DUR), of the pending prescription and prescriptions in the patient's profile. DUE is a condition of OBRA-90 that requires the pharmacist to make sure that the patient is not taking a medication that he or she may be allergic to, have drug interactions with, or that is contraindicated for the patient's condition. The majority of the time during the DUE process, potential problems do not appear, but in specific instances a warning may appear to the pharmacy technician. If a warning does appear, the technician must inform the pharmacist immediately. Under no circumstances should the technician continue with the prescription processing.

The pharmacist will investigate the cause of the warning and will make the appropriate decision regarding the processing of the prescription. This decision may involve contacting the physician, speaking to the patient, or allowing the prescription to be processed. It is the pharmacist's responsibility to decide the outcome of a DUE inquiry. Pharmacy technicians are not permitted to make judgment decisions. Situations indicating a DUE is required might include:

- A patient presenting a prescription for Cephalexin and he or she is allergic to penicillin.
- A patient having a prescription filled for Mephyton (Vitamin K) and he or she is taking Coumadin.
- A patient presenting a prescription for Zestril (lisinopril) and lisinopril has been previously filled.
- A female presenting a prescription for Triphasil and she has had a prescription filled for an antibiotic.

A pharmacy's computer system is unable to differentiate when a medication was processed. It is the responsibility of the pharmacist to make all decisions and to decide the actions to be taken due to drug utilization evaluation.

National Provider's Identifier

In May of 2008, pharmacies were required to submit a physician's National Provider's Identifier (NPI) when submitting prescriptions for reimbursement from a third-party provider. An NPI is a 10-digit intelligence-free numeric identifier that is required for all prescriptions to comply with HIPAA. Intelligence-free means that the numbers do not carry information about health care providers, such as the state in which they practice or their provider type or specialization.

NPIs provide:

- Simpler electronic transmission of HIPAA standard transactions
- Standard unique health identifiers for health care providers, health plans, and employers
- More efficient coordination of benefits transactions

All health care providers (e.g., physicians, suppliers, hospitals, and others) are eligible for NPIs. Health care providers are individuals or organizations that provide health care. All health care providers who are HIPAA-covered entities, whether they are individuals (such as physicians, nurses, dentists, chiropractors, physical therapists, or pharmacists) or organizations (such as hospitals, home health agencies, clinics, nursing homes, residential treatment centers, laboratories, ambulance companies, group practices, **health maintenance organizations (HMOs),** suppliers of durable medical equipment, pharmacies, etc.), must obtain an NPI to identify themselves in HIPAA standard transactions.

health maintenance organization (HMO) A managed-care organization that provides health care services to enrolled members for a fixed, prepaid fee.

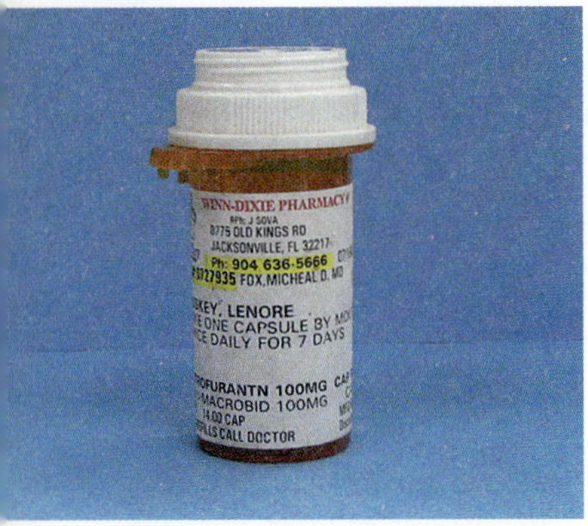

Figure 14-10 Prescription label.

Filling the Prescription

Once the prescription has been entered into the computer, the next step is to fill it. The pharmacy technician or pharmacist selects the print option, and the label will print out. Each computer system is different so the process of printing out prescription labels may differ (Figure 14-10).

The label will contain the following information:

- Pharmacy name
- Pharmacy address
- Pharmacy telephone number
- Patient's name
- Patient's address
- Prescription (serial) number
- Physician's name
- Date filled
- Drug name and strength
- Quantity
- Directions to the patient
- Expiration date of the prescription
- Number of refills

A drug monograph (literature) will be printed for the patient. The monograph is written in nontechnical language so the patient is able to understand the information. It will contain the name of the drug: brand and generic. It will state the drug's usage, possible side effects of the medication, and what one should do if the drug is not taken. It may list the NDC number of the drug.

The NDC (National Drug Code) number is assigned to every drug as a way to identify it. When you pull the drug from the shelf, you should always make sure you have the correct drug by checking all three components of the NDC number: the drug manufacturer, the active ingredient and strength of the drug, and the package size of the drug. If the middle number of the NDC number matches both the bottle and the monograph, circle and initial it to remind yourself and the pharmacist that you checked the drug.

National Drug Code Number.

NDC 00009-(7376)- 04 *LE*

Another safeguard used in the filling process to prevent medication errors involves the pharmacy technician scanning a new prescription into the computer system and then scanning the drug label from the manufacturer's bottle. This acts as a safety check to verify the medication being dispensed corresponds to the medication on the prescription. If the scanned drug label does not correspond to the drug, the scanner informs the pharmacy technician or pharmacist of the situation.

Pill Counting Some pharmacies may use automatic pill counters when counting out the medication. It is important that you pour the medication slowly or an error will occur that will require you to recount the medication. After you have pulled out the medication drawer, you must place the drawer back tightly or else medicine may be found under the machine. This means the patient did not receive all of the medication. The pill-counting machine should be cleaned several times during a shift to prevent

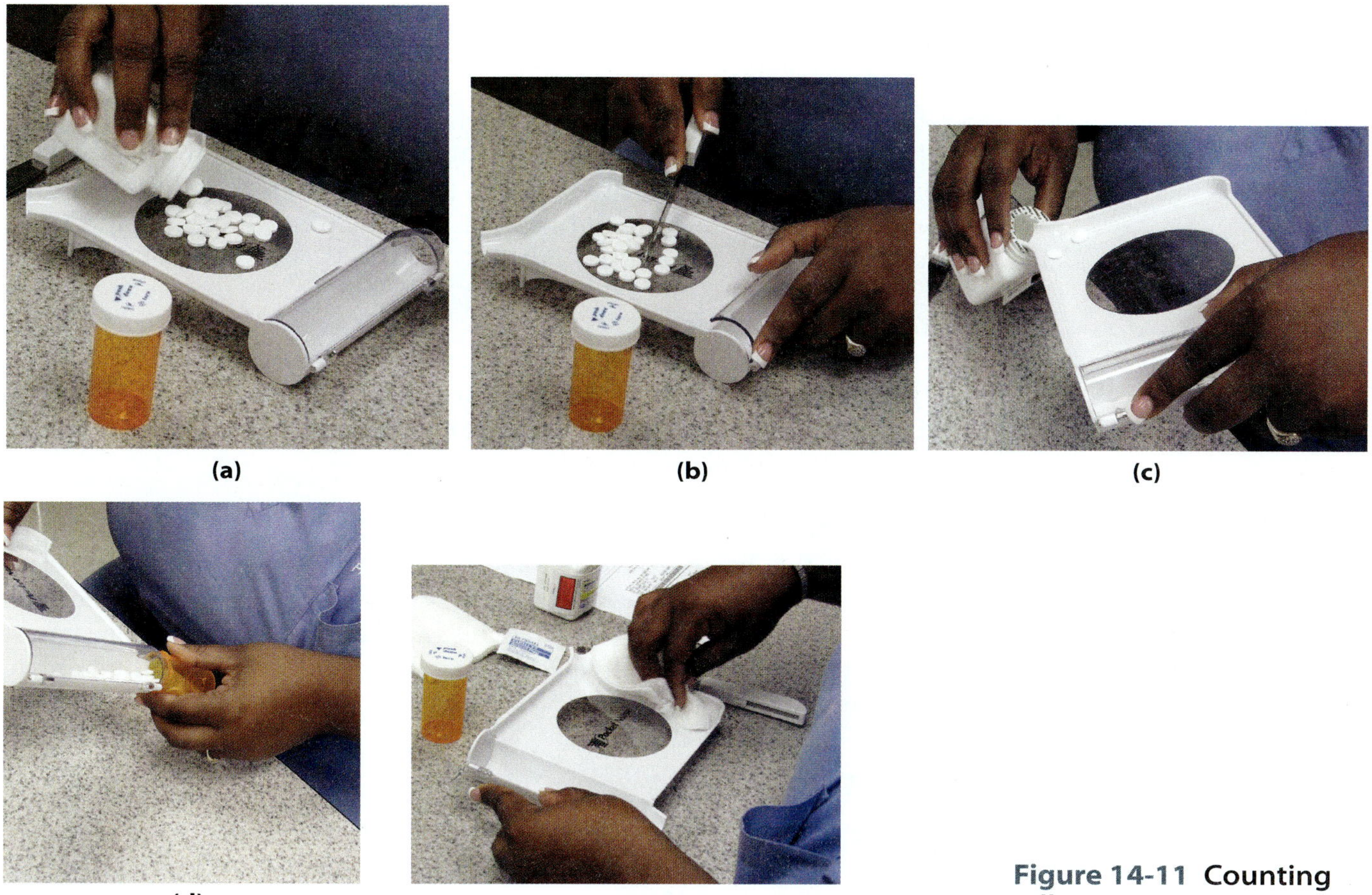

(a) (b) (c) (d) (e)

Figure 14-11 Counting pills.

medication residue from adhering to the drawer and coming in contact with other medications and possibly causing an adverse reaction for the patient.

When counting out pills, tablets, or capsules, the following steps should be followed (Figure 14-11):

a. Pour out the medication onto the counting tray.
b. Count the medication in multiples of fives with a spatula into the compartment on the side of the counting tray.
c. Once the medication has been counted out into the compartment, pour the remainder back into the bottle.
d. Pour the medication that is left in the compartment tray into a vial.
e. Clean the pill tray after counting out specific medications such as penicillin or sulfamethiazole/trimethoprim because the remaining residue may coat the next patient's medication. If the next patient is allergic to the medication, an allergic or anaphylactic reaction may occur.

The pharmacy technician in this figure has broken an OSHA rule. Do you see a problem? Look closely at her nails. They should be short, clean and without acrylic.

Container Once the medication is placed in the vial or bottle, apply the label and any necessary auxiliary labels. An auxiliary label provides additional information to the patient such as the route of administration (by mouth or topically), side effects (drowsiness or discoloration of urine), or how to store the medication (refrigerator). If a patient has requested an E-Z off cap, also referred to as a non-childproof cap, it should be a noted in the computer. Even though it is documented in the computer system, the pharmacist must stamp the back of the prescription, which will state that the patient has requested an E-Z off cap and the patient must sign his or her name to it. When the label prints, it will state on the monograph that there should be an E-Z off cap on the vial. Otherwise, place a childproof cap on the vial.

Patient Product Insert

Certain medications require that patients receive a Patient Product Insert (PPI) every time they receive a prescription. Examples of medications requiring PPIs include estrogens, injectable contraceptives, oral contraceptives, progestational drugs, and retinoids.

Completion

Once all of this has been completed, pass the completed (filled) prescription to the pharmacist with the written prescription and the medication bottle for the final check. The final check is performed by the pharmacist to verify that the work completed by the pharmacy technician is complete and accurate.

Prescription Pickup

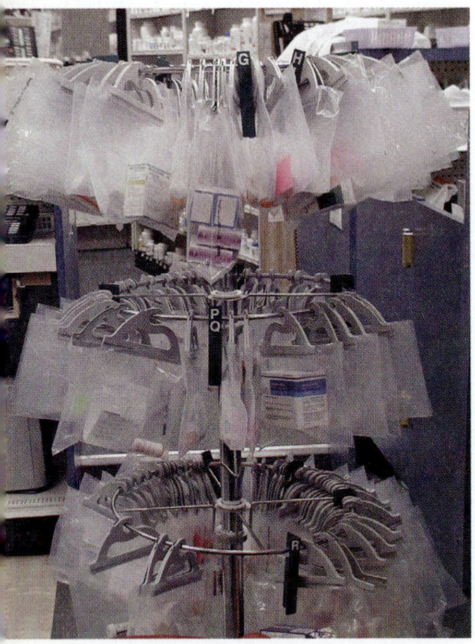

Figure 14-12 Alphabetized filing of completed prescriptions.

Once the pharmacist has made the final check, the prescription is placed in the pick up bins or hanging bags that are alphabetized by the patient's last name (Figure 14-12).

It is very important that filled prescriptions be filed properly. The failure to file prescriptions properly may result in the patient waiting longer for a prescription and cause poor customer service. The pharmacy team that knows their customers' names provides better customer service.

When a patient comes to pick up a prescription, always ask for first and last name. Ask the patient to spell out his or her name if you did not hear correctly. To verify it is the correct person, have the customer give you his or her address or date of birth. Never offer to give a prescription of a family member to a patient because this would be in violation of HIPAA.

After verifying the patient's identity, the technician should open the bag to ensure that the medication inside belongs to the patient, and that if it requires an E-Z off cap it is on the vial. This helps reduce prescription errors. Per OBRA-90, technicians must always ask if the patient has any questions for the pharmacist. Although the technician makes the initial offer to the patient, it is the responsibility of the pharmacist to counsel a patient. Examples of counseling include explaining:

- How the patient should take the medicine: on an empty stomach? with food?
- Which foods to avoid, if any, while taking the medication. For instance, green vegetables should be avoided when taking Coumadin; dairy products should not be taken with Tetracycline; wines, sherry, and beer as well as any foods that contain tyramine, should not be consumed if a patient is taking an MAO inhibitor.
- What to do if the patient forgets to take a dose of the medication.

- How to store the medication—whether at room temperature or in the refrigerator.
- Any side effects of a medication: drowsiness, diarrhea, constipation, etc.

Tech Check

3. Name two items found on a prescription.(LO 14.3)
4. What are the three components of an NDC number?(LO 14.5)
5. What is the purpose of DAW authorization codes?(LO 14.5)
6. What would hinder a pharmacy technician from continuing to fill a prescription?(LO 14.3, 14.4, 14.5, 14.7)
7. Are pharmacy technicians able to counsel customers?(LO 14.5)

Computer Usage in Retail Pharmacy(LO 14.7, 14.8, 14.12)

The usage of computers in the practice of pharmacy has simplified many of the tasks that pharmacists and pharmacy technicians must perform (Figure 14-13). Pharmacies have different computer systems but there are similarities among them all. All pharmacy computer systems allow you to enter patient, prescription, and physician data; they allow you to store the data and recall it at some other time. Pharmacy computers calculate the price of a prescription, bill the prescription to an insurance carrier, and are able to reorder medications from a warehouse or vendor.

The pharmacy technician may enter data into the computer system via a keyboard, mouse, or scanner. Pharmacies may utilize voice recognition technology or computerized physician order entry (CPOE), which will be explained in Chapter 15. Facsimiles (faxes) of a prescription may be accepted in a pharmacy depending on federal and state regulations. Technology and automation improve efficiency and reduce the possibility of errors.

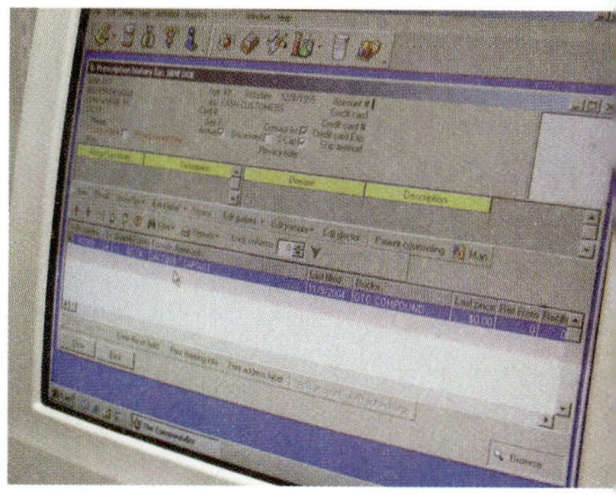

Figure 14-13 Computer usage in retail pharmacy has simplified many tasks.

Third-Party Providers

The different types of insurance companies include:

- Health maintenance organizations (HMOs)
- **Independent practice associations (IPAs)**
- **Preferred provider organizations (PPOs)**

A third-party payer means that three groups are involved in the payment process: the insurance companies that deal with the doctors, called clearance houses; the companies that deal with the pharmacies, called PBMs (prescription benefits managers); and finally, the customers. The majority of prescriptions filled today involve third-party providers.

Many PBMs utilize a formulary system, which is a list of approved drugs for which an insurance company will reimburse a pharmacy for payment of a prescription. Drugs that are not on the formulary (nonformulary drugs) may not be reimbursed or the patient may be responsible

independent practice association (IPA) A health maintenance organization in which individual physicians enter a nonexclusive contract to see both HMO and non-HMO patients.

preferred provider organization (PPO) A managed-care organization that provides health care services to enrolled members for a discounted fee.

for paying a higher portion of the cost of the prescription. A formulary is a cost-containment strategy used by PBMs. Terms used by third-party payers include:

- Co-pay—a predetermined amount of money or percentage of the cost of the prescription that the customer pays.
- Co-insurance—a percentage-based plan in which the customer must pay a certain percentage of the prescription price.
- Dual co-insurance—a lower percentage paid for generic and a higher percentage for brand.
- Multiple tiered co-payments—a specific amount of money paid for generics, brands, and nonformulary or lifestyle medications.

Each third-party plan is different and it is the responsibility of the pharmacy team to be familiar with each of them. A pharmacy technician who is familiar with various third-party plans is able to provide better customer service when issues arise.

Online Adjudication

When billing an insurance company electronically, the billing is completed within a matter of seconds. While the prescription is being processed, the computer sends a message to the insurance company by providing the company with specific prescription information. The provider responds with a message back to the pharmacy to tell how much to charge the patient. If the prescription may not be filled at this time an explanation is provided. This process is known as online adjudication, which is an active process for the online billing of a prescription.

It can be a challenge to input insurance information, because there are so many different third-party providers. The appearance of the card varies from provider to provider. Some cards may include the Rx symbol with the name of the company that you will bill the claim to. Third-party cards may contain the patient's ID number, a group number, and a bin number. The beneficiary identification number (bin) is an identification number for the prescription plan. Some insurance providers require a person code, which identifies the family member receiving the prescription, and must be included in the prescription claim (e.g., Jane Smith 01, John Smith 02).

Once the information has been entered into the computer and the prescription has been processed, the pharmacy will be notified if the prescription claim was paid and the amount being paid to the pharmacy. If the prescription is rejected, a rejection code is provided, and the pharmacy must resolve the issue before resubmitting the claim. For example, if the patient went to another pharmacy and tried to fill the same prescription the rejection code will read "Refill Too Soon" or "Filled At Other Pharmacy." If the patient says that is incorrect, the technician may call the insurance company (the telephone number may be found on the back of the card or it may appear on the screen) and find out where and when the prescription was filled. Some of the other rejections that technicians may encounter can be found in Table 14-3. Finding out that an insurance problem occurred and trying to fix is a part of the pharmacy technician's job.

Table 14-3 Common Causes of Rejection

PROBLEM	ACTION or CORRECTION
The pharmacy does not have a contract with the insurance company.	The patient would have to go to another pharmacy or the pharmacy would have to sign a contract with the insurance plan.
The ID, group number, or patient information does not match.	Always double-check that the information is entered correctly. If you do not find an error, call the insurance company to verify the information they have on record.
The drug is not covered by the insurance plan.	Tell the patient that the medication is not covered. The pharmacist may call the prescriber to ask for a different medication.
A refill request is not accepted because the refill is being requested too soon.	Verify with the patient when the medication was previously filled and where. If needed, call the insurance plan to verify when and where the previous prescription was filled and find out when it can be filled again. Exceptions may be allowed if a patient is going to be gone for an extended period of time. In some cases the patient may have to pay for the prescription.
The quantity or day's supply is limited by the insurance company, so the prescription is rejected.	Call the insurance plan to determine what quantity or day's supply is allowed.

Tech Check

8. Why is it important to understand insurance?(LO 14.7)

9. What is a bin number?(LO 14.8)

Customer Service(LO 14.6)

Today, there are many factors affecting a person's choice in selecting a pharmacy to fill their prescriptions. Some of these factors include prices, convenience, including the location and the hours of operation of a pharmacy, knowledgeable staff, and customer service. A pharmacy wishes to attract new customers and retain its current customers through superior customer service. Pharmacy is a customer service–oriented business.

A pharmacy technician is often the first person the customer encounters, so the way you greet a person is extremely important. Your body language sometimes speaks louder than your words. Poor posture, tapping on the counter, not making eye contact with the patient, or having your arms crossed in front of you may give the customer a negative impression. In addition, the tone of your voice is extremely important. For instance, you may say the correct thing to the customer, but the tone of your voice may make it seem as though you are acting hostile.

People come to the pharmacy to purchase medication for either an acute or a chronic condition. They may not be feeling well when they arrive. When an individual is not feeling well he or she may not act normally.

One of the easiest things for a technician to do for patients is to listen to what they have to say. Do not cut them off while they are talking. Do not assume that you know what they are going to say next. Let them say whatever is on their mind—most of the time this is enough to make them happy. Never argue with a customer; you may win the argument, but you will most likely lose a customer. Without the customer, the pharmacy will cease to exist. A more complete discussion on customer service is found in Chapter 3.

OTC (Over-the-Counter) Medications(LO 14.10, 14.11)

Over-the-counter medications (OTCs) are medications that do not require a physician's supervision. Patients may purchase them on their own. Many people self-medicate rather than go to the doctor, as it is less expensive. Pharmacy technicians are not permitted to counsel patients even though the medication is an OTC. When a customer asks the technician to recommend an OTC product, the technician must inform the pharmacist of the situation. The pharmacist will collect information from the patient before recommending an OTC medication.

A retail pharmacy may stock many different types of OTC drugs. Some of these classifications include:

- Cough and cold preparations, such as Robitussin, Dimetapp, or Afrin
- Allergy medications, such as Claritin or Benadryl
- Analgesics, antipyretics, and anti-inflammatory products, such as Tylenol, Motrin, or aspirin
- Antacids and stomach acids include such products as Prilosec, Pepcid AC, and Mylanta
- Antifungal agents such as Lotrimin AF, Lamisil AF, or Monistat 7
- Dietary supplements and herbal supplements, such as vitamin C, vitamin E, and melatonin
- Eye products such as contact lens products and Visine
- First-aid products include products such as Neosporin, hydrogen peroxide, and bandages
- Sleeping aids such as Sominex

There may be many other categories of OTC products that have not been mentioned. A more detailed discussion of OTC products is found in Chapter 8.

Tech Check

10. Should pharmacy technicians recommend OTC medications?(LO 14.11)

11. Is it the responsibility of the pharmacy technician to help a customer with OTC medications?(LO 14.11)

Chapter Summary

Understanding the pharmacy retail setting is vital to the pharmacy technician. Important points to know are:

- Retail pharmacy requires an individual to be able to multitask in a very busy setting.
- Pharmacy technicians must know the components required to process a prescription. These include the prescriber's information, the date the prescription was written, patient information, the inscription, the subscription, the signa, the signature of the prescriber on handwritten prescriptions, and a DEA number for controlled substances.
- Pharmacy technicians must be able to interpret a prescription, which may require them to know many pharmacy abbreviations.
- A pharmacy technician must be aware of the critical path of a prescription. The critical path of a prescription begins when the prescription is dropped off at the pharmacy. It is the responsibility of the technician to make sure the prescription is complete. The pharmacy technician must verify that the patient's information is correct and is in the pharmacy system. The technician may enter the prescription into the computer, bill the insurance company or the patient, and generate a prescription label. The technician will seek the pharmacist's attention if a DUE result and warning is being generated. The correct medication is selected and is verified by its NDC number. A pharmacy technician may count out the prescribed quantity of medication and package it in the proper-sized container. The prescription and auxiliary labels are affixed to the container. It is the responsibility of the pharmacist to perform the final check on the completed prescription. The prescription is placed in a prescription bag. The bag is placed in prescription bins waiting for its pickup by either the patient or the patient's representative. When the patient picks up the prescription, the technician may ring up the prescription on the cash register. The technician may ask the patient if he or she has any questions, but it is the responsibility of the pharmacist to answer these questions and to counsel the patient.
- Pharmacy technicians must be familiar with the various third-party plans in which their pharmacy participates. They may be required to troubleshoot any problems that arise in the billing of the prescription.
- Pharmacy is a customer service industry. It is the responsibility of the entire pharmacy staff to provide superior customer service to their patients. Pharmacy technicians may have the most contact with patients. It is normally the technician whom the patient sees first when dropping off a prescription and when picking it up. The success and profitability of a pharmacy is affected by the customer service it provides or fails to provide. Without the customer, a pharmacy cannot exist.

Chapter Review

Case Study Questions

1. Why is multitasking important?(LO 14.9)
2. Why is it important to know your computer system?(LO 14.7, 14.8)
3. What are some examples of customer service being observed in this retail pharmacy by Tina?(LO 14.6)

At Your Service Questions

1. What is the role of the pharmacy technician in a retail pharmacy?(LO 14.11)
2. What are some of the duties a pharmacy technician may be responsible for performing while working in a retail pharmacy?(LO 14.11)
3. Why is teamwork important in a retail pharmacy?(LO 14.11)

Multiple Choice

Select the best answer.

1. What makes a good technician?(LO 14.11)
   a. Knowing insurance plans
   b. Having great customer service skills
   c. Multitasking
   d. All of the above
2. In what area of the pharmacy would a patient drop off a prescription?(LO 14.2)
   a. Patient consultation area
   b. Out-window
   c. In-window
   d. None of the above
3. Which of the following would you ask a patient when taking a prescription request?(LO 14.1)
   a. Tag number
   b. Phone number
   c. Social Security number
   d. All of the above
4. What part of the NDC number should a technician check before counting a drug?(LO 14.5)
   a. First set of numbers
   b. Second set of numbers
   c. Third set of numbers
   d. All of the above
5. How are prescriptions filed in the pickup bins?(LO 14.1)
   a. By patient's last name
   b. By patient's first name
   c. By physician's last name
   d. By name of drug
6. What law states that you have to ask, "Do you have any questions for the pharmacist about your medication"?(LO 14.5)
   a. HICFA 1500
   b. HIPAA
   c. OBRA-90
   d. Adjudication
7. What information would you find on an insurance card?(LO 14.8)
   a. Patient's phone number
   b. Patient's address
   c. Patient's allergies
   d. Bin number
8. Which of the following is an OTC drug?(LO 14.10)
   a. Tylenol
   b. Prozac 20 mg
   c. Nexium
   d. None of the above
9. Which term refers to the online submission of a prescription claim to an insurance provider?(LO 14.5)
   a. Adjudication
   b. Reconstitution
   c. Manual submission
   d. None of the above
10. What is the inscription on a prescription? LO 14.3)
    a. Name, strength, and quantity of medication
    b. Directions to the pharmacist
    c. Instructions to the patient
    d. None of the above
11. What type of pharmacy has more than one location and will be run by an elected board of directors?(LO 14.2)
    a. Chain pharmacy
    b. Franchise pharmacy
    c. Independent pharmacy
    d. All of the above
12. Who designs, administers, and manages the prescription drug benefit?(LO 14.8)
    a. HMO
    b. IPA
    c. PBM
    d. PPO
13. Who may counsel a patient when picking up a prescription?(LO 14.5)
    a. Cashier
    b. Pharmacy aid
    c. Pharmacist
    d. Pharmacy technician
14. Which DAW code should be used if the physician is requesting a brand name medication for a patient?(LO 14.5)
    a. 0
    b. 1
    c. 2
    d. 3
15. How many days will the following prescription last a patient?(LO 14.5)

    cephalexin 500 mg #40

    i cap po qid

    a. 5 days
    b. 10 days
    c. 20 days
    d. 40 days

16. What route would the patient take the following prescription if it had the following signa?(LO 14.4)

    i supp pr q6–8h prn N&V

    a. Orally
    b. Rectally
    c. Sublingually
    d. Topically

17. What type of pharmacy weights would be used in a retail pharmacy?(LO 14.1)
    a. Apothecary
    b. Avoirdupois
    c. Household
    d. Metric

18. Which of the following tasks might a pharmacy technician perform in a retail pharmacy?(LO 14.11)
    a. Do extemporaneous compounding
    b. Order medications
    c. Enter patient information into the computer system
    d. Pharmacy technicians may perform all of the tasks mentioned

19. Who is required to have an NPI?(LO 14.5)
    a. Pharmacies
    b. Physicians
    c. Hospitals
    d. All of the above

20. When does a prescription require a DEA number?(LO 14.3, 14.4)
    a. For OTC medications that are written on a prescription blank by a physician
    b. For all prescription medications
    c. For all controlled substance prescriptions
    d. All of the above

Abbreviations

Print the meaning of the following pharmacy abbreviations.

ac ______________________________

bid ______________________________

caps ______________________________

elix ______________________________

mg ______________________________

mL ______________________________

pc ______________________________

po ______________________________

prn ______________________________

qs ______________________________

stat ______________________________

syr ______________________________

tab ______________________________

tid ______________________________

tsp ______________________________

Critical Thinking Questions

1. A patient presents a new prescription for Prilosec 20 mg, which is an OTC medication. The patient wants to have the prescription submitted to a their third-party provider. How would you handle the situation?(LO 14.6, 14.10)

2. A patient wishes to refill a prescription; however, it is rejected by the third-party provider with an explanation of "Refill Too Soon." The patient informs you that the physician has changed directions on the prescription. How would you handle the situation?(LO 14.7)

3. You are processing a new prescription for a patient and during the DUE phase, you receive a warning on the computer screen. What will you do and why?(LO 14.5)

4. A patient calls in a prescription to be refilled for hydrochlorothiazide 50 mg (a diuretic) on Saturday afternoon. There are no refills remaining on the prescription and you fax a refill request to the patient's physician. The patient comes in to the pharmacy to pick up their prescription but the physician has not approved a refill yet. You notice on the patient's prescription profile that the patient has been receiving this medication for the past 5 years. What will you do?(LO 14.5)

5. A patient is picking up a prescription for Coumadin (a blood thinner) and also picks up a bottle of Bayer aspirin? As a pharmacy technician, you know that a patient should never take aspirin while being prescribed Coumadin. What should you do?(LO 14.5, 14.6)

HIPAA Scenario

John, a pharmacy technician, used the pharmacy's computer system to access his wife Melissa's prescription information. During a conversation with his wife, John let it slip that he knew about a medication she was taking, and Melissa realized that he had accessed her medical information at work. She immediately called John's supervisor and asked if he had unlimited access to her medical records. The supervisor stated that while John, as an employee, had access to patient health care data, and that he was allowed to access patient's data only during the course of his duties as a pharmacy technician, as in filling or refilling a patient's prescription. He said that John should have accessed her medication profile only if he was filling or refilling a prescription for her, and assured Melissa that John would be disciplined.

Discussion Questions(PTCB II.73)

1. Should John be able to access his spouse's medical data without her consent?
2. Did John's access of Melissa's data appear to be in conjunction with providing health care?
3. What actions, if any, should be taken against John?

Internet Activities

1. Go to **www.nacds.com** and explore the Web site. What types of resources are available in the pharmacy section of this site? What type of opportunities are posted for pharmacy technicians?(LO 14.2)
2. Go to **www.medicineshoppe.com** and find out what one must do to obtain a franchise with Medicine Shoppe.(LO 14.2)

Hospital/Inpatient Setting

15

Learning Outcomes

Upon completion of this chapter, you will be able to:

15.1 Describe the hospital or inpatient setting.

15.2 Classify inpatient settings.

15.3 Identify organizations that regulate inpatient facilities.

15.4 Describe the policies and procedures manual.

15.5 Define *protocol* as it pertains to inpatient settings.

15.6 Define *formulary*.

15.7 Identify three types of medication orders.

15.8 Describe the role of the inpatient pharmacy technician.

PTCB

In preparation for the certification examination, you should understand and perform activities associated with the following PTCB Knowledge Statement:

PTCB Knowledge Statement

Domain I. Assisting the Pharmacist in Serving Patients

Knowledge of delivery system for distributing medications (43)
Knowledge of quality improvement methods (49)
Knowledge of infection control procedures (69)

Key Terms

aseptic technique
automation
centralized pharmacy
computerized physician order entry (CPOE)
decentralized pharmacy
drug order
formulary
hospital
intensive care unit (ICU)
medication administration record (MAR)
parenteral
Pharmacy and Therapeutics (P&T) Committee
policy and procedure manual
protocol
stat order
unit-dose

Case Study

Peter is 1 of 20 pharmacy technicians who work in a medical center with a decentralized pharmacy system. The satellite pharmacy where Peter usually works provides medications to the Emergency Department and Trauma Center of the medical center. Peter often has the duty of checking the crash carts.

While reading this chapter, keep the following questions in mind:

1. What is Peter looking for when he is checking the crash carts?(LO 15.1, 15.6, 15.7)
2. Why is this so important?(LO 15.6, 15.7)

hospital Also known as inpatient facility.

medication administration record (MAR) A document that includes when a patient received a medication ordered and who administered it.

intensive care unit (ICU) A patient care unit of a hospital where the patients are usually very ill and require special attention by the nurses and other medical staff.

cardiac care units (CCU) A patient care unit of a hospital where the patients are usually extremely ill and require special attention to care for conditions of their heart and vascular system.

Introduction to the Hospital Setting(LO 15.1)

Hospitals (many are called medical centers) are health care facilities where the care is focused on inpatients, or patients that are staying overnight in the facility. Many hospitals have outpatient clinics on the same campus. Institutional settings have inpatients as well but may be long-term care facilities designed for the rehabilitation of patients. The practice of pharmacy in the inpatient setting is critically important as there must be an medication order for every medication the patient receives, prescription or not. The medications must also be reconciled in the patient's chart. **Medication administration records (MARs)** document that the patient has received the medication, including identification of the nurse who administered the drug and the time the dose was received. As there are different types of facilities, there are also different types of pharmacy systems at work in hospitals to provide better service. Obviously, the inpatient pharmacy technician must be an integral part of the health care team to facilitate the provision of quality health care to patients. This chapter focuses on the role of the pharmacy technician in the inpatient setting.

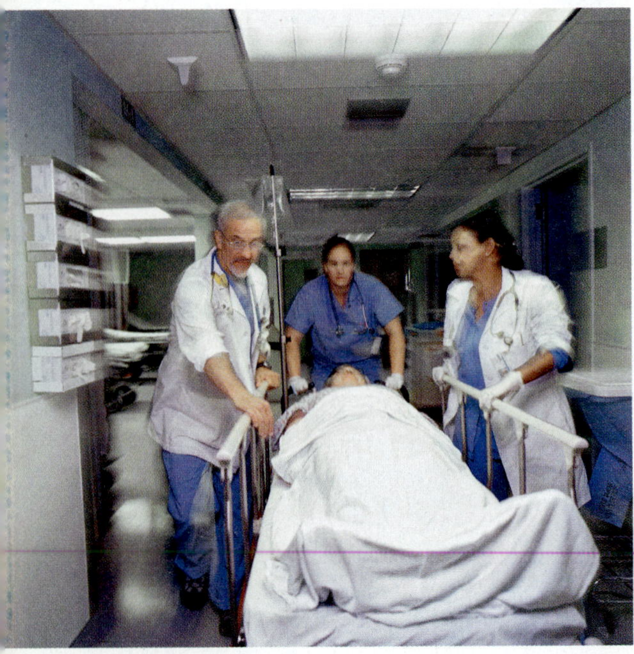

Inpatient Facility Classifications(LO 15.1, 15.2, 15.3)

One usually thinks of a hospital as being an acute care facility. Although this may be the case, inpatient facilities are of various types.

- Community hospitals typically have a small number of beds (25 to 100) and limited resources with respect to emergency care and surgery.
- Large hospitals, usually with more than 100 beds, may have specialty departments with an emergency department, **intensive care units (ICUs)**, and **cardiac care units (CCUs)**.
- Teaching hospitals are large hospitals that are affiliated with a medical school, and in addition to providing care for patients, also train medical and other allied health students, physicians, and pharmacists. Physicians and pharmacists who are being trained in these institutions are called residents.

At Your Service

Molly is an inpatient pharmacy technician who has been employed at the community hospital for 15 years. As she is one of the senior pharmacy technicians, she supervises other technicians as well as performing other pharmacy-specific duties in the hospital.

Yesterday, Molly noticed that one of the nurses was completing the medication administration record in a break room at the end of her shift. Molly questioned the nurse, who claimed to have committed the information to memory.

While reading this chapter, keep the following questions in mind:

1. What is wrong with what the nurse is doing?(LO 15.3, 15.4)
2. What potential problems might this create?(LO 15.3, 15.4)
3. What is Molly's responsibility?(LO 15.7)

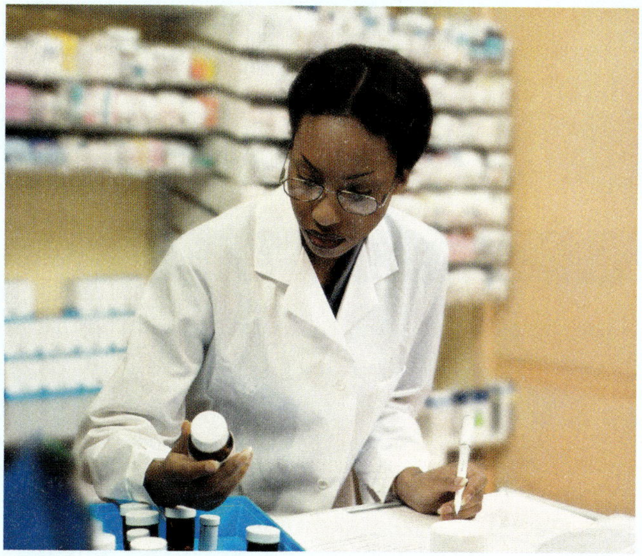

- Long-term care facilities may have any number of beds, but are not equipped for medical emergencies and surgeries.

With respect to pharmacy practice in these settings, the smaller the facility, the more likely it is to have a single **centralized pharmacy.** The larger the facility, the more likely it is that the facility has a **decentralized pharmacy** system. A decentralized pharmacy system using designated pharmacies to cover certain areas or departments more effectively provides medications to patients.

Inpatient Facility Standards

There are several regulatory agencies that have jurisdiction in the inpatient setting.

State Board of Pharmacy

The state board of pharmacy (BOP) licenses the pharmacies, pharmacists, and pharmacy technicians (depending upon the state). Each pharmacy within the same facility must have its own license.

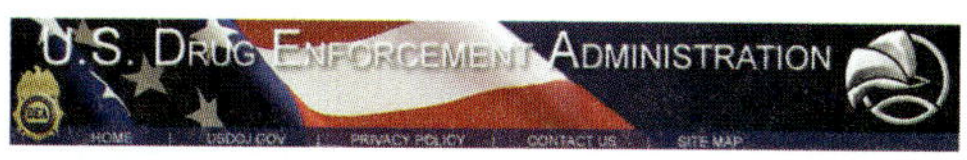

Drug Enforcement Administration

Each pharmacy must also have its own Drug Enforcement Administration (DEA) number if it stocks medications that are controlled substances.

The Joint Commission

The Joint Commission (TJC), formerly The Joint Commission on Accreditation of Healthcare Organizations (JCAHO), is the accrediting agency

centralized pharmacy One main pharmacy from which all medication orders are filled.

decentralized pharmacy Pharmacy system that includes multiple pharmacies serving various areas in a facility.

for hospitals. Periodically, TJC representatives pay visits to inpatient facilities and report their findings. It is important to note that TJC is concerned with the entire health care organization, and is not specific to pharmacy. TJC does make determinations as to whether or not the pharmacy is effectively working with other departments to reduce medication errors, complies with USP 797 and HIPAA, and provides quality.

The Centers for Medicare and Medicaid

The Centers for Medicare and Medicaid (CMS) inspects institutions, and as a result, determines whether the facility has the resources ability to provide service to those who receive health care that is paid for with federal funds (Medicare and Medicaid). Inpatient facilities may also be subject to inspections by county departments of health.

CMS Centers for **Medicare** & **Medicaid** Services

Tech Check

1. Which type of hospital trains physicians and medical students?[LO 15.1, 15.2]
2. Which organizations license both the inpatient pharmacies and pharmacists?[LO 15.3]
3. Which type of number is required for the pharmacy to handle controlled substances?[LO 15.3]

Policies and Procedures[LO 15.4, 15.5, 15.6]

Policy and Procedure Manual

The facility's **policy and procedure** manual provides information on the regulations (policies) of the organization and the steps or methods by which these rules are carried out (procedures). In other words, the rule is stated, followed by a series of steps that are to be taken to implement the rule. The policy and procedures manual contains information for very area of the facility and is updated periodically to reflect changes in the policies or in the structure of the facility. At least one policy and procedure manual is kept in each department, and every employee should be familiar with its location and with its contents, specifically as they pertain to an employee's particular area.

Information contained in the policy and procedures manual may include, but is not limited to, the following areas:

- Organization (including the mission and organizational chart)
- Administration (including organizational ethics, plan for provision of care)
- Human resources (including orientation, staffing, employee time and attendance)
- Safety
- Medical care (including admission, patient rights and responsibilities)
- Information management (including confidentiality, release of information, medical records)
- Medication use (including pharmacy services, formulary system, drug shortage)

policy and procedures manual
Manual containing regulations of the facility including how the regulations are performed.

Protocol

A **protocol** is a set of guidelines or standards, developed and approved by the **Pharmacy and Therapeutics (P&T) Committee**, a hospital committee chaired by a physician and composed of physicians, nursing staff, and pharmacists who establish and maintain a listing of approved drugs for use in a hospital. A protocol may be that a particular antibiotic is always given in the event of otitis media in children of a certain age. Or, it could be that patients with pneumonia are started with a particular antibiotic, which is discontinued only if the culture and sensitivity report indicates that the pathogen is resistant to the antibiotic.

The protocol may be developed as a result of demographic data, drug usage evaluation studies, literature review, or cost analysis. Adhering to the protocol is important in that it provides for standardized care throughout the facility.

Prior to adoption of a protocol, the P&T Committee invites presentations and comments from experts and stakeholders while reviewing data. After a protocol is approved, it is expected that all in the facility adhere to the protocol. The pharmacy technician needs to be aware of the protocol as it will impact medication processing and inventory management. The pharmacy technician should also be aware of any changes in a protocol to adjust medication ordering and medication processing accordingly.

Formulary

The **formulary** is a list of medications that are used in a facility and is determined and managed by the P&T Committee. Formularies may also be used by health maintenance organizations and insurance plans, so they may be encountered in outpatient pharmacy settings. The P&T Committee collects data and solicits comments prior to voting to put a drug onto the formulary. The committee also looks at drug utilization evaluation (DUE) studies to determine if an agent should be removed from the formulary.

Therapeutic substitutions are also approved by the P&T Committee. This limits the number of agents in the pharmacy inventory and helps contain costs. Therapeutic equivalence substitutions are not the same as generic substitutions. When a generic is substituted for the brand, the same chemical agent (drug) is given. With therapeutic equivalence substitutions, the substituted drug is in the same therapeutic class as the original agent, but is a different drug. The substituted agent also must share the same FDA-approved indication as the original agent.

Tech Check

4. What is the purpose of the policies and procedure manual?(LO 15.4)
5. What is a protocol?(LO 15.5)
6. Which group manages the formulary?(LO 15.6)

Medication Orders(LO 15.7)

Verbal Orders

The three types of medication or **drug orders** are verbal orders (also called oral orders), written orders, and electronic orders. Verbal orders

protocol Written guidelines for patient care given that criteria are met.

Pharmacy and Therapeutics (P&T) Committee A hospital committee chaired by a physician and composed of physicians, nursing staff, and pharmacists who establish and maintain a listing of approved drugs for use in a hospital.

formulary An approved list of medications to be used in an institution/facility or to be reimbursed by an insurance company health care plan as determined by the Pharmacy and Therapeutics (P&T) Committee.

drug order Prescription or medication order.

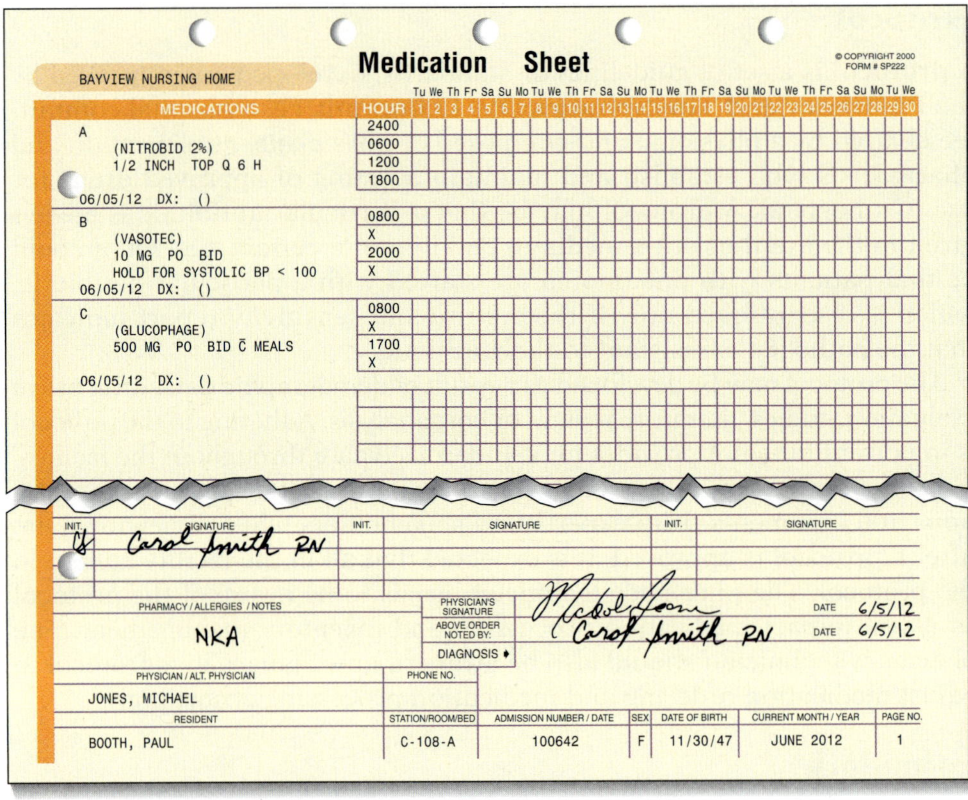

BAYVIEW NURSING HOME

Medication Sheet

© COPYRIGHT 2000 FORM # SP222

MEDICATIONS | HOUR

A
(NITROBID 2%)
1/2 INCH TOP Q 6 H
06/05/12 DX: ()
2400 / 0600 / 1200 / 1800

B
(VASOTEC)
10 MG PO BID
HOLD FOR SYSTOLIC BP < 100
06/05/12 DX: ()
0800 / X / 2000 / X

C
(GLUCOPHAGE)
500 MG PO BID C̄ MEALS
06/05/12 DX: ()
0800 / X / 1700 / X

INIT. SIGNATURE: CS Carol Smith RN

PHARMACY / ALLERGIES / NOTES: NKA

PHYSICIAN'S SIGNATURE: Michael Jones DATE 6/5/12

ABOVE ORDER NOTED BY: Carol Smith RN DATE 6/5/12

DIAGNOSIS

PHYSICIAN / ALT. PHYSICIAN: JONES, MICHAEL

PHONE NO.

RESIDENT: BOOTH, PAUL

STATION/ROOM/BED: C-108-A | ADMISSION NUMBER / DATE: 100642 | SEX: F | DATE OF BIRTH: 11/30/47 | CURRENT MONTH / YEAR: JUNE 2012 | PAGE NO.: 1

Figure 15-1 Medication Administration Record, hence M.A.R. (MAR).

involve a physician calling the pharmacy or telling a nurse to order a certain medication. Verbal orders must be documented in writing to meet BOP standards and to provide a record for the patient's chart. After the verbal order is processed, it becomes part of the MAR for documentation (Figure 15-1). Medication errors may result from inaccurate documentation of the verbal order, illegible handwriting, or lack of documentation of the order.

Written Orders

Written orders involve the physician writing a medication order. Often, nurses transcribe an oral or verbal order into written form to send to the pharmacy for processing. The inpatient pharmacy technician retrieves these orders from the floors and delivers them to the pharmacy for processing. Medication errors using this method may result from illegible handwriting, inappropriate drug or dose selection, or from the slips of paper being misplaced or lost (Figure 15-2). ASHP guidelines state that the following items are to be included on the written medication order:

- Patient's name and location
- Name of the medication
- Dose (expressed in the metric system)
- Frequency of administration
- Route of administration
- Signature of prescriber
- Date and time the order was written

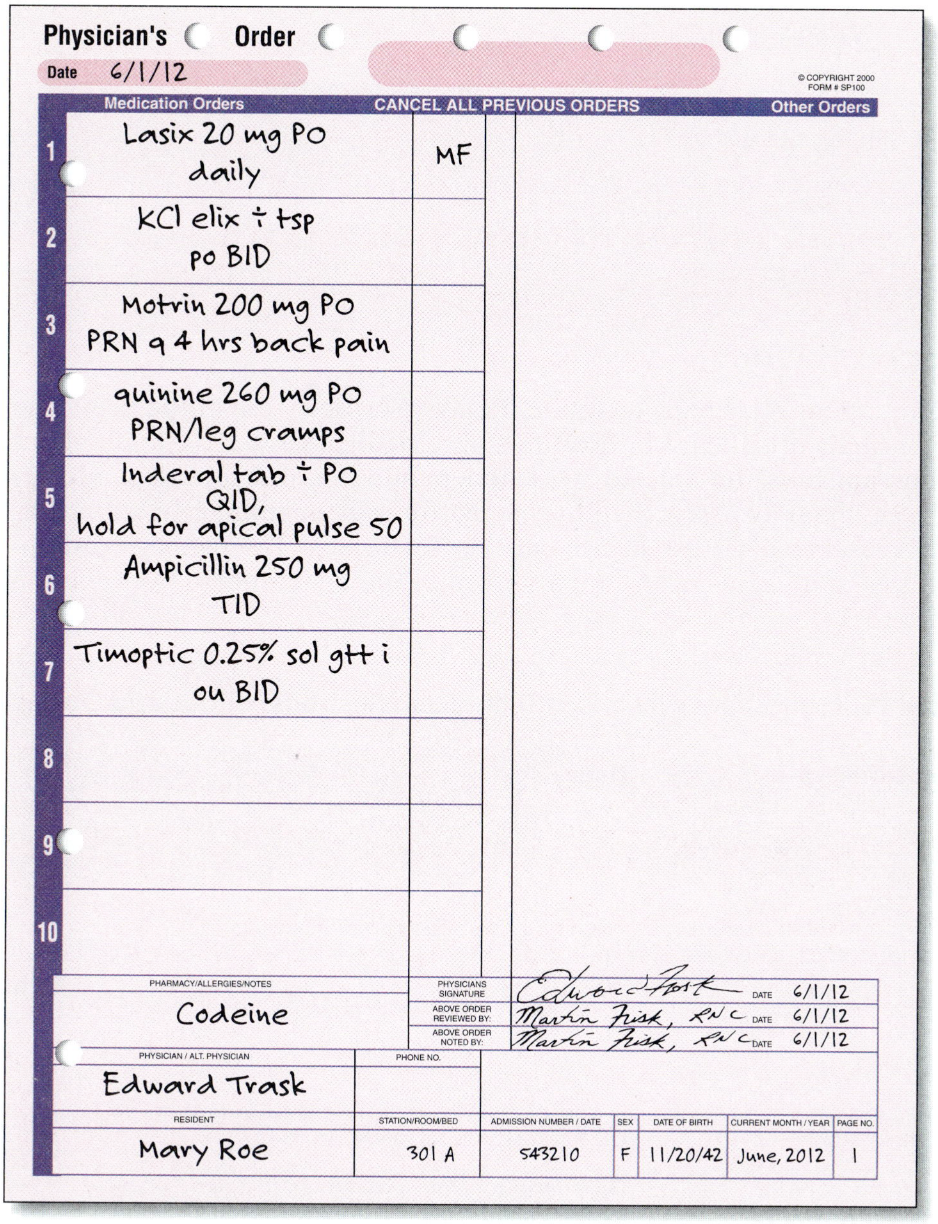
Physician's Order

Date 6/1/12

© COPYRIGHT 2000 FORM # SP100

	Medication Orders	CANCEL ALL PREVIOUS ORDERS		Other Orders
1	Lasix 20 mg PO daily	MF		
2	KCl elix $\dot{\bar{i}}$ tsp po BID			
3	Motrin 200 mg PO PRN q 4 hrs back pain			
4	quinine 260 mg PO PRN/leg cramps			
5	Inderal tab $\dot{\bar{i}}$ PO QID, hold for apical pulse 50			
6	Ampicillin 250 mg TID			
7	Timoptic 0.25% sol gtt i ou BID			
8				
9				
10				

PHARMACY/ALLERGIES/NOTES: Codeine

PHYSICIANS SIGNATURE: [signature] DATE 6/1/12

ABOVE ORDER REVIEWED BY: Martin Fisk, RNC DATE 6/1/12

ABOVE ORDER NOTED BY: Martin Fisk, RNC DATE 6/1/12

PHYSICIAN / ALT. PHYSICIAN: Edward Trask | PHONE NO.:

RESIDENT	STATION/ROOM/BED	ADMISSION NUMBER / DATE	SEX	DATE OF BIRTH	CURRENT MONTH / YEAR	PAGE NO.
Mary Roe	301 A	543210	F	11/20/42	June, 2012	1

Figure 15-2 Physician's order.

Source: ASHP Technical Assistance Bulletin on Hospital Drug Distribution and Control, **www.ashp.org**.

Electronic Orders

Electronic orders may be transmitted via fax or from a computer at the nurses' station or a physician's personal digital assistant (PDA) to the pharmacy's computer. Medication orders sent via fax need to be verified prior to the medication leaving the pharmacy. Other electronic order systems allow for order entry by the physician and the label is processed from the input. This is called **computerized physician order entry (CPOE)**. Medication errors are reduced using this method because only formulary items can be selected with appropriate dosing. Therapeutic equivalence substitutions and protocol guidelines are automatically entered. Errors may still occur—for example, incorrect agent selection—but the risk is reduced.

computerized physician order entry (CPOE) A paperless system in which medication orders are entered directly into the pharmacy computer system by the physician or prescriber.

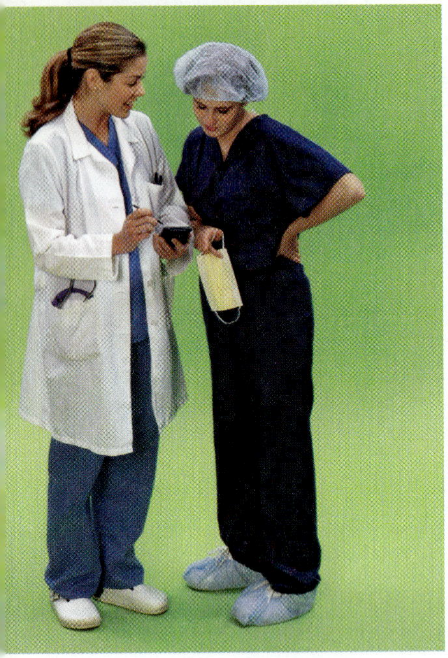

Tech Check

7. What are the three types of medication orders?(LO 15.7)

8. What is CPOE?(LO 15.7)

Pharmacy Technician–Inpatient Setting(LO 15.8)

Responsibilities

The inpatient pharmacy technician plays a critical role in the provision of pharmaceutical care in hospitals and medical centers. The inpatient technician must be able to work independently and interdependently as he or she may assist the pharmacist directly or indirectly, as well as work closely with other health care professionals. The primary responsibilities and duties of the inpatient pharmacy technician are listed in Table 15-1.

Table 15-1 Inpatient Pharmacy Technician Responsibilities and Duties

Responsibility	Duties
Assisting the pharmacist with DUR and cost-analysis studies	Assisting the pharmacist in collecting data
Chemotherapeutic agent compounding	Preparing chemotherapeutic agents
Communicating with other members of the health care team	Communicating effectively with other team members
Inspecting emergency cart and floor stock	Ensuring that the pharmaceutical agents are within date and stored properly
Managing inventory	Ordering, stocking, and removing items that have expired or are no longer on the formulary
Delivering/distributing medication	Delivering medications to the nursing station for administration
Processing medication orders	Taking an active role in all phases from computer data entry to preparation of the medication
Distributing narcotics	Retrieving the narcotic administration records and reconciling the forms with pharmacy orders and inventory
Repackaging and nonsterile compounding	Preparing medications from stock containers and extemporaneously compounding nonsterile products (refer to Chapter 11)
Sterile compounding	Employing aseptic technique and adhering to USP <797> guidelines while compounding sterile products, like intravenous solutions (refer to Chapter 11 for more information about sterile compounding)
Stocking automated systems	Ensuring that the correct medications are loaded into automated systems, like Pyxis

Processing Medication Orders

In the inpatient setting, medication orders are received by the pharmacy. Upon receipt of a written order, a pharmacy technician would review it for completeness and accuracy prior to entering the medication order into the computer system. It is important that the technician verify that all of the information being entered is correct. As this task of interpreting the medication order is critical and incorrect data entry increases the risk of medication errors, pharmacists must review all data entry prior to finalizing. Refer to Table 15-2 for TJC's Do Not Use List of Inappropriate Abbreviations.

After all of the information has been entered into the computer system, a label is generated. The label contains the following information:

- Patient's information
  - Name
  - Room number
  - Bed number
  - Medical record number
- Medication information
  - Drug name
  - Strength
  - Dosage form
  - Dosage regimen
- Physician's information
  - Name

Once the medication order is entered into the computer, generation of the label automatically adds the drug to the patient's medication profile. The patient's medication profile should include the following:

- Patient's information (full name, date hospitalized, date of birth, sex, weight, identification number, reason for admission)
- Laboratory test results
- Allergies, sensitivities, contraindications

Table 15-2 TJC's Official Do Not Use List of Abbreviations

Do Not Use	Use Instead
U (unit)	Write unit
IU (International Unit)	Write international unit
Q.D., QD, q.d., qd (daily)	Write daily
Q.O.D., QOD, q.o.d., qod (every other day)	Write every other day
Trailing zero (X.0 mg)	Write X mg
Lack of a leading zero (.X mg)	Write 0.X mg
MS	Write morphine sulfate
MSO4 and MgSO4	Write magnesium sulfate

Source: Adapted from **www.jointcommission.org/PatientSafety/DoNotUseList**.

- Other relevant medical information
- Drugs dispensed (dates of orders, strengths, dosage forms, dosage frequencies)
- Intravenous therapy information
- Blood products administered
- Number of doses dispensed
- Pharmacist's and/or pharmacy technician's initials

Source: Adapted from *ASHP Technical Assistance Bulletin on Hospital Drug Distribution and Control*, **www.ashp.org**.

The pharmacy technician then prepares the medication and affixes the label. Medications are processed on a 24-hour cycle. After the technician prepares the medication, it is checked by a pharmacist. After pharmacist review, the medication is then delivered to the nursing staff. Bar coding is often used in the pharmacy and on the patient floor to ensure that the right medication is prepared and administered to the right patient.

Stat and PRN Orders If a medication is needed **stat,** the medication must be prepared for administration within 10 to 15 minutes. A prn order is one in which the medication is given as needed. Once a medication is entered into the pharmacy computer system, the medication will appear on the medication administration record until the pharmacist receives an order to discontinue the medication or that the patient is being discharged.

Cassettes

Medication orders for oral medication may be filled using **unit-dose** packaged medications and a cassette (or drawer system). In this system, the cassettes (or drawers) are filled with the medications on the patient's MAR. Each patient (or each bed) has its own drawer. After the pharmacy technician finishes filling the cassettes, the technician's work is checked for accuracy by a pharmacist prior to delivery of the cassette to the nurses' station. Many inpatient facilities have moved away from the cassette system to **automation,** which is the use of electronic devices or robots to process drug orders.

Automation

Automated dispensing systems, such as Pyxis, Omnicell, and Suremed, use robotics to fill the drawers and as a result, aid in reducing medication errors and managing inventory (Figures 15-3 and 15-4). The pharmacy technician is responsible to ensure that these systems are properly stocked and has more time to complete other responsibilities. Although these automated systems do the bulk of the filling, the inpatient pharmacy technician must still physically fill orders for medicines not stocked in the automated dispensing system.

Parenteral Medications

Medication orders for **parenteral** medications are prepared in the same way as those for oral medications. The patient and drug data are entered into the pharmacy's computer system for label generation. Preparation of parenteral drugs requires the use of **aseptic technique** to avoid contamination of the drug with pathogens. The technician employs proper aseptic technique while preparing the medication in a laminar flow hood.

stat order A medication order for immediate administration.

unit-dose Medication packaged in a single dose.

automation The use of electronic devices or robotics to process drug orders.

parenteral Medication administration outside of the gastrointestinal tract, usually referring to intravenous administration.

aseptic technique Process that reduces the risk of contamination and helps ensure the sterility of a product.

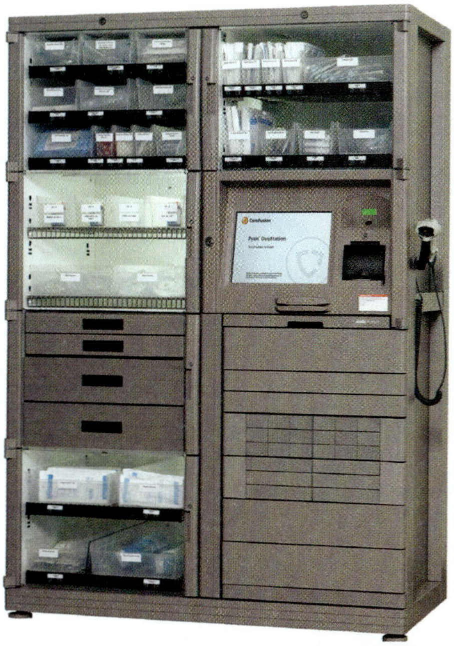

Figure 15-3 **Pyxis Duo Station System. Cardinal Health.**

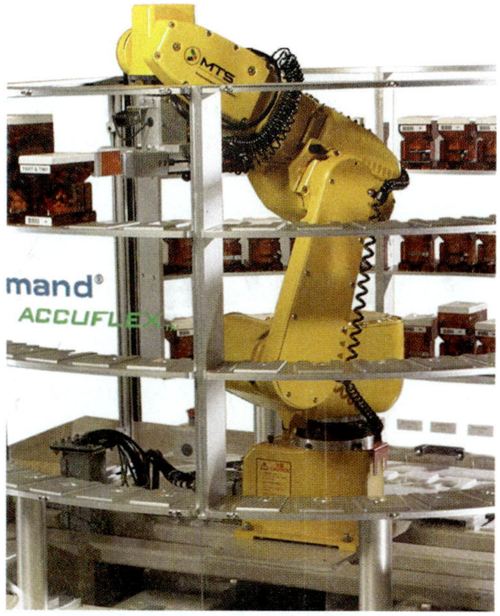

Figure 15-4 **Robotic arm. Cardinal Health. (Accufex® on Demand® by MTS medication Technologies®)**

The laminar flow hood is designed so that streams of air move toward the front of the hood (Figure 15.5). Pathogens and particles are kept away from the medication as it is being prepared. A label is affixed to the intravenous medication bag or syringe. The pharmacist checks the medication for accuracy and may ask the technician questions about the preparation process. The pharmacist also checks for particulate matter in the preparation, whether it is rubber from the punctured seal of a vial or a precipitate as a result of chemical incompatibilities. (Refer to Chapter 11 for more about sterile compounding.) The intravenous medication is delivered to the nurses' unit, in some cases with tubing required for administration, and always with additional information regarding handling and storage.

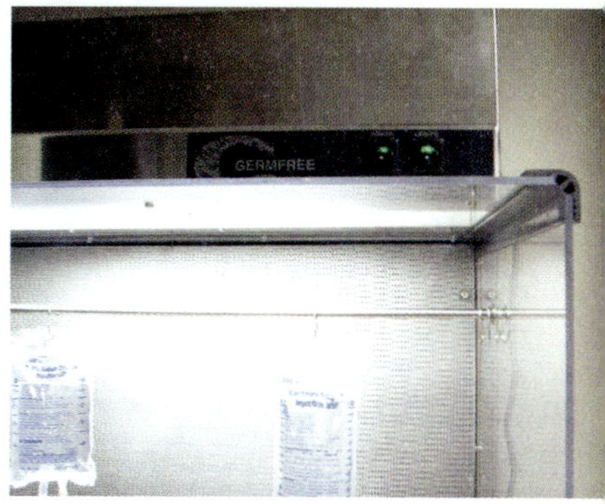

Figure 15-5 **Laminar flow hood.**

Tech Check

9. List the information that is included on the medication label.(LO 15.8)
10. List three automated dispensing systems.(LO 15.8)
11. What does prn mean?(LO 15.8)

Other Responsibilities of the Pharmacy Technician(LO 15.8)

Additional Duties

There may be additional duties that pharmacy technicians perform such as assisting with medication reconciliation (compilation of a complete list of all of a patient's medications, including OTC agents and those medicines transferred from another facility), participating in in-service training sessions, and possibly checking the work of other technicians.

As in any pharmacy setting, the pharmacist is ultimately responsible for the accuracy of the prescription or medication order. The technician prepares medications for review by the pharmacist, prior to the medications being distributed by the technician.

Compliance with OSHA Guidelines

Pharmacy technicians are included under the jurisdiction of OSHA (Occupational Safety and Health Administration). The technicians are at risk for various workplace accidents, and it is partially the responsibility of the technician to help maintain a safe pharmacy. The mission of OSHA is to ensure the safety and health of the workforce by setting and enforcing standards; providing training, outreach, and education; establishing partnerships; and encouraging continual improvement in workplace safety and health. In short, the purpose of OSHA is to prevent work-related injuries, illnesses, and deaths.

OSHA requires the use of appropriate personal protective equipment (PPE) to protect pharmacy technicians from hazardous drugs and chemicals. Examples of PPE include lab coats, gloves, masks, and goggles. Latex gloves without powder should be doubled and worn at all times while handling hazardous drugs. The pharmacy must stock hypoallergenic (nonlatex) gloves and liners for those who are allergic to latex. The proper technique with double gloving requires that the inner glove is placed under the sleeve of the lab coat, and the outer glove is placed over the sleeve of the lab coat. Gloves should be changed hourly during intravenous medication preparation, or immediately following contamination by spills. Removal of gloves should be performed in such a way as to avoid direct skin contact with the outside of the glove. Hands should be washed before donning and after removal of gloves. Lab coats should cover the clothing of the technician, be disposable with tight-fitting cuffs, and have a solid front. OSHA also requires the use of face and eye protection whenever splashes, sprays, or aerosols of hazardous drugs could result in eye, nose, or mouth contamination.

OSHA and the American Society of Health-System Pharmacists (ASHP) require that the area where hazardous drugs are prepared have restricted access and that signs are displayed indicating the restriction of access to authorized personnel. In addition, smoking, drinking, eating, and applying cosmetics where intravenous drugs are prepared, stored, or used is prohibited to reduce risk of exposure. All syringes and needles used in the course of preparation should be placed in sharps containers for disposal without being crushed, clipped, or capped. Any spills should be cleaned up immediately and placed in marked hazardous waste bags. (Refer to Chapter 2 for more details).

Communication with Nursing Staff

Effective communication among members of the health care team is critical for the provision of quality patient care. Ineffective communication increases the risk for medication errors and injuries to patients. Some medication errors have resulted in patient deaths. The pharmacy technician has many opportunities to communicate with nursing staff as the technician retrieves orders, delivers medications, and checks areas where medications are stored. It is important that the technician provide accurate information with respect and in a professional manner. The technician is often the primary link between the nurses and the pharmacy department. The inpatient pharmacy technician should communicate clearly and effectively to nursing staff to ensure the Five Rights of Medication Administration:

- Right patient
- Right drug
- Right dose
- Right time
- Right route

Specialization

Specialization refers to pharmacy technician involvement where higher levels of experience and expertise are required. Tasks performed in these areas may not be commonly performed by all pharmacy technicians. Specialty tasks may include:

- Preparing investigational medications
- Preparing nuclear pharmaceuticals
- Preparing chemotherapeutic agents
- Providing training to others regarding the use of automated dispensing systems
- Serving on committees
- Assisting the pharmacist in the preparation of reports
- Assisting in the training of pharmacy technician students and new hires

The inpatient pharmacy technician is an indispensable member of the health care team. These facilities could not provide quality patient care without the tasks performed by pharmacy technicians. From computer order entry to medication preparation, the pharmacy technician's role in the inpatient setting is one that will continue to expand as patient care needs increase.

Tech Check

12. List forms of personal protective equipment used by pharmacy technicians.(LO 15.8)

13. How should used needles and syringes be disposed of?(LO 15.8)

14. What are the Five Rights of Medication Administration?(LO 15.8)

Chapter Summary

Understanding the hospital setting is vital to the pharmacy technician. Important points to remember are:

- Hospitals, medical centers, or institutional settings are health care facilities where medical care is focused on inpatients, or patients that remain overnight in the facility.
- Classifications of inpatient settings include large medical centers, community hospitals, teaching hospitals, and long-term care facilities.

- Organizations that regulate inpatient facilities include The Joint Commission, Centers for Medicare and Medicaid, Drug Enforcement Administration, and state boards of pharmacy.
- The policy and procedures manual contains regulations of the facility, including the processes by which standards are met.
- A protocol is a set of guidelines or standards, developed and approved by the Pharmacy and Therapeutics (P&T) Committee, used in a given set of circumstances.
- The responsibilities and tasks of the inpatient pharmacy technician are vital to the provision of care in the inpatient setting.

Chapter Review

Case Study Questions

1. What is Peter looking for when he is checking the crash carts?(LO 15.1, 15.6, 15.8)
2. Why is this so important?(LO 15.1, 15.6, 15.8)

At Your Service Questions

1. What is wrong with what the nurse is doing?(LO 15.3, 15.4)
2. What potential problems might this create?(LO 15.3, 15.4)
3. What is Molly's responsibility?(LO 15.8)

Multiple Choice

Select the best answer.

1. MAR stands for _______ (LO 15.7)
   a. medications and regulations.
   b. medication administration record.
   c. medical administrators record.
   d. medicine and registration.
2. The formulary is determined by the _______ (LO 15.6)
   a. CEO.
   b. MAR.
   c. P&T Committee.
   d. board of directors.
3. The system that allows for medication order entry directly by the physician or prescriber is _______ (LO 15.7)
   a. DUR.
   b. TJC.
   c. CPOE.
   d. MAR.
4. Which of the following is *not* a responsibility of the inpatient pharmacy technician?(LO 15.8)
   a. Sterile compounding
   b. Medication distribution
   c. Writing of drug orders
   d. Repackaging and nonsterile compounding
5. Substituting one drug for another agent in the same class with the same indications is called _______ (LO 15.5)
   a. generic substitution.
   b. therapeutic equivalence.
   c. drug usage review.
   d. none of the above.
6. What is the pharmacy system that involves the use of satellite pharmacies?(LO 15.1, 15.2)
   a. Centralized pharmacy system
   b. Decentralized pharmacy system
   c. Computerized physician order entry system
   d. Formulary system
7. What contains the facility's regulations and methods by which regulations are executed?(LO 15.4)
   a. Policy and procedures manual
   b. Pharmacy and therapeutics committee
   c. Drug utilization review
   d. Protocol
8. What organization accredits hospitals?(LO 15.3)
   a. CMS
   b. TJC, formerly JCAHO
   c. BOP
   d. DEA

9. Standards for maintaining patients' privacy have been established by _______ (LO 15.3)
   a. TJC, formerly JCAHO.
   b. HIPAA.
   c. BOP.
   d. CMS.

10. Which of the following is *not* a duty of the inpatient pharmacy technician? (LO 15.8)
   a. Managing inventory
   b. Stocking automated systems with medications
   c. Entering data into the computer
   d. Transporting patients

Critical Thinking Questions

1. Recite the Five Rights of Medication Administration. Describe how advances in technology (bar coding, automated dispensing systems, and CPOE) contribute to the achievement of the Five Rights. (LO 15.8)
2. Review the abbreviations in the "Do Not Use List" included in this chapter. Identify other potential problem abbreviations. Describe what you would do if you received a written medication order you could not read due to illegible handwriting. (LO 15.3, 15.8)
3. Why is the relationship between pharmacy technicians and nursing staff so important? What other health care professionals must pharmacy technicians work and communicate with in the inpatient setting? (LO 15.8)

HIPAA Scenario

Mary is a compassionate hospital pharmacy technician who successfully battled breast cancer 5 years ago. She maintains contact with many agencies that provide support for those who have breast cancer.

During the course of filling prescriptions for one of the pharmacy's customers, Jeanne, Mary discovers that Jeanne has breast cancer. She forwards Jeanne's name to one of her support groups, who in turn mails Jeanne a brochure. When Jeanne inquired into how the support group obtained her name, she was told that Mary suggested she would be a good candidate for the group.

Jeanne later asked Mary why she forwarded her private medical history to the support group. She also made a formal complaint to the hospital's privacy officer and demanded that Mary give her an apology.

Discussion Questions (PTCB II. 73)

1. Are health care providers allowed to forward the names of patients being treated for specific diseases to groups who have no role in the provision of the patients' health care?
2. What actions should be taken in regard to Mary's role in the unlawful dissemination of Jeanne's PHI?

Internet Activities

1. Search for "The Joint Commission" on the Internet. Once you are on the Web site, click on "Accreditation Programs" and choose "Hospital." After the hospital page loads, click on "National Patient Safety Goals." Print out the list of goals and describe the potential role of the pharmacy technician in realizing this goals. (LO 15.3)
2. Go to your state board of pharmacy online. Choose a local hospital and check on the board of pharmacy site to see how many pharmacies are licensed within that facility. Be prepared to report your findings. (LO 15.3)

16 Other Environments

Learning Outcomes

Upon completion of this chapter, you will be able to:

16.1 Explain the need for pharmacy technicians in the various settings in the practice of pharmacy.

16.2 Clarify the services made available to patients in these settings.

16.3 Describe the processing of prescriptions in the various settings.

16.4 Compare and contrast the unique characteristics of each of these settings.

16.5 Explain the function of pharmacy benefit management firms.

16.6 Identify the payment process in each of these situations.

16.7 Distinguish specific skills necessary to be successful in each of these settings.

16.8 Recognize specific legislation that affects a specific pharmacy environment.

16.9 Identify the role, responsibilities, and duties of both the pharmacist and pharmacy technician in different pharmacy settings.

Key Terms

capitation
compounding record
disease management
Internet pharmacy
managed care pharmacy
nonresident pharmacy
total parenteral nutrition (TPN)
pharmaceutical care plan
Verified Internet Pharmacy Practice Site (VIPPS)

PTCB

In preparation for the certification examination, you should understand and perform activities associated with the following PTCB Knowledge Statements:

PTCB Knowledge Statement — *Domain I. Assisting the Pharmacist in Serving Patients*

Knowledge of federal, state, and/or practice site regulations, code of ethics, and standards pertaining to the practice of pharmacy (1)

Knowledge of therapeutic equivalence (6)

Knowledge of requirements for dispensing controlled substances (44)

PTCB Knowledge Statement — *Domain III. Participating in the Administration and Management Practice*

Knowledge of third-party reimbursement systems (31)

Case Study

Andrew, a recent graduate from a pharmacy technician training program, had submitted resumes to a long-term care pharmacy, a home infusion pharmacy, and a mail-order pharmacy. After reviewing his resume, each of these pharmacies had contacted Andrew for interviews. Andrew was busy conducting research in the computer lab on each of these employers when his instructor, Dr. Betyar, entered the room. Dr. Betyar asked Andrew what he was doing. After Andrew's response, Dr. Betyar emphasized to Andrew that each of these work environments have similarities and differences. Dr. Betyar informed Andrew that long-term care, home infusion, and mail-order pharmacy have specific patients with special needs to be addressed. Each of these settings requires special skills of both pharmacists and pharmacy technicians.

While reading this chapter, keep the following question in mind:

1 What should Andrew know before he goes on his first interview?(LO 16.1)

Introduction to Other Pharmacy Environments(LO 16.1)

Many individuals believe that pharmacy practice is restricted to retail or institutional (hospital) settings, but that belief is entirely false. Pharmacy has evolved greatly within the past 25 years. Numerous career opportunities have developed based upon a changing society with different needs. This chapter identifies various pharmacy environments, characteristics of them, the usage of pharmacy technicians, and the necessary skills to be successful.

At Your Service

Mary Ellen brings in a new prescription for a 90-day supply of Simvastatin. Andrew, the pharmacy technician, begins to fill the prescription for 90 days and bills it to Mary Ellen's prescription drug card. The third-party provider rejects the claim stating that it exceeds the day's supply according to the pharmacy benefit manager (PBM).

While reading this chapter, keep the following question in mind:

1. Andrew informs Mary Ellen of the situation and she would like to know how she is able to obtain a 90-day supply. What should Andrew tell her?(LO 16.3, 16.5, 16.7)

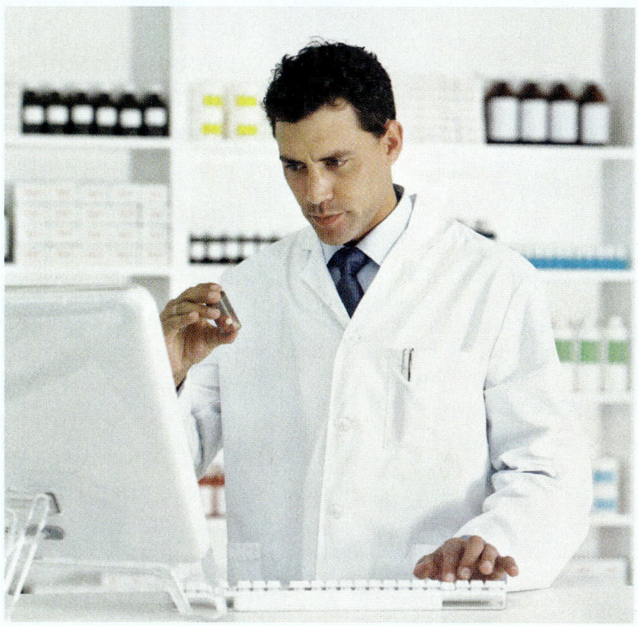

Long-Term Care Pharmacy (LO 16.1, 16.2, 16.4, 16.8, 16.9)

A long-term care facility is a facility or unit that is planned, staffed, and equipped to accommodate individuals who are chronically ill, aged or physically or mentally disabled. These patients do not require hospital care but need a wide range of medical, nursing, health, and social services. Long-term health care is intended to enable an individual to maintain the maximum possible level of functional independence (Figure 16-1). In 1999 there were 1,879,600 nursing home beds, which were located in 18,000 nursing homes.

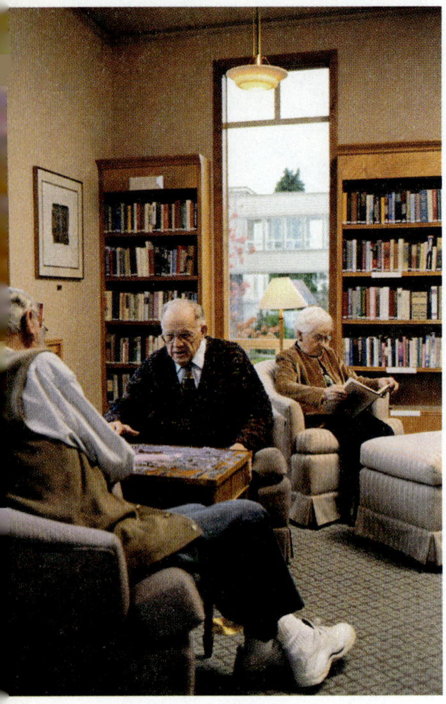

Figure 16-1 Assisted-living facility.

Examples of long-term care facilities include:

- Assisted-living facilities—a combination of housing, personalized support services, and health care
- Correctional facilities—long-term health care for individuals who have been incarcerated
- Extended-care facilities—nursing homes that qualify for participation in Medicare Part A
- Intermediate-care facilities—institutions recognized under the Medicaid program that are licensed under state laws to provide on a regular basis health-related care and services and that do not require the degree of care or treatment that a hospital or skilled nursing facility can provide
- Nursing facilities—provide a level of care between acute hospital care and community-based long-term care
- Personal care, shelter care, and board and care homes—nonmedical living arrangements for people who are elderly or mentally or physically disabled and who are not related to the owners of the homes
- Psychiatric hospitals—long-term care facilities that treat individuals with mental illness
- Skilled nursing facilities—nursing homes that meet requirements for the conditions for participation in both Medicare and Medicaid programs
- Special facilities for elderly people, which may include geriatric centers or institutes, apartments, or communities—continuous care retirement communities or naturally occurring retirement communities that provide an alternative to living and maintaining a home
- Subacute care units—health care that is less complex than that received in acute hospitals

Each of these facilities provides unique services for their residents who have specific needs that must be addressed. The level of care varies in each setting based upon residents' requirements.

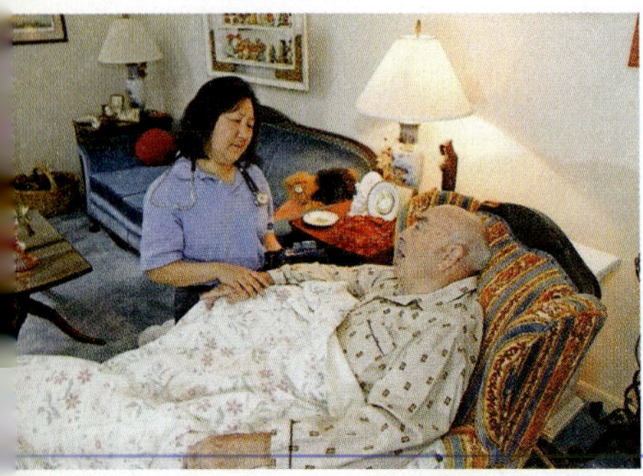

Figure 16-2 Residential care.

The major services found in long-term care facilities are nursing, personal, and residential care (Figure 16-2). Nursing care requires the professional services of a registered nurse or licensed practical nurse. These skills include the administration of medication, injections, catheterizations, and similar procedures ordered by a physician. Dispensing of pharmaceuticals is done under the supervision of the nursing staff. Personal care encompasses assisting residents in walking, getting in and out of bed, and bathing, dressing, and eating. Residential care includes providing residents with room and board in a protective environment that also nurtures their social and spiritual needs.

A long-term care pharmacy dispenses medications for residents in a long-term facility. A pharmacy may be either an open-shop pharmacy (one that provides medications to both residents and nonresidents of long-term care facilities) or closed-shop pharmacy (one that provides medications only to residents of long-term care facilities). The inventory found in a long-term care pharmacy resembles that of a community pharmacy. These pharmacies utilize special computer software necessary to provide specific reports required by a long-term care facility. A long-term care pharmacy may use automation and repackaging equipment.

All orders for residents in long-term care facilities are initiated by physicians who either write the orders in the charts or through verbal orders to nurses. The orders are transmitted to the pharmacy verbally or via a fax machine. The pharmacy processes the orders in the same manner as they would for any other prescription that includes identifying allergies, contraindications, and therapeutic duplications. The medication orders are packaged, labeled, and checked by the pharmacist prior to sending to the facilities.

The drug delivery system of a long-term care facility is a unit-dose system, which provides the medication in its final "unit-of-use" form. A unit-dose system is a safe and efficient method to dispense medication. Its advantages include:

- Less time for the nursing staff to administer medication
- A decrease in prescription errors
- Increased accountability of medication
- Built-in re ordering procedures

There are many different types of unit-dose systems. The modified unit-dose system combines unit-dose medications blister packaged onto a multiple-dose card (Figure 16-3). They are known as punch cards, bingo cards, or blister cards. A blended unit-dose system combines a "unit-of-use package" with a non-unit-dose drug distribution system. It may be in the form of a multiple medication package or a modular cassette.

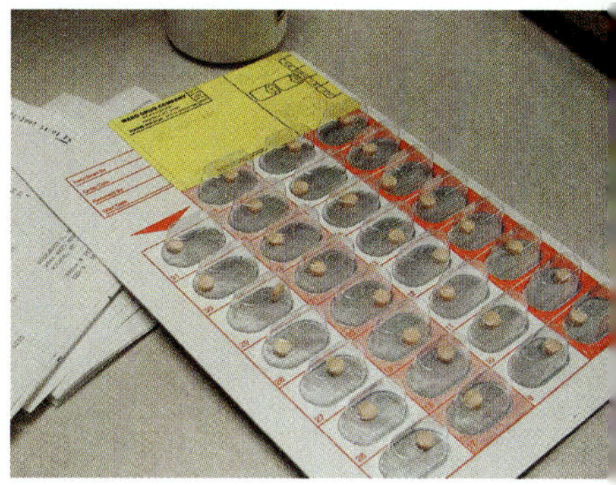

Figure 16-3 Blister card.

A resident's medication refill order may be initiated by the nurse as is seen in a turn-around system or using a cycle-fill system in which the pharmacy automatically refills the order. The long-term care pharmacy is responsible for transporting the medications to the facility. Upon receipt of the medications, a medication delivery record is signed by a facility staff member.

Legal Requirements of a Long-Term Care Pharmacy

OBRA-87 requires long-term care facilities to provide both routine and emergency medications to the residents. An emergency medication is one that can result in discomfort or distress or an acute or life-threatening condition if not administered to a patient within a reasonable period of time. A long-term care pharmacy provides emergency medications to the facility.

Examples of emergency medications include:

- Analgesics
- Antibiotics
- Anticoagulants
- Anticonvulsants
- Hyperglycemic agents
- Hypoglycemic agents

The emergency medications selected for a long-term care facility are determined by the pharmacist and the facility medical/nursing staff. A physician must provide an order before a medication can be administered to a patient. The emergency medication box is easily transferable and is sealed and stored in a secure location at the facility. After a medication is administered, it is the duty of the pharmacy to inventory what has been dispensed and provide a complete new emergency box to the facility.

Other OBRA requirements for a pharmacy include:

- Maintaining an infection control program to provide a safe and sanitary environment for residents that reduces the possibility of disease.
- Providing a resident with a comprehensive assessment at least once every 3 months to make sure that the patient's treatment is accurate and appropriate.
- Suppling a separately locked compartment for Schedule II medications except when a unit-dose system is being used.

The DEA allows the transmission of Schedule II medications by fax between the physician and the pharmacy. The faxed prescription is considered the written prescription and therefore a handwritten prescription does not need to be provided to the pharmacy. Note that some states still require the hard copy within a specified time frame. The DEA allows for the partial filling of a Schedule II medication. Partial prescriptions can be filled for up to 60 days from the date of issuance, but cannot exceed the original quantity. Again, states vary and the length of time a Schedule II can be filled is determined by the state board. The pharmacist must make a notation on the prescription that the patient is in a long-term care facility.

Caution

The laws regarding the filling of Schedule II medications varies from state to state. Know the laws in the state where you are practicing as a pharmacy technician. Check with your state's regulatory agency, which is usually the state board of pharmacy.

A long-term care pharmacy may accept the return of and reuse of medications in specific situations. These include:

- The returned medications are not controlled substances.
- The medications are dispensed in tamper-evident packaging and the packaging is intact when returned.
- The medications meet all federal and state requirements for product integrity.
- Policies and procedures are in place for the storage, transport, receipt, and security of medication from the long-term care facility to the pharmacy.
- A system is in place to track the reuse of medications.
- A system is in place for the patient to be credited for the return of these medications.

Pharmacy Technicians in a Long-Term Care Pharmacy

The American Society of Consultant Pharmacists (ASCP) supports the use of pharmacy technicians under the supervision of a licensed pharmacist in a long-term care pharmacy. Mechanisms must ensure that pharmacy technicians possess the skills and knowledge needed to perform their assigned tasks. These mechanisms include:

- Registration of pharmacy technicians by the state boards of pharmacy if such registration provides information to employers about an individual's suitability for employment as a pharmacy technician
- Certification of technicians by qualified certifying organizations
- Site-specific technician training

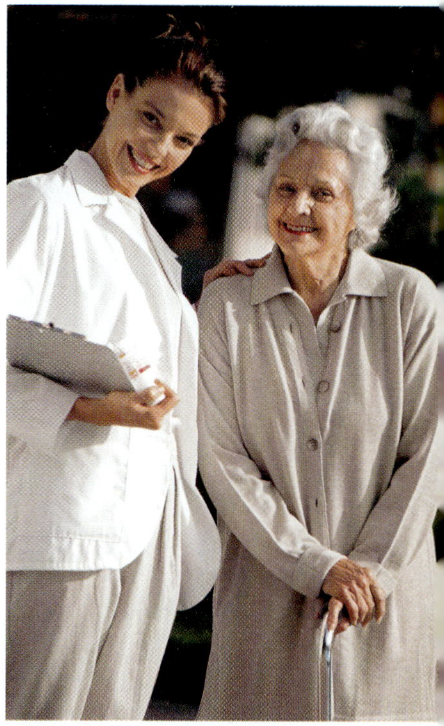

Figure 16-4 Pharmacy technician working in a long-term care facility must posses specialized skills.

The pharmacy technician working in a long-term care pharmacy must possess knowledge and skills associated with both community and institutional pharmacy (Figure 16-4). Requirements for a pharmacy technician working in a long-term care pharmacy include:

- Basic math and analytical skills
- Knowledge of drug names—both generic and trade
- The ability to work with at least one dispensing system
- Typing/keyboarding/computer skills
- Excellent interpersonal skills and well-developed communication skills
- Superior organizational skills and attention to detail
- Outstanding customer service skills
- A working knowledge of computer systems
- Ability—to work independently, meet deadlines, establish priorities, and be flexible
- Composure on the telephone when handling customer calls

A pharmacy technician working in a long-term pharmacy works under the supervision of a pharmacist and their primary task is to fill prescription orders. He or she must notate on each prescription the lot number, expiration date of the medication, and his or her initials. The technician prepares labels to include the name of the drug, its strength, the route of administration, quantity, and medication pass time, and packages and affixes the proper auxiliary labels to containers.

The pharmacy technician may reorder medications and supplies and may monitor back-order requests. The technician may help ensure that inventory stock levels of medications and equipment are maintained, and may check for overages, shortages, and damaged materials and report discrepancies to the supervisor or the appropriate personnel.

The pharmacy technician may prepare compounds after the pharmacist has verified the calculations. He or she may be responsible for filling bulk orders, preparing blister cards putting away the order, and staging deliveries. The technician may check the expiration dating of all medications on a scheduled basis or during each restocking period and provide the pharmacist with a list of expired drugs.

The pharmacy technician may replace emergency boxes of long-term care facilities as requested. He or she may replace medications in both interim and emergency medication boxes and check the expiration dates before sealing the boxes. The technician forwards all interim or emergency box requisitions for data entry.

The pharmacy technician may be responsible for maintaining any pharmacy-related equipment rental logs. He or she assists in maintaining all prescription logs, **compounding records**, or mixing reports, and any other related files as determined by the pharmacy. A long-term care pharmacy technician may remove and sort by work function the delivery bags or totes and equipment from the area inside the pharmacy. He or she helps ensure the proper dispensation of returned medication items to the proper outlet.

The pharmacy technician maintains a neat, clean, and organized work area at all times to avoid contamination. He or she assists in keeping the pharmacy clean and well organized (e.g., trash removal, daily cleaning), and refills bottles, vials, bags, and supplies.

Tech Check

1. What is a long-term care facility?(LO 16.2)
2. What type of drug distribution system is used in long-term care facilities?(LO 16.2)
3. What are three responsibilities of a long-term care pharmacy technician?(LO 16.9)

Home Infusion Pharmacy(LO 16.1, 16.2, 16.4, 16.7, 16.9)

A home infusion pharmacy prepares and dispenses infusion therapy to patients in a home or alternative site. Home infusion is a vital and growing element of our health care system. Annual growth for home infusion is expected to occur at a rate of 12.8% per year with a $4.87 billion market. The growth in the home infusion market can be attributed to an aging population due to the baby boomers, improvements in vascular access devices that allow for infusion lines to remain in place for longer periods with less monitoring by clinicians, and to an increase in the safety and design of infusion devices. Managed care has embraced home infusion therapies because the service is less expensive than having a patient hospitalized.

Home infusion therapy services are provided by a number of different organizations. A hospital may provide home infusion services to a patient upon discharge from the hospital. This provides a continuum of care deemed necessary for the transition of the individual from the institution to the home. A community pharmacy may provide infusion services in addition to their basic services. A home infusion company may provide specialized services for patients who have cancer, AIDS, or other terminal illnesses.

Home infusion pharmacy is a licensed pharmacy that provides comprehensive infusion therapy management, medications, nutritional support, infusion pumps, and supplies to patients in their homes or long-term care facilities. Depending on the patient's needs and the physician's orders, therapies are administered intravenously (into the bloodstream), subcutaneously (beneath the skin), or as an epidural (around the spinal cord). A patient receiving home infusion therapies may have diagnoses ranging from infections—multiple sclerosis, cancer, cancer-related pain, and gastrointestinal diseases—that may result in nutrition-related problems, congestive heart disease, and immune disorders. Home infusion therapy utilizes antibiotics,

compounding record A form that is used in the infusion pharmacy to document the compounding activities and is part of the patient's chart. It is also known as a mixing report.

Table 16-1 Commonly Used Medications in Home Infusion

• Analgesics to include fentanyl, fentanyl with bupivacaine, hydromorphone, meperidine, and morphine
• Antibiotics including amikacin, amphotericin B, ampicillin/sulbactam, cefotetan, cefazolin, cefoperazone, ceftriaxone, ganciclovir, nafcillin, oxacillin, penicillin G, ticarcillin/clavulanate, and vancomycin
• Antineoplastics such as 5-fluoruracil, adriamycin, cyclophosamide, taxol, vinblastine, and vincristine
• Biological response modifiers include erythropoietin, filgrastim, growth hormone, and interferon
• Parenteral therapy includes cimetidine, heparin, insulin, ranitidine, and vitamins

antineoplastics, analgesics, biological response modifiers, blood products/transfusions, colony-stimulating factors, and enteral and parenteral medications. Examples of these medications can be found in Table 16-1.

The Home Infusion Team

The home infusion team consists of physicians, clinical pharmacists, pharmacy technicians, registered nurses, registered dietitians, reimbursement specialists, patient service representatives, warehouse staff, and delivery staff.

Physician

The physician provides the direction of care, to which the home infusion team must adhere; any deviations from this care plan require the approval of the physician. The physician is responsible for signing the Certificate of Medical Necessity and Plan of Treatment. The medication orders may be transmitted to the pharmacist via verbal order or a written signed order by fax machine.

Pharmacist

The clinical pharmacist is responsible for scheduling the compounding of these medications. Proper scheduling will prevent a patient's supply from becoming depleted or overstocked. The pharmacist may recommend therapy options and medication dosing to the physician. He or she also may monitor the patient's response to therapy and lab values from tests given to the patient. The pharmacist provides valuable medication information to other members of the home infusion team. He or she screens the patient for duplicate therapies and drug-drug and food-drug interactions. In some instances the pharmacist may tailor a care plan to meet the patient's needs. The pharmacist is responsible for educating the patient regarding the storage and disposal of the medication and supplies.

Home infusion pharmacy requires the proper preparation, storage, and distribution of the medication, and the required supplies essential for the administration of the medication. A home infusion pharmacist is responsible for the calibration of home infusion devices, the calibration of catheter care supplies, and waste management issues. The nature of the compounds being used in an infusion pharmacy requires that the pharmacist be knowledgeable of all state and federal regulations regarding biohazardous substances and waste materials. In addition, infusion pharmacies need to receive accreditation from The Joint Commission (TJC), formerly the Joint Commission on Accreditation of Healthcare Organizations (JCAHO), to qualify for reimbursement from third-party payers.

Nurse

Registered nurses train the patients and their caregivers for infusion of ordered therapies. The registered nurse visits the patients intermittently to assess their situation and to monitor their compliance with the therapy. He or she assists the registered dietitians in screening patients who may be at nutritional risk. It is the nurse who inserts and maintains the peripheral, midline, or peripherally inserted central catheter. It is through the nurse's assessment of the patient's performance that a care plan for the patient is written.

Dietitian

Registered dietitians identify patients who are nutritionally at risk. This is accomplished by conducting serial nutritional assessments of the patient on a regular basis to ensure that the patient is meeting the nutritional needs and goals of the therapy. The dietitian consults with the pharmacist, nurse, and physician for enteral, parenteral, and oral nutritional supplements. Finally, a dietitian visits patients whom they have identified as requiring nutritional counseling.

Reimbursement Specialist

Reimbursement specialists verify a patient's eligibility for home infusion benefits with the insurer. These specialists determine the coverage available for each patient, and are responsible for the coordination and the collection of funds for services rendered. At times they may negotiate the pricing of services provided with the insurer and inform the insurer of the status of the patient and the therapeutic plan.

Patient Service Representative

Patient service representatives phone patients to inventory their medications and supplies on a weekly basis. They inform the patients of delivery plans. These representatives schedule and coordinate all deliveries, and they remind patients to rotate their products.

Warehouse and Delivery Staff

The warehouse staff manages both the drug and supply as well as the equipment inventory, including all preventative maintenance. The warehouse staff coordinates the delivery of medications and supplies to the patient, and the delivery staff delivers the medications and supplies to the patient in a timely manner. The delivery staff may remind the patient of specific storage requirements of the medications.

Home Infusion Pharmacist Responsibilities

A home infusion pharmacy carries a highly specialized drug inventory similar to that found in a hospital pharmacy. A home infusion pharmacy customizes the medication based upon the specifications of the medication order from the physician. The infusion pharmacy has designated areas where specific tasks are performed. The equipment found in an infusion pharmacy contains horizontal and vertical laminar flow hoods, automated compounding and dispensing machines, infusion pumps, and equipment essential for infusion pharmacy.

Pharmaceutical care is the responsible provision of drug therapy for the purpose of achieving specific outcomes to improve a patient's quality of life. The home infusion pharmacist must be knowledgeable of the patient's disease state and care plan to provide appropriate pharmaceutical services and to monitor the patient to ensure that the care plan and goals of therapy are attained. More specifically, the home infusion pharmacist must do the following:

1. The home infusion pharmacist must be certain that a thorough general assessment of the patient has been taken whether by an intake nurse or another individual. The information obtained through this evaluation is essential to develop an appropriate care plan for the patient. A home infusion pharmacist must complete his or her own assessment of the patient.
2. The home infusion pharmacist must evaluate the drug therapy proposed for the patient and develop monitoring parameters. This can be accomplished by a **pharmaceutical care plan.**

   A pharmaceutical care plan identifies:

   - The problems being treated with medications
   - The desired therapeutic outcomes (goals)
   - Pharmacy-related activities that can achieve the desired goals (interventions)
   - Information that can indicate if the interventions are producing the desired goals (monitoring)
   - If the problem or condition has been resolved (resolution)

The information contained in the pharmaceutical care plan must be shared with the other members of the home infusion team to ensure that common goals of the therapy are met.

3. It is the responsibility of the home infusion pharmacist to educate the patient regarding the drug therapy and the techniques associated with the administration of the medication. Areas to be covered in patient education include:

   - The medication (drug name, drug dose, dosing interval, and duration of therapy)
   - Medication administration (aseptic technique, catheter care, inspection of medications and the equipment)
   - Patient's response to therapy (adverse reactions, intolerances)
   - Troubleshooting (medication/supply outages and equipment malfunction)
   - Emergencies (contacting providers and emergency procedures)

4. The infusion pharmacist monitors the patient's IV therapy. This monitoring is a continuous process throughout the therapy and examines the patient's response to the drug, adverse reactions, and laboratory work. The home infusion pharmacist communicates with the other members of the team the results of the monitoring.
5. The infusion pharmacist performs a discharge assessment at the end of the IV therapy. It is hoped that the IV drug therapy results in the desired outcome. The pharmacist must document that the goals of the therapy have been met and that the patient is discharged from the therapy.

A physician writes the order for the infusion, which can be either transmitted by a fax machine or verbally through the use of the phone to the pharmacy. This prescription order must contain all of the required information for prescription orders per federal and state laws. The prescription is entered into the computer, which results in a label and a mixing report

pharmaceutical care plan A plan developed by the pharmacist at the beginning of therapy for a home infusion patient. The care plan is developed to accomplish the goals of the drug therapy and minimize drug-related problems. It is also known as a care plan.

(compound record). The prescription label must meet both federal and state requirements for an outpatient label.

Either a pharmacist or pharmacy technician can prepare an IV solution. Unlike an infusion prepared in the hospital for an inpatient, which is prepared prior to being infused, an outpatient order requires that multiple days be prepared simultaneously. An individual preparing outpatient IVs must possess excellent aseptic technique to prevent possible contamination. Either the pharmacist or pharmacy technician must document the activities on a compounding report. A lot number and expiration are assigned by the pharmacy. The expiration date is based on stability and sterility data of both the medication and vehicle used in compounding. The pharmacist performs the final check on the prescription order. The final product is stored in appropriate packaging, such as an insulated bag, until it is delivered to the patient.

The Pharmacy Technician in Home Infusion Pharmacy

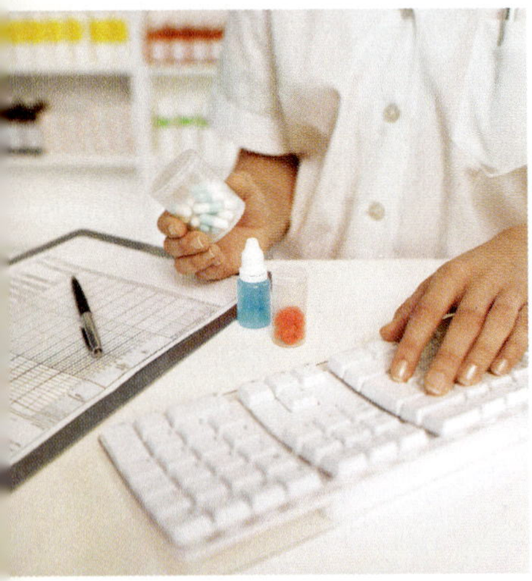

Figure 16-5 Pharmacy technicians must know the requirements for proper documentation and record-keeping.

A pharmacy technician may be responsible for the following tasks:

- Assists in the preparation of sterile mixtures including, but not limited to, antibiotics, antineoplastics, **total parenteral nutrition (TPN),** small- and large-volume parenterals, medications, ophthalmic preparations, and allergen extract preparations where applicable
- Prepares aseptically all sterile mixture requests for members upon receipt of a physician order
- Assists the IV pharmacist in receiving prescription orders for oncology infusion therapy both for internal and external referrals
- Maintains patient profile records and prescription files where appropriate
- Apprises the pharmacist of patient problems or problems in the operation of the service

The pharmacy technician working in a home infusion pharmacy must have the following competencies:

- Experience with computerized pharmacy systems and using both IV manual and automated equipment
- Knowledge of aseptic technique
- Knowledge of medial terminology, pharmaceutical dosage forms, and nomenclature
- Basic accounting and purchasing skills
- Pharmacy calculations involving dosages, dilutions, flow rates, and mEq
- Ability to read and interpret prescriptions/medication orders
- Knowledge and understanding of the pharmacology of medications being used (i.e., antibiotics and oncology agents)
- Knowledge of both federal and state pharmacy laws affecting home infusion (i.e., OBRA-90, FDA Safe Medical Device Act of 1990, usage of Category II medications in home infusion patients)
- Comprehension of OSHA requirements involving home infusion pharmacy
- Knowledge of TJC regulations affecting home infusion pharmacy
- Knowledge of proper documentation and record-keeping requirements for home infusion pharmacy (Figure 16-5)

total parenteral nutrition (TPN)
A combination of amino acids, dextrose, fats, vitamins, minerals, electrolytes, and water administered intravenously.

- Familiarity of nutrition therapy (enteral and parenteral)
- Experience in reading and completing a compounding record
- Knowledge of equipment used in home infusion (i.e., vascular access devices, infusion devices, and home infusion supplies)
- General reimbursement knowledge to include durable medical equipment (DME)
- Excellent oral and written communication skills
- Strong computer skills

A pharmacy technician working in an infusion environment orders and maintains appropriate stock levels of IV drugs and supplies in compliance to contracts. He or she assists with the proper accounting and transfer of IV pharmaceuticals to infusion therapy and oncology cost centers. A technician works cooperatively to identify the special needs or changing demands in drugs and medical supplies.

The technician maintains appropriate logs and cleaning records of biomedical (pumps) equipment and a arranges for preventative maintenance and inspects and maintains the necessary records as required by the FDA Safe Medical Devices Act of 1990. The technician may assist in various quality assurance procedures including the laminar flow hood cleaning, repairs, and inspection to include biological laboratory testing. He or she may be accountable for maintaining the cleanliness of the admixture machinery and keeping the IV room properly stocked with supplies

The pharmacy technician may arrange the packing, shipping, and delivery or the pick up of home infusion products, and coordinates the efficient operation of the IV admixture service. He or she may be asked to take part in the aseptic training of new pharmacy trainees.

A home infusion pharmacy is responsible for the proper preparation, storage, and distribution of medication and supplies. It is the responsibility of the pharmacist to ensure that stability, compatibility, and safety of injectable medications are maintained.

Tech Check

4. Who are the members of a home infusion team?(LO 16.9)
5. What types of duties will a pharmacy technician have in a home infusion pharmacy?(LO 16.9)
6. What are three skills required by a pharmacy technician working in a home infusion pharmacy?(LO 16.9)

Managed Care Pharmacy(LO 16.1, 16.2, 16.3, 16.5, 16.6, 16.9)

Managed care has been defined by the Academy of Managed Care Pharmacy as "the indirect supervision of the financial management of a patient's medical care . . . performed by the ultimate reimbursement entity, commonly known as the 'payer.' Payers use 'utilization review'—a medical professional oversees the treating physician's decisions to determine if the most financially efficient method is being used." Managed care offers a coordinated, integrated system of care that emphasizes prevention and cost restraints while increasing value for the patient.

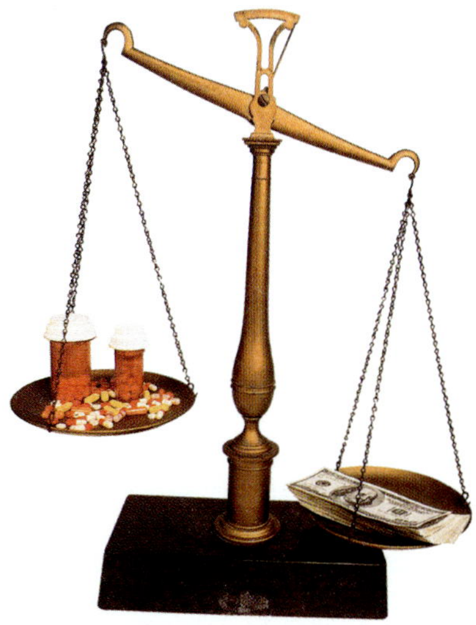

Figure 16-6 Managed-care has greatly impacted the practice of pharmacy in recent years.

In recent years the practice of pharmacy has been greatly impacted by the presence of managed care (Figure 16-6). National enrollment in HMO plans stood at 80.1 million people in 2000. In 2003, 63% of the American population was participating in some form of managed care that contained a prescription drug benefit. A prescription drug benefit is defined as prescription drug coverage provided as an employee benefit. In the managed-care arena, a member of prescription plans would pay the pharmacy a copayment when a prescription is dispensed and the remainder of the cost of the prescription would be paid by the insurance company.

A **managed care pharmacy** is part of a network of pharmacies that are linked together through a benefit to provide pharmaceutical services. A member pharmacy has signed a contract with a pharmacy benefit manager (PBM) or insurer based upon specific conditions to be met for reimbursement. A managed care pharmacy network may consist of independent, franchise, chain pharmacies, or an in-house pharmacy operated by an HMO or a mail-order pharmacy.

Regardless of the pharmacy setting, managed care pharmacy will have an impact on that practice. Pharmacists and pharmacy technicians involved in managed care pharmacy are employed by various managed care organizations, including HMOs and PBMs, as well as retail pharmacies, hospitals, integrated health systems, and the pharmaceutical industry.

Managed Care Organizations

Managed care pharmacy consists of various managed care organizations (MCOs) each having a special niche in the market place. A managed care organization is a health care organization that both insures and provides health care services. These include:

- Pharmacy benefit manager (PBM)
- Health maintenance organization (HMO)
- Preferred provider organization (PPO)
- Individual practice association (IPA)
- Medicare
- Medicaid

Pharmacy Benefit Manager

A pharmacy benefit manager (PBM) is an organization responsible for designing, administering, and managing the prescription drug benefit. In addition to the drug benefit portion of managed care the PBM is involved in **disease management** (which includes behavioral modification), outcomes reporting, and patient education. A PBM develops relationships with its members, employers, pharmacies, and drug manufacturers. The PBM designs the prescription drug benefit based upon the conditions established by the employer.

In addition, PBMs perform the following:

- Develop and manage the drug formulary
- Establish rebates from drug manufacturers
- Extend the pharmacy network
- Process prescription claims data
- Maintain member eligibility
- Provide pharmacy data reports (develop and monitor pharmacy reports, conduct DUE, and provide profile report cards)

managed care pharmacy The practice of pharmacy that involves clinical and administrative activities performed in a managed care organization by a pharmacist.

disease management A coordinated approach to treat a specific disease that involves the entire health care team.

- Conduct DUE (review patient prescription utilization and physician prescribing patterns by geographic location, product, and other characteristics)
- Present patient and health care provider education

Health Maintenance Organization

Health maintenance organizations (HMOs) are a managed care organization that provides health care services to members on a **capitation**-based reimbursement system. Under a capitation reimbursement system the provider is paid a predetermined amount of money on a yearly basis to keep the patient healthy regardless of the number of visits to the provider.

The goal of HMOs is to keep the patient healthy rather than be faced with expenses after a situation has developed in a patient, which in the long run will be more expensive.

There are several different types of HMO and they include:

- Staff model HMO: An HMO in which salaried staff physicians treat patients at facilities owned by the HMO.
- Group model HMO: Patient care is provided through one or more large, multispecialty group practices under contract with the HMO. These are often owned by the physician group practice that provides care exclusively for that group of HMO enrollees, often for a fixed capita fee.
- Independent practice association: This managed care plan allows patients to receive physician services from independent doctors in individual or small group practices. Payment may either be a fee-for-service or on a capitated basis.
- Network model HMO: An HMO that contracts with both physician group practices and independently practicing physicians to provide health care, including a combination of two or more types of HMO plans.

The differences among these models involve the types of physicians retained by the HMO, the type of contract, whether or not private patients are seen by the HMO, and the form of payment system. In most situations, the HMO system is the least costly to the patient. One disadvantage of the HMO system is that a patient may be required to see his or her primary care physician and obtain a referral to see a specialist.

Preferred Provider Organization

A preferred provider organization (PPO) is a type of a managed care plan in which patients receive physician services from independent doctors in individual or small group practice. The payment for a PPO may either be a fee-for-service or capitated basis. A point-of-service (POS) plan permits patients to use providers outside the plan network for an increased deductible and/or copayment.

Medicare

Medicare is a federally funded program for those individuals older than the age of 65 or who have permanent disabilities, such as dialysis patients. Prior to 2003, there were three different parts of Medicare: Part A, Part B, and Part C—none of these provided prescription coverage. The Medicare Modernization Act of 2003 established a fourth component: Medicare Part D. In Part D, a patient subscribes to a particular plan and the pharmacy bills the patient's prescriptions to the plan.

capitation A health care reimbursement system in which a flat, prepaid fee is paid for a range of health care service.

Medicaid

Medicaid is a federal program administered by the states for individuals with low income. Each state has its own set of eligibility requirements. These individuals may already be receiving public assistance either in the form of welfare or other social programs. Other individuals who qualify may be blind, disabled, or have families with dependents younger than the age of 18 who do not have resources available to them from the parents. Prescription coverage is provided where the individual pays a predetermined fee (often \$1) for the service rendered unless they are younger than the age of 18 or are receiving prenatal care.

Cost-Containment Strategies of Managed Care Organizations

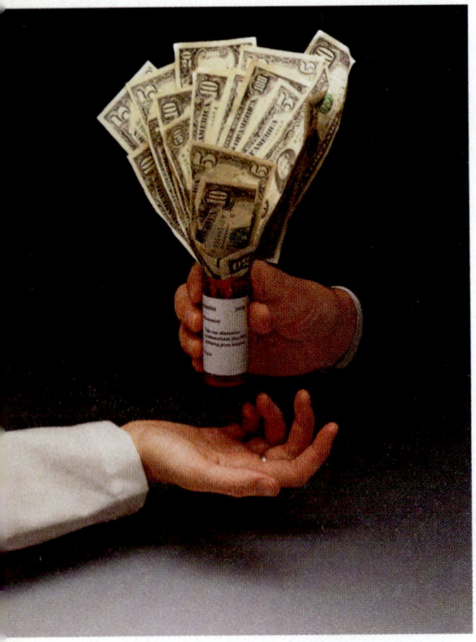

Figure 16-7 Managed care companies contain costs associated with prescription drug benefits.

Within the past decade consumers have seen the cost of their prescription drug benefit skyrocket yearly with double-digit increases (Figure 16.7).

This can be attributed to:

- An increase in senior citizens who in turn take more medications than younger adults do. This can be credited to the number of chronic conditions that elderly people experience.
- An increase in the number of people covered under a drug benefit plan.
- A desire from individuals to use the newest pharmaceutical product available on the market. Newer pharmaceuticals cost more than older established medicines.
- Direct advertising by the drug manufacturers.
- The cost associated in the development of new products.

Formulary

In order for the managed care companies to control costs, various safeguards may be utilized. A managed care organization may adopt the use of a formulary (an approved listing of drugs). The formulary is developed by the Pharmacy and Therapeutics (P&T) Committee of the managed care organization and is used to promote high-quality medical care that is affordable to patients. Formularies are a revised list of prescription medications that represent the current clinical judgment of providers in hospitals, health plans, and physician groups under contract with health plans.

The P&T Committee decides if therapeutic interchange will be permitted. In therapeutic interchange, a patient receives a medication that is the therapeutic equivalent of the drug originally prescribed. Two or more drugs are considered therapeutically equivalent if they can be expected to produce identical levels of clinical effectiveness and outcomes in patients. Therapeutic interchange can occur only if the patient's prescriber approves it. Therapeutic interchange differs from generic interchange in which one drug in the same therapeutic class is substitute; generic interchange involves medications that contain the same active ingredients with the same strength, concentration, dosage form, and route of administration. Therapeutic interchange provides quality drug care in a cost-effective manner.

The formulary system may be open, closed, or restricted. Open formularies allow for any medication to be dispensed, closed formularies are extremely limited, and a restricted formulary allows for nonformulary medications to be dispensed through use of the exception process. The exception process normally requires documentation from the physician stating the rationale for a specific medication to be dispensed.

A managed care pharmacy collects a copayment fee from the patient and bills the remainder of the cost to the insurer. This copayment may be in the form of a fixed or percentage copayment. A fixed copayment is a predetermined fee for either a brand or generic drug. A percentage copayment is based upon predetermined percentage of the reimbursement formula. The percentage copayment is an incentive for the patient to request a generic medication. In some situations the patient is charged a higher copayment if a nonformulary lifestyle medication is dispensed. If a patient requests a brand name medication when the physician has approved the use of a generic drug, the patient maybe charged copayment for what is associated with a brand name drug.

Limitations

Another cost-containment strategy used in managed care pharmacy is the use of limitations. In most plans honored by retail pharmacies, there is a maximum of a 30-day supply of medication; mail-order pharmacies will allow for up to a 90-day supply of medicines. In both of these cases the prescription must be written as such. A less frequently used limitation is based upon a predetermined dollar amount that a patient has available for medications during the calendar year.

Online Adjudication

Prescription claims are submitted electronically today and the process is known as online adjudication. Online adjudication informs the pharmacy that the prescription claim has been approved before the prescription leaves the pharmacy. A prescription claim can be rejected because a patient is not covered under the plan, information regarding the patient was incorrect, the medication is not covered under the insurance plan, or the patient was attempting to refill the prescription earlier than the insurance carrier would approve payment.

Other methods to control costs in the managed care arena of pharmacy is the use of networks of pharmacies, the use of mail-order pharmacies for maintenance medications (the patient is able to obtain a 90-day supply of medication instead of a 30-day quantity), and mandatory generic substitution that is utilized by many HMOs. Managed care may utilize both multiple-tiered and higher copayments.

The Role of the Pharmacist and Pharmacy Technician

Pharmacists and pharmacy technicians may be involved in the Pharmacy and Therapeutics (P&T) Committee of the managed care organization to provide integral information regarding the adaptation or modification of the formulary (Figure 16-8). They may work on the disease management programs that are beneficial to all parties in a managed-care setting because of the goal to control the cost associated with the disease. A major component of prescription processing is drug utilization evaluation (DUE). DUE can identify drug allergies, drug interactions, contraindications, and both under- and over usage of a medication.

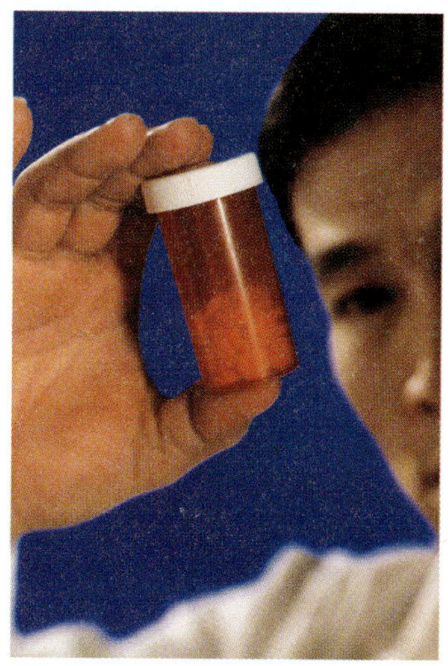

Figure 16-8 Pharmacy technicians may be involved with the P & T committee.

The retail pharmacist and pharmacy technician are responsible not only for providing pharmaceutical care but also for processing the prescription and sending information to the managed care organization or pharmacy benefit manager. Both pharmacists and pharmacy technicians make face-to-face contact with patients, and give input on the administration of the pharmacy benefit and of the care patients receive.

The pharmacy technician working in a managed care pharmacy should have the following qualifications:

- Strong organizational, communications, and mathematical skills
- A strong knowledge of commonly prescribed medications to include their indications and drug classifications
- Pharmacy claims processing computer system experience
- Experience in a retail pharmacy and/or managed care or pharmacy benefit environment
- Comprehensive understanding of third-party pharmacy benefits
- Ability to understand the importance of and respect the confidentiality of information
- Computer literacy with proficiency in general word processing activities

A pharmacy technician, working under the supervision of a pharmacist, has the following responsibilities:

- Handles the ongoing pharmacy benefit telephone calls from members, pharmacy providers, and physicians
- Troubleshoots third-party prescription claims questions with a strong understanding of online rejections and plan parameters
- Develops and maintains an electronic service log on all telephone calls with a complete follow-up history
- Assists in developing a trending report on the aforementioned service calls with an eye toward forecasting possible trends in the pharmacy service
- Provides needed and administrative support for the department
- Maintains current information on the pharmacy benefit
- Maintains drug information references
- Assists in pharmacy patient educational programs

Tech Check

7. What type of problems can be identified by drug utilization evaluation?(LO 16.3)

8. What is a disease management program?(LO 16.2)

9. Which part of Medicare allows for the billing of prescriptions in the future?(LO 16.5)

10. What are four characteristics of a pharmacy technician working in managed care pharmacy?(LO 16.9)

Mail-Order Pharmacy(LO 16.1, 16.2, 16.4)

A mail-order pharmacy dispenses maintenance medications through the mail to a patient (Figure 16-9). Ninety percent of HMO members have the option of receiving their medication from a mail-order pharmacy. Mail-order pharmacies may either be a traditional or specialty mail-order company. A specialty mail-order company focuses on specific diseases such as AIDS or cancer.

In addition to the tasks normally occurring in a community pharmacy, a mail-order pharmacy may be responsible for the development of disease management programs, formulary management, adherence monitoring, and patient education. Disease management programs are developed to prevent acute incidents of chronic disease from occurring in a patient. Formulary management includes involvement in the P&T Committee and informing physicians of appropriate usage of the drug formulary system. Adherence monitoring is used to identify patients who may not be taking the medication as prescribed from the physician. Patient nonadherence may raise the cost of therapy over a period of time. The pharmacist may develop patient education programs, such as the use of behavior modification in the treatment of a chronic condition.

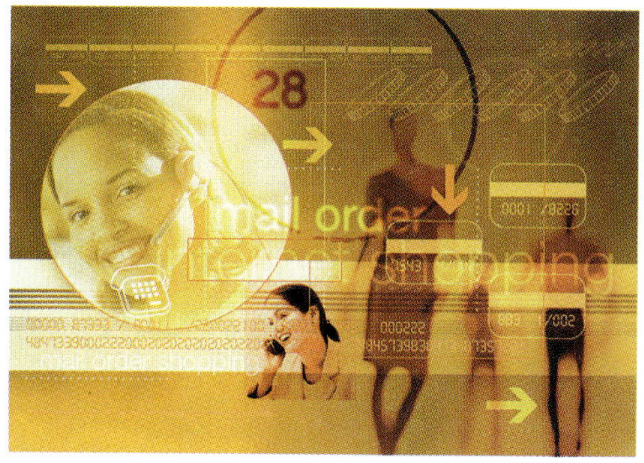

Figure 16-9 Mail-order pharmacy provides cost saving to the patient.

Advantages

A mail-order pharmacy has the advantage of providing a cost savings to the patient, which enables the patient to purchase a larger quantity of medication in terms of day's supply compared to a community pharmacy. Mail-order pharmacy offers a convenience to the patient where the prescription is mailed to an address selected by the patient (Figure 16-10).

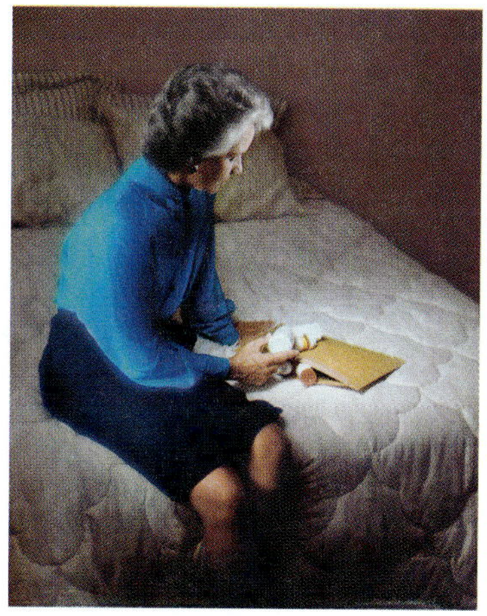

Figure 16-10 Mail-order pharmacy can be convenient for the patient.

This saves the patient time since he or she does not need to drive to a pharmacy to purchase the prescription. Mail-order pharmacies are open 24/7, 365 days a year, and a pharmacist is always available to speak to the patient. A patient's adherence to the therapy is improved because the mail-order pharmacy is capable of providing electronic reminders to the patient as to the availability of a prescription refill. Prescription errors decrease due to organized workflow, an increase in the utilization of automation, and fewer distractions that may occur in a traditional retail pharmacy. A mail-order pharmacy is capable of stocking a wider range of medications than a community pharmacy due to its increased prescription volume. A patient is capable of refilling a prescription through the Internet and able to track it upon being mailed.

Disadvantages

There are two major disadvantages of a mail-order pharmacy. First, there is a delay in the delivery of the completed prescription. In most situations, the patient must mail the new prescription to the mail-order pharmacy and wait for its delivery. Many mail-order pharmacies will not accept a new prescription verbally or a fax of the prescription from the physician's office. The second disadvantage of a mail-order pharmacy is that a patient may feel that he or she may not be receiving the personal attention or face-to-face contact that the person receives in a community pharmacy.

Workflow

An interesting characteristic of a mail-order pharmacy is its organized workflow. Specific tasks are accomplished in a clearly defined manner and in areas of the pharmacy. The workflow in a mail-order pharmacy includes the following steps:

- Order entry—basic patient and insurance information is entered into the computer system. A patient's profile is entered at the same time.
- Prescription item entry—the prescription is entered into the computer system.
- Screening—prescription is verified to ensure that it has been entered correctly. DUE is performed and if problems are discovered during this process, they can be resolved.
- Adjudication—prescription claims are submitted to the insurance carrier for reimbursement. If the claim is approved, the prescription label is printed; if the claim is rejected, corrections are initiated for resubmission of the claim. A prescription claim may be rejected if it is being refilled too soon, a medication is not part of the drug formulary, or if generic substitution or therapeutic substitution is required.
- Dispensing—the medication is selected either manually or through automation based upon the prescription label. Dispensing includes selecting, counting, labeling (includes auxiliary labels), and packaging of the prescription. A delay in the dispensing could result from not having the medication in stock.
- Quality assurance check—the pharmacist verifies that the work performed during the dispensing phase is accurate. The pharmacist employs technology such as bar code scanning and images of medication to ensure that the correct medication and strength are dispensed. The pharmacist is responsible for patient counseling literature to be provided.
- Packing and shipping—the medication is packaged and shipped. In most situations, the U.S. Postal Service is used, but another company such as UPS or FedEx may be used.

Technology

Mail-order pharmacy utilizes technology effectively to reduce labor-intensive activities that in the past have been performed by pharmacists and pharmacy technicians. Technology has been effective in reducing prescription errors in a mail-order pharmacy. Imaging systems are employed to scan written prescriptions as they are received and to provide the pharmacists an image of the prescribed medication. Bar code scanning devices assist the pharmacy personnel to ensure that correct drug has been dispensed. Automatic pill-counting machines are used to count out the correct quantity of medication in an expedient manner and can assist in inventory management activities. Some mail-order pharmacies employ robotics to retrieve medication from the shelf.

Licensure

A mail-order pharmacy is licensed and regulated by the state board of pharmacy in the state in which it practices. A mail-order pharmacy located outside a state where it wishes to practice must register with the board of pharmacy as a **nonresident pharmacy.** A nonresident pharmacy must provide patient counseling to patients. A mail-order pharmacy must be aware of the generic substitution laws for each state in which it practices. Patient records and prescription must be readily retrievable for inspection if requested.

nonresident pharmacy A pharmacy that is located outside a particular state that mails, ships, or delivers prescriptions to patients inside that particular state.

A type of mail-order pharmacy that fills prescriptions for other pharmacies is known as a central fill pharmacy. Central fill pharmacies may be used to process prescription refills. These refills are either transported to a particular pharmacy or mailed to the patient. A pharmacy technician must have a strong knowledge of the regulations for a central fill pharmacy in the state.

Internet

The practice of pharmacy has expanded into the vast world of the Internet. Chain pharmacies have developed Web sites that allow patients to purchase their medications online. The National Association of Boards of Pharmacy (NABP) enacted regulations to ensure the safety of the practice of pharmacy. An **Internet pharmacy** is an established commercial Web site that allows a patient to obtain prescription and over-the-counter (OTC) products via the Internet. An internet pharmacy is certified by the NABP is recognized as being a **Verified Internet Pharmacy Practice Site (VIPPS)** (Figure 16-11). This credential protects consumers from unscrupulous Web site developers.

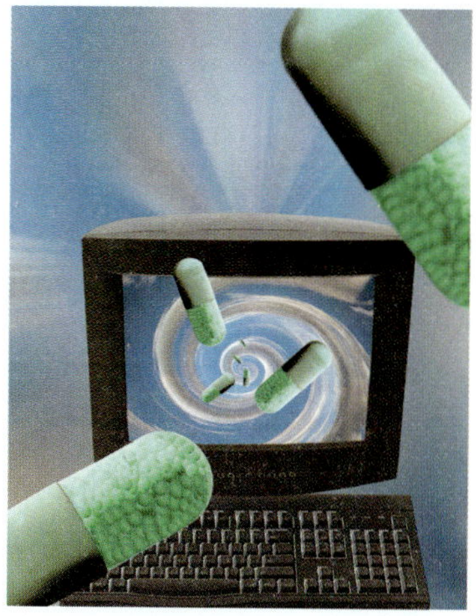

Figure 16-11 An Internet pharmacy certified by the NABP is recognized as being a VIPPS.

The Pharmacy Technician in a Mail-Order Pharmacy

A pharmacy technician working in a mail-order pharmacy requires the following skills:

- Familiarity of the prescription filling process in a retail pharmacy
- Ability to interpret prescription orders from a physician
- Knowledge of commonly prescribed prescription medications
- Use of automated filling systems and knowledge of the required documentation to be used in these systems
- Understanding of both federal and state legislation affecting the practice of pharmacy as an in-state or out-of-state pharmacy
- Computer skills
- Communication skills

A pharmacy technician working in a mail-order pharmacy assists the pharmacist with duties. The technician is highly specialized because of the workflow of a mail-order pharmacy. His or her duties may include performing any of the following:

- Order entry process
- Prescription entry
- Adjudication
- Dispensing process
- Packing and shipping of prescriptions

Tech Check

11. What are the seven steps in processing a prescription in a mail-order program?(LO 16.3)

12. What advantages does a mail-order pharmacy have over a traditional community pharmacy?(LO 16.4)

13. What is a nonresident pharmacy?(LO 16.4)

Internet pharmacy An established commercial Web site that allows a patient to obtain prescription and over-the-counter (OTC) products via the Internet.

Verified Internet Pharmacy Practice Site (VIPPS) A program developed by the National Association of Boards of Pharmacy (NABP) to direct the safety of the practice of pharmacy.

Federal Pharmacy (LO 16.1, 16.2, 16.4)

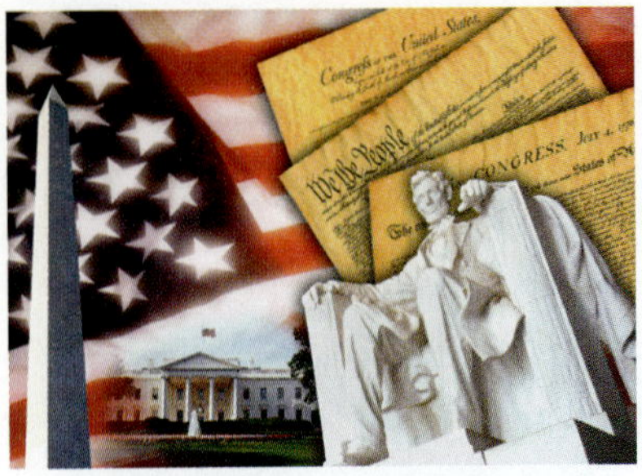

Figure 16-12 Federal pharmacy is the practice of pharmacy within the federal government.

Federal pharmacy is the practice of pharmacy within the federal government (Figure 16-12). The federal agencies that offer career opportunities are the Department of Defense, through the Army, Navy, and Air Force, U.S. Public Health Service, and the Department of Veterans Affairs.

Pharmacists and pharmacy technicians are given greater responsibilities than have been discussed with long-term care, managed care, mail-order, or home infusion pharmacy. Federal pharmacy is not regulated by the state boards of pharmacy but by the federal government. Pharmacists in the federal government must have a minimum of a baccalaureate degree from an institution accredited by the American Council on Pharmaceutical Education and be licensed to practice in at least one of the states or territories of the United States. Federal pharmacy allows for federal pharmacy technicians to dispense and counsel without the presence of a pharmacist.

Department of Defense

The Air Force commissions pharmacists as members of the Biomedical Service Corps; in the Army and Navy pharmacists are associates of Medical Service Corps. Both the military and civilians are employed as pharmacists and pharmacy technicians in the various military settings. Army and Air Force pharmacy personnel support the medical facilities throughout the world. Both the Army and Air Force pharmacy personnel support military medical centers and hospitals similar to those found in the private sector. Pharmacists in the Navy provide health support to and readiness for active-duty naval and marine forces throughout the world. Pharmacists in all three branches of the military may either follow a traditional role as a pharmacist or specialize in other health-related areas.

Pharmacy technicians in the Army, Navy, and Air Force undergo rigorous educational programs. All three branches utilize programs developed by the American Society of Health-System Pharmacists (ASHP). Pharmacy technicians in the Army, Navy, and Air Force are allowed to check the work of another pharmacy technician. This is known as "tech-check-tech". Pharmacy technicians are essential in the operation of pharmacy in the military. For example, the Army dispenses 60,000 ambulatory care prescriptions and 40,000 medication orders daily and the Air Force dispenses more than 63,000 prescriptions daily.

U.S. Public Health Service

The Department of Health and Human Services oversees the U.S. Public Health System (PHS), which is another career possibility for pharmacy technicians. The U.S. Public Health System is responsible for protecting and advancing the health care of the American public. It is responsible for the following organizations:

- The Agency for Health Care Policy Research (AHCPR)—conducts broad-based outcomes and quality research through the awarding of grants to researchers.
- The Centers for Disease Control and Prevention (CDC)—provides leadership in the control and prevention of disease and monitors immunization status of the population.

- The Food and Drug Administration (FDA)—is responsible for protecting the nation's health as it relates to foods, pharmaceuticals, biologicals, vaccine products, medical devices, radioactive health products, cosmetics, food additives, poisons, and certain pesticides.
- The Health Resource and Services Administration (HRSA)—provides leadership in the identification and deployment of health personnel and in the educational, physical, financial, and organizational resources to achieve optimal health services for all citizens.
- The National Institutes of Health (NIH)—provides leadership and direction in advanced areas of medical and biomedical research.
- The Substance Abuse and Mental Health Services Administration (SAMSHA)—focuses its efforts on substance abuse prevention and treatment, and provides funding for programs that have linkages between drug treatment activities and primary care programs.
- The Indian Health Service (IHS)—provides direct health services to American Indians and native Alaskans.

Department of Veterans Affairs

The Veterans Health Administration is the health care branch of the Department of Veterans Affairs. The VHA dispenses in excess of 57 million ambulatory care prescriptions yearly, 300 million doses of inpatient medication, 2 million units of IV admixtures, and 10 million piggybacks. In a VHA setting the ratio of pharmacists to pharmacy technicians is one-to-one.

Federal service offers the unique opportunity to pursue a career in which one's seniority and retirement program remains intact throughout one's career. The pharmacist and pharmacy technician hold values and educational backgrounds oriented toward patient care and public health.

Tech Check

14. Who oversees the U.S. Public Health System?(LO 16.4)

15. Who develops the program for pharmacy technician training in the military services?(LO 16.4)

16. What group or groups of individuals benefit from the IHS?(LO 16.2)

Pharmaceutical Industry(LO 16.1, 16.2, 16.4)

The U.S. pharmaceutical industry is relatively young compared to other industries in the United States, but unlike more established industries the pharmaceutical industry shows very strong growth in the future (Figure 16-13). This growth can be attributed to a strong commitment by the pharmaceutical industry for research and development. The industry continues to discover, develop, produce, and market life-enhancing, life-lengthening, and life-saving medications to improve patients' quality of life.

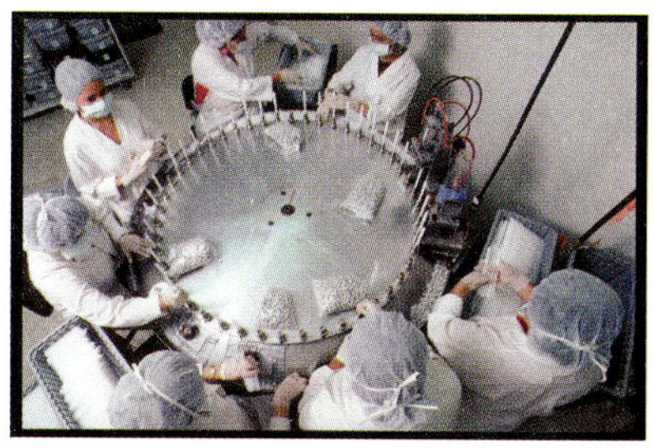

Figure 16-13 Pharmaceutical manufacturer.

The pharmaceutical industry has several strengths that will fuel its continued growth. These include an ever-growing science base, especially in biotechnology and gene therapy. Pharmaceuticals produce a positive impact on the health of individuals; in some cases medications have shown to lower the cost associated with other health care costs. The pharmaceutical industry provides reasonable returns for its investment in research and development and will continue to do so.

The pharmaceutical industry does have several obstacles to overcome, however. They include a continuing health care cost-containment effort. The FDA has been under attack in recent years due to a lack of strong leadership and direction. Drug product recalls continue to plague the FDA. Congress continues to seek an explanation for the continual high prices associated with medications. Another issue the pharmaceutical companies are battling involves the reimportation of medications.

Pharmaceutical Sales

There are two areas of the pharmaceutical industry where pharmacy technicians have an opportunity to participate. First, pharmaceutical sales are a pathway for an individual to enter the pharmaceutical industry. Sales representatives, also known as medical service representatives or detail men and women, call on physicians, dentists, pharmacists, and veterinarians. The purpose of their calls is to provide them with complete information on products and to encourage their use.

Many pharmaceutical companies are seeking individuals who either have experience in pharmacy or a science background. Professional sales representatives should have a congenial personality, effective oral communication skills, and a strong interest in selling.

Marketing

A second pharmaceutical opportunity lies in the marketing of a drug product. The marketing department is responsible for implementing marketing plans to promote the company's products to the appropriate target audience. Marketing includes conducting marketing research, marketing planning, product management, and new product development.

A strong knowledge of pharmaceutical sales; an understanding of the health care delivery system; general business principles; and a basic knowledge of pharmaceutical research and development, manufacturing, quality assurance, and drug distribution can be extremely beneficial to a marketing candidate. Possessing pharmacy experience may be helpful as well. A pharmaceutical marketing specialist needs to have a strong comprehension of the drug-approval process, patent activity, and the importance of pharmaceutical research.

Tech Check

17. What personal traits are essential in procuring a pharmacy sales position?(LO 16.9)

18. What is the marketing department in a pharmaceutical company responsible for?(LO 16.2, 16.4)

Chapter Summary

Understanding the other pharmacy environments is vital to the pharmacy technician. Important points to know are:

- Pharmacy technicians are used in a variety of health care facilities. Each of these facilities requires special technical skills and knowledge to be proficient in them.
- A long-term care pharmacy dispenses medications to patients in long-term facilities such as assisted-living facilities, nursing facilities, sub acute care, or hospice care. Long-term care pharmacies utilize a unit-dose delivery system to provide medications to the residents.
- A home infusion pharmacy provides infusion therapy to patients residing in a variety of settings. These medications are infused parenterally and encompass analgesics, antibiotics, antineoplastic agents, and biological-response modifiers. A home infusion pharmacy utilizes aseptic technique in the preparation of these medications.
- A managed care pharmacy provides both clinical and administrative activities in a managed care organization. A managed care pharmacy may provide services to patients from a variety of managed care organizations. A managed care pharmacy is faced with minimizing costs, providing access to patients, and providing quality pharmaceutical services to its patients.
- Mail-order pharmacies dispense maintenance medications to a patient using a mail delivery service. A mail-order pharmacy may be an option of a managed care organization. The mail-order pharmacy employs a systematic process of filling prescriptions where specific tasks are performed at specific locations of a pharmacy.
- The U.S. Public Health System, the Department of Defense, and the Department of Veterans Affairs use pharmacy technicians in various settings.
- The pharmaceutical industry shows an extremely strong potential for growth in the future; pharmacy technicians have the potential to find positions either in sales or marketing.

Chapter Review

Case Study Question

1. What should Andrew know before he goes on his first interview?(LO 16.1)

At Your Service

1. Andrew informs Mary Ellen of the situation and she would like to know how she is able to obtain a 90-day supply? What should Andrew tell her?(LO 16.3, 16.5, 16.7)

Multiple Choice

Select the best answer.

1. What type of refill in a long-term care facility is initiated by the nurse?(LO 16.4)
   a. Cycle-fill
   b. Prn refill
   c. Turn-around fill
   d. All of the above

2. Which pharmacy environment would utilize aseptic technique?(LO 16.4)
   a. Home infusion
   b. Long-term
   c. Mail-order
   d. Managed care

3. Which of the following is an advantage for mail-order pharmacy (may select more than one)?(LO 16.4)
   a. Cost savings
   b. Patient convenience
   c. Improved compliance
   d. All of the above

4. Which of the following managed care programs are federal programs administered to patients who are elderly or have permanent disabilities?(LO 16.4, 16.6)
   a. CHAMPVA
   b. Medicaid
   c. Medicare
   d. Tricare

5. What is another name for a pharmacy sales representative?(LO 16.9)
   a. Detail men and women
   b. Medical services representatives
   c. Professional sales representatives
   d. All of the above

6. Which of the following is an example of a long-term care facility?(LO 16.4)
   a. Assisted-living facility
   b. Board and care homes
   c. Psychiatric hospital
   d. All of the above

7. Which of the following is the electronic submission of a prescription claim to an insurer?(LO 16.3, 16.5, 16.6)
   a. Adjudication
   b. Capitation
   c. Fee-for-service
   d. None of the above

8. Which of the following is *not* a goal of managed care?(LO 16.4)
   a. Maximize costs
   b. Provide access to a pharmacy
   c. Provide quality medications to a patient
   d. All of the above are goals of managed care

9. What organization is responsible for accrediting home infusion pharmacies to allow them to participate in Medicare?(LO 16.x)
   a. BOP
   b. DEA
   c. FDA
   d. TJC

10. Which of the following drug classifications would be found in an emergency box in a long-term care facility?(LO 16.2)
    a. Anticonvulsants
    b. Hypoglycemic agents
    c. Nitroglycerin
    d. All of the above

11. Which of the following drug classifications would be used in the practice of home infusion pharmacy?(LO 16.2, 16.4)
    a. Analgesics
    b. Antibiotics
    c. Antineoplastics
    d. All of the above

12. Which of the following is an explanation for an increase in the cost of prescription drug benefits?(LO 16.5)
    a. An decrease in the number of individuals under a drug benefit plan
    b. An increase in pediatric patients
    c. Use of older medications instead of recently developed drugs
    d. An increase in senior citizens

13. What type of technique is used in the preparation of home infusion medications?(LO 16.7)
    a. Aseptic technique
    b. Punch method
    c. Sifting
    d. Trituration

14. Which of the following is *not* a function of a pharmacy benefit management firm?(LO 16.5)
    a. Administering the drug benefit
    b. Designing the drug benefit
    c. Managing the drug benefit
    d. All of the above

15. What may drug utilization evaluation reveal to a pharmacist?(LO 16.3)
    a. Drug-drug interactions
    b. Duplicate drug therapy
    c. Underutilization of the medication
    d. All of the above

16. Who is responsible for developing a formulary for a managed care organization?(LO 16.4)
    a. BOP
    b. DEA
    c. NABP
    d. P&T Committee

17. Which of the following is *not* a method to control costs in managed care?(LO 16.5)
    a. Mandatory generic substitution
    b. Manual submission of prescription claims
    c. Usage of pharmacy networks
    d. Use of plan limitations

18. What are the hours of operation for a mail-order pharmacy?(LO 16.4)
    a. 6 am to 12 midnight
    b. 6 am to 10 pm.
    c. 7 am to 12 midnight
    d. Open 24 hours a day, 7 days a week, 365 days a year

19. Which practice of pharmacy utilizes tech-check-tech?(LO 16.4)
    a. Army, Navy, and Air Force pharmacies
    b. Home infusion pharmacy
    c. Long-term care pharmacy
    d. Managed care pharmacy

20. Which of the following is an example of a modified unit-dose system?(LO 16.3, 16.4)
    a. Bingo cards
    b. Blister cards
    c. Punch cards
    d. All of the above

Acronyms

Print the meaning of the following acronyms.

ASHP ____________________________
CDC ____________________________
FDA ____________________________
IHS ____________________________
NABP ____________________________
NIH ____________________________
P&T ____________________________
PHS ____________________________
SAMSHA ____________________________
VIPPS ____________________________

Critical Thinking Questions

1. How would you explain to a current pharmacy customer the advantages of mail-order pharmacy?(LO 16.4)
2. Why do managed-care organizations need to use a formulary system?(LO 16.4, 16.5)
3. Will the need for long-term care facilities increase or decrease in the future? Why?(LO 16.1)

HIPAA Scenario

Gale Johnson of Austin, Texas, received a package from her mail-order pharmacy. She was expecting her maintenance prescription for legend drug glyburide. Instead, she received a box for a natural hormone replacement therapy (vaginal skin cream) with a label for a patient named Gail Johnston. The packaging label had Gale Johnson's correct name and address, but the prescription container had the incorrect name and wrong medication. If this medication had been shipped to Gail Johnston of Houston, Texas, then it would have gone to the right patient.

Discussion Questions (PTCB II.73)

1. What HIPAA laws were broken if any?
2. What is the ethical thing for the patient to do?
3. What should the pharmacist or director of pharmacy do?)
4. What other ethical questions does this raise?

Internet Activities

- Go to **www.cvs.com** to determine what type of products can be purchased. Can prescriptions be refilled? Are OTCs available? If so, what type? Is **www.cvs.com** a VIPPS pharmacy?(LO 16.4)
- Go to a managed care pharmacy Web site such as **www.caremark.com** and find out what type of services it offers?(LO 16.2)

17 Inventory Management

Learning Outcomes

Upon completion of this chapter, you will be able to:

17.1 Justify the importance of inventory management in the practice of pharmacy.

17.2 Discuss the principles of inventory management.

17.3 Give reasons for the importance of a formulary system in institutional pharmacy.

17.4 Describe the function of a group purchasing organization.

17.5 List the steps in ordering medication for the pharmacy.

17.6 Explain the processes in ordering of controlled substances.

17.7 Demonstrate the steps in receiving medication from a supplier.

17.8 Justify the importance of rotating stock upon receipt of new products.

17.9 Describe the storage of medications in a pharmacy.

17.10 Calculate inventory turnover rate.

17.11 Explain the processes involved in the destruction of controlled substances.

17.12 Describe the importance and preparation of a yearly physical inventory.

17.13 Contrast the various types of inventories found in pharmacy practice.

17.14 Explain the handling of "unsalable" merchandise.

17.15 Disclose the procedures involved with the development of new drug products.

17.16 Explain the methods in obtaining investigational new drug products.

17.17 Describe the drug recall process.

Key Terms

bid (also known as contract compliance)

Pharmacy and Therapeutics (P&T) Committee

product rotation

reverse distributor

velocity report

PTCB

In preparation for the certification examination, you should understand and perform activities associated with the following PTCB Knowledge Statement:

PTCB Knowledge Statement

Domain II. Maintaining Medication and Inventory Control Systems

Knowledge of drug product laws and regulations and professional standards related to obtaining medication supplies, durable medical equipment, and products (1)

Knowledge of pharmaceutical industry procedures for obtaining pharmaceuticals (2)

Knowledge of purchasing policies, procedures, and practices (3)

Knowledge of formulary and approved stock list (5)

Knowledge of PAR and reorder levels and drug usage (6)

Knowledge of inventory receiving process (7)

Knowledge of the DEA controlled substance ordering forms (9)

Knowledge of regulatory requirements regarding record keeping for repackaged products, recalled products, and refunded products (10)

Knowledge of policies, procedures, and practices for inventory procedures (11)

Knowledge of the FDA's classifications of recalls (14)

Knowledge of systems to identify and return expired and unsalable products (15)

Knowledge of rules and regulations for removal and disposal of products (16)

Knowledge of regulatory requirements and professional standards (18)

Knowledge of medication distribution and controlled systems for controlled substances, investigational drugs, and hazardous materials and wastes (23)

Knowledge of quality assurance policies, procedures, and practices for medication, and inventory control systems (25)

Case Study

A warehouse delivery is coming in on Tuesday. However, Sharon, the inventory specialist, has noticed that many of the items there were supposed to have been on the shelf are not there. Sharon knew that the order was not checked in properly while she was on vacation. The pharmacy was charged for many items that were never received.

On Tuesday, Sharon took her time going through the entire pharmacy with the Telazon (a handheld device used in the ordering process), before the warehouse delivery arrived. Once it arrived, she checked it in by going through each tote and initialing each item. After the warehouse items were put away, she went back and checked the invoices that came in while she was on vacation and called the warehouse for credits. Now that this was done, she went back through the shelves to find that people were not rotating the bottles.

While reading this chapter, keep the following questions in mind:

1. There were three open bottles of Diflucan 100 mg sitting on the shelf. What should Sharon do?(LO 17.7)
2. Should she talk with the pharmacy manager to let him or her know what is going on with the inventory, or should she just take care of the problem?(LO 17.1)

Introduction to Inventory Management(LO 17.1)

An inventory is a listing of goods or items available for use in a normal business operation. A pharmacy's inventory is one of its largest expenses. It is the pharmacist's responsibility to ensure that the pharmacy stocks the correct medications needed by patients. A pharmacy that maintains a proper inventory of medications provides excellent customer service to its customers.

At Your Service

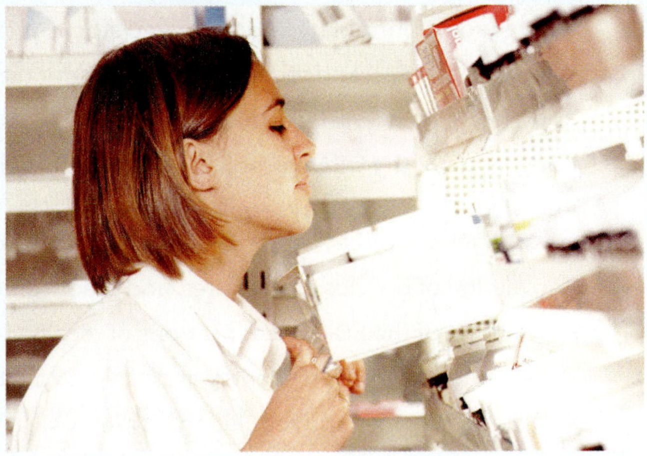

Betty Johnson called the pharmacy with a prescription refill on Monday morning. It was to be picked up on Wednesday at 5 pm When she arrived on Wednesday, she informed the pharmacy technician that she was picking up a prescription refill. The technician looked through the bins of completed prescriptions but was unable to find it. The pharmacy technician looked up Ms. Johnson's name in the computer system to see if a refill had been filled for her. The computer indicated a prescription had not been filled.

The pharmacy technician went to the on-order bin in the pharmacy to see if the pharmacy was waiting for medication to arrive from the wholesaler. The technician asked the pharmacist about the status of the prescription. The pharmacy technician was told the wholesaler did not have the medication in stock when it was ordered for Tuesday. The pharmacy had reordered the medication for today but the order had not arrived yet.

The technician returned to Ms. Johnson and informed her of the situation. Ms. Johnson became upset that she had not been notified by the pharmacy on the status of her refill, since she had given the pharmacy her home, work, and cell phone numbers. Also, it bothered her that this was not the first time this situation had occurred at this pharmacy regarding her medication.

While reading this chapter, keep the following questions in mind:

1. Was Ms. Johnson correct about being upset with this situation?(LO 17.1)
2. What may have caused the situation?(LO 17.7, 17.8)
3. What could the pharmacy have done to prevent this from happening?(LO 17.7, 17.8)

Overview of Inventory Management(LO 17.2, 17.5, 17.10, 17.12, 17.13)

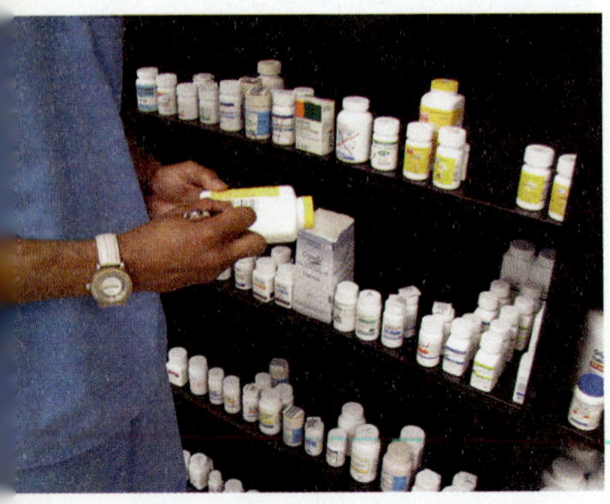

Figure 17.1 Pharmacy inventory.

One of the greatest challenges that faces pharmacists and their staff is maintaining an appropriate inventory in the pharmacy at all times (Figure 17.1). Inventory management is important for these reasons:

- It provides for an adequate stock of pharmaceuticals and supplies at all times.
- It reduces unexpected stock-outs and temporary shortages that ultimately affect patient care.
- It minimizes shrinkage, breakage, and obsolescence of inventory.
- It minimizes the time spent on purchasing functions.
- It minimizes the costs associated with placing orders to the wholesaler.
- It reduces the carrying cost (financial investment) in drug products.
- It reduces the capital charge on the average inventory.

All members of the pharmacy team must understand the importance of proper inventory management. Both pharmacists and pharmacy technicians need to know when, where, and how to order medications.

Once the order is received, the staff must know the procedures to handle the medication and the invoice that accompanies the product. An invoice is a bill for the merchandise purchased. This paperwork must be submitted to the accounts payable department of the company to ensure proper payment to the vendor. Also, invoices for controlled substances must be maintained in the pharmacy for a minimum of 2 years. A pharmacy that fails to maintain proper records may face legal action.

A pharmacy may purchase medications from several different sources including drug manufacturers and prime vendors, such as wholesalers. Purchasing medications directly from the drug manufacturer is the most economical method for a pharmacy, but it requires a commitment of time and effort. Contracts will need to be initiated with the manufacturer to ensure the drug is available. Multiple manufacturers will be required to supply a pharmacy with medications. Drug orders must be placed in advance and the pharmacy staff must be able to anticipate product movement based upon past prescribing practices.

Pharmacies that use a wholesaler or prime vendor are able to maintain smaller inventories. A wholesaler is a company that sells merchandise to a business and may require the pharmacy to purchase the majority of its pharmaceuticals from the company. Wholesalers provide a range of services the pharmacy to include a high in-stock position, a 24-hour emergency service computer hardware, and software for ordering. The wholesaler provides a very competitive pricing structure.

PAR

Many retail and hospital pharmacies have initiated systems to link their physical inventory to their computer system (Figure 17-2). A pharmacy establishes a preset quantity for each medication to be maintained on its shelves. The pharmacy computer system automatically reorders the medication when it reaches a specific quantity.

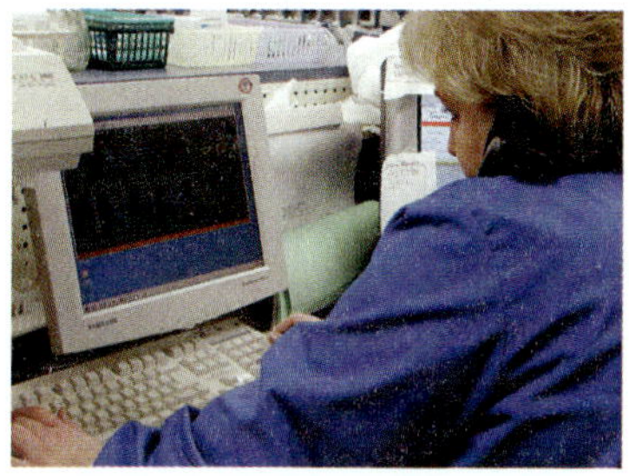

Figure 17-2 Physical inventory can be linked to computer systems.

This concept is known as periodic automatic replenishment, or PAR. PAR is used in all pharmacy settings, whether it is retail or hospital pharmacy. Some of the factors affecting PAR include:

- The number of times the medication has been dispensed within a given time period
- The seasonality of a product, such as allergy products and antibiotics
- Current trends in a pharmacy, whether it is filling more or fewer prescriptions
- The average number of units dispensed per prescription order
- The number of new prescriptions and refills of the drug during the time being examined

The PAR quantity is determined by calculating a fixed number of day's supply of medication to be stocked on the shelf.

When a prescription is processed, the quantity dispensed will automatically be deducted from the inventory and reordered. This process eliminates the pharmacy staff from guessing the amount to be ordered. The major drawback is the system is unable to detect increasing or decreasing trends of a medication. An increasing trend will need to be adjusted manually by the pharmacy staff to ensure enough medication is available to fill patients' prescriptions. If the pharmacy team is not aware of fewer prescriptions being dispensed for a medication, a potential overstock situation may occur resulting in extra dollars being spent on the pharmacy's inventory.

Physical Inventory

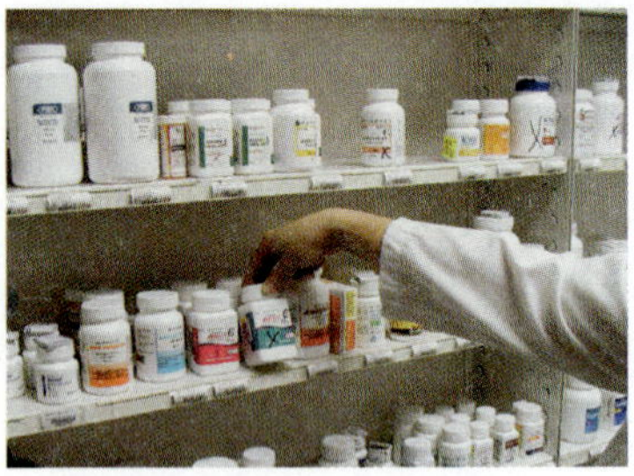

Figure 17-3 Physical inventory.

Pharmacies conduct physical inventories of salable merchandise once or twice a year, often during its fiscal year. A fiscal year is an accounting period that is 365 days in length but does not need to be the calendar year. A physical inventory demonstrates the financial status of the pharmacy.

Preparing for a physical inventory requires the pharmacy staff to make certain that all opened bottles of medication are marked with an X on the label to indicate that the container is not a full container (Figure 17-3). If the staff does not do this, the value of the medications will be inaccurate. The physical inventory is performed by an outside company with no relationship to the facility being inventoried. The inventory may be conducted when the pharmacy is closed or when it first opens in the morning; however, a pharmacist must be present during the entire inventory. The physical inventory by a member of the inventory team involves either performing an exact count of medication or an estimate of the number of tablets, capsules, or milliliters present in a container.

The quantity of each kind of inventory is listed on inventory summary sheets. Each section of the pharmacy, whether it is particular sections or shelves, is identified with a specific dollar value. This allows for a verification of the inventory by the pharmacist and the inventory member. If there is a large discrepancy in a particular section, the inventory team leader recounts the particular areas. The physical inventory must be accurate due to its impact on the profitability of the pharmacy.

Prior to the physical inventory, all purchases and credits must be posted for the inventory. The inventory of the pharmacy is reconciled by comparing the ending inventory value of the last physical inventory and the ending value of the current physical inventory. It takes into consideration all purchases (cost), credits, and sales (cost) during the period. Theoretically:

Beginning inventory + Purchases − Credits − Sales = Ending inventory

This formula does not consider all drug manufacturers' price changes, which occur on a daily basis. Often, price changes result in an increase of the cost of the product. If the value of the pharmacy is greater than what is calculated at that moment of time, the business realizes a profit. On the other hand, if the value of the pharmacy is less than what is computed, the pharmacy loses money.

The results of a physical inventory are used to calculate the inventory turnover rate, which is an accounting tool used to evaluate the flow of inventory dollars. Inventory turnover rate is the number of times the entire stock is used and replenished each year and can be expressed by the following formula:

Inventory turnover rates = Total annual purchases / Inventory value

An application of this can be seen using the following data:

Total purchases of $5,000,000 and an Inventory value of $500,000

Inventory turnover rate = $5,000,000 / $500,000

Table 17-1 Perpetual Inventory for Oxycodone/Acetaminophen

Date	Rx Number	Quantity Dispensed	Invoice Number	Quantity Received	Ending Count
8/1/12			N08011234	500	500
8/1/12	123456	30			470
8/1/12	123502	50			420
8/2/12	123597	75			345
8/3/12	123782	30			315
8/4/12	123952	50			265

The inventory turnover rate for this pharmacy would be equal to 10.

Decreasing the physical inventory and maximizing the number of inventory turns has been proved to reduce costs and provide sources of funds for the institution. The inventory turnover rate is inversely proportional to the inventory value: the higher the turnover rate, the lower the inventory. By decreasing the inventory of the pharmacy, lower financial investment values in inventory will be observed resulting in lower capital interest and lower incidences of waste, shrinkage, and inventory obsolescence.

Other Types of Inventories(LO 17.13)

A pharmacy may be required to maintain perpetual inventories on specific medications, such as Schedules II, III, IV, and V drugs. A perpetual inventory is a detailed record of each purchase and sale of a particular medication. A perpetual inventory provides a "snapshot" of how much of a particular drug is on hand at any given time (see Table 17-1). In some states, a pharmacy may be required to report this inventory to the state board of pharmacy twice a month.

There are two other types of inventories that a pharmacy is required to perform according to the DEA. They are the initial inventory and a biennial inventory. An initial inventory must be taken prior to the opening of a pharmacy before its first day of business or when a new pharmacist-in-charge takes over a pharmacy. A biennial inventory must be taken every 2 years. Both of these records must be maintained in a pharmacy for a minimum of 2 years.

Tech Check

1. Why is inventory management important?(LO 17.1)
2. What term is defined as the total annual purchases divided by the inventory value?(LO 17.10)
3. What are four types of inventories that may be conducted in a pharmacy?(LO 17.13)
4. What is the inventory turnover rate for a pharmacy with average inventory of $250,000 and purchases of $4,000,000?(LO 17.13)
5. If you had an inventory turnover rate of 15.5 and purchases of $3,750,000 what is your average inventory value?(LO 17.13)

Retail Inventory Management (LO 17.2, 17.5, 17.7, 17.8, 17.9, 17.11, 17.14)

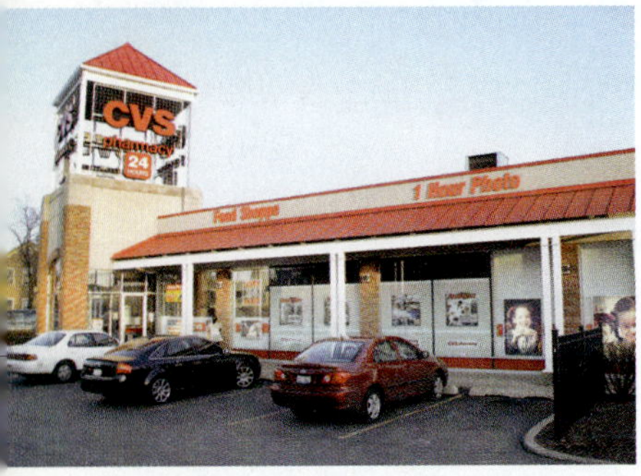

Figure 17-4 CVS is a retail pharmacy.

Many of the inventory management tools are used in both retail and hospital pharmacies to maintain proper inventory levels.

A retail pharmacy can be either a chain, franchise, or independently owned (Figure 17-4). A chain pharmacy maintains a purchasing department or buyers who deal directly with drug manufacturers for the entire company. These pharmaceutical buyers negotiate prices and rebates with the drug manufacturers and arrange for shipment to their warehouses (distribution centers) or directly to the stores. The purchasing department is able to obtain medications at a lower price because of the volume of business. The individual pharmacies in a chain obtain their medications directly from the warehouse based upon a predetermined schedule.

At most chain pharmacies, the pharmacy receives a warehouse order once a week, but an extremely busy pharmacy may receive multiple warehouse deliveries during this time. Every pharmacy has a "want-book." The want-book lists any item that needs to be ordered from the wholesaler or vendor for the next scheduled delivery day. A wholesale order may be placed Monday through Friday. If an error has occurred with the original order or there has been a sudden increase of a specific medication by a change in the physician's prescribing habits, a pharmacy may place an order with its wholesaler.

A franchise pharmacy will operate in much the same way as a chain pharmacy but on a much lower scale. The franchise negotiates prices for its franchisers and may arrange for the distribution of the product. The franchise may select the wholesaler where medications can be ordered. An independent pharmacy will not have a warehouse to stock medications. An independent pharmacy may buy some of the medications directly from the drug manufacturer, as in the case of antibiotics for the cough and cold season. The independent pharmacy signs a contract with a wholesaler that establishes the wholesaler as a "prime vendor" for the pharmacy.

Wholesalers

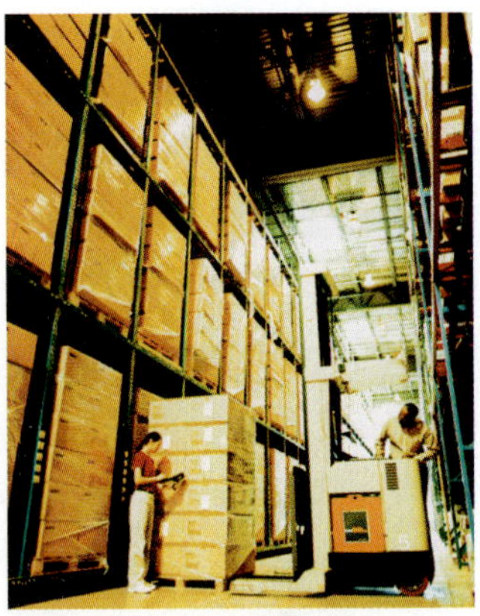

Figure 17-5 Wholesalers provide a range of services to the pharmacy.

All pharmacies sign agreements with wholesalers to obtain medications and OTC products. The pharmacy assures the wholesaler it will purchase the majority of pharmaceuticals from the wholesaler; in some cases, this may be as high 80% to 95% of the total purchase. Because of this agreement, the wholesaler provides the pharmacy with a range of services (Figure 17-5).

These services may include:

- A 95% to 98% delivery rate of the items on a timely schedule
- A 24-hour emergency service for ordering medications
- A computer system for ordering medications
- An electronic order entry device
- Bar-coded labels
- A highly competitive servicing fee ranging from 1% to 5% above cost and contract pricing
- Purchasing history reports, such as contract compliance and velocity reports
- Pricing information
- Notification of drug recalls

An advantage of a prime vendor relationship is that it allows a pharmacy to purchase its pharmaceuticals shortly before they are needed creating a "just-in-time" (JIT) ordering system. A JIT situation results in a shorter turnaround time, smaller physical inventories, higher inventory stock turns, and fewer dollars invested in the pharmacy.

Placing an Order

Each company has its own way of ordering medications, therefore it is important for an individual to be familiar with the policies and procedures manual. Technology plays an important role in medications ordering, and pharmacies have implemented PAR numbers to assist in the process. Often, a pharmacy's computer system will monitor the movement of product from the shelves and place an order to replenish needs.

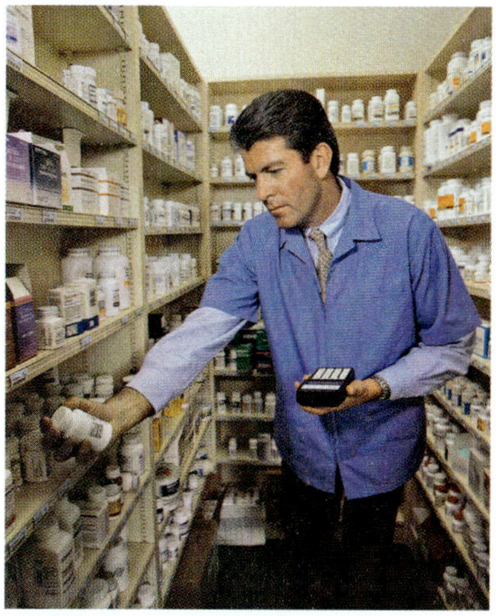

Figure 17-6 A Telazon may be used to place medication orders.

In other situations, it may be the responsibility of the pharmacy technician or pharmacist to use a Telazon (Figure 17-6). With the Telazon you may go through the pharmacy and scan the bar code on the medication bottle and enter the desired quantity to be ordered. This is a variation of an inventory management tool known as Min/Max, where you order up to a predetermined quantity of each medication. Upon completion of entering your order, you should go back and check the quantities ordered to prevent ordering excessive inventory.

The pharmacy team needs to know when the order must be placed (time and day) for it to be delivered during that week. The failure to place an order on time may result in an order not being received that week and can have a serious impact on customer service. The individual responsible for medications should take his or her time and not be rushed; ordering should be done when distractions or interruptions are less likely to occur. It is extremely important to be accurate and thorough when writing a pharmacy order, and interruptions can increase the possibility of errors.

Ordering from a wholesaler is very similar to ordering from the warehouse, with a few exceptions. You may use a Telazon to place an order and, in some situations, may telephone the order in to the wholesaler. To begin the ordering process, first look at the want-book and find the corresponding number to that item in the wholesaler's catalog. Record that number in the book. After finding all of the items to be ordered, make sure that the Telazon has been cleared from the previous day's order; failure to do so may result in unnecessary merchandise being ordered. Enter the medication's item number followed by the quantity to be ordered. Similar to ordering from the warehouse the order must be placed prior to the day's deadline in order to receive it on the next business day.

Orders for a wholesaler are normally processed Monday through Friday; deliveries on the weekend are an exception to the rule. Patients should be informed of the time of day when a special order or the remaining quantity of a prescription will be available for pick-up. Ordering from a wholesaler should be held to a minimum. Every pharmacy has been assigned an inventory budget to maintain; if ordering the medication can wait until the next warehouse delivery or can be borrowed from another pharmacy, you should explore these possibilities first, but customer service should not be jeopardized by being out of stock of a specific medication.

Receiving the Order/Rotating Stock

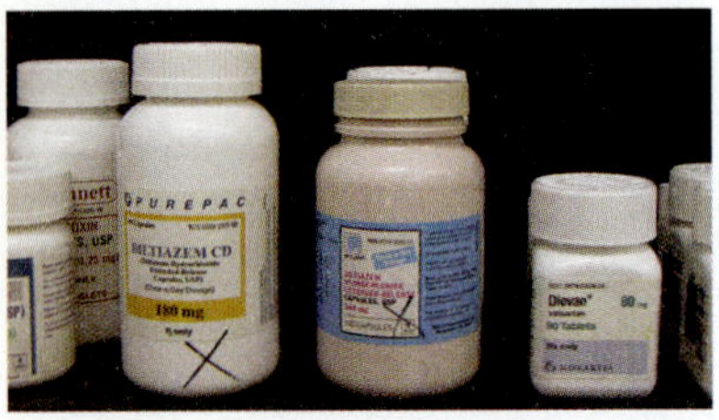

Figure 17-7 Medications must be rotated based on expiration dates.

When the order comes in to the pharmacy, the pharmacy technician must check in the order. To do this you need to have the invoice or packing slip. A packing slip is a document that accompanies a shipment indicating what has been shipped. The technician verifies what has been sent with the invoice or packing slip. Before you place the medication on the shelf, it should be checked off on the invoice as being received. When checking off a medication from an invoice it is important to check the product name, dosage form, strength, package size, and quantity. This can be done by placing a check mark next to the name of the medication or placing your initials next to the name of the medication.

It is important that the medication is placed in its proper spot on the shelf or in the refrigerator. It should be placed behind all of the other medications in that location, so that the product with the shortest amount of time before manufacturer's expiration is in the front to be used or purchased first, which is known as **product rotation** (Figure 17-7). The reason for stock rotation is to prevent patients from receiving short-dated medications and to eliminate the wastage of expired medications. Also, if you place a new bottle of medication in the front of a bottle that has already been opened, there may be two bottles opened. A member of the pharmacy staff may make a false assumption about the amount of a drug in stock. As stated earlier, all opened bottles should be marked with a black X on the label to indicate that it has been opened. The X should not block any important information on the bottle such as drug name, strength, NDC number, expiration date, lot number, or bar code.

As mentioned, you should always make sure that you check in every order that you receive. Failing to check in the order may result in the pharmacy being charged for a medication it did not receive. If the pharmacy is charged for an unreceived item, you must notify the wholesaler, who may do one of the following:

- Send the medication on the next shipment or the next day
- Issue a credit to the pharmacy

Sometimes a pharmacy order contains damaged merchandise. Upon receipt of receiving damaged medication, it is imperative that you notify the warehouse or wholesaler immediately. In many situations, a wholesaler contract might specify that credit will be given only if the company is notified within a specified period of time, such as within 24 hours of delivery. The wholesaler may either issue a credit for the merchandise or send out a replacement for the damaged medication. It will indicate what is to be done with the damaged medication, whether it is to be returned or destroyed.

When a company provides credit for an item, it provides a confirmation number to the pharmacy so that the credit can be tracked. This confirmation number should be placed on the invoice with the name of the individual with whom you spoke. If the pharmacy does not receive a credit, the technician can phone the wholesaler and refer to the confirmation number. Keeping up with the credits in a pharmacy is very important because it helps in managing the budget.

product rotation Placing the merchandise with the shortest amount of time remaining before the manufacturer's expiration in a location to be purchased and used before the product expires.

Outdated and Damaged Stock

Every medication has an expiration date. An expiration date is a guarantee from the drug manufacturer that a medication is good until the last day of the month or the date indicated on the package. A medication that has expired may or may not produce the therapeutic effects as intended. An expired medication can be harmful or even fatal to the patient, as has occurred with tetracycline. Selling short-dated or outdated medication is unethical.

Checking expiration dates can be done when the pharmacy order is received and is being placed on the shelf. Finding an expired bottle of medication on the shelf may indicate the product has not have been rotated properly. Second, it may indicate that the movement of that product has slowed down and the pharmacy should reconsider the quantity of that product to be maintained. Third, it may indicate that the vendor sent a product with short dating.

Every pharmacy will have procedures to outline its processes in checking for outdated or soon-to-expire medication. The volume of the prescriptions being filled may affect the frequency of checking the medications. For instance, a pharmacy may require the pharmacy technicians to check their shelves every month (for high-volume pharmacies) to every 6 months (for low-volume pharmacies) for outdated medication. Other pharmacies may require that a colored dot be placed on the front of a bottle of medication to indicate which month a medication would expire.

When checking for outdated medication, look at the expiration date of the medicine and automatically pull any medication that has expired. Place this medication in a specially designated area. Federal and state laws require that outdated medication do not co-mingle with medication that is in date. It is best to check with the pharmacist if there is any question regarding pulling soon-to-expire medications from the shelf.

Inventory that is outdated or damaged is known as reclamation. Reclamation is unsalable medication and every pharmacy will have procedures explaining the process of handling these expired medications. Please note that separate procedures exist for controlled substances. Once the medication has been pulled from the shelves it may be returned to the warehouse or wholesaler for credit. Depending on the procedures of the pharmacy, you may need to separate the expired medication by drug manufacturer. At that point, you may be required to provide either an estimate (e.g., 1/4, 1/2, or 3/4 bottles) or actual count of the medication being returned. When credit is issued, the pharmacy will receive only a small percentage of value of the outdated medication.

Packaging and Storage of Medications

All medications must be packaged and stored properly to ensure their maximum life span. The failure to store a medication properly may result in the breakdown of the active ingredient. The USP has addressed the packaging and storage of all medications. The packaging cannot interact physically or chemically with the medication placed in it to alter strength, quality, or purity of the medication. The USP has defined the various types of packaging and containers used for storing medications. Refer to Table 17-2.

Table 17-2 Types of Packaging

Tamper-Evident Packaging	The container or individual carton of a sterile article intended for ophthalmic or otic use, except where extemporaneously compounded for immediate dispensing on prescription, shall be so sealed that the contents cannot be used without obvious destruction of the seal.
Light-Resistant Packaging	A light-resistant container protects the contents from the effects of light by virtue of the specific properties of the material of which it is composed, including any coating applied to it.
Well-Closed Container	A well-closed container protects the contents from extraneous solids and from loss of the article under the ordinary or customary conditions of handling, shipment, storage, and distribution.
Tight Container	A tight container protects the contents from contamination by extraneous liquids, solids, or vapors from efflorescence, deliquescence, or evaporation under the ordinary or customary conditions of handling, shipment, storage, and distribution. Where a tight container is specified, it may be replaced by a hermetic container for a single dose of an article. A gas cylinder is a metallic container to hold a gas under pressure.
Hermetic Container	A hermetic container is impervious to air or any other gas under ordinary or customary conditions of handling, shipment, storage, and shipment
Single-Unit Container	A single-unit container is one that is designed to hold quantity of drug product intended for administration as a single dose or a single finished device intended for use promptly after the container is opened.
Single-Dose Container	A single-dose container is a single-unit container for articles intended for parenteral administration only.
Unit-Dose Container	A unit-dose container is a single-unit container for articles intended for administration by other than the parenteral route as a single dose from the container.
Unit-of-Use Container	A unit-of-use container is one that contains a specific quantity of a drug product that is to be dispensed as such without further modification except for the addition of appropriate labeling.
Multiple-Unit Container	A multiple-unit container is a container that permits withdrawal of successive portions of the contents without changing the strength, quality, or purity of the remaining portion.
Multiple-Dose Container	A multiple-dose container for articles intended for parenteral administration only.

In every drug monograph, specific directions are provided as to the proper temperature and humidity for that specific product. Definitions are explained in Table 17-3.

It is extremely important that all medications are stored under the proper conditions. Failing to do so may result in the medication losing its potency and therefore not providing its therapeutic effect on the individual.

Table 17-3 Temperature and Humidity

Temperature	Definition
Freezer	A place in which the temperature is maintained thermostatically between −25° and −10°C (−13° and 14°F).
Cold	Any temperature not exceeding 8°C (46°F). A refrigerator is a cold place in which the temperature is maintained between 2° and 8°C (36° and 46°F).
Cool	Any temperature between 8° and 15°C (46° and 59°F).
Room Temperature	The temperature prevailing in a working area.
Controlled Room Temperature	A temperature maintained that encompasses the usual and customary working environment of 20° to 25°C (68° to 77°F). It does allow temperatures to vary between 15° and 30°C (59° and 86°F) that are experienced in pharmacies, hospitals, and warehouses.
Warm	Any temperature between 30° and 40°C (86° to 104°F).
Excessive Heat	Any temperature above 40°C (104°F).
Protect from Freezing	In addition to the risk of breakage of the container, freezing medication leads to loss of strength, potency, or destructive alterations.
Dry Temperature	A place that does not exceed 40% average relative humidity at controlled room temperature.

Tech Check

6. What is the purpose of a want-book?(LO 17.2, 17.5)
7. What are three advantages of developing a wholesaler relationship?(LO 17.2,)
8. What are four advantages of just-in-time?(LO 17.2)
9. What does one call unsalable merchandise?(LO 17.14)
10. Why is it important to rotate stock?(LO 17.8)
11. Why is it important to check in an order?(LO 17.7)

Hospital Inventory Management(LO 17.2, 17.3, 17.4)

A major difference between retail and hospital pharmacy is the presence of a formulary system in a hospital. As stated in an earlier chapter, a formulary is a list of approved drugs for use by the **Pharmacy and Therapeutics (P&T) Committee.** Formularies are established for hospitals, long-term care facilities, and managed care organizations. Medications approved for

Pharmacy and Therapeutics (P&T) Committee A hospital committee chaired by a physician and composed of physicians, nursing staff, and pharmacists who establish and maintain a listing of approved drugs for use in a hospital.

inclusion in the drug formulary are based upon safety, best therapeutic effect, and the least-expensive alternative. Medications may be added or deleted from the formulary based upon the policies and procedures of an institution. If a doctor writes a prescription for a prescription drug that is not on the formulary, the pharmacist contacts the doctor to ask him or her to order a medication that is on the formulary.

The P&T Committee controls the number of medications available for use in a hospital. As new drugs are approved for formulary usage, current medications are evaluated for therapy duplication. Products are evaluated to determine if they are therapeutically equivalent, which means they contain the same.

- Active ingredient(s)
- Strength or concentration
- Dosage form
- Route of administration

Therapeutic-equivalent drugs must possess the same clinical effect and safety profile when they are administered to patients.

The P&T Committee may approve the use of therapeutic interchange for certain medications. A therapeutic interchange is a substitution of one medication that is not generically equivalent but has the same therapeutic effect. A therapeutic interchange is a cost-effective substitution. Some pharmacists are not required to contact the doctor if a drug that is not on the formulary is prescribed; they may change the drug as long as it is appropriate for the patient's therapy. A therapeutic interchange must be communicated effectively to all affected parties, especially the pharmacy so it is able to ensure proper inventory levels of medication. Note that therapeutic interchange may not be legal in all states, therefore you must be familiar with your state pharmacy regulations.

Contracts and Pricing

Many hospitals and health-system pharmacies belong to a group purchasing organization (GPO). The GPO is responsible for negotiating discounted drug prices and developing contracts directly with the vendors. Once a contract has been negotiated, the GPO offers its members the option to purchase these medications at the contracted or **bid** price. The GPO negotiates prices for the hospital, but it is the hospital that makes the purchase.

The GPO, wholesaler, or prime vendor may provide to the hospital pharmacy a compliance or bid report (see Table 17-4), which summarizes medications that were not purchased on the bid is also know as the contract compliance report. The compliance report indicates dollars lost by the pharmacy by not ordering contracted items. It is the responsibility of the pharmacy director to ensure that medications are being purchased on bid. Failing to order bid medications may be caused by inaccurate shelf labels, items temporarily out of stock, manufacturer back orders, or poor purchasing habits. It is important that the pharmacy director carefully updates quantities for each item, whether increasing or decreasing, during the bid roll process (the period when the contract changes).

bid (also known as contract compliance) The ability to purchase contract items with a group purchasing organization (GPO).

A hospital will order the majority of its medications through one wholesaler. This practice is similar to that of a retail pharmacy, whereby

Table 17-4 Compliance (Bid) Report

Drug	Strength	Manufacturer	Award Status	Quantity	Unit Cost	Extd. Cost	Savings
Morphine sulfate	0.5 mg/mL	Baxter	None	40	$6.89	$275.60	
Morphine sulfate	0.5 mg/mL	Lederle	Primary	40	$1.27	$ 50.80	$224.80
Morphine sulfate	1 mg/mL	Baxter	None	20	$7.38	$147.60	
Morphine sulfate	1 mg/mL	Abbott	Primary	20	$1.41	$ 28.20	$119.40

Table 17-5 80/20 Report*

Trade Name	Generic Name	Cost	Strength	Ship	Total Dollars	%	Total %
Nebcin	Tobramycin sulfate	$ 182.71	1.2 gm	60	$10,962.60	7.71%	7.7%
Claforan	Cefotaxime	$ 118.60	10 gm	55	$ 6,523.00	4.58%	12.29%
Procrit	Epoetin alfa	$ 801.36	10,000 units	8	$ 6,410.88	4.51%	16.8%
Retavase	Reteplase	$2,872.40		2	$ 5,744.80	4.04%	20.84%
Levaquin	Levofloxacin	$ 43.82	25 mg/mL	125	$ 5,477.50	3.80%	24.64%
Propofol	Propofol	$ 31.88	10 mg/mL	105	$ 3,347.40	2.35%	26.99%
							79.99%

*This is a partial report. A complete report would account for 80% of the pharmacy drug purchases.

a wholesaler is selected by the pharmacy. A prime vendor relationship allows a pharmacy the ability to track its purchasing history to identify those areas needed to focus its inventory control efforts. Most prime vendor agreements provide the pharmacy with a **velocity report** (80/20 report). The 80/20 report lists is a detailed summary of purchasing history, where 80% of purchasing dollars are spent on 20% of the products. The 80/20 report. (see Table 17-5) summarizes top purchases by dollar in descending order.

Similar to the pharmacy buyers for a chain drug store, a hospital may have multiple buyers or purchasing agents. It is important that the pharmacy staff provide accurate information in a timely manner to the buyers, allowing them to make appropriate purchases for the pharmacy.

As is seen in a retail setting, the pharmacy may find that it is completely out of a medication and it must obtain it quickly. A hospital pharmacy will also maintain a want-book that allow the hospital to either borrow the medication from a nearby pharmacy or purchase it from a wholesaler. A hospital pharmacy can obtain medications from the wholesaler on Monday through Friday. The staff will follow the same steps when receiving an order as is observed in a retail pharmacy setting. The failure to maintain appropriate inventory levels in a hospital is crucial because it may adversely affect an individual's life. There are many similarities between retail and hospital inventory as seen on table 17.6.

velocity report Also known as an 80/20 report, which is a detailed summary of purchasing history, where 80% of purchasing dollars are spent on 20% of the products.

Table 17-6 Inventory

	Retail Pharmacy	Hospital Pharmacy
Source of medications	Direct from manufacturer, warehouse, or wholesaler	Direct from manufacturer and wholesaler
Formulary system	No	Yes
Group purchasing organization	No	Yes
Pharmacy and Therapeutics (P&T) Committee	No	Yes
Use of want-book	Yes	Yes
PAR system	Yes	Yes
Delivery from wholesaler	Monday through Friday	Monday through Friday
Rotation of drug products	Yes	Yes
Ordering of controlled substances	Yes	Yes
DEA Form 222 required for Schedule II medications	Yes	Yes
DEA Form 41 required for destruction of controlled substances	Yes	Yes
Blanket authorization for destruction of controlled substances	No	Yes
Investigational medications	No	Yes
Inventory management required	Yes	Yes

Tech Check

12. What is the purpose of a formulary?(LO 17.3)

13. What does a GPO do for a hospital pharmacy?(LO 17.4)

14. What is a therapeutically equivalent drug?(LO 17.3)

Controlled Substances (LO 17.6, 17.11)

Controlled substances need to be ordered, stocked, and dispensed from a pharmacy regardless of the setting. Ordering controlled substances requires the pharmacy to register with the DEA. The pharmacy registers with the DEA using a DEA Form 224 and indicates which schedules (C-II, C-III, C-IV, or C-V) it wishes to stock. Once a pharmacy has registered with the DEA, it is able to procure controlled substances from a wholesaler.

Schedule II medications can be ordered only with a DEA Form 222 (Figure 17-8).

This must be done by the pharmacist-in-charge (PIC) or an individual who has obtained a power-of-attorney to order Schedule II medications. A DEA Form 222 allows for a pharmacy to order up to 10 different Schedule II medications at a time; quantities ordered are based upon the need of the pharmacy. A DEA Form 222 is a triplicate form and must be completed in either ink or indelible ink. The pharmacy retains the bottom copy of this form and forwards the other two copies to the wholesaler.

Figure 17-8 Sample DEA Form 222.

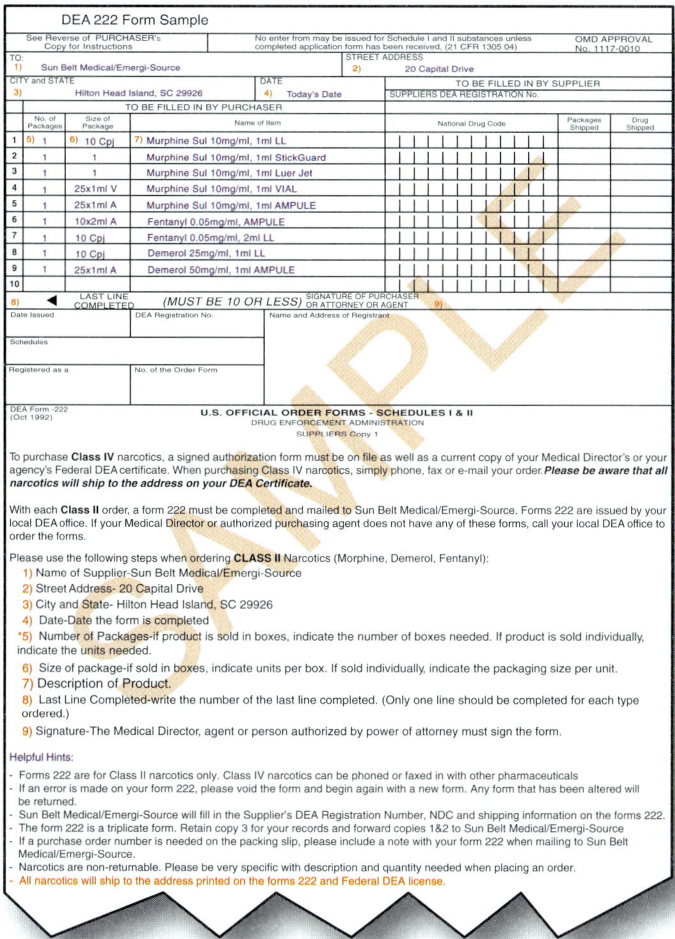

DEA 222 Form Sample

See Reverse of PURCHASER's Copy for Instructions | No enter from may be issued for Schedule I and II substances unless completed application form has been received, (21 CFR 1305 04) | OMD APPROVAL No. 1117-0010

TO: 1) Sun Belt Medical/Emergi-Source | STREET ADDRESS 2) 20 Capital Drive

CITY and STATE 3) Hilton Head Island, SC 29926 | DATE 4) Today's Date | TO BE FILLED IN BY SUPPLIER — SUPPLIERS DEA REGISTRATION No.

TO BE FILLED IN BY PURCHASER

	No. of Packages	Size of Package	Name of Item	National Drug Code	Packages Shipped	Drug Shipped
1	5) 1	6) 10 Cpj	7) Murphine Sul 10mg/ml, 1ml LL			
2	1	1	Murphine Sul 10mg/ml, 1ml StickGuard			
3	1	1	Murphine Sul 10mg/ml, 1ml Luer Jet			
4	1	25x1ml V	Murphine Sul 10mg/ml, 1ml VIAL			
5	1	25x1ml A	Murphine Sul 10mg/ml, 1ml AMPULE			
6	1	10x2ml A	Fentanyl 0.05mg/ml, AMPULE			
7	1	10 Cpj	Fentanyl 0.05mg/ml, 2ml LL			
8	1	10 Cpj	Demerol 25mg/ml, 1ml LL			
9	1	25x1ml A	Demerol 50mg/ml, 1ml AMPULE			
10						

8) ◀ LAST LINE COMPLETED (MUST BE 10 OR LESS) SIGNATURE OF PURCHASER OR ATTORNEY OR AGENT 9)

Date Issued | DEA Registration No. | Name and Address of Registrant

Schedules

Registered as a | No. of the Order Form

DEA Form -222 (Oct 1992)

U.S. OFFICIAL ORDER FORMS - SCHEDULES I & II
DRUG ENFORCEMENT ADMINISTRATION
SUPPLIERS Copy 1

To purchase **Class IV** narcotics, a signed authorization form must be on file as well as a current copy of your Medical Director's or your agency's Federal DEA certificate. When purchasing Class IV narcotics, simply phone, fax or e-mail your order. ***Please be aware that all narcotics will ship to the address on your DEA Certificate.***

With each **Class II** order, a form 222 must be completed and mailed to Sun Belt Medical/Emergi-Source. Forms 222 are issued by your local DEA office. If your Medical Director or authorized purchasing agent does not have any of these forms, call your local DEA office to order the forms.

Please use the following steps when ordering **CLASS II** Narcotics (Morphine, Demerol, Fentanyl):

1) Name of Supplier-Sun Belt Medical/Emergi-Source
2) Street Address- 20 Capital Drive
3) City and State- Hilton Head Island, SC 29926
4) Date-Date the form is completed
*5) Number of Packages-if product is sold in boxes, indicate the number of boxes needed. If product is sold individually, indicate the units needed.
6) Size of package-if sold in boxes, indicate units per box. If sold individually, indicate the packaging size per unit.
7) Description of Product.
8) Last Line Completed-write the number of the last line completed. (Only one line should be completed for each type ordered.)
9) Signature-The Medical Director, agent or person authorized by power of attorney must sign the form.

Helpful Hints:

- Forms 222 are for Class II narcotics only. Class IV narcotics can be phoned or faxed in with other pharmaceuticals
- If an error is made on your form 222, please void the form and begin again with a new form. Any form that has been altered will be returned.
- Sun Belt Medical/Emergi-Source will fill in the Supplier's DEA Registration Number, NDC and shipping information on the forms 222.
- The form 222 is a triplicate form. Retain copy 3 for your records and forward copies 1&2 to Sun Belt Medical/Emergi-Source
- If a purchase order number is needed on the packing slip, please include a note with your form 222 when mailing to Sun Belt Medical/Emergi-Source.
- Narcotics are non-returnable. Please be very specific with description and quantity needed when placing an order.
- All narcotics will ship to the address printed on the forms 222 and Federal DEA license.

If an error occurs when completing a DEA Form 222, the form becomes void and must be retained in the pharmacy for a minimum of 2 years.

When the order arrives from the wholesaler, its receipt must be signed by the pharmacist. The pharmacist must check in the order, verifying the medication received against the invoice and against the pharmacy copy of the DEA Form 222. The pharmacist indicates on the DEA Form 222 the number of bottles received of each medication, dates each line, and signs his or her name on each line. The pharmacist cannot use ditto marks as substitutes for the date or a personal signature. If a medication that has been ordered on the DEA Form 222 is out of stock and the pharmacy is not billed for it, the wholesaler has 60 days to deliver the medication or the order for medication becomes void. In many situations, the wholesaler will ask that the pharmacy submit another DEA Form 222 for that medication. Schedule II, also known as C-II, medications must be stored in a locked safe or drawer. If the pharmacy purchases refrigerated C-IIs, there must be a dedicated locked refrigerator for these medications.

Schedules III, IV, and V may be ordered by the same means as noncontrolled substances, whether it is by a Telazon or verbally over the phone. The C-III through C-V controlled drugs may be delivered with the noncontrolled order and the pharmacy technician can sign for them. The pharmacist may allow a technician to check in Schedules III through V, but this may depend on state laws or company policies. Once the C-III through

C-V drugs have been checked in, the pharmacist must sign and date the invoice; it should be stamped with a red "C" to indicate that controlled substances were in the order. These invoices need to be maintained for a minimum of 2 years, similar to Schedule II medications. The C-III through C-V controlled drugs may be dispersed throughout the pharmacy with the noncontrolled drugs or they may be locked in a safe or drawer, depending on state laws or company policy.

The pharmacy may hire an outside firm to inventory, package, and arrange for the transfer of its controlled substances to another pharmacy, supplier, or manufacturer. The pharmacy is responsible for the actual transfer of the controlled substances and for the accuracy of the inventory and records. The pharmacy may also transfer the drugs to a distributor registered with the DEA to destroy drugs (**reverse distributor**). The pharmacy may not turn over any controlled substances to a distributor unless the reverse distributor is registered to destroy controlled substances. The pharmacy is responsible for verifying that the reverse distributor is registered with the DEA.

If a pharmacy goes out of business or is acquired by a new pharmacy, it may transfer the controlled substances to another pharmacy, supplier, manufacturer, or distributor registered to dispose of controlled substances. To transfer Schedule II substances, the receiving registrant must issue an Official Order Form (DEA Form 222, U.S. Official Order Forms–Schedules I and II) to the registrant transferring the drugs.

The transfer of Schedules III through V controlled substances must be documented in writing to show the drug name, dosage form, strength, quantity, and date transferred. The document must include the names, addresses, and DEA registration numbers of the parties involved in the transfer of the controlled substances.

On the day the controlled substances are transferred, a complete inventory must be taken that documents the drug name, dosage form, strength, quantity, and date transferred. In addition, DEA Form 222 (Official Order Form) must be prepared to document the transfer of Schedule II controlled substances. This inventory serves as the final inventory for the registrant going out of business and transferring the controlled substances. It also serves as the initial inventory for the registrant acquiring the controlled substances. A copy of the inventory must be included in the records of each pharmacy. It is not necessary to send a copy of the inventory to the DEA. The person acquiring the controlled substances must maintain all records involved in the transfer of the controlled substances for a minimum of 2 years.

Any pharmacy may transfer controlled substances to a supplier or a manufacturer. The pharmacist must maintain a written record showing:

- The date of the transaction
- The name, strength, form, and quantity of the controlled substance
- The supplier's or manufacturer's name, address, and, if known, registration number
- The DEA Form 222 will be the official record for the transfer of Schedule II substances

reverse distributor A pharmacy wholesaler capable of accepting expired controlled substances for destruction.

Any pharmacy may forward controlled substances to DEA-registered reverse distributors who handle the disposal of drugs. The DEA recommends that any pharmacy seeking to dispose of controlled substances first

Figure 17-9. Sample DEA Form 41.

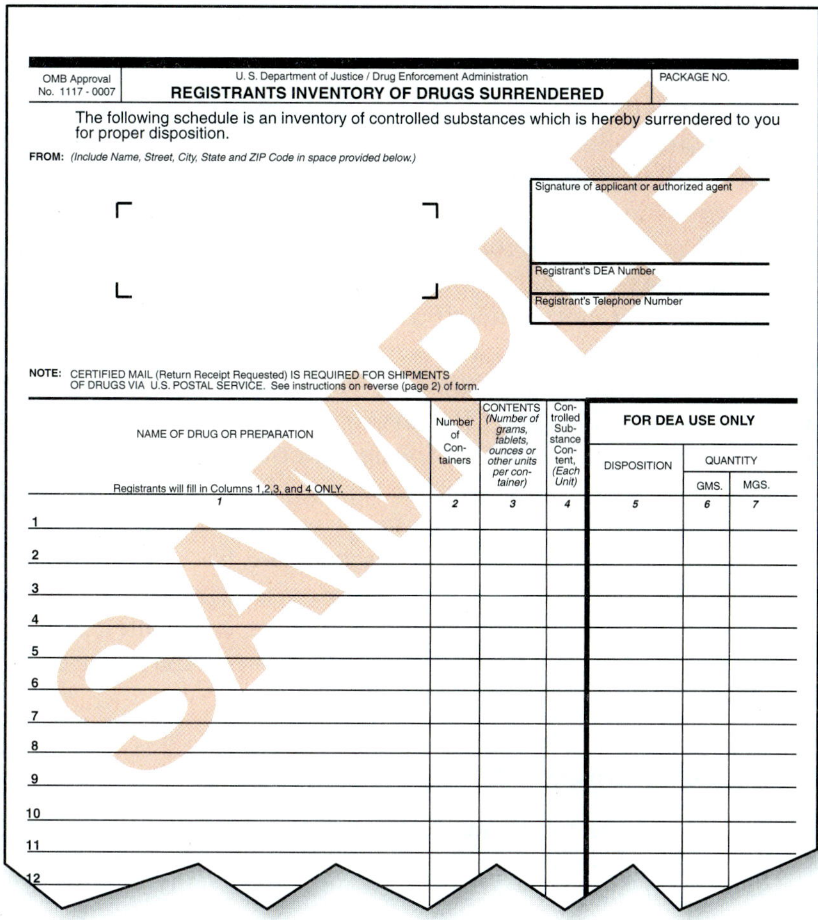

OMB Approval No. 1117 - 0007 | U. S. Department of Justice / Drug Enforcement Administration | PACKAGE NO.

REGISTRANTS INVENTORY OF DRUGS SURRENDERED

The following schedule is an inventory of controlled substances which is hereby surrendered to you for proper disposition.

FROM: *(Include Name, Street, City, State and ZIP Code in space provided below.)*

Signature of applicant or authorized agent

Registrant's DEA Number

Registrant's Telephone Number

NOTE: CERTIFIED MAIL (Return Receipt Requested) IS REQUIRED FOR SHIPMENTS OF DRUGS VIA U.S. POSTAL SERVICE. See instructions on reverse (page 2) of form.

NAME OF DRUG OR PREPARATION Registrants will fill in Columns 1,2,3, and 4 ONLY.	Number of Containers	CONTENTS (*Number of grams, tablets, ounces or other units per container*)	Controlled Substance Content, (*Each Unit*)	FOR DEA USE ONLY DISPOSITION	QUANTITY GMS.	 MGS.
1	2	3	4	5	6	7
1						
2						
3						
4						
5						
6						
7						
8						
9						
10						
11						
12						

SAMPLE

contact the nearest DEA Diversion Field Office for disposal instructions. In no case should drugs be forwarded to the DEA unless the registrant has received prior approval from the DEA. DEA procedures take precedence unless state regulations are more stringent. Requests from registrants seeking authorization to destroy controlled substances without DEA presence or requests from nonregistrants desiring to dispose of controlled substances will be handled as follows:

Once each calendar year, retail pharmacies may request DEA authorization to destroy damaged, outdated, or otherwise unwanted controlled substances. The pharmacy must complete DEA Form 41 (Figure 17-9) listing all drugs to be destroyed. In addition, the pharmacy must prepare a letter requesting permission to destroy the controlled substances, proposing a date and method of destruction, and listing the names of at least two people who will witness the destruction.

The witnesses should be a licensed physician, pharmacist, mid-level practitioner, nurse, or a state or local law enforcement officer. Both documents must be received by the nearest DEA Diversion Field Office at least 2 weeks prior to the proposed destruction date. After reviewing all available information, the DEA office will then notify the registrant in writing of its decision. Once the controlled substances have been destroyed, signed copies of the DEA Form 41 must be forwarded to DEA. The pharmacist should contact local environmental authorities prior to implementing the proposed method of destruction to ascertain that hazards are not associated with the destruction.

Prior DEA authorization to destroy controlled substances is not necessary when an authorized member of a state law enforcement authority or regulatory agency witnesses the destruction. Copies of a DEA Form 41 or state controlled substance destruction form must be forwarded to the local DEA Diversion Office after the destruction.

A pharmacy may at any time forward controlled substances to the DEA via a registered reverse distributor who handles the disposal of drugs. The pharmacist may contact a local DEA Diversion Field Office for an updated list of those reverse distributors in the area. When a pharmacy transfers Schedule II substances to a reverse distributor for destruction, the distributor must issue an Official Order Form (DEA Form 222) to the pharmacy. When Schedules III through V controlled substances are transferred to a reverse distributor for destruction, the pharmacy should document in writing the drug name, dosage form, strength, quantity, and date transferred. The DEA-registered reverse distributor who will destroy the controlled substances is responsible for submitting a DEA Form 41 to DEA when the drugs have been destroyed. A DEA Form 41 should not be used to record the transfer of controlled substances between the pharmacy and the registered reverse distributor disposing of the drugs.

Controlled Substances in a Hospital

In a hospital setting, the pharmacist handles the counts on all of the controlled substances and is ultimately responsible for these drugs. However, it is the pharmacy technician who delivers controlled substances to the nursing stations throughout the hospital. Hospitals use a controlled substance delivery inventory sheet to indicate the quantity of these drugs being delivered and to acknowledge receipt of the drugs to the hospital department or nursing unit. Only a registered nurse can sign for the receipt of controlled substances. At no time should a pharmacy technician leave controlled substances unattended at a nursing station while seeking the nurse. If something should happen to the drugs while being delivered, the technician is held responsible for the them.

The DEA issues a "blanket authorization" for destruction of controlled substances on a very limited basis to registrants who are associated with hospitals, clinics, or other registrants having to dispose of used needles, syringes, or other injectable objects only. This limited exception is granted because of the probability that those objects have been contaminated by hazardous body fluids. The pharmacist should contact the local DEA Diversion Field Office for information about how to request such an authorization. The DEA evaluates requests for a blanket authorization based on the following guidelines:

- Frequency of destruction (i.e., daily, weekly) and volume of drugs involved that warrant such authorization
- Method of destruction—drugs must be destroyed in such a manner that they are beyond reclamation
- Registrant's past history
- Security at the pharmacy or registered location
- Name and position of the individual responsible for the destruction

Registrants who are granted blanket authorization to destroy controlled substances must complete DEA Form 41.

Tech Check

15. Why would controlled substances need to be signed for by a registered nurse?(LO 17.6)

16. What form is used to order Schedule II medications?(LO 17.6)

17. What form is used to request the destruction of controlled substances?(LO 17.11)

Investigational Drugs(LO 17.15, 17.16)

An individual or pharmaceutical company, governmental agency, or academic institution may bring a new drug to market. An Investigational New Drug (IND) application is used to provide data indicating that it is reasonable to begin tests of a new drug on humans (Figure 17.10).

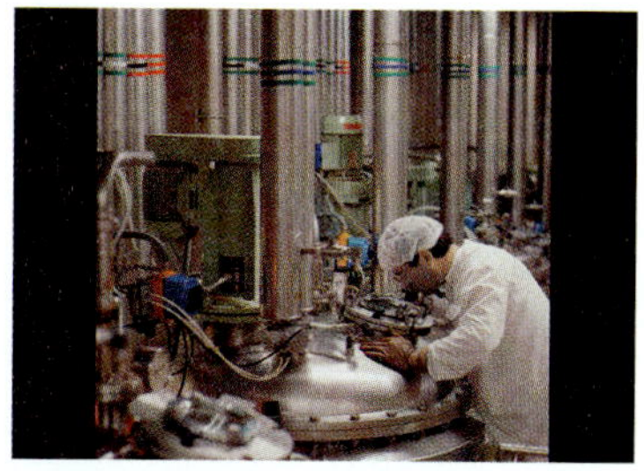

Figure 17-10 **Investigational drugs are regulated by Federal law.**

Federal law requires that a drug be the subject of an approved marketing application before it is transported or distributed across state lines. The drug sponsor will want to ship an investigational drug to clinical investigators in many states and therefore an exemption from federal law must be obtained. The IND application is the vehicle through which the sponsor obtains an exemption.

The following terms are used in the IND process:

- Clinical investigation: any experiment in which a drug is administered or dispensed to a subject.
- Investigator: an individual under whose immediate direction the drug is administered or dispensed to a subject.
- Sponsor: a person who takes responsibility for and initiates a clinical investigation.
- Sponsor-investigator: an individual who both initiates and conducts an investigation, and under whose immediate direction the investigational drug is administered or dispensed.

During a new drug's early preclinical development, the sponsor's primary goal is to determine if the product is reasonably safe for initial use in humans, and if the compound exhibits pharmacological activity to validate the commercial development. When a drug is identified as a possible entity for further development, the sponsor collects data and information necessary to prove that the product will not expose humans to unreasonable risks in the early clinical studies.

Under FDA requirements, a sponsor must first submit data showing that the drug is reasonably safe for use in initial, small-scale clinical studies. Depending on whether the compound has been studied or marketed previously, the sponsor may have several options for fulfilling this requirement:

- Compiling existing nonclinical data from past in vitro laboratory or animal studies on the compound.
- Compiling data from previous clinical testing or marketing of the drug in the United States or another country whose population is relevant to the U.S. population.

- Undertaking new preclinical studies designed to provide the evidence necessary to support the safety of administering the compound to humans.

During preclinical drug development, a sponsor evaluates the drug's toxic and pharmacologic effects through in vitro (nonliving organism) and in vivo (living organism) laboratory testing. Genotoxicity screening is performed, as well as investigations on drug absorption and metabolism, the toxicity of the drugs metabolites, and the speed with which the drug and its metabolites are excreted from the body. During the preclinical stage, the FDA will ask at a minimum that sponsors:

- Develop a pharmacological profile of the drug
- Determine the acute toxicity of the drug in at least two species of animals
- Conduct short-term toxicity studies ranging from 2 weeks to 3 months, depending on the proposed duration of use of the substance in the proposed clinical studies

There are three different types of INDs:

- An Investigator IND is submitted by a physician who both initiates and conducts an investigation, and under whose immediate direction the investigational drug is administered or dispensed. A physician might submit a research IND to propose an unapproved drug, or an approved product for a new indication or in a new patient population.
- An emergency Use IND allows the FDA to authorize use of an experimental drug in an emergency that does not allow time for submission of an IND. The FDA may authorize shipment of the drug for a specified use in advance of submission of an IND. A request for such authorization may be transmitted to the FDA by telephone or other rapid communication. An Emergency Use IND may be used for patients who do not meet the criteria of an existing study protocol or, if an approved study, protocol does not exist.
- Treatment IND is submitted for experimental drugs showing promise in clinical testing for serious or immediately life-threatening conditions while the clinical work is conducted and the FDA review take place.

INDs fall into two categories: commercial and noncommercial. A commercial IND application is used by a company whose ultimate goal is to obtain marketing approval for a new product. A noncommercial IND is used to conduct research.

A sponsor submits an IND to the FDA if the sponsor intends to conduct a clinical investigation with an IND. A sponsor must not begin a clinical trial until the investigation is subject to an approval IND application. A sponsor must submit a separate IND for any clinical investigation involving an exception from informed consent.

An IND may be submitted for one or more phases of an investigation. The clinical investigation of a previously untested drug is generally divided into three phases. Although in general the phases are conducted sequentially, they may overlap. The three phases of an investigation are as follows:

- Phase 1 includes the initial introduction of an investigational new drug into humans. These studies are usually conducted in healthy volunteer subjects. The studies are designed to determine the metabolic and pharmacological actions of the drug in humans, the side effects associated with increasing doses, and if possible, evidence on effectiveness. Phase I studies evaluate drug metabolism, structure activity relationships, and the mechanism of action in humans. The total number of subjects included in phase 1 studies is generally in the range of 20 to 80.

- Phase 2 includes the early controlled clinical studies conducted to obtain some preliminary data on the effectiveness of the drug for a particular indication or indications in patients with the disease or condition. This phase of testing also helps determine the common short-term side effects and risks associated with the drug. Phase 2 studies involve several hundred people.
- Phase 3 studies are intended to gather the additional information about effectiveness and safety that is needed to evaluate the overall benefit-risk relationship of the drug. Phase 3 studies provide an adequate basis for extrapolating the results to the general population and transmitting that information in the physician labeling. Phase 3 studies include several hundred to several thousand people.

A hospital pharmacy may be involved in an evaluation program utilizing investigational drugs. Investigational drugs may be used in a hospital setting due to the presence of a laboratory, and other medical facilities may be required for the study. The Pharmacy and Therapeutics (P&T) Committee will establish policies and procedures regarding the handling and control of investigational drugs in the hospital.

There are many problems associated with the use of investigational drugs in a hospital setting and some of them include:

- Legal problems may result if a hospital fails to exercise due care in the handling of these medications.
- Nurses administer investigational drugs to patients and there must be sufficient information regarding the proper dosage, route of administration, possible toxic reactions, side effects, precautions, and labeling of these medications.
- Investigational drugs are made available from the manufacturer to the principle investigator (the hospital) and may not be labeled in a manner to reduce an error in the administration to the patients.
- Investigational drugs are considered part of research and legal implications maybe present requiring written consent by the patient.
- The FDA has set legal requirements forth by the FDA and in case of a drug recall; records must be available and include the lot numbers of investigational drugs being used.
- If investigational drugs are used on outpatients, they must be labeled to conform to legal requirements, such as child-resistant containers. Information regarding these medications must be available to physicians.
- An adequate supply of the medication must be available to the patient to ensure that interrupted dosage schedules do not occur.

Before an investigational drug is used on a patient, the physician must obtain written consent from the patient. The hospital pharmacist must maintain adequate dispensing records for all investigational drugs dispensed. The pharmacist may be required to provide patient education to the patient receiving the investigational drug. Upon completion of the study all unused investigational medication must be returned to the manufacturer.

Tech Check

18. How many phases must a drug undergo before it is available as a prescription item?(LO 17.15)
19. What type of pharmacy may stock an investigational drug?(LO 17.16)
20. What types of problems are associated with investigational drugs?(LO 17.16)

Drug Recalls(LO 17.17)

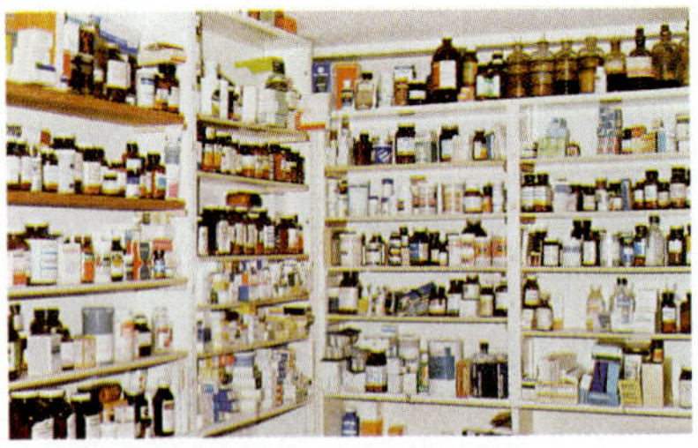

Figure 17-11 Drug recalls ensure patient safety.

The role of the FDA is to ensure that all food and drugs are safe for consumption. Every year many drug products are either recalled or withdrawn from the market. These actions may be initiated by the drug manufacturer, the FDA, or by FDA order under statutory authority (Figure 17.11).

The following terms are associated with the recall/withdrawal process:

- Class I recall: a situation in which there is a reasonable probability that the use of or exposure to a violative product will cause serious adverse health consequences or death.
- Class II recall: a situation in which use of or exposure to a violative product may cause temporary or medically reversible adverse health consequences or where the probability of serious adverse health consequences is remote.
- Class III recall: a situation in which use of or exposure to a violative product is not likely to cause adverse health consequences.
- Market withdrawal: occurs when a product has a minor violation that would not be subject to FDA legal action. The firm removes the product from the market or corrects the violation. For example, a product removed from the market due to tampering, without evidence of manufacturing or distribution problems would be a market withdrawal. In the 1980s, McNeil Laboratories had a market withdrawal for its Tylenol products.
- Medical device safety alert: issued in situations where a medical device may present an unreasonable risk or substantial harm. In some situations, they are considered recalls. Table 17-7 identifies the major reasons for a medication to be recalled.

In most situations the drug recall begins with the drug manufacturer proceeding to the drug wholesaler to the pharmacy and finally to the patient.

Once a drug recall has been initiated, the following steps are observed:

1. Receiving the initial notification
2. Listing further action steps
3. Carrying out further notification
4. Responding to the initial notification
5. Handling the products
6. Receiving reimbursement

The pharmacy may learn of a drug recall or withdrawal from the drug manufacturer, a wholesaler, or from a chain pharmacy headquarters via letter, fax, telephone voice mail, a pharmacy journal, an Internet Web page, mass media, or even from the patient. The particular product is identified by a lot or batch number with its expiration date. A lot number is an

Table 17-7 Common Reasons for a Drug Recall

Reason	Description of Recall	Percentage of Total Recalls
Potency	Failure to maintain potency at certain times during the in-date period	30%
Labeling/packaging mix-ups	Incorrect strength on label, wrong product in bottle	25%
Miscellaneous product problems	Discoloration, leaking bottles, particulate matter, etc	20%
Dissolution	Failure to dissolve at certain time during the in-date period	10%
Manufacturing discrepancies	Deviations from official manufacturing procedures	10%
Contamination	Contamination with bacteria, or general lack of sterility	5%

alphanumeric combination that identifies a specific batch of medication produced at a specific time. All drug products must have a lot number.

Upon notification, the pharmacy staff should follow the procedures outlined in the company policies and procedures manual regarding drug recalls. In some situations, a sub-recall may be issued where the pharmacy staff needs to identify all of the patients who have received the recall product and communicate those instructions to the patient. It is important that patients are notified immediately to prevent any additional or possible injuries. It is critical that the pharmacy also respond back to the issuer of the notification. Very often, the notifying party will enclose a prepaid card or provide the pharmacy with a fax number to respond back with the amount of medication present in the pharmacy. If the pharmacy does not possess any of the recalled medication, it is important the pharmacy relay this information to the issuing party. Once the medication has been identified, located, isolated, and returned to the pharmacy from patients, the pharmacy must follow the procedure outlined by the issuer of the recall. On the financial side, it is essential that the pharmacy watch for any reimbursement from the manufacturer. In many situations, a pharmacy will refund the amount the patients paid for the prescriptions. Table 17-7 identifies the major reasons for a medication to be recalled.

Chapter Summary

Understanding inventory is vital to the pharmacy technician. Important points to know are:

- Inventory management is fundamental to the success of any pharmacy regardless of the setting.
- There are four types of inventories that occur in a pharmacy regardless of the setting: initial, biennial, perpetual, and physical.
- A pharmacy may obtain its medications directly from the manufacturer or a wholesaler.
- The USP has defined specific terms used for the packaging and storage of medications.
- There are many inventory similarities between retail and hospital pharmacy as identified in Table 17-6.
- The FDA has implemented a system whereby a new medication can be introduced into the marketplace after various studies have been conducted.

Chapter Review

Case Study Questions

1. There were three open bottles of Diflucan 100 mg sitting on the shelf. What should Sharon do?(LO 17.7)
2. Should she talk with the pharmacy manager to let him or her know what is going on with the inventory, or should she just take care of the problem?(LO 17.1)

At Your Service

1. Was Ms. Johnson correct about being upset with this situation?(LO 17.1)
2. What may have caused the situation?(LO 17.7, 17.8)
3. What could the pharmacy have done to prevent this from happening?(LO 17.7, 17.8)

Multiple Choice

Select the best answer.

1. Which form do you use to order C-II drugs?(LO 17.6)
   a. DEA Form 41
   b. DEA Form 106
   c. DEA Form 222
   d. DEA Form 363
2. What temperature classification has a temperature range of 20° to 25°C (68° to 77°F)?(LO 17.9)
   a. Controlled room temperature
   b. Cool
   c. Dry temperature
   d. Warm
3. Which form is used to request the destruction of controlled substances in a retail pharmacy?(LO 17.11)
   a. DEA Form 41
   b. DEA Form 106
   c. DEA Form 222
   d. DEA Form 363
4. During which phase in the development of a new drug product is the medication tested on healthy individuals?(LO 17.15)
   a. Phase I
   b. Phase II
   c. Phase III
   d. All of the phases
5. As the size of the inventory decreases, which of the following are at an increased risk?(LO 17.1, 17.2)
   a. Obsolescence
   b. Shrinkage
   c. Unexpected stock-outs
   d. All of the above
6. Which of the following may cause inventory to become obsolete?(LO 17.2)
   a. Changes in physician prescribing habits
   b. New knowledge of drugs, disease states, and transient states
   c. Technological changes
   d. All of the above
7. Who is responsible for negotiating prices of pharmaceutical drugs for a hospital?(LO 17.4)
   a. Accounting
   b. Drug manufacturers
   c. GPO
   d. Hospital buyers
8. Which pharmacy setting may utilize a blanket authorization for the destruction of controlled substances?(LO 17.12)
   a. Chain pharmacy
   b. Franchise pharmacy
   c. Hospital pharmacy
   d. Independent pharmacy
9. Which pharmacy setting may be able to use investigational drugs?(LO 17.16)
   a. Chain pharmacy
   b. Franchise pharmacy
   c. Hospital pharmacy
   d. Independent pharmacy
10. What type of container protects the integrity of the medication from light?(LO 17.9)
    a. Hermetic container
    b. Light-resistant container
    c. Tamper-evident container
    d. Tight container

11. Which of the following is an advantage of just-in-time ordering?(LO 17.1, 17.2)
 a. Fewer dollars invested in inventory
 b. Higher inventory stock turns
 c. Smaller physical inventories
 d. All of the above
12. What is another name for an 80/20 report?(LO 17.2)
 a. Bid report
 b. Compliance report
 c. Velocity report
 d. All of the above
13. Who establishes a formulary for an institution?(LO 17.3)
 a. GPO
 b. P&T Committee
 c. PAR committee
 d. Physicians
14. Why is inventory management important in the practice of pharmacy?(LO 17.1)
 a. To minimize shrinkage, breakage, and obsolescence of medication
 b. To provide appropriate levels of medication in stock
 c. To reduce the carrying cost of excess medications
 d. All of the above
15. What type of report summarizes the top purchases made by an organization?(LO 17.2)
 a. Bid report
 b. Compliance report
 c. Velocity report
 d. All of the above
16. Who may be responsible for bringing a new drug entity to market?(LO 17.15)
 a. Academic institution
 b. Governmental agency
 c. Pharmaceutical company
 d. All of the above
17. The IND process includes how many phases of investigation?(LO 17.15)
 a. One phase
 b. Two phases
 c. Three phases
 d. Four phases
18. Which of the following is an example of a problem associated with the use of investigational new drugs (may select more than one)?(LO 17.15, 17.16)
 a. The pharmacy must have an adequate supply of medication on hand to prevent any interruption in therapy.
 b. Investigational drugs are part of the research process and therefore will require written permission by the patient.
 c. Legal issues may occur if the facility does not exercise proper care in handling medications.
 d. All of the above.
19. What type of drug recall results when either serious adverse effects or death occurs from a drug product?(LO 17.17)
 a. Class I
 b. Class II
 c. Class III
 d. Class IV
20. What is the greatest cause for a drug recall?(LO 17.17)
 a. Contamination
 b. Dissolution
 c. Labeling/packaging
 b. Potency

Acronyms

Print the meaning of the following acronyms.

1. DEA ______________________
2. FDA ______________________
3. GPO ______________________
4. IND ______________________
5. JIT ______________________
6. PAR ______________________
7. PIC ______________________
8. P&T Committee ______________
9. USP ______________________

Critical Thinking Questions

1. Go to your local pharmacy and identify yourself as a pharmacy technician student. Ask the pharmacist what the procedures are when a drug recall is issued.(LO 17.17)
2. What would you say and do if a patient returned a container of medication that had been recently recalled by the drug manufacturer?(LO 17.17)
3. What would you do if a patient returned a container of medication that was recently dispensed and he or she informed you that the medication was out of date?(LO 17.14)

HIPAA Scenario

A particular pharmacy is under investigation for the lack of proper maintenance of controlled substance prescriptions and accurate accounting of controlled substances. The pharmacy technician Robert Yoo, CPhT, is approached by a person at the pickup window who identifies herself as a DEA agent: diversion investigator Blackburn. Blackburn asks Robert for access to all C-II through C-V prescriptions on file for the last 5 years.

Discussion Questions(PTCB II. 73)

1. Is the pharmacy technician by law allowed or required to give the DEA diversion investigator access to the controlled substance prescription files and subsequently PHI?
2. Does the technician have to get approval from the pharmacist first?
3. What precautions should the technician and/or pharmacist take?

Internet Activities

1. Go to **www.fda.gov** and identify the two most recent recalled medications. Include the name of the medication, the NDC number, the lot number, and the reason for the recall.(LO 17.17)
2. Search the Internet and identify the local drug wholesaler servicing your geographical area.(LO 17.2)

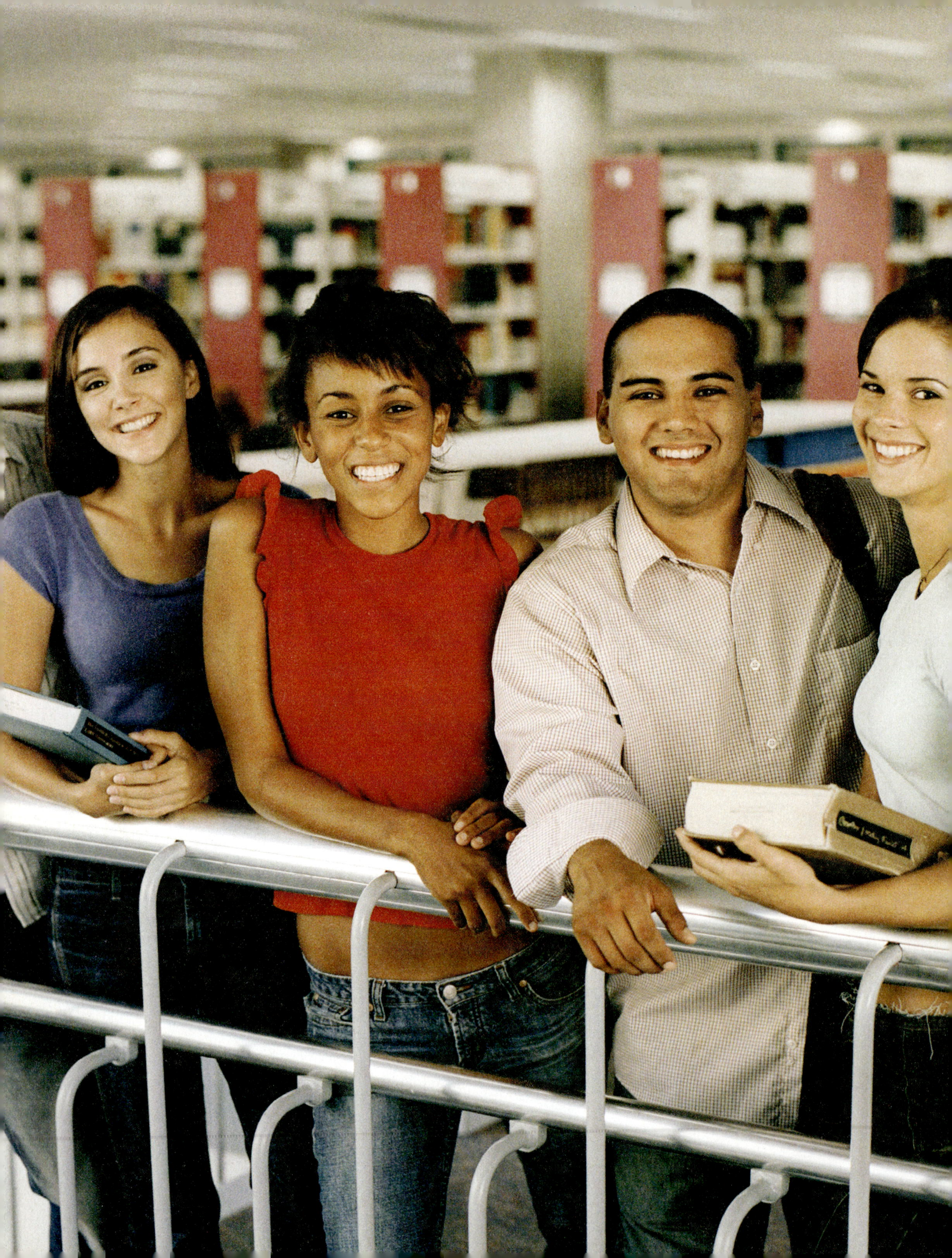

Unit 5

Transition from Student to Technician

Chapter 18 Preparing for Your Career as a Pharmacy Technician

Chapter 19 Career Development

18 Preparing for Your Career as a Pharmacy Technician

Learning Outcomes

Upon completion of this chapter, you will be able to:

18.1 Define *externship* and explain its significance.

18.2 Define *professionalism*

18.3 Identify expectations of the pharmacy technician student during the externship.

18.4 Differentiate between national certification and state board of pharmacy requirements.

18.5 Describe methods by which the pharmacy technician can seek employment.

18.6 List the components of a resume.

18.7 Describe pre-employment requirements.

18.8 List positive interviewing strategies for the job applicant.

Key Terms

clinical coordinator
externship
networking
preceptor
professionalism
program director
resume

PTCB

In preparation for the certification examination, you should understand and perform activities associated with the following PTCB Knowledge Statement:

PTCB Knowledge Statement

Domain III. Participating in the Administration and Management of Pharmacy Practice

Knowledge of productivity, efficiency, and customer satisfaction (4)

Knowledge of roles and responsibilities of pharmacists, pharmacy technicians, and other pharmacy employees (7)

Case Study

Mary is finishing up her pharmacy technician training program and is currently doing her externship at Better Care Pharmacy. Mary has a 2-year-old son who is frequently ill, so she has been receiving two or three phone calls daily from her mother who babysits while Mary is in school, and from her son's doctor. Mary has to stay up nights while her son is sick, so she often arrives late for her externship. Sometimes she leaves early because she has to run errands or take her son to the doctor. Joe, the pharmacist at Better Care Pharmacy, is displeased with Mary's attendance and with her progress as it relates to competencies. He has complained to the program director and is considering not accepting any other students from this particular technician program.

While reading this chapter, keep the following question in mind:

1. What should Mary do in this situation? (LO 18.3)

Introduction to Preparing for Your Career (LO 18.1)

As you are nearing completion of your pharmacy technician training program, you are preparing to embark upon your professional life as a pharmacy professional. You have dedicated many hours of hard work and study, so you will also want to take the necessary steps to ensure a successful career as a pharmacy technician. Many of those steps take place now, prior to your completion of the training program. The purpose of this chapter is to identify steps and strategies to prepare you for a career as a pharmacy technician.

Pharmacy Technician Training Programs (LO 18.1, 18.2, 18.3)

The American Society of Health-System Pharmacists (ASHP), the accrediting body for pharmacy technician training programs, states that technician training programs must include three components: didactic, laboratory, and experiential.

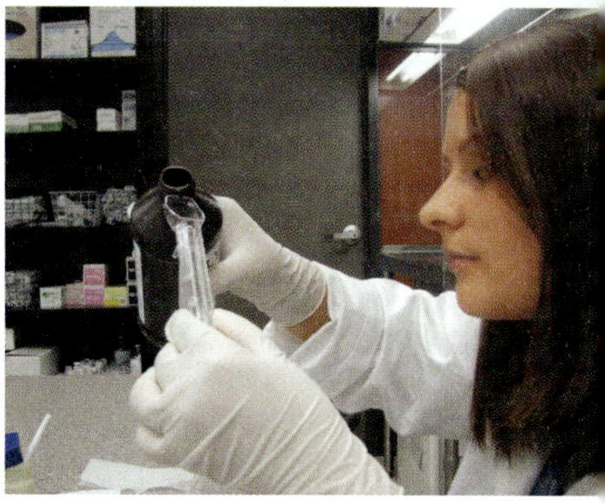

Figure 18-1 Pharmacy technician student in school lab.

- The didactic component of the program includes courses held in a classroom setting, where information is presented and the student is assessed based upon his or her understanding of the material. The pharmacology course or module in a pharmacy technician training program is an example of the didactic component.
- The laboratory component includes work performed in pharmacy labs, where information or techniques are presented to the student and the student is assessed based upon his or her ability to perform or complete a task or series of tasks (Figure 18-1). Students compounding ointments in the pharmacy lab is an example of the laboratory component of pharmacy technician education.
- The experiential component of a pharmacy technician training program is sometimes called an externship or an internship. Externship implies the experiential component occurs after the student has completed the

At Your Service

Joshua has completed the pharmacy technician program with honors. He has state registration and is certified as a result of taking the Pharmacy Technician Certification Examination. He saw an ad in yesterday's paper indicating an open position for pharmacy technician at the local community hospital pharmacy. He would like to apply for this position.

While reading this chapter, keep the following questions in mind:

1. What should Joshua do first? (LO 18.5)
2. Assuming he is called for an interview, how should he prepare for the interview? (LO 18.8)

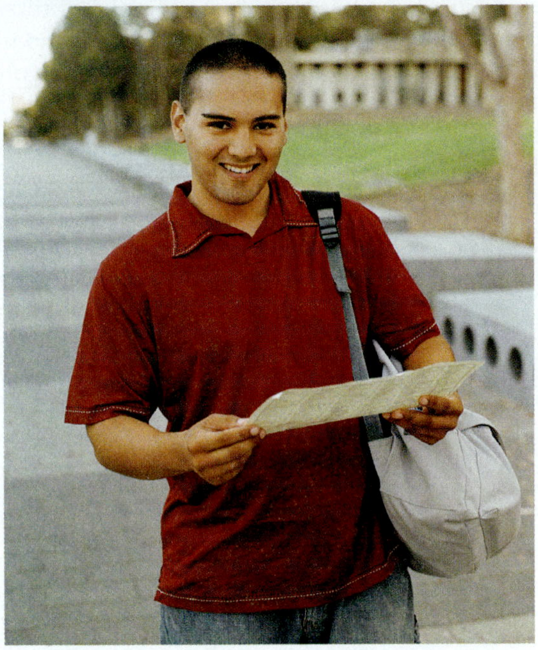

classroom requirements of the course of study. Internship usually refers to experiential education obtained prior to completion of classroom requirements of the course of study.

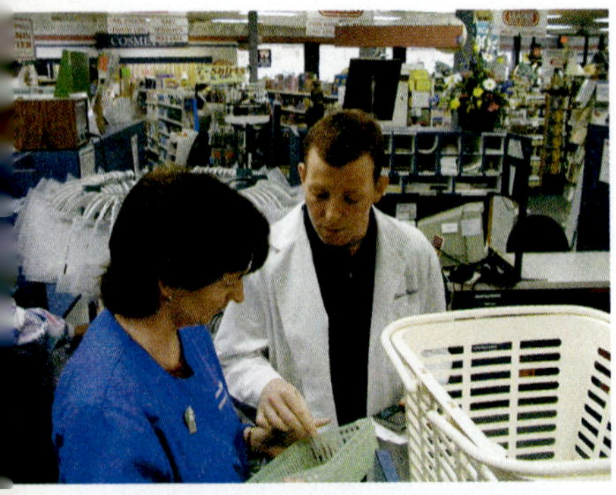

Figure 18-2 Student in externship facility.

externship Final component of a pharmacy technician program, consisting of experiential learning experiences that support the program objectives.

program director Individual responsible for the administration of the pharmacy technician program.

preceptor Pharmacist or pharmacy technician that supervises students on a daily basis during the externship.

clinical coordinator Individual responsible for organizing and facilitating experiential education.

Externship

Most pharmacy technician programs offer **externships** as the experiential education component. The externship is usually the final step in the completion of the pharmacy technician training program as it builds upon the knowledge and skills learned in didactic and laboratory courses. It allows the student to apply these tools in a "real-world" environment (Figure 18-2).

During the externship, the student demonstrates competencies outlined by ASHP and coordinated by the **program director** and the **preceptor** for a specified number of hours. The program director is responsible for the administration of the pharmacy technician program, and the preceptor is a pharmacist or pharmacy technician that supervises students on a daily basis during the externship. This training takes place in a pharmacy setting, whether community, hospital, or long-term care facility pharmacy. Depending upon the length of the pharmacy technician training program and state board of pharmacy regulations, the externship may consist of anywhere between 50 and 320 hours. The student is supervised by the preceptor on a daily basis and periodically by the program director or **clinical coordinator** (also referred to as externship coordinator). Each competency the student meets is signed off by the preceptor and verified by the program director. The student also completes time sheets that are signed by the preceptor.

Pharmacy settings used for the externship must be in compliance with federal and state laws and demonstrate high professional standards to qualify as appropriate training sites. Activities performed by the student in the externship must coincide with the educational goals of the technician training program. Although it is the responsibility of the preceptor to supervise the student, it is the student's responsibility to report any deficiency in meeting the standards and guidelines of the externship immediately to the program director.

It is important for the student to understand that the externship is an important final part of the pharmacy technician training program. It should not be considered "free labor" or optional. The pharmacy technician student should participate in the externship as if it is his or her job (being on time and professional) while reinforcing the concepts learned in the didactic and laboratory components of the technician program.

While some pharmacy technician training programs allow students to choose from a list of approved externship sites, others allow students to find sites to be approved later by the program director. Other programs place students in required sites for the externship portion of the program. The externship is an opportunity for the pharmacy technician student to practice knowledge and skills learned in the training program while developing professional skills and obtaining experience in a pharmacy. Programs may require that students obtain the majority of the externship hours in community and inpatient pharmacies while offering additional externship hours in other pharmacy settings (mail-order pharmacy, long-term care pharmacy, etc.). It is important that the pharmacy technician student know and understand the requirements of the training program as they relate to externships.

As the externship component of a program consists of educational training, all involved parties must keep documentation of the activities of the student at the training site. The student is responsible for meeting competencies during the required number of hours. The preceptor documents the activities and competencies met by the student and keeps a record of the number of hours the student spends at the externship. The student must be proactive, meaning being assertive when it comes to making certain that the competencies the students demonstrated are documented. In the practice of pharmacy, one often hears the saying, "If it is not documented, it did not happen." The student also keeps time sheets, identifying days and time periods spent in the pharmacy setting. Time sheets are to be completed on a regular basis. The student should not neglect or delay submitting time sheets. The program director may require that time sheets are submitted to the program on a weekly basis. Again, it is important for the student to know the requirements.

Expectations of Student Externship Candidates

The expectations of student externship candidates are numerous. The primary expectation is that the student, after learning about the practice of pharmacy and gaining skills employed by pharmacy technicians, is eager to hone those skills and become part of the health care professional community.

Professionalism

Professionalism is the quality of being a professional (positive, proactive, competent). Professionalism while on externship means that the student acts as if he or she is a pharmacy technician at work. It also means that the

professionalism The quality of being a professional (positive, proactive, competent).

opportunity to successfully complete the externship is taken seriously and as a positive step in the process of developing one's career.

Professionalism is demonstrated through arriving and leaving at the agreed upon times, being courteous to the patients and preceptor, using discretion when encountering problems or conflicts, and having a positive attitude with a strong work ethic. It also means performing one's work accurately and efficiently, paying attention to detail, maintaining a neat and orderly working space, and being willing to learn.

Professionalism should be reflected in one's appearance as well. The externship experience is not the occasion to explore fashion trends and it is wise to be conservative in dress. Clothes and lab coats are clean and pressed, hair is conservatively groomed, and jewelry and cosmetics are kept to a minimum. The technician student is wise to remember that he or she is an image of pharmacy technicians being represented to the public.

Attitude

Attitude is an intangible quality and although it cannot be touched, it can be seen. A poor attitude can destroy a professional image. One problem with a poor attitude is that it not only ruins the professional image of the person displaying this attitude, but also may reflect on the pharmacy setting in which the person is working.

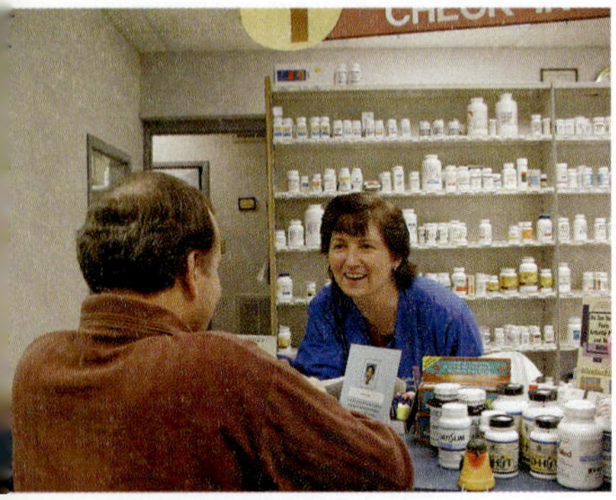

Figure 18-3 A positive attitude is part of being professional.

Some customers never return to a pharmacy where they were rudely addressed or ignored by only one person. On a larger scale, a poor attitude reflects poorly on the entire profession of pharmacy, and may cause the individuals we wish to serve to distrust or discredit the contributions of pharmacy professionals to health care. Remember, your attitude is showing when you greet a new customer, take a complaint, are corrected by the preceptor, work with other students and technicians, and deal with other professionals. Your attitude toward your work will dictate whether or not you will take the initiative and be a self-starter, or whether you will wait to be told to do tasks you routinely perform. Your attitude toward others will dictate whether or not you are perceived as a professional (Figure 18-3).

Professional Relationship

It is important to bear in mind that there might be an open position at your externship site and your preceptor may be considering whether or not to hire you as a technician once you complete your program. Even if the preceptor is not looking to fill any positions at this time, he or she may be able to provide you with a letter of reference or even refer you to another potential employer on an informal basis. In any case, the externship is often the initial professional contact the pharmacy technician student makes. It is wise to nurture and preserve this professional relationship.

Tech Check

1. What are the three components of technician training programs? (LO 18.1)
2. The externship is part of the _____ component of a pharmacy technician training program. (LO 18.1)
3. Describe the externship. (LO 18.1)

Finding a Position (LO 18.5)

After completing your training program, you will want to find a postition as a pharmacy technician. There are several ways of finding employment as a pharmacy technician.

Networking

Networking involves meeting pharmacists, pharmacy technicians, and potential employers at professional meetings, conferences, or events and becoming familiar with these individuals and their practice sites (Figure 18-4). It may be that a position is open, but it is through this social interaction that you may become aware of an employment opportunity. Again, professionalism is important, regardless of the setting, no matter how informal it may be. For example, you may meet a potential employer at a golf tournament that may be a fund-raiser for a worthy cause. Although you may be casually attired, a pleasant greeting with a firm handshake is appropriate.

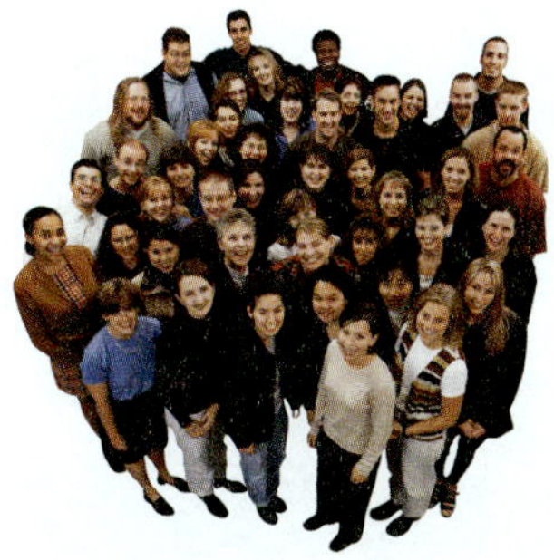

Figure 18-4 Networking may lead to employment.

Classifieds

Other means of finding positions include classified ads (either in print or electronic), employment agencies or services, and directly contacting a potential employer (Figure 18-5). With newspaper ads and advertisements on Web sites, it is important that the applicant read the ad carefully to determine if he or she qualifies for the position, and if so, what the preferred response to the ad is. Ads may ask that the interested applicant call, send a letter with a resume, fax a resume, or e-mail a resume. Read the instructions.

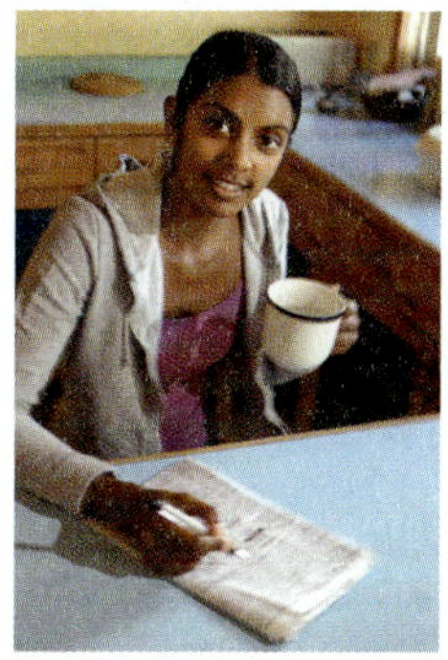

Figure 18-5 Classified ads list employment opportunities.

Employment Agencies

Employment agencies or services have a listing of available positions for the job applicant to review. It is important to note that employment agencies may have a "finder's fee" and benefit financially from your successful placement. A pharmacy technician may also find a position by accessing the Web site of a potential employer. Many company Web sites contain a link to employment opportunities.

Word of Mouth

Word of mouth is another way that pharmacy technicians can learn about employment opportunities. It is similar to networking, but tends to be much more informal. An example of word of mouth is that your friend went to a local pharmacy to pick up a prescription and mentioned that you just graduated from a pharmacy technician program. The pharmacist in charge then indicated that he may need another technician and is interested in hiring a new graduate.

Your Resume (LO 18.6)

Your **resume** is a professional document that consists of a listing of your education and employment history, and personal experiences that qualify your for employment. You should always keep your resume current. You should always be working on your resume, in one way or another.

networking Establishing and maintaining professional relationships with colleagues and others in one's discipline and related disciplines.

resume Professional document consisting of a listing of an individual's educational, work, and personal experiences qualifying that person for a job.

Resume Components

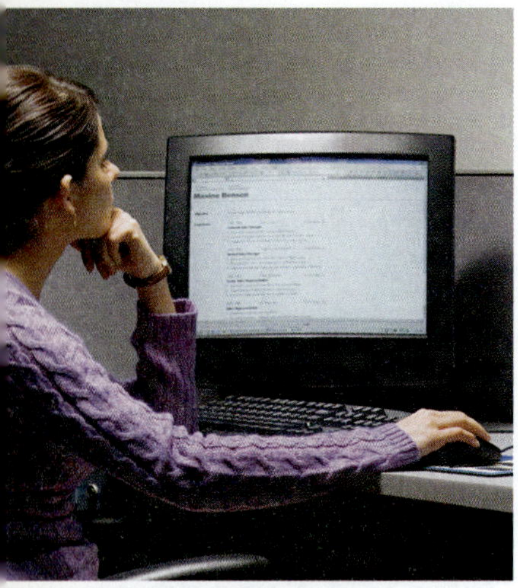

Figure 18-6 Completing an electronic resume

As you begin to work on your resume, remember that you are applying for a position as a pharmacy technician. Your resume should reflect your professionalism, accomplishments, and commitment to the profession. The basic components of a resume are listed in Table 18-1.

Some applicants may also wish to include a brief statement regarding a career objective including short term and long term goals, major qualifications, and professional information. Because your resume may be the first impression you provide to a prospective employer, it should show your strengths clearly. In other words, if you have just completed a pharmacy technician program, achieved high marks, and received an award but have little work experience, the education component of the resume should be listed first. If you have strong experience from your externship sites and have worked as a pharmacy clerk prior to completing your technician program, you may wish to list experience first.

Resume style should reflect the profession and the position for which you are seeking employment. Since the pharmacy profession is focused on patient care with accuracy and efficiency, your resume in hard-copy form should be printed in black ink on white or light-colored high-quality paper. Some job applicants may even wish to have the resume typeset and professionally printed. For electronic transmission of a resume, make certain you have saved a read-only copy using the type of software requested by the prospective employer (Figure 18-6). Regardless of the vehicle for the resume, the information should be accurate and the document should be free of spelling, grammatical, and typographical errors. In addition, the resume should be brief, at no more than one to two pages. If your resume is outstanding, you will have the opportunity to describe more about yourself in an interview. The content of your resume is limited to the facts.

Table 18-1 Basic Resume Components

Name and contact information of the applicant	State clearly at the top center of the first page.
Education	List in reverse chronological order (starting with the most recent educational experience and working backward). Identify degrees, diplomas, or certificates earned including the school or institution and the date.
Employment	As with education, in reverse chronological order list employers, positions held, duties, and specifies periods of employment.
License, registration, and certification	Identify license, registration, or certification status with corresponding dates.
Professional involvement	List involvement in pharmacy or other professional organizations while specifying periods of involvement.
Awards and honors	List awards and honors including the type of award, the granting agency, and the date of the award.
References	List individuals who have already agreed to provide a reference for you, with their contact information. Or, use the following statement: "References available upon request."

Figure 18-7 **Sample resume.**

Annie B. Public
123 Market Street
Localtown, Anystate
(999)555-5555
abpublic@email.com

Career Objective:	To work as a pharmacy technician in an inpatient pharmacy setting and assist with the training of pharmacy technician students during their externships.
Major Qualifications:	Graduate of XYZ Pharmacy Technician Program; possess state registration and national certification
Education:	XYZ Pharmacy Technician Program, 2005–2006 Diploma — August 2006 City High School 2002–2005 High School Diploma — June 2005
Experience:	Nice Store, Stock Clerk 2004–present Duties: stock shelves, manag inventory on a part-time basis
Licensure:	Anystate registration: TCH 0000 October 2006 PTCB Certification: CPhT XXX November 2006
Professional Involvement:	Anystate Pharmacists Association, Technician Division, member since 2006
Awards:	Student Service to the Community Award Anystate Pharmacists Association, Technician Division, May 2006
References:	Simon Pharmacist, Pharm.D., Director XYZ Pharmacy Technician Program Susie Storeowner Owner Nice Store Inc. Samuel Leader, RPh, President Anystate Pharmacists Association

Basic tips to writing a resume are:

- Refrain from embellishing your document to make you seem like a better applicant. Resumes are frequently verified.
- Correct any grammatical, spelling, or typographical errors
- Clearly state accomplishments.
- Keep it simple and brief.
- Use bold print for headings and indent for specification.
- Keep style consistent.

After completing your resume, ask yourself, "Would I hire this person? Why or why not?" See Figure 18-7 for a sample resume.

Tech Check

4. List basic components of a resume. (LO 18.6)
5. Education and employment are listed in ________. (LO 18.6)

The Application Process (LO 18.5, 18.6)

Your Cover Letter

When sending a resume to a prospective employer, it is appropriate to include a cover letter to introduce yourself and describe your interest in a position. A cover letter is also an opportunity to indicate your interest, enthusiasm, and commitment to the profession of pharmacy and how these qualities contribute to making you a qualified candidate for the position, whereas the resume is a document based solely upon facts.

The cover letter should be printed on the same high-quality paper as the resume, using similar fonts and style. If a prospective employer requests a faxed resume, include a fax cover sheet identifying the person or department for whom the document is intended with a cover letter followed by the resume. When the employer requests an electronic (or e-mail) transmission of a resume, include a cover letter and resume as attachments to a brief e-mail message. Unless the employer specifically states that a cover letter not be sent, include a cover letter.

If you are applying for multiple positions at different organizations, each cover letter should be specific to the position and the employer. It is appropriate to address the letter to a specific individual (if one is indicated in the advertisement) or to the holder of a position identified in the advertisement (for example, the Director of Human Resources).

The cover letter should:

1. Identify the purpose for the letter.
2. Indicate how the applicant's educational, experiential, and personal attributes contribute to making the person a good candidate for the job.
3. Request some action from the employer; for example, a request for an interview or future contact.

It is important to include your contact information in the cover letter, as well as in the resume, in case the two documents are separated during review. See Figure 18-8 for a sample cover letter format.

Distributing a Resume

A resume may be distributed in person, by mail, by fax, or by e-mail. Each method requires professionalism on the part of the applicant. For example, if you are attending a job fair, it is wise to have copies of your resume available; although you may not have a cover letter, have a large envelope or folder in which to place your resume prior to handing it to the prospective employer. Likewise, when mailing your resume and cover letter, use a large envelope so that you do not need to fold your documents. When mailing, make certain you have included sufficient postage for delivery of your document. Fax transmission is a quick method by which documents are

Figure 18-8 Cover letter format.

Your Street Address
City, State, Zip Code

Date

Name of person to whom you are writing
Title
Company or Organization
Street Address
City, State, Zip Code

Dear Dr., Mr., Mrs., Miss, or Ms. ____________:

1st Paragraph: Tell why you are writing. Name the position or general area of work that interests you. Mention how you learned about the job opening. State why you are interested in the job.

2nd Paragraph:Refer to the enclosed (or attached if e-mailing) resume and give some background information Indicate why you should be considered as a candidate, focusing on how your skills can fulfill the needs of the company. Relate your experiences to the company's needs and mention results and achievements. Do not restate what is said on your resume—you want to pull together all the information and tell how your background fits the position.

3rd Paragraph: Close by making a specific request for an interview. Say that you will follow up with a phone call to arrange a mutually convenient interview time. Offer to provide any additional information that may be needed. Thank the employer for his or her time and consideration.

Sincerely,

(your handwritten signature if not e-mailing)

Type your name

Enclosure

transferred. Make certain you include a fax cover sheet, your cover letter, and your resume when faxing documents. You may wish to call the recipient immediately prior to faxing the document or immediately after to ensure receipt of letter and resume. For e-mail transmission, attach the cover letter and resume to a brief e-mail message. Be certain you have complied with the electronic format requests from the prospective employer.

Your Personal Portfolio

Your personal portfolio is a record of all of your professional accomplishments and activities. It is important to maintain this collection of documents because it serves as documentation of your commitment to the profession and supports the information contained within your resume. Your portfolio will expand as you mature in your career as a pharmacy technician. It will need to be updated and kept current accordingly. A personal portfolio includes, but is not limited to:

- Resume
- Diplomas and certificates
- Copies of your licenses, registrations, and certification
- Proof of membership in professional organizations
- Copies of letters of recommendation
- Copies of letters of appreciation or acknowledgment of service
- Certificates of completion for continuing education
- Proof of community service and or volunteerism

Tech Check

6. What is the name of the document that should accompany a resume? (LO 18.5, 18.6)

7. What is one way to ensure receipt of your faxed cover letter and resume? (LO 18.5)

8. What is the purpose of the personal portfolio? (LO 18.5)

Pre-Employment Requirements (LO 18.7)

Proof of State Registration or Licensure

Prior to being employed as a pharmacy technician, you will need to show proof that you are registered or licensed as a technician in your state and/or provide proof of certification. The processes for registration and certification should be initiated prior to your search for employment. If you find yourself in the position of being offered a position prior to obtaining registration and certification, be honest with the prospective employer and let him or her know where you are in the process. Refer to your state board of pharmacy for state requirements for registration or licensure, accessible at **www.nabp.org.**

Successful completion of the Pharmacy Technician Certification Examination (PTCE) provides for certification and the use of the credential CPhT after the certified technician's name. The PTCB certified technician must complete 20 hours of continuing education in each certification period to maintain certified status. For more information on certification, see Chapter 19 or go to **www.ptcb.org.** The National Center for Competency Testing (NCCT) also provides an examination for certification of pharmacy technicians and the use of the credential NCPhT after the certified technician's name. NCCT offers examinations for certification of other health care professionals as well. For more information about NCCT, access **www.ncctinc.com.**

Completing the Application Form

After you have submitted your resume and cover letter, you may need to go through a process at the institution's human resources department. One component of the process is that you may be asked to complete a job application (Figure 18-9).

This is a legal document that is signed and dated by you attesting to the accuracy of your statements. As with your resume, be truthful. Do not leave any section blank. Indicate "N/A" or "not applicable" if an area does not apply to you. Ask questions if you are unclear as to the meaning of a particular question. Prior to submitting this document, make sure you make a copy for your records. You may also need to complete other documents including health history, allowing background and credit checks, and providing emergency contact information.

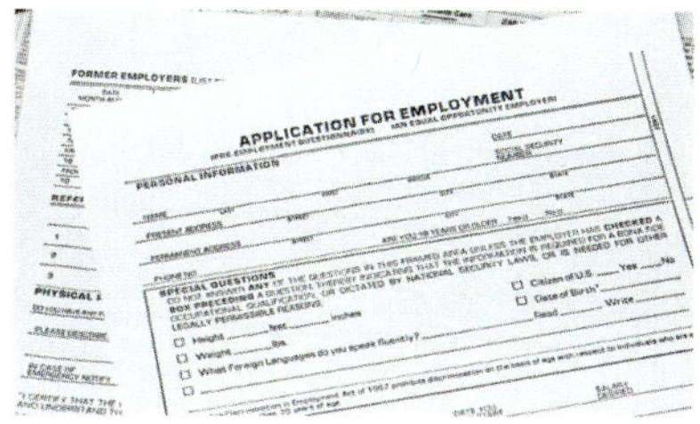

Figure 18-9 Application form.

Drug Screening

Drug screening is routinely required in pharmacy positions due to access to pharmaceutical agents. It is important for you to state and provide documentation of any medications you are taking or have taken recently prior to the drug test. Many individuals have lost potential positions as a result of failing a drug screening test.

Physical Exam

Many employers also require a pre-employment physical exam. This exam may not consist of a complete physical. It may be closer to an assessment including checking vital signs and taking a complete medical history by a physician assistant, nurse practitioner, or nurse. Depending upon the setting, the pharmacy technician applicant may be requested to provide his or her immunization record. As a job applicant, it is your responsibility to be aware of the pre-employment requirements of the employer.

Interviewing

Although resume submission, the human resources process, and interviewing may occur in various sequences, it is rare that an individual is hired without an interview.

Strong interviewing skills contribute to success in obtaining employment positions (Figure 18-10). If you are asked for an interview after the prospective employer has had an opportunity to review your resume, remember that this is your chance to make a positive impact on your chances of securing employment. Depending upon the organization and its structure,

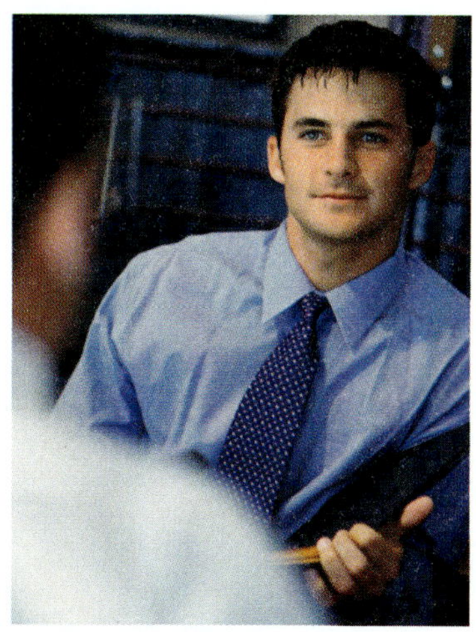

Figure 18-10 Interviewing.

you may be called for multiple interviews, panel interviews, and/or one-on-one interviews. You must always present a professional image when meeting anyone in the company where you are seeking employment.

When preparing for an interview, do some research on the prospective employer's organization. It is not advisable to memorize everything you can about the organization, but it is helpful to know key facts about the organization to identify how you in your proposed role could contribute to the success of the employer. You may wish to access the company's Web site, if it has one, to find information about the organization's history, mission, milestones, and accomplishments. Spend time thinking about how you would contribute to the mission and focus of the employer.

To continue to prepare for your interview, rehearse answers to questions you are likely to be asked. You are likely to address items similar to the following:

- "Why did you choose a career as a pharmacy technician?"
- "Why did you apply for this position at our pharmacy?"
- "Where do you see yourself in 5 years?"
- "Identify your three strengths and weaknesses."
- "How would you describe your working style?"
- "What was your most challenging work experience, and how did you handle it?"

You may wish to write down some of these questions and address them using two or three bullet points. Although you will have thought about and rehearsed your answers, during the interview, try not to sound as if you memorized the answers to the questions. Be aware that there are some questions that are inappropriate for the interviewer to ask you. Questions regarding religious, racial, and ethnic background are inappropriate, as well as questions relating to age, marital status, parenthood, and sexual orientation.

Prior to your interview, write down a few questions you would like to ask your prospective employer. Writing questions ahead of time contributes to clear development of thought and will enable you to articulate your questions clearly. Acceptable questions include:

- "How do you see the role of pharmacy technicians in this pharmacy?"
- "What are your expectations of leadership by pharmacy technicians?"
- "What qualities characterize the successful employee in your organization?"
- "What benefits do you provide?"

Enlist the help of a classmate or friend to do a "mock" interview (Figure 18-11). It is helpful to get feedback prior to the real event.

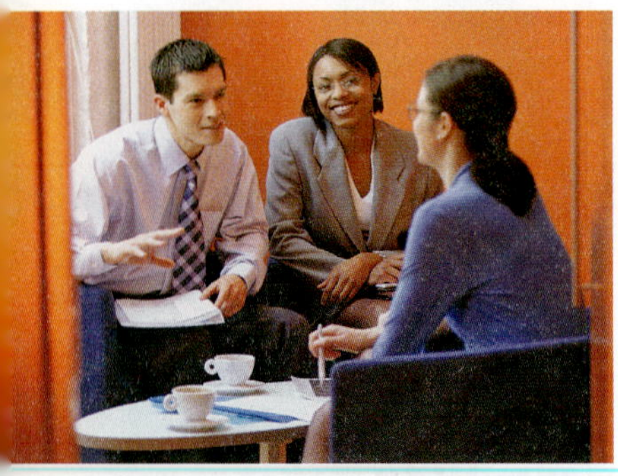

Figure 18-11 Mock interview.

You may also wish to speak your responses aloud while looking in a mirror to have an idea of what your interviewer might see.

Reviewing the previous items will help you mentally prepare for your interview. Remember, this is your big opportunity to present yourself as a professional.

All of these skills involve mental preparation for your interview. Now the focus turns to physical preparation.

- Start early.
- Wear clean and ironed conservative clothing. A dark sport coat or suit and a conservative tie with a white or light shirt project a professional

image for male applicants. Female applicants as well should dress conservatively, avoiding fashion extremes.

- Practice good hygiene and keep colognes, perfumes, and other cosmetics to a minimum.
- Do not chew gum.
- Because your focus is on projecting a professional appearance, cover any tattoos as well as multiple piercings.
- Remember, as always, show a positive attitude.
- Arrive at your interview appointment 10 to 15 minutes early, this gives you time to complete an employment application if requested. Bring a few extra copies of your resume in an envelope or folder.

When greeting your interviewer or interviewers, establish eye contact and offer to shake hands (Figure 18-12).

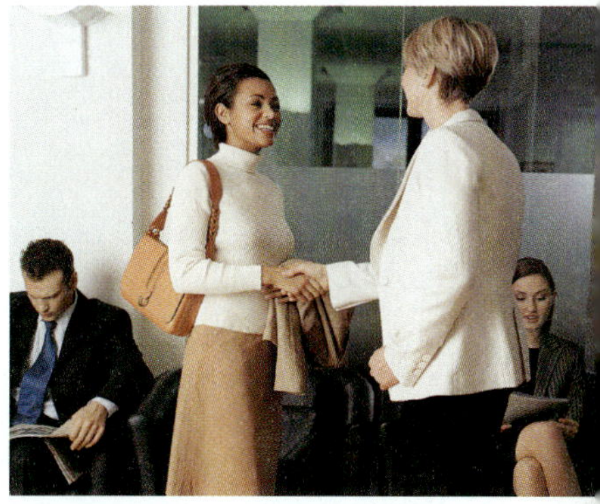

Figure 8-12 **Eye contact, hand shake, and smile.**

Be pleasant and smile, and try to appear relaxed. If you are nervous, you may wish to mention it in a positive way to diffuse the tension. After being asked a question, pause briefly to think about your answer, respond thoughtfully, and speak clearly. Keep in mind that your responses should match your expressions. For example, if you are asked what you would do in the event that you discovered that your coworker was stealing, do not smile while answering the question.

Usually, in an initial interview, the prospective applicant will not ask directly about salary, but you may wish to use your own discretion. It may already be published in the advertisement or in the job description. If you are called for a second interview, it may be appropriate at that time to ask about salary range and benefits packages. Benefits are a component of compensation and include sick leave, paid holidays, health insurance, life insurance, and retirement plans. Before leaving your interview, be certain to thank the interviewer (or interviewers) for taking time to meet with you. Occasionally, the interviewer will indicate how and when you will be notified of the final decision. This may be good final question for you to ask your interviewer if the information is not offered.

After your interview, you may receive a call or a letter indicating that you are hired. Congratulations! On the other hand, it may be the case that although you were very well prepared for your interview and presented a professional image, you were not hired. It is critical that the experience is not viewed as a failure but as an opportunity to build your skills and apply for other positions. It is possible that there was a freeze on hiring, or that you were competing with many other applicants for the position, or that the employer was looking for someone with more experience. It could also be that although you might have had all of the qualifications, you may not have been a good "fit" for the organization. Do not be discouraged. Although you may not have gotten the job, you still have the chance to increase your visibility as a professional. It is appropriate to send a letter to thank the employer for the opportunity for an interview. Doing so may result in the employer calling you for the next open position or recommending you to someone else when a position opens at another pharmacy. Remember, you are building the foundation for your career with every contact. Make the most of it.

Pharmacy technician students must consider that every aspect of the training program is preparation for a career. This is most evident in the externship phase of education, where the pharmacy technician student has the opportunity to learn in the real world. The externship may also be the first networking experience, which may lead to future employment.

Professionalism is the common thread through resume writing, interviewing, and networking to contribute to the pharmacy technician's success.

Tech Check

9. Aside from submitting a resume, what other items may be required prior to employment? (LO 18.7)

10. What are some things a pharmacy technician should not do during an interview? (LO 18.8)

Chapter Summary

Understanding how to prepare for a career is vital to the pharmacy technician student. Important points to remember are:

- The externship experience is significant to the pharmacy technician student as it is a curricular component of the educational program and is preparation for entering the workforce.
- Professionalism is reflected in one's attitude, dress, interpersonal interactions, and work.
- While on the externship experience, the pharmacy technician should behave as if it were his or her job.
- It is the pharmacy technician student's responsibility to ensure that all hours at the externship site are properly recorded and communicated to the program director.
- Although registration requirements of state boards of pharmacy vary, requirements for obtaining and retaining national certification are consistent throughout the United States.
- The resume should be neat, accurate, complete, and printed on high-quality white paper.
- The cover letter should accompany the resume to provide the potential employer with additional information related to the applicant's qualifications for the position.
- Pre-employment requirements may include drug screening, physical examination, and completion of an application form.
- Positive interviewing strategies for the job applicant include arriving early, being professionally attired, maintaining eye contact, and presenting a professional image.

Chapter Review

Case Study Question

1. What should Mary do in this situation? (LO 18.3)

At Your Service Questions

1. What should Joshua do first? (LO 18.5)
2. Assuming he is called for an interview, how should he prepare for the interview? (LO 18.8)

Multiple Choice

Select the best answer.

1. Pharmacy technicians obtain experiential training primarily in the_______ of the pharmacy technician program. (LO 18.1)
   a. didactic courses
   b. laboratory courses
   c. externship
   d. none of the above
2. The accrediting body for pharmacy technician programs is the _______ (LO 18.1)
   a. Food and Drug Administration.
   b. Pharmacy Technician Certification Board.
   c. American Pharmacist Association.
   d. American Society of Health-System Pharmacists.
3. Networking involves _____ (LO 18.5)
   a. meeting colleagues.
   b. participating in professional events.
   c. meeting potential employers.
   d. all of the above.
4. Which of the following displays professionalism? (LO 18.2, 18.3)
   a. Asking your preceptor about your progress
   b. Arriving on time 90% of the time
   c. Matching wits with your preceptor
   d. Submitting your time sheets before the time is worked
5. Which of the following is a component of the resume? (LO 18.6)
   a. Health history
   b. Education
   c. Salary
   d. Introduction
6. Which of the following is included in a cover letter? (LO 18.5, 18.6)
   a. Registration card numbers
   b. Resume
   c. Salary requirements
   d. Introduction
7. Which of the following is *not* a part of the personal portfolio? (LO 18.5)
   a. Resume
   b. Letters of recommendation
   c. Immunization records
   d. Copy of registration card
8. Which of the following should a pharmacy technician do to prepare for an interview? (LO 18.8)
   a. Research the prospective employer organization
   b. Determine responses to appropriate interview questions
   c. Draft a few questions to ask the interviewer
   d. All of the above
9. Which of the following should be brought to the interview? (LO 18.8)
   a. Cell phone
   b. Extra copies of the resume
   c. Immunization records
   d. Chewing gum
10. Which of the following is *not* appropriate during an interview? (LO 18.8)
    a. Maintaining eye contact
    b. Responding to questions clearly
    c. Identifying future career goals
    d. Attempting to entertain the interviewers

Critical Thinking Questions

1. Imagine you are an employer looking to hire a new pharmacy technician. What qualities would you value in a prospective employee? What qualities would you consider undesirable? Why? (LO 18.2, 18.3)
2. What are qualities you possess that make you a good pharmacy technician extern? What specific skills do you want to develop or improve upon? How can you assist the preceptor and program director in making your externship experience more valuable? (LO 18.1, 18.2, 18.3)
3. In what ways can pharmacy technician students increase the professional status of pharmacy technicians? What specific activities may increase community awareness of the role of pharmacists and pharmacy technicians? (LO 18.2)
4. What can pharmacy technicians students do to get the most out the externship experiences? (LO 18.1, 18.2, 18.3)

HIPAA Scenario

Larry Rowles is the owner of a small independent pharmacy. His employee health care expenses are outrageous, and he is considering reducing medical benefits. At the same time, Larry is attempting to hire new technicians in preparation for an expansion.

Jason Johnson is an excellent technician who is looking for employment. He also has a chronic illness and must secure employment soon or risk losing valuable health care benefits. After interviewing Jason, Larry wants to hire him. However, prior to offering Jason a job, Larry has a contact at the insurance company run a "check" on Jason. He discovers his ongoing treatment for a chronic illness and decides he cannot afford to provide Jason health care coverage. He does not offer Jason the job.

Discussion Questions (PTCB II. 73)

1. What violations of HIPAA did Larry commit?
2. Is he guilty of an ethical violation as well?

Internet Activities

1. Go to **www.careerpharm.com** or **www.monster.com.** Type in the key words "pharmacy technician." Print out three job announcements and bring them to class for presentation and discussion. Identify the job you find most desirable, and list the steps you would take to pursue that employment opportunity. (LO 18.5)
2. Go to the American Society of Health-System Pharmacists Web site at **www.ashp.org.** Click on "Technician" and go to the chronology. Identify for the class three key events you believe contributed to increasing the professional status of pharmacy technicians. (LO 18.2)

Career Development

19

Learning Outcomes

Upon completion of this chapter, you will be able to:

19.1 Identify stress management strategies.

19.2 Identify time management strategies.

19.3 Describe the role of the employee evaluation in career development.

19.4 Differentiate between certification and registration.

19.5 Describe the role of continuing education in the maintenance of professional status.

19.6 List pharmacy organizations and describe their purposes.

Key Terms

certification
continuing education
employee evaluation
orientation
probation

PTCB

In preparation for the certification examination, you should understand and perform activities associated with the following PTCB Knowledge Statement:

PTCB Knowledge Statement

Domain III. Participating in the Administration and Management of Pharmacy Practice

Knowledge of required operational licenses and certificates (6)

Knowledge of employee performance evaluation (37)

Case Study

Mike, CPhT, has recently been hired as a pharmacy technician at JK Drug Store. Mike was thrilled to get this position because he was aware that five other technicians applied for the same job and he was the only one hired. The store is very busy and Mike finds that he sometimes feels stressed when there are so many things to handle at once. Mike has been working at the store for 3 weeks. Yesterday, the lead pharmacy technician broke his arm at home, and called to say he will be out for a few weeks. The pharmacist in charge told Mike that he will have to "pick up the slack" in the meantime. Mike is now worried as he is a new employee and is still learning about working in the store.

While reading this chapter, keep the following questions in mind:

1. How can Mike handle this situation professionally?(LO 19.1, 19.2)
2. What should he not do?(LO 19.1, 19.2)
3. What would you do if you were Mike?(LO 19.1, 19.2)

Introduction to Career Development

Your first position as a pharmacy technician is an important one because it will be the experience by which you benchmark all future pharmacy-related jobs and experiences. As in any field, it is unlikely that anyone starts at the top. However, this is only the beginning of developing your career as a pharmacy technician. This chapter will acquaint you with various aspects of career development including handling on-the-job issues, maintaining registration and **certification,** and being involved in professional organizations.

On the Job(LO 19.3)

You have reached a milestone in obtaining your new position. You have completed the **orientation** through human resources and are now an employee. As you begin work, you are excited to have this new opportunity and (finally) a paycheck! Your position may also include benefits like health insurance, life insurance, vacation time, sick pay, personal holidays, and paid holidays. You will want to keep your position since you have invested much time and energy to earn it.

Professionalism may contribute to job security. The better employee you are, the less likely you are to be laid off or fired. It is possible to be "let go" due to downsizing, but as this is something you do not have control over, it is wise to maintain your connection to other pharmacy professionals through networking and involvement in professional organizations.

A large part of professionalism is responsibility. A good pharmacy technician arrives at work on time, completes assigned tasks, provides excellent customer service, and works as a team member with the pharmacist. As a member of a team your work, or lack of work, affects the entire team. For example, although sick time is a benefit, it is not to be used if you are not sick and just want to take a day off. If you are experiencing difficulties at work, it is best to attempt to resolve conflict

certification Proof of knowledge and competence.

orientation The process of educating the new hire about the company and area of work.

At Your Service

Aimee has been working for a mail-order pharmacy for the past 3 years. She likes her job, although she is sometimes bored. Sometimes she has to stay an extra 10 or 15 minutes because she wants to leave things neat and orderly for the next shift. Because she stays late, she routinely comes to work 10 to 15 minutes late.

Last week, Aimee's supervisor reprimanded her for being frequently late and not finishing her work in a timely manner. Aimee is thinking of quitting because she thinks her supervisor is being unfair.

While reading this chapter, keep the following questions in mind:

1. Is Aimee's supervisor being unfair?(LO 19.3)
2. How might this situation have been avoided?(LO 19.2)
3. What is Aimee's responsibility as an employee?(LO 19.2)

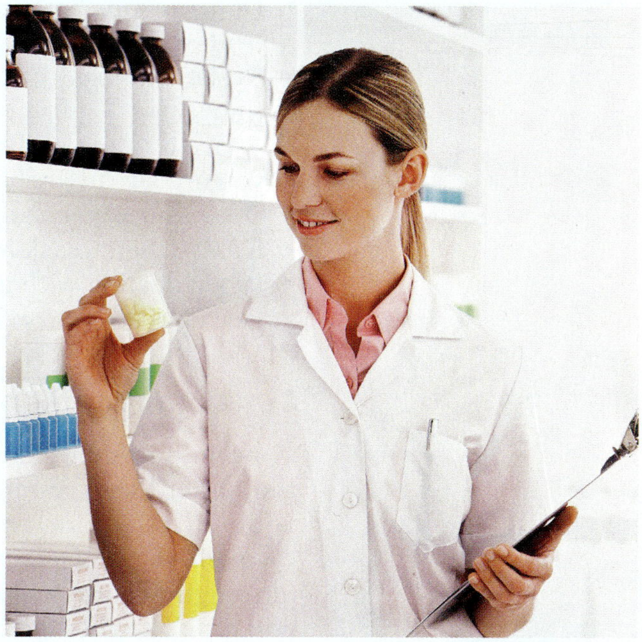

through open communication. If you are actually sick or are experiencing an emergency or delay, contact your supervisor as soon as possible. If you wish to leave your position of employment, provide your supervisor with at least 2 weeks written notice. Do not simply stop coming to work. Unprofessional behavior will be noted and may haunt you when seeking future positions.

As a pharmacy technician, your responsibilities of assisting the pharmacist with prescription processing, insurance billing, and inventory management are combined with another major responsibility—providing customer service. In the field of pharmacy our patients are our customers. Pharmacy technicians are the "front line," or seen first by customers in the pharmacy. It may be a challenge in a busy store to answer phones, process prescriptions, accept inventory orders, and provide efficient and courteous service. In an inpatient setting, it may be a challenge to process medication orders, deliver medications to the floors, and be courteous to other health care professionals with whom you have contact. The pharmacy technician who is able to manage time and stress effectively will be more productive in any pharmacy setting.

Stress Management

Managing stress is critical to working efficiently in any work environment. Effectively managing stress not only increases efficiency, but also helps maintain professionalism in the pharmacy setting (Figure 19-1). Pharmacy technicians who manage stress are able to maintain good working

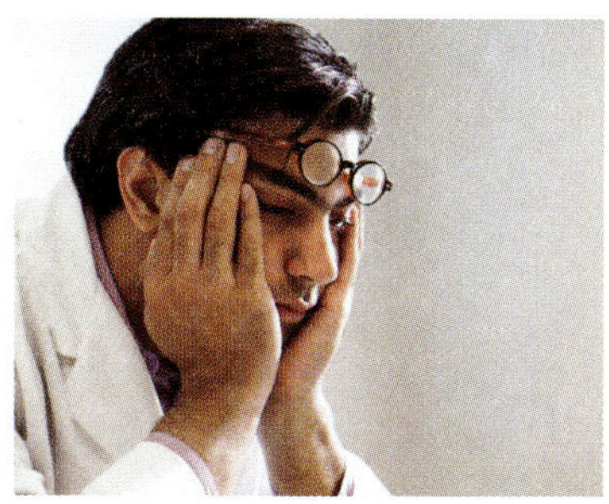

Figure 19-1 Stress management helps maintain professionalism.

relationships with their coworkers and provide customer service to patients. Several keys to stress management are:

- Know your job. Clearly understand your responsibilities and duties.
- Do your job. Procrastinating and neglecting duties lead to reprimands from your supervisor and complaints from the customers.
- Resist the urge to take on too much too soon. You cannot do everything.
- Arrive on time and be ready to work. Coming in late increases stress as you are already behind as you start the day.
- Take your breaks and lunch periods.
- Know when to ask for help.
- When dealing with a difficult or angry patient, remember to provide service as best you can but consider referring the person to the pharmacist.

Time Management

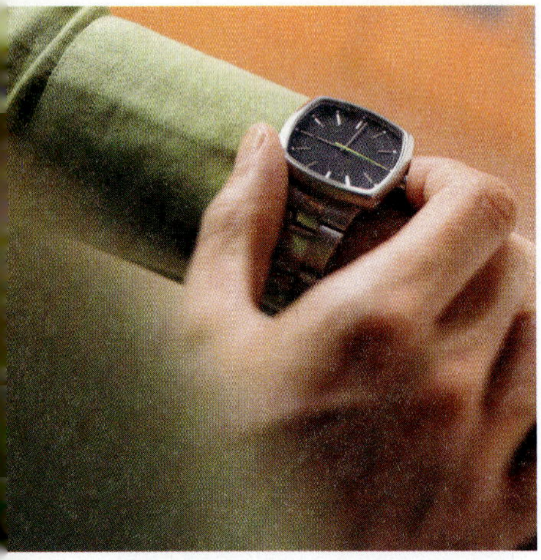

Figure 19-2 **Time management can reduce stress.**

Time management may contribute to stress management. In other words, the better you are at managing time in the pharmacy, the more stress you may relieve or avoid at work (Figure 19-2). As you have progressed through the pharmacy technician program, you will have noticed that although accuracy is emphasized, efficiency in performing tasks is encouraged. This is the reason that tablets and capsules are usually counted by fives and not one at a time. This is also why typing 35 to 40 words per minute is a requirement for being hired in many pharmacies. Rushing is not the answer, because you may be more prone to make errors. Working efficiently means effective work is performed using a minimal amount of time. Getting work done accurately and quickly is a good quality for any pharmacy technician to possess.

How time is managed may vary from one pharmacy to another depending upon the division of labor and the type of pharmacy setting. Technicians working in pharmacies with few personnel will have to manage time more effectively than technicians working in busy stores that are well staffed. Although somewhat similar to the points for stress management, the following are keys to time management:

- Be on time. Starting late eliminates some of the time you have to perform your job.
- Pace yourself. Trying to do everything at once leads to disaster. Also, do not spend an inordinate amount of time doing one thing.
- Focus. Start a task and follow it through to completion. Time is wasted when the technician has multiple unfinished tasks.
- Plan how you use your time. In some stores, lunchtime is very busy. In other settings, first thing in the morning is the busiest time. Free yourself by doing other tasks, like processing refills, before or after this busy period.
- Do not waste time. If it is "slow" (not busy) in the pharmacy, use the time to check for expired medications on the shelf, follow-up on will-call items, and so on.
- Take your breaks and lunch periods. If you are tired and hungry, you will not be able to work as efficiently.
- Prioritize. Perform the most critical tasks first.

These are some methods of managing time and stress. Stress management and time management are necessary in every area of life. If there is a lack of stress and/or time management in other parts of your life, it may impact your professional life. Other resources for stress management and time management include:

- Blonna, R. *Coping with Stress in a Changing World,* 4th ed., 2007. ISBN: 978073026602
- Colbert, Bruce J. *Navigating Your Future: An Interactive Journey to Personal and Academic Success,* 2009. ISBN: 9780131960848
- Greenberg, JS. *Your Personal Stress Profile and Activity Workbook,* 4th ed., 2006. ISBN: 9780073106755
- Lamberton, L, Minor-Evans, L. *Human Relations: Strategies for Success,* 3rd ed., 2006. ISBN: 9780073522319
- Mancini, M. *Time Management,* 2003. ISBN: 7780071406109
- Yena, DJ. *Career directions,* 4th ed., 2007. ISBN: 9780073123141
- Zeigler, K. *Getting Organized at Work: 24 Lessons to Set Goals, Establish Priorities, and Manage Your Time,* 2005. ISBN: 9780071457798

Employee Evaluations

Employee evaluations, sometimes called performance appraisals, are used to assess an employee's work performance. The employee evaluation is an important tool to help an employee do a better job and to improve the organization through clearly communicated expectations to employees. Although employee evaluations are usually performed on an annual basis, employees may be evaluated after a few weeks or months on the job following a **probation** period. Employee evaluations involve more than just the completion of a form.

There are three phases to an employee evaluation: planning, feedback, and assessment. Items included in the employee evaluation may be taken from the job description the employee received when hired for the position. The employee evaluation contains aspects of the employee's conduct that can be measured. It is wise to discuss components of the assessment with your employer to get input on how you might improve your performance. The employee evaluation form is completed by the employee's immediate supervisor. After the form is completed, the supervisor presents the completed evaluation form to the employee for feedback and comment (Figure 19-3). The employee then signs the form and retains a copy for his or her record. A copy is also kept in the employee's work record.

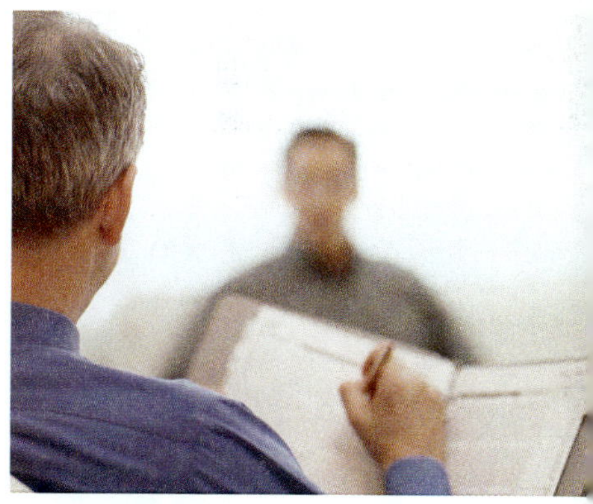

Figure 19-3 Employee evaluation.

Evaluations should be taken seriously as they may affect whether an employee retains his or her position, gets a raise, or gets a promotion. It becomes part of the permanent employee's work record. A sample of an employee evaluation form is included in Figure 19-4.

Tech Check

1. Identify three ways to help manage stress.(LO 19.1)
2. Identify three ways to manage time.(LO 19.2)
3. What is another term for employee evaluation?(LO 19.3)

employee evaluation Periodic review of work performance, also known as performance appraisal.

probation Trial period that often must be completed prior to permanent hiring.

Figure 19-4 Sample employee evaluation.

QRS Pharmacy Employee Evaluation

Employee Last Name	First Name	Middle Initial
Title		Date
From	To	

Period covered by evaluation

[ ] Initial [ ] Annual [ ] Transfer [ ] Other

Reason for this evaluation

Name of Supervisor

QRS Pharmacy Employee Evaluation Program provides the opportunity for the supervisor and employee to participate in work performance evaluation. The form assists supervisors in determining whether to continue employment, raise salaries, or promote employees.

Procedures:

1. Employee is informed by the supervisor of a pending employee evaluation.
2. Supervisor prepares the evaluation using the job description.
3. Supervisor reviews evaluation with employee allowing for employee comment within three (3) days.
4. Final evaluation is completed by the supervisor. Both the supervisor and the employee must sign the final evaluation.
5. Supervisor must keep one copy of the signed evaluation in the employee's file, and provide employee with a copy for his/her records.

QRS Pharmacy Employee Evaluation

3	2	1	N/A	Competency
				Completes tasks with accuracy and efficiency
				Organizes and plans work
				Prioritizes tasks appropriately

3	2	1	N/A	Initiative
				Works effectively as a member of the team
				Completes assignments independently
				Offers assistance when available

3	2	1	N/A	Safety
				Maintains equipment according to policies
				Monitors pharmacy for possible hazards
				Appropriately uses Personal Protective Equipment

3	2	1	N/A	Other
				Reports to work on-time
				Adheres to policies and procedures
				Meets customer expectations

3 = Above Average; 2 = Average; 1 = Below Average; N/A = Not Applicable

Identify areas needing improvement including agreed upon actions to be taken to achieve improvement.

In previous appraisal period, what areas were identified as needing improvement, and what progress has been made?

Overall, employee :
( ) Exceeds expectations
( ) Meets expectations
( ) Partially meets expectations
( ) Does not meet expectations.

Employee Signature ____________ Date ____________

Supervisor Signature ____________ Date ____________

Continuing Education (LO 19.4, 19.5)

As newer agents are approved, newer techniques are developed, and innovative ways to manage common diseases are designed, pharmacy technicians need to obtain continuing education to keep their practice current with emerging trends. **Continuing education** is also a requirement to maintain certification. Continuing education is measured in hours or in units.

For example, 1 hour of continuing education is equivalent to 0.1 CEU (continuing education unit). Continuing education units are available at professional meetings or conferences, at the worksite in larger health care facilities, in professional journals, through pharmaceutical company sponsored presentations, and on the Internet (Figure 19-5). Some boards of pharmacy offer continuing education for attending a board meeting. Check your state board of pharmacy for more information.

Several Web sites offering continuing education to pharmacy technicians include:

- American Society of Health-System Pharmacists: **www.ashp.org**
- Free Online Education for the Healthcare Profession: **www.freece.com**
- PharmaCE: **www.pharmace.com**
- Pharmacy Choice: **www.pharmacychoice.com**
- Pharmacy Now: **www.pharmacynow.com**
- National Pharmacy Technician Association: **www.pharmacytechnician.org**

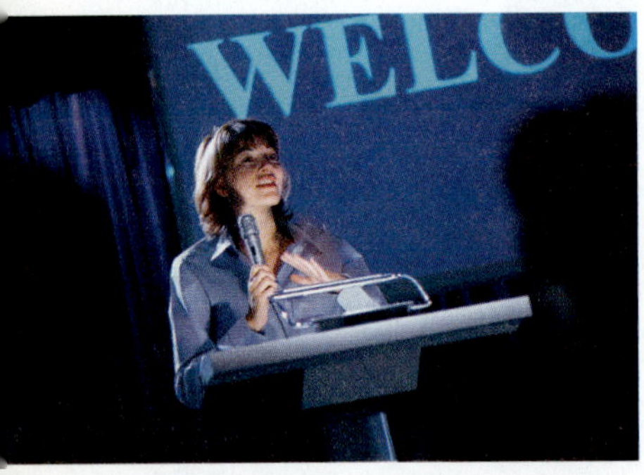

Figure 19-5 Continuing education credits may be earned by attending a professional conference.

continuing education Coursework or study to keep the pharmacy technician current in practice; may be required to maintain certification, licensure, and/or registration.

- Powerpak C.E.: **www.powerpak.com**
- Rxinsider.com: **www.rxinsider.com**
- U.S. Pharmacist: **www.uspharmacist.com**

The Accreditation Council for Pharmacy Education (ACPE) accredits its continuing education providers. It is important to look for the ACPE logo when considering a continuing education program. Providers not indicating ACPE accreditation may offer continuing education, but it may not be recognized by the certification agency.

Certification

National certification is achieved through successful completion of knowledge- and competency-based examinations (Figure 19-6). One method of certification is through taking the Pharmacy Technician Certification Examination (PTCE) administered by Professional Examination Service.

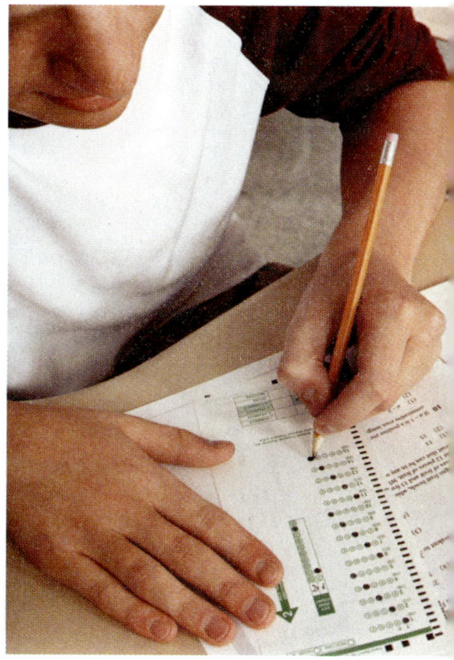

Figure 19-6 Certification examination.

The examination consists of 140 multiple choice questions based on the following three areas:

1. Assisting the pharmacist in serving patients
2. Maintaining medication and inventory control systems
3. Participating in the administration and management of pharmacy practice

Certification must be renewed every 2 years. The PTCB certified pharmacy technician is required to complete 20 hours of continuing education, with at least 1 hour of education focused on pharmacy law. Technicians with current certification may use the initials CPhT following their names. Some states require certification of pharmacy technicians, while others do not. Review the requirements for your state. Access the Pharmacy Technician Certification Board Web site (**www.ptcb.org**) for more information.

Pharmacy technicians may also be certified by taking the Exam for the Certification of Pharmacy Technicians (ExCPT), which is recognized by the National Community Pharmacists Association (NCPA) and the National Association of Chain Drug Stores (NACDS). This exam is administered by the Institute for the Certification of Pharmacy Technicians (ICPT) and is available in several states. Certification is renewable every 2 years with a continuing education requirement of 20 hours for each certification cycle. For more information on the ExCPT, visit **www.nationaltechexam.org.**

The National Center for Competency Testing (NCCT) administers competency examinations for allied health professionals, among which are pharmacy technicians. Certification is renewable annually with a continuing education requirement of 14 hours per year. For more information on certification through NCCT, access **www.ncctinc.com.**

Registration

State boards of pharmacy may require that pharmacy technicians are registered or licensed. For registration, a pharmacy technician must provide proof of eligibility through completing a pharmacy technician training program and/or obtaining certification. A photograph, fingerprints, and/or a background check may also be prerequisites for registration. As requirements vary by state, it is important for the pharmacy technician to know the requirements in his or her own state. A technician must keep registration current in order to practice. The certificate or registration card must be displayed in the pharmacy where the technician works. Access the National Association of Boards of Pharmacy at **www.nabp.net** for links to specific boards of pharmacy.

Tech Check

4. Which organization accredits continuing education providers? (LO 19.5)
5. How many hours of continuing education are needed every 2 years to maintain certification through PTCB? (LO 19.4)
6. Which organization is responsible for registering pharmacy technicians? (LO 19.4)

Professional Organizations (LO 19.6)

Participation in professional organizations is critical for keeping current, networking, and increasing the knowledge of one's profession. The pharmacy technician needs to be abreast of changes in the profession of pharmacy. Those changes may involve changes in legislation, professional standards, educational requirements, licensure requirements, and scope of practice. Professional organizations provide a context for the discussion and opportunities to contribute to outcomes. Some professional organizations are primarily focused on pharmacy technicians. Additionally, most of the pharmacists' associations have technician divisions or academies. There are a number of types of organizations with which to be involved.

Some of the benefits of participation in professional organizations include, but are not limited to:

- Employment opportunities
- Exchange of ideas
- Networking
- Opportunities for advocacy for the profession
- Opportunities for leadership
- Recognition among peers
- Scholarships and awards
- Support for the development of new programs

Several professional pharmacy organizations are described in Table 19-1. Although they do not all directly focus on the profession of the pharmacy technician, they all are related to the pharmacy profession. Most hold at least one annual meeting, while the larger organizations—for example, ASHP—hold several meetings annually. Some of the organizations described have state affiliate organizations, for more local involvement.

Of course, there are other professional organizations seeking technician involvement and input. Only the pharmacy technician can provide this perspective. As you gain membership (and hopefully assume a leadership role) in any of these organizations, your involvement benefits both your present and future career. It is critical that you also consider the future role of pharmacy technicians and what you can contribute to raise current awareness and advocacy for the profession.

Table 19-1 Professional Pharmacy Organizations

Organization	Description
American Pharmacists Association (APhA) **www.aphanet.org**	• Founded in 1852 and is dedicated to advancing the profession of pharmacy. • Originally named the American Pharmaceutical Association, it is the first established association of pharmacists in the United States. • The mission of APhA is to "provide information, education, and advocacy to empower its members to improve medication use and advance patient care." • Some state affiliates sponsor legislation days for the members to meet with lawmakers in the state capitols. • Although the emphasis is not primarily on pharmacy technicians, APhA contributed to the founding of the Pharmacy Technician Certification Board. More information about APhA can be obtained through the Web site at **www.aphanet.org**.
American Society of Health-System Pharmacists (ASHP) **www.ashp.org**	• The mission is "to advance and support the professional practice of pharmacists in hospitals and health systems and serve as their collective voice on issues related to medication use and public health." • ASHP is also the accrediting agency for pharmacy technician programs for pharmacy residency programs. • ASHP has a technician division with Web site links to resources for pharmacy technician training programs and pharmacy technicians. • ASHP also offers Web site continuing education. • Many of the state affiliate organizations have technician divisions. For more information on the American Society of Health-System Pharmacists, access the Web site at **www.ashp.org**.
American Association of Pharmacy Technicians (AAPT) **www.pharmacytechnician.com**	• Began in 1979. • Its mission is: "Provides leadership and represents the interests of its members to the public as well as health care organizations; promotes the safe, efficacious, and cost effective dispensing, distribution, and use of medications; provides continuing education programs and services to help technicians update their skills to keep pace with changes in pharmacy services; and, promotes pharmacy technicians as an integral part of the patient care team." • The association offers continuing education through its Web site. Access **www.pharmacytechnician.com** for more information.
Pharmacy Technician Certification Board (PTCB) **www.ptcb.org**	• PTCB "develops, maintains, promotes and administers a high-quality certification and recertification program for pharmacy technicians." • The PTCB seeks to provide high standards for the certification of pharmacy technicians. More information about PTCB may be obtained at **www.ptcb.org**.
National Pharmacy Technician Association (NPTA) **www.pharmacytechnician.org**	• Committed to increasing the value of pharmacy technicians while recognizing their role in providing pharmaceutical care. • The focus of this organization is primarily the practice of pharmacy technicians. • The association offers resources and continuing education to its members. More information about the NPTA may be obtained on the Web site at **www.pharmacytechnician.org**.

(Continued)

Table 19-1 Professional Pharmacy Organizations *(Continued)*

Organization	Description
Pharmacy Technician Educators Council (PTEC) **www.rxptec.org**	• Held its first conference in 1989. • The mission of the organization is: "To assist the profession of pharmacy in preparing high quality well-trained technical personnel through education and practical training; and, to promote the profession of pharmacy through professional activities and dissemination of information and knowledge to members, pharmacy organizations, and other specialists and professions." • The Pharmacy Technician Educators Council mostly consists of technician educators, although membership is open to pharmacists, pharmacy technicians, and other professionals who desire to promote high standards for the education of pharmacy technicians. For more information about PTEC, access **www.rxptec.org**.

Tech Check

7. Which organizations are primarily focused on pharmacy technicians?(LO 19.6)

8. Which organization focuses on the education of pharmacy technicians?(LO 19.6)

9. Which organization accredits pharmacy technician programs?(LO 19.6)

Chapter Summary

Understanding how to excel in their career is vital to the pharmacy technician. Important points to keep in mind are:

- Pharmacy technicians may utilize stress management strategies to optimize productivity while maintaining a professional image.
- Time management strategies may be utilized to ensure that work is completed efficiently and on time.
- Stress management and time management are related in that if either is not properly managed, the impact will be evident in the other.
- The employee evaluation is a supervisor's regular assessment of the performance of an employee.
- Certification is governed by national organizations, while registration is the purview of state boards of pharmacy.
- Continuing education is designed to keep pharmacy technicians abreast of current pharmacy practices and regulation, and is a requirement for the maintenance of certification.
- Pharmacy organizations present opportunities for involvement, leadership, education, and advocacy for pharmacy technicians.

Chapter Review

Case Study Questions

1. How can Mike handle this situation professionally?(LO 19.1. 19.2)
2. What should he not do?(LO 19.1, 19.2)
3. What would you do if you were Mike?(LO 19.1, 19.2)

At Your Service Questions

1. Is Aimee's supervisor being unfair? (LO 19.3)
2. How might this situation have been avoided? (LO 19.2)
3. What is Aimee's responsibility as an employee? (LO 19.2)

Multiple Choice

Select the best answer.

1. What must a pharmacy technician do to obtain certification? (LO 19.4)
   a. Get fingerprinted
   b. Finish a technician program
   c. Pass the certification examination
   d. Complete an externship
2. How many hours of pharmacy law continuing education are needed to maintain PTCB certification? (LO 19.4)
   a. 1
   b. 14
   c. 20
   d. None
3. Which of the following is *not* an effective stress management strategy? (LO 19.1)
   a. Know when to ask for help
   b. Know your job
   c. Leave early
   d. Do not take on more than you can handle
4. Which of the following is *not* an effective time management strategy? (LO 19.2)
   a. Arrive at work on time
   b. Stay late
   c. Pace yourself
   d. Plan your time at work
5. Which of the following is responsible for accrediting continuing education providers? (LO 19.6)
   a. AAPT
   b. APhA
   c. ASHP
   d. ACPE
6. Which of the following is *not* true regarding employee evaluations? (LO 19.3)
   a. It is a periodic review of the employee's performance.
   b. It is not kept on record.
   c. The employee and the supervisor sign the evaluation.
   d. It may also be called a performance appraisal.
7. Which of the following pharmacy organizations is involved with the certification of pharmacy technicians? (LO 19.6)
   a. NPTA
   b. ASHP
   c. PTEC
   d. PTCB
8. Which of the following pharmacy organizations accredits pharmacy technician programs? (LO 19.6)
   a. APhA
   b. ASHP
   c. AAPT
   d. ACPE
9. Which of the following pharmacy organizations is focused on the role of pharmacy technician educators? (LO 19.6)
   a. PTCB
   b. PTEC
   c. ICPT
   d. NACDS
10. Which of the following organizations is *not* primarily focused on an aspect of pharmacy technician education, certification, or practice? (LO 19.6)
    a. NPTA
    b. NCPA
    c. AAPT
    d. PTCB

Acronyms

Print the meaning of the following acronyms.

AAPT ______________________________
ACPE ______________________________
APhA ______________________________
ASHP ______________________________
CEU ______________________________
CPhT ______________________________
ExCPT______________________________
NACDS ______________________________
NPTA ______________________________
PTCB ______________________________
PTCE ______________________________

Critical Thinking Questions

1. What constitutes professional behavior in pharmacy technicians?(LO 19.3)
2. You work with another pharmacy technician who is habitually late. This person also often leaves work behind after her shift. How would you handle this problem? Whom would you speak with first, your coworker or your supervisor?(LO 19.2, 19.3)
3. Would you be interested in participating in a professional organization? If so, in which of the organizations do you have an interest? How do you think you might be able to get involved now?(LO 19.6)
4. If you were an employer, what qualities would you look for in a pharmacy technician? If your state does not require certifications, would you prefer a certified technician or not? Why? If your state does require certification, what other criteria would you use to evaluate whether or not to hire a particular pharmacy technician?(LO 19.3)
5. Do you think of pharmacy technicians as professionals or simply as workers? Why? What can you do to increase the professional image of pharmacy technicians?(LO 19.3, 19.5)

HIPAA Scenario

Angela Graham is a pharmacy technician who genuinely cares about the pharmacy's patients. One elderly lady who comes in to have her prescriptions filled can barely afford her medications. Thinking that she is helping, Angela enrolls the patient in one of the programs sponsored by drug manufacturers that assist people with inadequate health insurance. The following month the patient is informed that she will receive one of her medications, her most expensive prescription, at a very low cost. When the patient inquires about the change in price, Angela informs her that the medication is being purchased for her through the drug manufacturer's program. The patient becomes very angry, stating that she does not take handouts, and demands to see Angela's supervisor.

Discussion Questions (PTCB II. 73)

1. Should Angela have taken the liberty of enrolling the patient in the drug manufacturer's program?
2. Did Angela disseminate PHI to unauthorized entities?
3. What could Angela have done instead to assist the patient?

Internet Activities

1. Go to **www.napb.net.** Find and click the link to your state board of pharmacy on the Web site. Does your state recognize pharmacy technicians? If so, what are the requirements for registration for pharmacy technicians in your state?(LO 19.4)
2. Access **www.ptcb.org.** Find the section for statistics. How many pharmacy technicians are currently certified in the United States? In your state?(LO 19.4)

The 50 Most Common Drugs by Prescriptions Dispensed (2007)

Drug Name	Trade or Generic Equivalents	Category
Lipitor	atorvastatin	Antilipidemic
Singulair	montelukast	Antiasthmatic
Lexapro	escitalopram	Antidepressant
Nexium	esomeprazole magnesium	Antiulcer
Synthroid	levothyroxine sodium	Hormone replacement
Plavix	clopidogrel bisulfate	Platelet aggregation inhibitor
Toprol XL	metoprolol succinate	Antihypertensive
Prevacid	lansoprazole	Antacid/antiulcer
Vytorin	ezetimibe/simvastatin	Antilipidemic
Advair Diskus	fluticasone propionate/ salmeterol	Antiasthmatic
Zyrtec	cetirizine hydrochloride	Antihistamine
Effexor XR	venlafaxine hydrochloride	Antidepressant
Protonix	pantoprazole sodium	Antacid/antiulcer
Diovan	valsartan	Antihypertensive
Fosamax	alendronate sodium	Bone-reabsorption inhibitor
Zetia	ezetimibe	Antilipidemic
Crestor	rosuvastatin	Antilipidemic
Levaquin	levofloxacin	Antibiotic
Diovan HCT	valsartan	Antihypertensive
Klor-Con	potassium chloride	Potassium supplement
Cymbalta	duloxetine hydrochloride	Antidepressant
Actos	pioglitazone hydrochloride	Antidiabetic
Premarin Tabs	conjugated estrogens	Hormone replacement
ProAir HFA	albuterol	Antiasthmatic

Drug Name	Trade or Generic Equivalents	Category
Celebrex	celecoxib	Anti-inflammatory (NSAID)
Flomax	tamsulosin hydrochloride	Treats benign prostatic hyperplasia
Seroquel	quetiapine fumarate	Antidepressant
Norvasc	amlodipine besylate	Antihypertensive
Nasonex	mometasone furoate monohydrate	Anti-inflammatory corticosteroid (nasal spray)
TriCor	fenofibrate	Antilipidemic
Lantus	insulin glargine (rDNA origin)	Aormone replacement
Viagra	sildenafil citrate	Treats erectile dysfunction
Altace	ramipril	Antihypertensive
Yasmin 28	drospirenone and ethinyl estradiol	Oral contraceptive
Levoxyl	levothyroxine Sodium	Hormone replacement
Adderall XR (extended release)	amphetamine aspartate, amphetamine sulfate, dextroamphetamine saccharate, dextroamphetamine sulfate	Amphetamine; treats attention hyperactivity disorder (ADHD) and narcolepsy
Lotrel	amlodipine besylate and benazepril hydrochloride	Antihypertensive
Actonel	risedronate sodium	Treats and prevents osteoporosis
Ambien CR (extended release)	zolpidem tartrate	Hypnotic (sleep aid)
Cozaar	losartan potassium	Antihypertensive
Coreg	carvedilol	Antihypertensive
Valtrex	valacyclovir hydrochloride	Antiviral
Lyrica	pregabalin	Anticonvulsant
Concerta	methylphenidate	Central nervous system stimulant
Ambien	zolpidem tartrate	Hypnotic (sleep aid)
Risperdal	risperidone	Antipsychotic
Digitek	digoxin	Antiarrhythmic
Topamax	topiramate	Anticonvulsant
Chantix	varenicline	Antismoking
Avandia	rosiglitazone maleate	Antidiabetic

Source: Adapted from "The Top 300 Prescriptions for 2007 by Number of U.S. Prescriptions Dispensed," Rx List: The Internet Drug Index, **www.rxlist.com**.

Common Look-Alike and Sound-Alike Medications

Drug names listed in the column on the left may look or sound like the drug names found in the column on the right.

Accupril	Aciphex Accolate Accutane Altace Aricept Monopril
Acetaminophen and codeine	Acetaminophen and hydrocodone Acetaminophen and oxycodone
Acetohexamide	Acetazolamide
Aciphex	Accupril Adipex-P Aricept
Actos	Actonel
Acyclovir	Acetazolamide Famciclovir
Adderall	Inderal
Advair	Advicor
Albuterol	Acebutolol
Allegra	Adalat CC Allegra-D Asacol Viagra
Allegra-D	Allegra AlleRx-D
Allopurinol	Apresoline
Alprazolam	Clonazepam Diazepam Lorazepam
Altace	Accupril Amaryl Artane Norvasc
Amaryl	Altace Avandia Reminyl Symmetrel
Ambien	Amen Ativan Coumadin

Amicar	Omacor
Amiodarone	Trazodone Amantadine Amlodipine Amrinone (former nomenclature for inamrinone)
Amitriptyline	Aminophylline Imipramine Nortriptyline
Amoxicillin	Amoxil Ampicillin Atarax Augmentin
Amoxil	Amoxicillin
Aricept	Accupril Aciphex Anzemet
Atacand	Antacid Avandia
Atarax	Ativan
Atenolol	Metoprolol
Augmentin	Amoxicillin Ampicillin
Avandia	Amaryl Atacand Avelox Coumadin Prandin
Avapro	Anaprox Avelox
Avelox	Avandia Avapro Cerebyx
Bactrim	Biaxin
Bactrim DS	Bancap HC
Benadryl	Benazepril Bentyl
Benazepril	Benadryl Benzonatate Donepezil Lisinopril
Benzonatate	Benazepril Benztropine
Biaxin	Bactrim
Bisoprolol	Bisacodyl Fosinopril
Bupropion	Buspirone
Butalbital, acetaminophen, and caffeine	Butalbital, aspirin, and caffeine
Capoten	Catapres

Captopril	Carvedilol
Cardizem CD	Cardizem SR
Cartia XT (Diltiazem in U.S.)	Diltia XT Procardia XL Cartia (aspirin in New Zealand)
Cataflam	Catapres
Cefaclor	Cephalexin
Ceftin	Cefzil Rocephin
Cefzil	Cefol Ceftin Kefzol
Celebrex	Celexa
Celexa	Zyprexa
Cephalexin	Cefaclor
Chlorhexidine	Chlorpromazine
Ciprofloxacin	Cephalexin Levofloxacin Ofloxacin
Claritin	Claritin-D
Clomiphene	Clomipramine
Clonazepam	Alprazolam Clonidine Clorazepate Diazepam Lorazepam
Clonidine	Colchicine Cardizem Klonopin
Cosopt	Trusopt
Coumadin	Avandia Cardura Cordarone Ambien
Cozaar	Corgard Hyzaar Zocor
Cyclobenzaprine	Cetirizine Cyproheptadine
Danazol	Dantrium
Danocrine	Dantrium
Darvocet	Percocet
Darvocet-N	Darvon Darvon-N
Depakene	Depakote
Depakote	Senokot

Depakote (delayed release)	Depakote ER (extended release)
Detrol	Datril Dextrostat
DiaBeta	Zebeta
Diazepam	Alprazolam Clonazepam Ditropan Ditropan XL Lorazepam Midazolam
Dicyclomine	Demeclocycline Diphenhydramine Doxycycline
Diflucan	Dilantin Diprivan
Digoxin	Doxepin
Dilantin	Diflucan
Diovan	Darvon Zyban
Diphenhydramine	Dicyclomine Dipyridamole
Ditropan	Diazepam Diprivan
Docusate calcium	Docusate sodium
Doxazosin	Terazosin Donepezil
Doxepin	Digoxin Doxycycline
Doxycycline	Dicloxacillin Dicyclomine Doxepin
Effexor	Effexor XR
Elidel	Eligard
Enalapril	Eldepryl Lisinopril
Ephedrine	Epinephrine
Erythromycin	Azithromycin
Esomeprazole	Omeprazole
Estradiol	Ethinyl estradiol Risperdal
Estratest	Estratab Estratest HS
Evista	Avinza
Famotidine	Fluoxetine Furosemide
Fioricet	Fiorinal

Flomax	Flonase Flovent Fosamax Volmax
Flovent	Atrovent Flomax Flonase
Fluocinolone	Fluocinonide
Fluoxetine	Fluphenazine Fluvoxamine Famotidine Fluvastatin Furosemide Paroxetine
FML Forte	FML S.O.P.
Folinic acid (leucovorin calcium)	Folic acid
Fosinopril	Bisoprolol Furosemide Lisinopril Minoxidil
Furosemide	Famotidine Fluoxetine Fosinopril Torsemide
Glucophage XR	Glucotrol XL Glucophage XR Glucophage
Glucotrol	Glucotrol XL Glyburide
Glyburide	Glipizide
Haldol	Halcion
Heparin	Hespan
Humalog	Humalog mix
Humalog	Humulin
Humulin 70/30	Humulin N Humulin R
Humulin N	Humulin 70/30 Humulin R Humulin U Novolin N Humulin L
Hydralazine	Hydroxyzine
Hydrochlorothiazide	Hydralazine Hydroxychloroquine
Hydrocortisone	Cortisone Hydralazine Hydrocodone
Hydroxychloroquine	Hydrochlorothiazide
Hydroxyzine	Hydralazine Hydroxyurea

Hyzaar	Cozaar
Idarubicin	Doxorubicin Daunorubicin
Inderal LA	IMDUR
Indocin	Imodium
Isosorbide Mononitrate	Isosorbide Dinitrate
K-Lor	K-Dur K-Lyte
Lamictal	Labetalol Lamisil Lomotil Ludiomil
Lamisil	Lamicel Lamictal Lomotil
Lamivudine	Lamotrigine
Lanoxin	Levothyroxine Inapsine Lasix Lomotil Levoxyl Levsin Lonox Lovenox Xanax
Lantus, insulin human	Lente, insulin human
Leukeran	Leucovorin calcium
Levaquin	Heparin Lovenox Tequin
Levothyroxine	Lanoxin Leucovorin Liothyronine
Levoxyl	Lanoxin Luvox
Lexapro	Loxapine
Lipitor	Zocor
Lisinopril	Benazepril Enalapril Fosinopril Quinapril Risperdal
Lomotil	Lamictal Lamisil Lanoxin Lasix
Loratadine	Losartan

Lorazepam	Alprazolam Clonazepam Diazepam Loperamide Midazolam Temazepam
Lortab	Lorabid
Lovastatin	Lotensin
Medroxyprogesterone	Methylprednisolone Metolazone
Metformin	Metronidazole
Methotrexate	Methohexital Metolazone
Methylprednisolone	Medroxyprogesterone Prednisone
Metoclopramide	Metolazone Metoprolol Metronidazole
Metoprolol	Atenolol Metoclopramide Metolazone Metronidazole Misoprostol
MetroGel	MetroGel-Vaginal
Metronidazole	Metformin Methazolamide Metoclopramide Metoprolol Miconazole
Miacalcin	Micatin
MiraLAX	Mirapex
Mobic	Moban
Morphine	Hydromorphone Meperidine
MS Contin	OxyContin
Mucinex	Mucomyst
Naprosyn	Naprelan Niaspan
Nasacort	Azmacort
Neurontin	Neoral Noroxin
Niaspan	Naprosyn Niacin
Nifedipine	Felodipine Nicardipine Nimodipine
Nitroglycerin	Glycerin

NitroQuick	Nitro-Dur
Nortriptyline	Amitriptyline Desipramine Norpramin
Norvasc	Altace Navane Nolvadex Norflex Vasotec
Novolin	Novolog
Novolin 70/30	Novolog mix
Omeprazole	Esomeprazole
Opium tincture	Paregoric (camphorated opium tincture)
Ortho Tri-Cyclen	Ortho-Cyclen Tri-Levlen
Oxycodone	Oxazepam OxyContin Hydrocodone
OxyContin	MS Contin Oxybutynin Oxycodone
Paroxetine	Fluoxetine Paclitaxel Pyridoxine
Paxil	Paclitaxel Plavix Taxol
Penicillin	Penicillamine
Percocet	Percodan
Phenazopyridine	Promethazine
Phenobarbital	Pentobarbital
Phenytoin	Fosphenytoin Phenylephrine
Plavix	Elavil Paxil
Plendil	Pindolol Pletal Prilosec Prinivil
Potassium chloride	Potassium acetate Potassium citrate Sodium chloride
Pravachol	Prevacid Prinivil Propranolol
Pravastatin	Atorvastatin

Prednisone	Methylprednisolone Potassium Prednisolone Prilosec Primidone Pseudoephedrine
Premarin	Prempro Prevacid Primaxin Provera
Premphase	Prempro
Prempro	Premarin Premphase
Prevacid	Prinivil Pepcid Pravachol Premarin Prilosec
Prinivil	Plendil Pravachol Prevacid Prilosec Prinzide Proventil
Promethazine	Phenazopyridine Prochlorperazine
Promethazine w/codeine	Promethazine VC w/codeine
Proscar	Procan SR ProSom Prozac ProSom Provera
Protonix	Lotronex
Prozac	Prilosec
Pulmicort	Pulmozyme
Quinine	Quinidine
Ranitidine	Amantadine Rimantadine Felodipine
Retrovir	Ritonavir
Rifampin	Rifabutin
Risperdal	Estradiol Lisinopril Pediapred Requip Reserpine Risperidone Restoril

Risperidone	Reserpine Risperdal Risedronate Ropinirole
Robitussin AC	Robitussin DAC
Serevent Diskus	Serevent
Seroquel	Serentil Serzone Symmetrel Sinequan Sertraline
Singulair	Sinequan
Soma Compound	Soma
Synthroid	Symmetrel
Tamoxifen	Tamiflu Tamsulosin
Temazepam	Flurazepam Lorazepam Oxazepam
Terazosin	Prazosin Doxazosin
Tetracycline	Tetradecyl sulfate
Timoptic	Timoptic-XE
Tizanidine	Nizatidine Tiagabine
Tobrex	TobraDex
Topamax	Toprol-XL
Topiramate	Torsemide
Toprol-XL	Tegretol-XR Topamax
Tramadol	Toradol Trandolapril Trazodone Voltaren
Trazodone	Amiodarone Tramadol
Trileptal	Tegretol
Ultracet (acetaminophen/tramadol hydrochloride in U.S.)	Ultracef (Cefadroxil in other countries)
Valtrex	Valcyte
Vancenase AQ	Vanceril DS
Vanceril	Vancenase
Vanceril DS	Vancenase AQ
Verapamil	Verelan
Viagra	Allegra

Vicodin	Vicodin ES
Vinblastine	Vincristine
Wellbutrin XL	Wellbutrin SR
Xalatan	Xalcom (latanoprost/timolol in other countries)
Xanax	Lanoxin Zanaflex Zantac Zyrtec
Zantac	Xanax Xanax Zofran Zyrtec
Zestril	Zetia Zyprexa
Zithromax	Zinacef
Zocor	Zyrtec Cozaar Lipitor Yocon Zestril Ziac Zoloft
Zoloft	Zocor Zyloprim
Zyprexa	Celexa Zaroxolyn Zyprexa Zydis Zyrtec
Zyrtec	Xanax Zestril Zyprexa

Source: Information obtained from The Joint Commission, National Patient Safety Goal: Identify and, at a minimum, annually review a list of look-alike/sound-alike drugs used in the organization, and take action to prevent errors involving the interchange of these drugs. 2006–2008 and *USP Quality Review*, No. 79, April 2004.

All drug names have been capitalized for purposes of this table.

Appendix C

Selected Drug Categories

Drug Category	Action of Drug	Generic (Trade Name) Examples
Analgesic	Relieves mild to severe pain	Acetaminophen (Tylenol) Acetylsalicylic acid, or aspirin Morphine sulfate (MS Contin) Oxycodone HCl (Percocet)
Anesthetic	Prevents sensation of pain (generally, locally, or topically)	Lidocaine HCl (Xylocaine, Lidoderm) Tetracaine HCl (Pontocaine)
Antacid/Antiulcer	Neutralizes stomach acid	Calcium carbonate (Tums) Esomeprazole (Nexium) Lansoprazole (Prevacid) Protonix (pantoprazole sodium)
Anthelmintic	Kills, paralyzes, or inhibits the growth of parasitic worms	Mebendazole (Vermox) Pyrantel pamoate (Combantrin, Antiminth)
Antiarrhythmic	Normalizes heartbeat in cases of certain cardiac arrhythmias	Disopyramide phosphate (Norpace) Propafenone hydrochloride (Rythmol) Propranolol HCl (Inderal)
Antiasthmatic	Treats or prevents asthma attacks	Montelukast (Singulair) Fluticasone propionate and salmeterol (Advair Diskus) Albuterol (ProAir HFA)
Antibiotic (Anti-infective)	Kills microorganisms or inhibits or prevents their growth	Amoxicillin (Amoxil) Azithromycin (Zithromax) Cefprozil (Cefzil) Ciprofloxacin (Cipro) Clarithromycin (Biaxin XL) Levofloxacin (Levaquin)
Anticholinergic	Blocks parasympathetic nerve impulses	Atropine sulfate (Isopto Atropine) Dilomine HCl (Bentyl)
Anticoagulant	Prevents blood from clotting	Enoxaparin sodium (Lovenox) Heparin sodium (Hep-Lock) Warfarin sodium (Coumadin)
Anticonvulsant	Relieves or controls seizures (convulsions)	Clonazepam (Klonopin) Divalproex (Depakote) Phenobarbital sodium (Luminol Sodium) Phenytoin (Dilantin)

Drug Category	Action of Drug	Generic (Trade Name) Examples
Antidepressant (four types)	Relieves depression	
Tricyclic		Amitriptyline HCl (Elavil) Doxepin HCl (Sinequan)
Monoamine oxidase (MAO) inhibitor		Phenelzine sulfate (Nardil) Tranylcypromine sulfate (Parnate)
Selective serotonin reuptake inhibitor (SSRI)		Escitalopram (Lexapro) Fluoxetine HCl (Prozac) Paroxetine (Paxil) Sertraline HCl (Zoloft)
Serotonin-norepinephrine reuptake inhibitor (SNRI)		Venlafaxine hydrochloride (Effexor XR) Duloxetine hydrochloride (Cymbalta)
Antidiabetic	Treats diabetes by reducing glucose	Metformin (Glucophage) Glipizide (Glucotrol) Glyburide (Micronase) Pioglitazone hydrochloride (Actos)
Antidiarrheal	Relieves diarrhea	Bismuth subsalicylate (Pepto-Bismol) Kaolin and pectin mixtures (Kaopectate) Loperamide HCl (Imodium)
Antidote	Counteracts action of specific drug class	Acetylcysteine (Mucosil) for acetaminophen (Tylenol) Flumazenil (Romazicon) for benzodiazepines, such as diazepam (Valium) or alprazolam (Xanax) Naloxone HCl (Narcan) for narcotics, such as morphine
Antiemetic	Prevents or relieves nausea and vomiting	Prochlorperazine (Compazine) Promethazine (Phenergan) Trimethobenzamide HCl (Tigan)
Antifungal	Kills or inhibits growth of fungi	Amphotericin B (Fungizone) Fluconazole (Diflucan) Nystatin (Mycostatin) Terbinafine (Lamisil)
Antihistamine	Counteracts effects of histamine and relieves allergic symptoms	Cetirizine HCl (Zyrtec) Diphenhydramine HCl (Benadryl) Fexofenadine (Allegra) Desloratadine (Clarinex)
Antihypertensive	Reduces blood pressure	Amlodipine (Norvasc) Diltiazem hydrochloride (Cartia XL) Quinapril (Prinivil) Metoprolol succinate (Toprol XL) Valsartan (Diovan)
Anti-inflammatory (two types) Nonsteroidal (NSAID)	Reduces inflammation	Naproxen (Aleve) Colchicine (Goutnil or Colchicindon) Ibuprofen (Motrin, Advil) Celecoxib (Celebrex)
Steroid		Dexamethasone (Decadron) Methylprednisolone (Medrol) Prednisone (Deltasone) Triamcinolone (Kenalog)

Drug Category	Action of Drug	Generic (Trade Name) Examples
Antilipidemic	Lowers blood lipids such as triglycerides	Gemfibrozil (Lopid) Atorvastatin (Lipitor) Fenofibrate (TriCor) Ezetimibe/simvastatin (Vytorin) Ezetimibe (Zetia) Rosuvastatin (Crestor)
Antineoplastic	Poisons cancerous cells	Bleomycin sulfate (Blenoxane) Dactinomycin (Cosmegen) Paclitaxel (Taxol) Tamoxifen citrate (Nolvadex)
Antipsychotic	Controls psychotic symptoms	Chlorpromazine HCl (Thorazine) Clozapine (Clozaril) Haloperidol (Haldol) Risperidone (Risperdal) Thioridazine HCl (Mellaril)
Antipyretic	Reduces fever	Acetaminophen (Tylenol) Acetylsalicylic acid, or aspirin (Bayer aspirin)
Antiseptic	Inhibits growth of microorganisms	70% Isopropyl alcohol (Isopropyl alcohol 70%) Povidone-iodine (Betadine) Chlorhexidine gluconate (PerioChip)
Antitussive	Inhibits cough reflex	Codeine (Codeine Sulfate) Dextromethorphan hydrobromide (component of Robitussin DM)
Bronchodilator	Dilates bronchi (airways in the lungs)	Albuterol (Proventil) Epinephrine (Epinephrine Mist) Salmeterol (Serevent)
Cathartic (laxative)	Induces defecation, alleviates constipation	Bisacodyl (Dulcolax) Casanthranol (Peri-Colace) Magnesium hydroxide (Milk of Magnesia)
Contraceptive	Reduces risk of pregnancy	Ethinyl estradiol and norgestimate (Ortho Tri-Cyclen) Norethindrone and ethinyl estradiol (Ortho-Evra) Norgestrel (Ovrette)
Decongestant	Relieves nasal swelling and congestion	Oxymetazoline HCl (Afrin) Phenylephrine HCl (Neo-Synephrine) Pseudoephedrine HCl (Sudafed)
Diuretic	Increases urine output, reduces blood pressure and cardiac output	Bumetanide (Bumex) Furosemide (Lasix) Hydrochlorothiazide (Hydrodiuril) Mannitol (Mannitol IV)
Expectorant	Liquefies mucus in bronchi; allows expectoration of sputum, mucus, and phlegm	Guaifenesin (component of Robitussin)
Hemostatic	Controls or stops bleeding by promoting coagulation	Aminocaproic acid (Amicar) Phytonadione or vitamin K1 (Mephyton) Thrombin (Thrombogen)
Hormone replacement	Replaces or resolves hormone deficiency	Insulin (Humulin) for pancreatic deficiency Levothyroxine sodium (Synthroid) for thyroid deficiency Conjugated estrogens (Premarin Tabs)

Drug Category	Action of Drug	Generic (Trade Name) Examples
Hypnotic (sleep-inducing) or sedative	Induces sleep or relaxation (depending on drug potency and dosage)	Chloral hydrate (Noctec) Ethchlorvynol (Placidyl) Secobarbital sodium (Seconal Sodium) Zolpidem (Ambien)
Muscle relaxant	Relaxes skeletal muscles	Carisoprodol (RelA or Soma) Cyclobenzaprine HCl (Flexeril)
Mydriatic	Constricts vessels of eye or nasal passage, raises blood pressure, dilates pupil of eye in ophthalmic preparations	Atropine sulfate (Allergan) for ophthalmic use Phenylephrine HCl (Alcon Efrin) for ophthalmic use or (Neo-Synephrine HCl) for nasal use
Stimulant (central nervous system)	Increases activity of brain and other organs, decreases appetite	Amphetamine sulfate (Benzedrine) Caffeine (No-Doz); also component of many analgesic formulations and coffee
Vasoconstrictor	Constricts blood vessels, increases blood pressure	Dopamine HCl (Intropin) Norepinephrine bitartrate (Levophed)
Vasodilator	Dilates blood vessels, decreases blood pressure	Enalapril (Vasotec) Lisinopril (Prinivil) Nitroglycerin (Nitrostat, NitroQuick)

Note: Some drugs have a secondary category. When in doubt, check the *PDR* or other drug reference.

Appendix D

Measurements, Abbreviations, and Formulas

Metric to Metric Equivalents

Metric Weight Measure

1 kilogram (kg) = 1000 grams (g)
1 gram (g) = 0.001 kilogram (kg)
1 gram (g) = 1000 milligrams (mg)
1 milligram (mg) = 0.001 gram (g)
1 milligram (mg) = 1000 micrograms (mcg)
1 microgram (mcg) = 0.001 milligram (mg)

Metric Fluid Measure

1 liter (L) = 1000 milliliters (mL)
1 milliliter (mL) = 0.001 liter (L)
1 milliliter (mL) = 1 cubic centimeter

Common Approximations

1 milliliter (mL) = 15 to 20 drops (gtts) (droppers vary)
5 milliliters (mL) = 1 teaspoon (tsp)
15 milliliters (mL) = 1 tablespoon (tbsp)
30 milliliters (mL) = 1 ounce (oz)
1 kilogram (kg) = 2.2 pounds (lb)
1 tablespoon (tbsp) = 3 teaspoons (tsp)
1 ounce (oz) = 2 tablespoons (tbsp)
1 cup (c) = 8 ounces (oz)
1 pint (pt) = 2 cups (c) = 16 ounces (oz)
1 grain (gr) = 60 or 65 milligrams (mg)

Determine the Total Number of Tablets/Capsules to Dispense

1 tab/cap daily for 1 month = 30 tab/cap
(1/2 tab daily = 15 tablets)

1 tab/cap bid/q12h for 1 month = 60 tab/cap
(1/2 tab bid/q12h = 30 tablets)

1 tab/cap tid/q8h for 1 month = 90 tab/cap
(1/2 tab tid/q8h = 45 tablets)

1 tab/cap qid/q6h for 1 month = 120 tab/cap
(1/2 tab qid/q6h = 60 tablets)

1 tab/cap daily for 3 months = 90 tab/cap
(1/2 tab daily = 45 tablets)

1 tab/cap bid/q12h for 3 months = 120 tab/cap
(1/2 tab bid/q12h = 60 tablets)

1 tab/cap tid/q8h for 3 months = 180 tab/cap
(1/2 tab tid/q8h = 90 tablets)

1 tab/cap qid/q6h for 3 months = 240 tab/cap
(1/2 tab qid/q6h = 120 tablets)

Determine the Total Amount of Liquid Medication to Dispense

1 oz = 30 mL	5 oz = 150 mL	9 oz = 270 mL
2 oz = 60 mL	6 oz = 180 mL	10 oz = 300 mL
3 oz = 90 mL	7 oz = 210 mL	11 oz = 330 mL
4 oz = 120 mL	8 oz = 240 mL	12 oz = 360 mL

1 tsp/5 mL bid/q12h (10 mL/day) for 10 days = 100 mL = 3.33 oz

1 tsp/5 mL tid/q8h (15 mL/day) for 10 days = 150 mL = 5 oz

1 tsp/5 mL qid/q6h (20 mL/day) for 10 days = 200 mL = 6.66 oz

1 tsp/5 mL q4h/six times a day (30 mL/day) for 10 days = 300 mL 10 oz

2 tsp/10 mL bid/q12h (20 mL/day) for 10 days = 200 mL = 6.66 oz

2 tsp/10 mL tid/q8h (30 mL/day) for 10 days = 300 mL = 10 oz

2 tsp/10 mL qid/q6h (40 mL/day) for 10 days = 400 mL = 13.33 oz

2 tsp/10 mL q4h/six times a day (60 mL/day) for 10 days = 600 mL = 20 oz

Alligation

The concentration of the **higher** concentrated solution		Parts of the **higher** concentrated solution needed**
	The **desired** concentration needed	
The concentration of the **less** concentrated solution*		Parts of the **lesser** concentrated solution needed***

*When you are diluting with water, the less concentrated solution has a concentration of *ZERO*.

The difference between the concentration needed and the concentration of the LESSER concentrated solution (the **diagonal difference).

***The difference between the concentration needed and the concentration of the HIGHER concentrated solution (the **diagonal** difference).

Math Formulas

The Fraction Proportion Method

$$\frac{\text{Dosage unit}}{\text{Dose on hand}} = \frac{\text{Amount to ad minister}}{\text{Desired dose}} \quad \textbf{Or} \quad \frac{Q}{H} = \frac{A}{D}$$

The Ratio Proportion Method

Dosage unit: Dose on hand::Amount to dispense: Desired dose

Or

$Q{:}H{::}A{:}D$

The Formula Method

$$\frac{D}{H} \times Q = A$$

Common Abbreviations Used in Pharmacy

Frequency

Abbreviation	Meaning	Abbreviation	Meaning
ac, a.c., AC, $\overline{ac}$	before meals	**prn, p.r.n., PRN**	when necessary, when required, as needed
ad lib, ad. lib.	as desired, freely	**qam, q.a.m.**	every morning
bid, b.i.d., BID	twice a day	**qpm, q.n.**	every night
biw	twice a week	**qh, q.h.**	every hour
h, hr	hour	**q_h, q_hrs**	every __ hour(s)
LOS	length of stay	**qhs, q.h.s.**	every night, at bedtime
min	minute	**qid, q.i.d., QID**	4 times a day
non rep, nr	do not repeat	**rep, rept**	repeat
n, noc, noct	night	**SOS, s.o.s.**	once if necessary, as necessary
od	every day	**stat**	immediately
pc, p.c., PC, $\overline{pc}$	after meals	**tid, t.i.d., TID**	3 times a day

Common Abbreviations Used in Pharmacy

Form of Medication

Abbreviation	Meaning	Abbreviation	Meaning
cap, caps	capsule	**lot**	lotion
comp, cmpd	compound	**MDI**	metered-dose inhaler
dil	dilute	**sol, soln.**	solution
EC	enteric-coated	**SR**	slow-release
elix	elixir	**supp**	suppository
ext	extract	**susp**	suspension
fl, fld.	fluid	**syr, syp.**	syrup
gtt	drop(s)	**syr**	syringe
H_2O	water	**tab**	tablet
LA	long-acting	**tr, tinct, tinc.**	tincture
liq	liquid	**ung, oint**	ointment

PTCB Correlation

	CH 1	2	3	4	5	6	7	8	9	10	11	12	13	14	15	16	17	18	19
PTCB KNOWLEDGE STATEMENTS I. Assisting the Pharmacist in Serving Patients	**Overview, Practice Settings, and Organizations**	**Basic Safety and Standards**	**Communication and Customer Service**	**Ethics, Law, and Regulatory Agencies**	**Measurements and Calculations**	**Introduction to Pharmacology**	**Drug Classifications**	**Over-the-Counter Agents**	**Complementary and Alternative Modalities**	**Dosage Forms, Abbreviations, and Routes of Administration**	**Extemporaneous and Sterile Compounding (IV Admixtures)**	**Medication Errors**	**Referencing**	**Retail Setting**	**Hospital/Inpatient Setting**	**Other Environments**	**Inventory Management**	**Preparing for Your Career as a Pharmacy Technician**	**Career Development**
1. Knowledge of federal, state, and/or practice site regulations, codes of ethics, and standards pertaining to the practice of pharmacy.		X		X				X	X		X				X	X		X	X
2. Knowledge of pharmaceutical, medical, and legal developments which impact on the practice of pharmacy.				X				X	X									X	
3. Knowledge of state-specific prescription transfer regulations.				X															
4. Knowledge of pharmaceutical and medical abbreviations and terminology.										X	X			X					
5. Knowledge of generic and brand names of pharmaceuticals.							X	X											
6. Knowledge of therapeutic equivalence.						X	X	X								X			
7. Knowledge of epidemiology.		X																	
8. Knowledge of risk factors for disease.		X									X								
9. Knowledge of anatomy and physiology.							X	X											

	CH 1	2	3	4	5	6	7	8	9	10	11	12	13	14	15	16	17	18	19
PTCB KNOWLEDGE STATEMENTS I. Assisting the Pharmacist in Serving Patients	**Overview, Practice Settings, and Organizations**	**Basic Safety and Standards**	**Communication and Customer Service**	**Ethics, Law, and Regulatory Agencies**	**Measurements and Calculations**	**Introduction to Pharmacology**	**Drug Classifications**	**Over-the-Counter Agents**	**Complementary and Alternative Modalities**	**Dosage Forms, Abbreviations, and Routes of Administration**	**Extemporaneous and Sterile Compounding (IV Admixtures)**	**Medication Errors**	**Referencing**	**Retail Setting**	**Hospital/Inpatient Setting**	**Other Environments**	**Inventory Management**	**Preparing for Your Career as a Pharmacy Technician**	**Career Development**
10. Knowledge of signs and symptoms of disease states.		X					X	X											
11. Knowledge of standard and abnormal laboratory values.																			
12. Knowledge of drug interactions (such as drug disease, drug-drug, drug-laboratory, drug-nutrient).						X	X	X	X										
13. Knowledge of strengths/dose, dosage forms, physical appearance, routes of administration, and duration of drug therapy.							X	X			X								
14. Knowledge of effects of patient's age (e.g., neonates, geriatrics) on drug and non-drug therapy.						X		X	X										
15. Knowledge of drug information sources including printed and electronic reference materials.													X						
16. Knowledge of pharmacology (e.g., mechanism of action).						X	X	X											

	CH 1	2	3	4	5	6	7	8	9	10	11	12	13	14	15	16	17	18	19
PTCB KNOWLEDGE STATEMENTS I. Assisting the Pharmacist in Serving Patients	**Overview, Practice Settings, and Organizations**	**Basic Safety and Standards**	**Communication and Customer Service**	**Ethics, Law, and Regulatory Agencies**	**Measurements and Calculations**	**Introduction to Pharmacology**	**Drug Classifications**	**Over-the-Counter Agents**	**Complementary and Alternative Modalities**	**Dosage Forms, Abbreviations, and Routes of Administration**	**Extemporaneous and Sterile Compounding (IV Admixtures)**	**Medication Errors**	**Referencing**	**Retail Setting**	**Hospital/Inpatient Setting**	**Other Environments**	**Inventory Management**	**Preparing for Your Career as a Pharmacy Technician**	**Career Development**
17. Knowledge of common and severe side or adverse effects, allergies, and therapeutic contraindications associated with medications.						X	X	X											
18. Knowledge of drug indications.						X	X	X											
19. Knowledge of relative role of drug and nondrug therapy (e.g., herbal remedies, lifestyle modification, smoking cessation).							X	X	X										
20. Knowledge of practice site policies and procedures regarding prescriptions or medication orders.		X									X				X				
21. Knowledge of information to be obtained from patient/patient's representative (e.g., demographic information, allergy, third-party information).				X															
22. Knowledge of required prescription order refill information.				X											X				
23. Knowledge of formula to verify the validity of a prescriber's DEA number.				X															

	CH 1	2	3	4	5	6	7	8	9	10	11	12	13	14	15	16	17	18	19
PTCB KNOWLEDGE STATEMENTS I. Assisting the Pharmacist in Serving Patients	**Overview, Practice Settings, and Organizations**	**Basic Safety and Standards**	**Communication and Customer Service**	**Ethics, Law, and Regulatory Agencies**	**Measurements and Calculations**	**Introduction to Pharmacology**	**Drug Classifications**	**Over-the-Counter Agents**	**Complementary and Alternative Modalities**	**Dosage Forms, Abbreviations, and Routes of Administration**	**Extemporaneous and Sterile Compounding (IV Admixtures)**	**Medication Errors**	**Referencing**	**Retail Setting**	**Hospital/ Inpatient Setting**	**Other Environments**	**Inventory Management**	**Preparing for Your Career as a Pharmacy Technician**	**Career Development**
24. Knowledge of techniques for detecting forged or altered prescriptions.				X															
25. Knowledge of techniques for detecting prescription errors (e.g., abnormal doses, early refill, incorrect quantity, incorrect patient ID #, incorrect drug).												X							
26. Knowledge of effects of patient's disabilities (e.g., visual, physical) on drug and nondrug therapy.																			
27. Knowledge of techniques, equipment, and supplies for drug administration (e.g., insulin syringes and IV tubing)".															X				
28. Knowledge of nonprescription (over-the-counter [OTC]) formulations.								X	X										
29. Knowledge of monitoring and screening equipment (e.g., blood pressure cuffs, glucose monitors).								X											

	CH 1	2	3	4	5	6	7	8	9	10	11	12	13	14	15	16	17	18	19
PTCB KNOWLEDGE STATEMENTS I. Assisting the Pharmacist in Serving Patients	**Overview, Practice Settings, and Organizations**	**Basic Safety and Standards**	**Communication and Customer Service**	**Ethics, Law, and Regulatory Agencies**	**Measurements and Calculations**	**Introduction to Pharmacology**	**Drug Classifications**	**Over-the-Counter Agents**	**Complementary and Alternative Modalities**	**Dosage Forms, Abbreviations, and Routes of Administration**	**Extemporaneous and Sterile Compounding (IV Admixtures)**	**Medication Errors**	**Referencing**	**Retail Setting**	**Hospital/Inpatient Setting**	**Other Environments**	**Inventory Management**	**Preparing for Your Career as a Pharmacy Technician**	**Career Development**
30. Knowledge of medical and surgical appliances and devices (e.g., ostomies, orthopedic devices, pumps).											X								
31. Knowledge of proper storage conditions.		X									X				X				
32. Knowledge of automated dispensing technology.															X				
33. Knowledge of packaging requirements.		X						X	X					X					
34. Knowledge of NDC number components.				X										X					
35. Knowledge of purpose for lot numbers and expiration dates.																	X		
36. Knowledge of information for prescription or medication order label(s).														X	X				
37. Knowledge of requirements regarding auxiliary labels.							X							X	X				
38. Knowledge of requirements regarding patient package inserts.														X					

	CH 1	2	3	4	5	6	7	8	9	10	11	12	13	14	15	16	17	18	19
PTCB KNOWLEDGE STATEMENTS I. Assisting the Pharmacist in Serving Patients	**Overview, Practice Settings, and Organizations**	**Basic Safety and Standards**	**Communication and Customer Service**	**Ethics, Law, and Regulatory Agencies**	**Measurements and Calculations**	**Introduction to Pharmacology**	**Drug Classifications**	**Over-the-Counter Agents**	**Complementary and Alternative Modalities**	**Dosage Forms, Abbreviations, and Routes of Administration**	**Extemporaneous and Sterile Compounding (IV Admixtures)**	**Medication Errors**	**Referencing**	**Retail Setting**	**Hospital/Inpatient Setting**	**Other Environments**	**Inventory Management**	**Preparing for Your Career as a Pharmacy Technician**	**Career Development**
39. Knowledge of special directions and precautions for patient/patient's representative regarding preparation and use of medications.				X			X	X		X									
40. Knowledge of techniques for assessing patient's compliance with prescription or medication order.							X												
41. Knowledge of action to be taken in the event of a missed dose.							X												
42. Knowledge of requirements for mailing medications.				X															
43. Knowledge of delivery systems for distributing medications (e.g., pneumatic tube, robotics).															X				
44. Knowledge of requirements for dispensing controlled substances.				X			X									X			
45. Knowledge of requirements for dispensing investigational drugs.																	X		

	CH 1	2	3	4	5	6	7	8	9	10	11	12	13	14	15	16	17	18	19
PTCB KNOWLEDGE STATEMENTS I. Assisting the Pharmacist in Serving Patients	**Overview, Practice Settings, and Organizations**	**Basic Safety and Standards**	**Communication and Customer Service**	**Ethics, Law, and Regulatory Agencies**	**Measurements and Calculations**	**Introduction to Pharmacology**	**Drug Classifications**	**Over-the-Counter Agents**	**Complementary and Alternative Modalities**	**Dosage Forms, Abbreviations, and Routes of Administration**	**Extemporaneous and Sterile Compounding (IV Admixtures)**	**Medication Errors**	**Referencing**	**Retail Setting**	**Hospital/Inpatient Setting**	**Other Environments**	**Inventory Management**	**Preparing for Your Career as a Pharmacy Technician**	**Career Development**
46. Knowledge of record-keeping requirements for medication dispensing.				X							X				X				
47. Knowledge of automatic stop orders.															X				
48. Knowledge of restricted medication orders.															X				
49. Knowledge of quality improvement methods (e.g., matching NDC number, double-counting narcotics).												X		X					
50. Knowledge of pharmacy calculations (e.g., algebra, ratio and proportions, metric conversions, IV drip rates, IV admixture calculations).					X						X								
"51. Knowledge of measurement systems (e.g., metric and avoirdupois)".					X						X								
52. Knowledge of drug stability.						X					X								
53. Knowledge of physical and chemical incompatibilities.		X					X				X								

	CH 1	2	3	4	5	6	7	8	9	10	11	12	13	14	15	16	17	18	19
PTCB KNOWLEDGE STATEMENTS I. Assisting the Pharmacist in Serving Patients	**Overview, Practice Settings, and Organizations**	**Basic Safety and Standards**	**Communication and Customer Service**	**Ethics, Law, and Regulatory Agencies**	**Measurements and Calculations**	**Introduction to Pharmacology**	**Drug Classifications**	**Over-the-Counter Agents**	**Complementary and Alternative Modalities**	**Dosage Forms, Abbreviations, and Routes of Administration**	**Extemporaneous and Sterile Compounding (IV Admixtures)**	**Medication Errors**	**Referencing**	**Retail Setting**	**Hospital/Inpatient Setting**	**Other Environments**	**Inventory Management**	**Preparing for Your Career as a Pharmacy Technician**	**Career Development**
54. Knowledge of equipment calibration techniques.											X								
55. Knowledge of procedures to prepare IV admixtures.											X								
56. Knowledge of procedures to prepare chemotherapy.											X								
57. Knowledge of procedures to prepare total parenteral nutrition (TPN) solutions.											X								
58. Knowledge of procedures to prepare reconstituted injectable and noninjectable medications.											X								
59. Knowledge of specialized procedures to prepare injectable medications (e.g., epidurals and patient controlled analgesic [PCA] cassettes).											X								
60. Knowledge of procedures to prepare radiopharmaceuticals.		X																	

	CH 1	2	3	4	5	6	7	8	9	10	11	12	13	14	15	16	17	18	19
PTCB KNOWLEDGE STATEMENTS I. Assisting the Pharmacist in Serving Patients	**Overview, Practice Settings, and Organizations**	**Basic Safety and Standards**	**Communication and Customer Service**	**Ethics, Law, and Regulatory Agencies**	**Measurements and Calculations**	**Introduction to Pharmacology**	**Drug Classifications**	**Over-the-Counter Agents**	**Complementary and Alternative Modalities**	**Dosage Forms, Abbreviations, and Routes of Administration**	**Extemporaneous and Sterile Compounding (IV Admixtures)**	**Medication Errors**	**Referencing**	**Retail Setting**	**Hospital/ Inpatient Setting**	**Other Environments**	**Inventory Management**	**Preparing for Your Career as a Pharmacy Technician**	**Career Development**
61. Knowledge of procedures to prepare oral dosage forms (e.g., tablets, capsules, liquids) in unit-dose or non–unit-dose packaging.															X				
62. Knowledge of procedures to compound sterile noninjectable products (e.g., eyedrops).											X								
63. Knowledge of procedures to compound nonsterile products (e.g.. ointments, mixtures, liquids, emulsions).											X								
64. Knowledge of procedures to prepare ready-to-dispense multidose packages (e.g., ophthalmics, otics, inhalers, topicals, transdermals).							X												
65. Knowledge of aseptic techniques (e.g., laminar flow hood, filters).		X									X								
66. Knowledge of infection control procedures.		X									X								

	CH 1	2	3	4	5	6	7	8	9	10	11	12	13	14	15	16	17	18	19
PTCB KNOWLEDGE STATEMENTS I. Assisting the Pharmacist in Serving Patients	**Overview, Practice Settings, and Organizations**	**Basic Safety and Standards**	**Communication and Customer Service**	**Ethics, Law, and Regulatory Agencies**	**Measurements and Calculations**	**Introduction to Pharmacology**	**Drug Classifications**	**Over-the-Counter Agents**	**Complementary and Alternative Modalities**	**Dosage Forms, Abbreviations, and Routes of Administration**	**Extemporaneous and Sterile Compounding (IV Admixtures)**	**Medication Errors**	**Referencing**	**Retail Setting**	**Hospital/Inpatient Setting**	**Other Environments**	**Inventory Management**	**Preparing for Your Career as a Pharmacy Technician**	**Career Development**
67. Knowledge of requirements for handling hazardous products and disposing of hazardous waste.		X		X							X								
68. Knowledge of documentation requirements for controlled substances, investigational drugs, and hazardous wastes.		X																	
69. Knowledge of pharmacy-related computer software for documenting the dispensing of prescriptions or medication orders.															X				
70. Knowledge of manual systems for documenting the dispensing of prescriptions or medication orders.															X				
71. Knowledge of customer service principles.			X															X	X
72. Knowledge of communication techniques.			X															X	X
73. Knowledge of confidentiality requirements.			X	X														X	X
74. Knowledge of cash handling procedures.														??					

	CH 1	2	3	4	5	6	7	8	9	10	11	12	13	14	15	16	17	18	19
PTCB KNOWLEDGE STATEMENTS I. Assisting the Pharmacist in Serving Patients	**Overview, Practice Settings, and Organizations**	**Basic Safety and Standards**	**Communication and Customer Service**	**Ethics, Law, and Regulatory Agencies**	**Measurements and Calculations**	**Introduction to Pharmacology**	**Drug Classifications**	**Over-the-Counter Agents**	**Complementary and Alternative Modalities**	**Dosage Forms, Abbreviations, and Routes of Administration**	**Extemporaneous and Sterile Compounding (IV Admixtures)**	**Medication Errors**	**Referencing**	**Retail Setting**	**Hospital/Inpatient Setting**	**Other Environments**	**Inventory Management**	**Preparing for Your Career as a Pharmacy Technician**	**Career Development**
75. Knowledge of reimbursement policies and plans.														X					
76. Knowledge of legal requirements for pharmacist counseling of patient/patient's representative.								X						X					
PTCB KNOWLEDGE STATEMENTS II. Maintaining Medication and Inventory Control Systems																			
1. Knowledge of drug product laws and regulations and professional standards related to obtaining medication supplies, durable medical equipment, and products (e.g., Food, Drug and Cosmetic Act; Controlled Substances Act; Prescription Drug Marketing Act;-NF; NRC standards).									X		X						X	X	X
2. Knowledge of pharmaceutical industry procedures for obtaining pharmaceuticals.																	X		

	CH 1	2	3	4	5	6	7	8	9	10	11	12	13	14	15	16	17	18	19
PTCB KNOWLEDGE STATEMENTS II. Maintaining Medication and Inventory Control Systems	**Overview, Practice Settings, and Organizations**	**Basic Safety and Standards**	**Communication and Customer Service**	**Ethics, Law, and Regulatory Agencies**	**Measurements and Calculations**	**Introduction to Pharmacology**	**Drug Classifications**	**Over-the-Counter Agents**	**Complementary and Alternative Modalities**	**Dosage Forms, Abbreviations, and Routes of Administration**	**Extemporaneous and Sterile Compounding (IV Admixtures)**	**Medication Errors**	**Referencing**	**Retail Setting**	**Hospital/Inpatient Setting**	**Other Environments**	**Inventory Management**	**Preparing for Your Career as a Pharmacy Technician**	**Career Development**
3. Knowledge of purchasing policies, procedures, and practices.																	X		
4. Knowledge of dosage forms.				X			X	X	X	X									
5. Knowledge of formulary or approved stock list.														X			X		
6. Knowledge of par and reorder levels and drug usage.																	X		
7. Knowledge of inventory receiving process.																	X		
8. Knowledge of bioavailability standards (e.g., generic substitutes).						X	X	X											
9. Knowledge of the use of DEA controlled substance ordering forms.				X			X										X		
10. Knowledge of regulatory requirements regarding record-keeping for repackaged products, recalled products, and refunded products.												X					X		
11. Knowledge of policies, procedures, and practices for inventory systems.																	X		

	CH 1	2	3	4	5	6	7	8	9	10	11	12	13	14	15	16	17	18	19
PTCB KNOWLEDGE STATEMENTS II. Maintaining Medication and Inventory Control Systems	**Overview, Practice Settings, and Organizations**	**Basic Safety and Standards**	**Communication and Customer Service**	**Ethics, Law, and Regulatory Agencies**	**Measurements and Calculations**	**Introduction to Pharmacology**	**Drug Classifications**	**Over-the-Counter Agents**	**Complementary and Alternative Modalities**	**Dosage Forms, Abbreviations, and Routes of Administration**	**Extemporaneous and Sterile Compounding (IV Admixtures)**	**Medication Errors**	**Referencing**	**Retail Setting**	**Hospital/Inpatient Setting**	**Other Environments**	**Inventory Management**	**Preparing for Your Career as a Pharmacy Technician**	**Career Development**
12. Knowledge of products used in packaging and repackaging (e.g., child-resistant caps and light-protective unit-dose packaging).											X			X					
13. Knowledge of risk management opportunities (e.g., dress code, personal protective equipment [PPE], needle recapping).		X									X				X				
14. Knowledge of the FDA's classifications of recalls.																	X		
15. Knowledge of systems to identify and return expired and unsalable products.																	X		
16. Knowledge of rules and regulations for the removal and disposal of products.		X															X		
17. Knowledge of legal and regulatory requirements and professional standards governing operations of pharmacies (e.g., prepackaging, difference between compounding and manufacturing).											X				X				

	CH 1	2	3	4	5	6	7	8	9	10	11	12	13	14	15	16	17	18	19
PTCB KNOWLEDGE STATEMENTS II. Maintaining Medication and Inventory Control Systems	**Overview, Practice Settings, and Organizations**	**Basic Safety and Standards**	**Communication and Customer Service**	**Ethics, Law, and Regulatory Agencies**	**Measurements and Calculations**	**Introduction to Pharmacology**	**Drug Classifications**	**Over-the-Counter Agents**	**Complementary and Alternative Modalities**	**Dosage Forms, Abbreviations, and Routes of Administration**	**Extemporaneous and Sterile Compounding (IV Admixtures)**	**Medication Errors**	**Referencing**	**Retail Setting**	**Hospital/Inpatient Setting**	**Other Environments**	**Inventory Management**	**Preparing for Your Career as a Pharmacy Technician**	**Career Development**
18. Knowledge of legal and regulatory requirements and professional standards (e.g., FDA, DEA, state Board of Pharmacy, TJC [formerly JCAHO]) for preparing, labeling, dispensing, distributing, and administering medications.		X		X					X		X				X		X		
19. Knowledge of medication distribution and control systems requirements for the use of medications in various practice settings (e.g., automated dispensing systems, bar coding, nursing stations, crash carts).															X				
20. Knowledge of preparation, storage requirements, and documentation for medications compounded in anticipation of prescriptions or medication orders.											X				X				

	CH 1	2	3	4	5	6	7	8	9	10	11	12	13	14	15	16	17	18	19
PTCB KNOWLEDGE STATEMENTS II. Maintaining Medication and Inventory Control Systems	**Overview, Practice Settings, and Organizations**	**Basic Safety and Standards**	**Communication and Customer Service**	**Ethics, Law, and Regulatory Agencies**	**Measurements and Calculations**	**Introduction to Pharmacology**	**Drug Classifications**	**Over-the-Counter Agents**	**Complementary and Alternative Modalities**	**Dosage Forms, Abbreviations, and Routes of Administration**	**Extemporaneous and Sterile Compounding (IV Admixtures)**	**Medication Errors**	**Referencing**	**Retail Setting**	**Hospital/Inpatient Setting**	**Other Environments**	**Inventory Management**	**Preparing for Your Career as a Pharmacy Technician**	**Career Development**
21. Knowledge of repackaging, storage requirements, and documentation for finished dosage forms prepared in anticipation of prescriptions or medication orders.																	X		
22. Knowledge of policies, procedures, and practices regarding storage and handling of hazardous materials and wastes (e.g., Materials Safety Data Sheet [MSDS].		X		X															
23. Knowledge of medication distribution and control systems requirements for controlled substances, investigational drugs, and hazardous materials and wastes.		X															X		
24. Knowledge of the written, oral, and electronic communication channels necessary to ensure appropriate follow-up and problem resolution (e.g., product recalls, supplier shorts).		X	X																

	CH 1	2	3	4	5	6	7	8	9	10	11	12	13	14	15	16	17	18	19
PTCB KNOWLEDGE STATEMENTS II. Maintaining Medication and Inventory Control Systems	**Overview, Practice Settings, and Organizations**	**Basic Safety and Standards**	**Communication and Customer Service**	**Ethics, Law, and Regulatory Agencies**	**Measurements and Calculations**	**Introduction to Pharmacology**	**Drug Classifications**	**Over-the-Counter Agents**	**Complementary and Alternative Modalities**	**Dosage Forms, Abbreviations, and Routes of Administration**	**Extemporaneous and Sterile Compounding (IV Admixtures)**	**Medication Errors**	**Referencing**	**Retail Setting**	**Hospital/ Inpatient Setting**	**Other Environments**	**Inventory Management**	**Preparing for Your Career as a Pharmacy Technician**	**Career Development**
25. Knowledge of quality assurance policies, procedures, and practices for medication and inventory control systems.											X						X		
PTCB KNOWLEDGE STATEMENTS III. Participating in the Administration and Management of Pharmacy Practice																			
1. Knowledge of the practice setting's mission, goals and objectives, organizational structure, and policies and procedures.											X				X				
2. Knowledge of lines of communication throughout the organization.		X	X												X			X	X
3. Knowledge of principles of resource allocation (e.g., scheduling, cross training, work flow).																		X	X
4. Knowledge of productivity, efficiency, and customer satisfaction measures.																		X	X

	CH 1	2	3	4	5	6	7	8	9	10	11	12	13	14	15	16	17	18	19
PTCB KNOWLEDGE STATEMENTS III. Participating in the Administration and Management of Pharmacy Practice	**Overview, Practice Settings, and Organizations**	**Basic Safety and Standards**	**Communication and Customer Service**	**Ethics, Law, and Regulatory Agencies**	**Measurements and Calculations**	**Introduction to Pharmacology**	**Drug Classifications**	**Over-the-Counter Agents**	**Complementary and Alternative Modalities**	**Dosage Forms, Abbreviations, and Routes of Administration**	**Extemporaneous and Sterile Compounding (IV Admixtures)**	**Medication Errors**	**Referencing**	**Retail Setting**	**Hospital/ Inpatient Setting**	**Other Environments**	**Inventory Management**	**Preparing for Your Career as a Pharmacy Technician**	**Career Development**
5. Knowledge of written, oral, and electronic communication systems.			X															X	X
6. Knowledge of required operational licenses and certificates.	X														X			X	
7. Knowledge of roles and responsibilities of pharmacists, pharmacy technicians, and other pharmacy employees.	X	X						X			X			X	X			X	X
8. Knowledge of legal and regulatory requirements for personnel, facilities, equipment, and supplies (e.g., space requirements, prescription file storage, cleanliness, reference materials, storage of radiopharmaceuticals).		X									X			X	X				
9. Knowledge of professional standards (e.g., JCAHO) for personnel, facilities, equipment, and supplies.	X	X									X				X				

	CH 1	2	3	4	5	6	7	8	9	10	11	12	13	14	15	16	17	18	19
PTCB KNOWLEDGE STATEMENTS III. Participating in the Administration and Management of Pharmacy Practice	**Overview, Practice Settings, and Organizations**	**Basic Safety and Standards**	**Communication and Customer Service**	**Ethics, Law, and Regulatory Agencies**	**Measurements and Calculations**	**Introduction to Pharmacology**	**Drug Classifications**	**Over-the-Counter Agents**	**Complementary and Alternative Modalities**	**Dosage Forms, Abbreviations, and Routes of Administration**	**Extemporaneous and Sterile Compounding (IV Admixtures)**	**Medication Errors**	**Referencing**	**Retail Setting**	**Hospital/Inpatient Setting**	**Other Environments**	**Inventory Management**	**Preparing for Your Career as a Pharmacy Technician**	**Career Development**
10. Knowledge of quality improvement standards and guidelines.															X				
11. Knowledge of state Board of Pharmacy regulations.				X			X	X	X					X	X			X	
12. Knowledge of storage requirements and expiration dates for equipment and supplies (e.g., first-aid items, fire extinguishers).		X																	
13. Knowledge of storage and handling requirements for hazardous substances (e.g., chemotherapeutics, radiopharmaceuticals).		X																	
14. Knowledge of hazardous waste disposal requirements.		X																	
15. Knowledge of procedures for the treatment of exposure to hazardous substances (e.g., eyewash).		X																	

	CH 1	2	3	4	5	6	7	8	9	10	11	12	13	14	15	16	17	18	19
PTCB KNOWLEDGE STATEMENTS III. Participating in the Administration and Management of Pharmacy Practice	**Overview, Practice Settings, and Organizations**	**Basic Safety and Standards**	**Communication and Customer Service**	**Ethics, Law, and Regulatory Agencies**	**Measurements and Calculations**	**Introduction to Pharmacology**	**Drug Classifications**	**Over-the-Counter Agents**	**Complementary and Alternative Modalities**	**Dosage Forms, Abbreviations, and Routes of Administration**	**Extemporaneous and Sterile Compounding (IV Admixtures)**	**Medication Errors**	**Referencing**	**Retail Setting**	**Hospital/Inpatient Setting**	**Other Environments**	**Inventory Management**	**Preparing for Your Career as a Pharmacy Technician**	**Career Development**
16. Knowledge of security systems for the protection of employees, customers, and property.																			
17. Knowledge of laminar flow hood maintenance requirements.											X								
18. Knowledge of infection control policies and procedures.		X									X								
19. Knowledge of sanitation requirements (e.g., handwashing, cleaning counting trays, countertop, and equipment).		X									X			X	X				
20. Knowledge of equipment calibration and maintenance procedures.											X				X				
21. Knowledge of supply procurement procedures.																			
22. Knowledge of technology used in the preparation, delivery, and administration of medications (e.g., robotics, Baker cells, automated TPN equipment, Pyxis, infusion pumps).											X				X				

	CH 1	2	3	4	5	6	7	8	9	10	11	12	13	14	15	16	17	18	19
PTCB KNOWLEDGE STATEMENTS III. Participating in the Administration and Management of Pharmacy Practice	**Overview, Practice Settings, and Organizations**	**Basic Safety and Standards**	**Communication and Customer Service**	**Ethics, Law, and Regulatory Agencies**	**Measurements and Calculations**	**Introduction to Pharmacology**	**Drug Classifications**	**Over-the-Counter Agents**	**Complementary and Alternative Modalities**	**Dosage Forms, Abbreviations, and Routes of Administration**	**Extemporaneous and Sterile Compounding (IV Admixtures)**	**Medication Errors**	**Referencing**	**Retail Setting**	**Hospital/Inpatient Setting**	**Other Environments**	**Inventory Management**	**Preparing for Your Career as a Pharmacy Technician**	**Career Development**
23. Knowledge of purpose and function of pharmacy equipment.											X				X				
24. Knowledge of documentation requirements for routine sanitation, maintenance, and equipment calibration.		X									X								
25. Knowledge of the Americans with Disabilities Act requirements (e.g., physical accessibility).				X															
26. Knowledge of manual and computer-based systems for storing, retrieving, and using pharmacy-related pharmacy information (e.g., drug interactions, patient profiles, generating labels).				X										X					
27. Knowledge of security procedures related to data integrity, security, and confidentiality.																		X	X
28. Knowledge of downtime emergency policies and procedures.		X																	

	CH 1	2	3	4	5	6	7	8	9	10	11	12	13	14	15	16	17	18	19
PTCB KNOWLEDGE STATEMENTS III. Participating in the Administration and Management of Pharmacy Practice	**Overview, Practice Settings, and Organizations**	**Basic Safety and Standards**	**Communication and Customer Service**	**Ethics, Law, and Regulatory Agencies**	**Measurements and Calculations**	**Introduction to Pharmacology**	**Drug Classifications**	**Over-the-Counter Agents**	**Complementary and Alternative Modalities**	**Dosage Forms, Abbreviations, and Routes of Administration**	**Extemporaneous and Sterile Compounding (IV Admixtures)**	**Medication Errors**	**Referencing**	**Retail Setting**	**Hospital/Inpatient Setting**	**Other Environments**	**Inventory Management**	**Preparing for Your Career as a Pharmacy Technician**	**Career Development**
29. Knowledge of backup and archiving procedures for stored data and documentation.																			
30. Knowledge of legal requirements regarding archiving.				X															
31. Knowledge of third-party reimbursement systems.																X			
32. Knowledge of healthcare reimbursement systems (e.g., home health, respiratory medications, eligibility and reimbursement).																			
33. Knowledge of billing and accounting policies and procedures.																			
34. Knowledge of information sources used to obtain data in a quality improvement system (e.g., the patient's chart, patient profile, computerized information systems, medication administration record).																			

	CH 1	2	3	4	5	6	7	8	9	10	11	12	13	14	15	16	17	18	19
PTCB KNOWLEDGE STATEMENTS III. Participating in the Administration and Management of Pharmacy Practice	**Overview, Practice Settings, and Organizations**	**Basic Safety and Standards**	**Communication and Customer Service**	**Ethics, Law, and Regulatory Agencies**	**Measurements and Calculations**	**Introduction to Pharmacology**	**Drug Classifications**	**Over-the-Counter Agents**	**Complementary and Alternative Modalities**	**Dosage Forms, Abbreviations, and Routes of Administration**	**Extemporaneous and Sterile Compounding (IV Admixtures)**	**Medication Errors**	**Referencing**	**Retail Setting**	**Hospital/Inpatient Setting**	**Other Environments**	**Inventory Management**	**Preparing for Your Career as a Pharmacy Technician**	**Career Development**
35. Knowledge of procedures to document occurrences such as medication errors, adverse effects, and product integrity (e.g., FDA Med Watch Program).		X																	
36. Knowledge of staff training techniques.																		X	X
37. Knowledge of employee performance evaluation techniques.																			X
38. Knowledge of employee performance feedback techniques.																			X

Glossary

absorption Process by which a drug enters the bloodstream.

accreditation Process by which a private association, organization, or government agency, after initial and periodic evaluations, grants recognition to an organization that has met certain established criteria.

acid Substance that yields hydrogen atoms when dissolved in water. It has a pH less than 7.

active transport Selective process that requires energy to take place, where a substance goes from a lower to a higher concentration.

adjudication Electronic online billing of prescriptions, ensures prompt payment to the pharmacy and reduces the number of rejected prescriptions.

ADME process Absorption, distribution, metabolism, and elimination.

adulteration Contamination of a substance with other agents.

adverse effect Physical effect that occurs for a longer period than a side effect and can be more intense. Negative nontherapeutic effect associated with medication use.

aerosol Product that is packaged under pressure and contains therapeutically active ingredients that are released upon activation of an appropriate valve.

affinity Ability of a cell to bind to the cell structure.

agonist Drug that binds to a specific receptor and produces a specific drug action.

alligation Mathematical method to determine the respective percentages of a compounded product.

alternative medicine Type of nontraditional medical therapy that is used in place of conventional medicine treatments.

analgesic Agent that relieves pain.

anhydrous Free from water, especially water that is chemically combined in a crystalline substance.

antagonism Process where a drug blocks the effects of a medication.

antagonist Drug that does not bind to a specific site.

antipyretic Agent that reduces fever.

antiretroviral Agent used in the management of HIV.

antiseptic Antimicrobial substance applied to skin to reduce microbial flora.

Arabic numbers Commonly used system of writing numbers, using the 10 digits from 0 to 9.

aseptic technique Processes that reduce the risk of contamination and help ensure the sterility of a product.

automation Use of electronic devices or robotics to process drug orders.

Ayurvedic medicine An entire medical system originating in India that utilizes many therapies (yoga, meditation, massage, herbal preparations); also known as Ayurveda.

base Substance that yields hydroxide atoms when dissolved in water. It has a pH greater than 7.

bid (also known as contract compliance) Ability to purchase contract items with a group purchasing organization.

bioavailability Rate and extent to which an active drug is absorbed into the body.

biological Medicinal preparation made from living organisms and their products, including serums and vaccines.

biotechnology Field of study that combines the sciences of biology, chemistry, and immunology to produce synthetic, unique drugs with specific therapeutic effects.

bloodborne Pathogens or disease carried in blood and other body fluids.

bloodstream infection Bacteria from infected site in the body invade bloodstream.

brand name Proprietary or trade name assigned by the drug manufacturer and protected under trademark law; also known as a trade name.

broad spectrum Exhibits activity against a wide variety of bacteria.

buccal Medication placed between the cheek and gum

capitation Health care reimbursement system in which a flat fee is prepaid for a range of health care services.

capsule Solid dosage form in which the drug substance is enclosed in either a hard of soft soluble container or shell.

carcinogenesis Production of a cancer.

Cardiopulmonary Resuscitation (CPR) To provide ventilations (breaths) and chest compressions (blood circulation) for a person who shows no signs of breathing or having a heartbeat.

CDC See Centers for Disease Control and Prevention.

census Number of inpatients.

Centers for Disease Control and Prevention (CDC) The Centers for Disease Control and Prevention is the primary organization concerned with controlling disease transmission to prevent its spread and impact on society.

centralized pharmacy One main pharmacy from which all medication orders are filled.

central nervous system (CNS) Consists of the brain and the spinal cord.

certification Process by which a nongovernmental agency or association grants recognition to an individual who has met certain predetermined qualifications specified by that agency or association.

certification Proof of knowledge and competence.

chain pharmacy Retail unit containing prescription departments that are centrally owned by individuals or organizations with 11 or more units.

chemical name Description of the chemical structure of a drug.

Chinese medicine Entire medical system that evolved over thousands of years in China and is based on the concept of balanced "qi" (pronounced "chee") or vital energy. Herbal therapies, diet, and massage are utilized to restore balance in the vital energy.

Clark's Rule Method of calculating a child's dose based upon the child's weight and the recommended adult dose of a particular drug.

clinical coordinator Individual responsible for organizing and facilitating experiential education.

central nervous system (CNS) Brain and the spinal cord. See *central nervous system*.

colloid State of matter composed of single, large molecules or a collection of smaller molecules of a solid, liquid, or gas in a continuous medium.

compassion Sympathetic consciousness of others' distress together with a desire to alleviate it.

competitive antagonist Drug that competes for a specific site on a cell that an agonist is attempting to use.

complementary medicine Any nontraditional medical treatment that is used in combination with conventional medicine.

compounding record A form used in the infusion pharmacy to document the compounding activities and is part of the patient's chart; also known as a mixing report.

computerized physician order entry (CPOE) Paperless system in which medication orders are entered directly into the pharmacy computer system by the physician or prescriber.

contamination Presence of impurities, microorganisms, pesticides, or radioactive substances in a product.

continuing education Coursework or study to keep the pharmacy technician current in practice; may be required to maintain certification, licensure, and/or registration.

contraindication Situation in which a particular drug should not be used.

controlled substance A drug that has been declared illegal for sale or use but may be dispensed by a physician's prescription.

conversion factor Fraction made up of two values that are equal to one another but that are expressed in different units of measurement.

cosmeceuticals Preparation that contains both pharmaceutical and cosmetic properties.

CPOE See *computerized physician order entry*.

CPR See *cardiopulmonary resuscitation*.

Cream A Semisolid dosage form containing one or more drug substances dissolved in an appropriate base.

credentialing General process of formally recognizing professional or technical competence.

customer service Meeting the needs of the patient or customer.

decentralized pharmacy Pharmacy system involving multiple pharmacies serving various areas in a facility.

demulcent Soothing moist and sticky application.

denominator Value written in the bottom part of a fraction.

density Mass per unit volume of a substance.

desired dose Amount of drug to be administered at a single time.

dietary supplement Any product intended for ingestion that is designed to supplement the diet and contains at least one of the following agents: vitamin, mineral, herb or other botanical, amino acid, or dietary substance used to increase total daily intake of a constituent, metabolite, or extract.

Dietary Supplement Health and Education Act (DSHEA) of 1994 Legislation defining dietary supplements and outlining their regulation.

diffusion Process in which a substance goes from a higher to a lower concentration.

diluent Inert substance that reduces the strength of a substance.

dilution Process of reducing the strength of a substance through the addition of an inert substance.

disease management Coordinated approach to treat a specific disease that involves the entire health care team.

dosage form Vehicle into which a drug is incorporated to enable administration.

dosage ordered Amount of drug to be administered and frequency it is to be given.

douche Aqueous solution directed against a part or into a body cavity.

drug Any chemical agent that affects living processes.

drug contraindication Condition where a drug is not indicated and should not be prescribed.

drug-disease contraindication Condition where administration of a drug should be avoided because it may worsen the patient's condition.

Drug Enforcement Administration (DEA) Agency that is part of the U.S. Department of Justice, whose mission is to enforce controlled substance laws and regulations.

drug orders Prescription or medication orders.

drug utilization evaluation (DUE) Process that examines whether prescription drugs are being used efficiently and appropriately within a prescription drug benefit.

ED50 Effective dose 50; amount of drug needed to produce one-half of the maximum response.

efficacy Describes how successful a drug is able to produce its effect.

elixir Clear, pleasantly flavored, sweetened hydro-alcoholic liquid for oral use.

emesis Vomiting.

empathy Action of understanding, being aware of, and being sensitive to the feelings, thoughts, and experience of another.

emulsion A two phase system in which one liquid is dispersed throughout another liquid in the form of small droplets.

employee evaluation Periodic review of work performance; also known as performance appraisal.

encoding Process of converting information from one system of communication to another system.

enema Rectal dosage form used to evacuate the bowel or to affect a local disease.

enteral administration Oral administration of a drug.

error Failure of a planned action to be completed as intended or the use of a wrong plan to achieve an aim.

ethics Set of moral principles or values that govern the conduct of an individual or group.

etiology Science dealing with the causes of disease.

excipient Inactive ingredient incorporated into a dosage form.

exempt narcotic Schedule V medication, which does not require a prescription from a prescriber, but does have specific conditions in order to receive the medication.

extemporaneous compounding Manufacture of pharmaceutical products in a nonsterile environment.

externship Final component of a pharmacy technician program, consisting of experiential learning experiences that support the program objectives.

flow rate Comparison of two measurements with different types of units. In the practice of pharmacy, one of the units compared is time.

Food and Drug Administration (FDA) Federal administrative agency that administers and enforces the federal Food, Drug and Cosmetic Act and other federal consumer protection laws.

formulary Approved list of medications to be used in an institution.

franchise pharmacy Pharmacy where the owner of a trademark, a patent, or a product licenses another party to sell products or services under the franchisor.

gel (jellies) A semisolid dosage form consisting of small particles suspended in a liquid.

generic name Nonproprietary name given to a drug by its manufacturer.

half-life (t1/2) Amount of time for one-half of the drug present to be eliminated from the body.

hand hygiene Hand washing, antiseptic hand rub, antiseptic hand wash.

health maintenance organization (HMO) Managed-care organization that provides health care services to enrolled members for a fixed, prepaid fee.

hepatic Referring to the liver.

hospital Also known as inpatient facility.

ICU See *intensive care unit*.

incident report Document used for internal reporting of injury or accident.

independent pharmacy Privately owned pharmacy, whose function is to serve society's need for both drug products and pharmaceutical services.

independent practice association Health maintenance organization in which individual physicians enter a nonexclusive contract to see both HMO and non-HMO patients.

indication Purpose for which a specific medication is approved for use.

infection control Methods used to decrease contamination and disease due to pathogens.

inhalant Drugs or combinations of drugs that, due to its high vapor pressure, can be carried by an air current into the respiratory system.

Institute for Safe Medication Practices (ISMP) Nonprofit organization educating the health care community and consumers about safe medication practices.

integrative medicine Combination of components of Western (traditional) medicine with complementary and alternative medicine modalities with scientific evidence of efficacy.

intensive care unit (ICU) A patient care unit of a hospital where the patients are usually very ill and require special attention by the nurses and other medical staff.

interaction Event occurring as a result of two or more agents being used together.

international time (military time) Time based on the 24-hour clock.

Internet pharmacy Established commercial Web site that allows patients to obtain prescriptions and over-the-counter (OTC) products via the Internet.

internship Practical experience obtained while an individual is obtaining education or training.

Intrademal Injection administered between the upper layer of the skin.

intramuscular Injection into the skeletal muscles.

intravenous Aqueous solutions injections directly into the patient's vein.

ionized Process by which an atom or group of atoms has acquired an electrical charge by gaining or losing one or more electrons.

ISMP See *Institute for Safe Medication Practices*.

isotonicity Relating to or exhibiting equal osmotic pressure.

IV Intravenous, intravenously; medication administration into the vein.

IV piggyback Small-volume intravenous medication (usually containing an antibiotic) that is added to an existing catheter site through the tubing.

kinesics Systematic study of the relationship between nonlinguistic body motions (as blushes, shrugs, or eye movement) and communication.

laminar flow hood Apparatus used in sterile compounding that employs air jets to assist in providing a sterile environment.

LD50 Lethal dose 50; dose of a drug that will kill 50% of the animals it is tested on.

legend drug Prescription medication bearing the federal legend (Federal law prohibits the dispensing of this medication without a prescription).

levigation Gradual circular motion used to incorporate solid particles into a diluent.

licensure Process by which government grants permission to an individual to engage in a given occupation based upon finding that the applicant has attained the minimal degree of competency necessary to ensure that the public health, safety, and welfare will be reasonably well protected.

loading dose Larger initial dose compared to the subsequent doses.

maintenance dose Dose given after the loading dose to maintain a therapeutic concentration of the drug in the body.

malpractice Act of continuing conduct of a professional that does not meet the standard of professional competence and results in provable damages to his or her client or patient.

managed-care pharmacy Practice of pharmacy that involves clinical and administrative activities performed in a managed-care organization by a pharmacist.

MAR See *medication administration record.*

mechanism of action Explanation of how a drug produces its effects.

Medicare Program of the Social Security Administration, which provides medical care to people who are elderly.

medication administration record (MAR) A document that includes when a patient received a medication ordered and who administered it.

medication error Any preventable event that may cause or lead to inappropriate medication use or patient harm while the medication is in the control of health care professional. Includes health care products, procedures, and systems; prescriptions; order communication; product labeling, packaging, nomenclature; compounding; dispensing; distribution; administration; education; monitoring; and use.

MEDMARX National, Internet-accessible database that hospitals and health care systems use to track and trend adverse drug reactions and medication errors. Hospitals and health care systems participate in MEDMARX voluntarily and subscribe to it on an annual basis.

MedWatch FDA Safety Information and Adverse Event Reporting Program serves both health care professionals and the medical product–using public.

misidentification Mislabeling a preparation as containing agents not included in the preparation.

monoclonal antibodies Antibodies derived from a single cell.

monograph Essay or treatise on one subject.

multidrug-resistant pathogens Bacteria impervious to multiple antibacterial agents.

mutagenesis Induction of a genetic mutation.

mydriasis Dilation of the pupil.

narcotic An addictive drug that dulls the senses, reduces pain, alters mood or behavior, and usually induces sleep or stupor.

National Drug Code (NDC) An 11-digit number identifying a particular medication. The first 5 digits identify the drug manufacturer, the next 4 digits represent a particular medication, and the last 2 digits identify the packaging of the product.

negligence The failure to do something that a reasonable person would do, or doing something that a reasonable person would not do.

networking Establishing and maintaining professional relationships with colleagues and others in one's discipline and related disciplines.

nonionized A substance that has have an electrical charge.

nomogram A chart using the weight and height of a patient to calculate the correct dose for the patient.

nonproprietary drug Medication that is not protected by a patent; also referred to as a generic drug.

nonresident pharmacy Pharmacy that is located outside a particular state that mails, ships, or delivers prescriptions to patients inside that particular state.

nosocomial Originating or taking place in a hospital or other health care facility.

numerator Value written in the top part of a fraction.

nutraceuticals Foodstuff (as a fortified food or dietary supplement) that is held to provide health or medical benefits in addition to its basic nutritional value.

Occupational Safety and Health Administration (OSHA) Organization responsible for developing standards for safety in the workplace.

oculesics Use of the eyes in a communication setting. In most Western cultures, the use of direct eye contact symbolizes listening and attention.

ointment A semisolid preparations intended for external application to the skin or mucous membranes.

onside effect Not necessarily harmful; may include nausea, vomiting, headaches, constipation, and diarrhea.

on-the-job training Training obtained from working in a specific job. This form of training is informal in nature and may lack structure.

Ophthalmic Agents used to treat surface or intraocular conditions of the eyes or eyelids.

oral Most convenient route of medication administration, taken by mouth and/or swallowed.

orientation Process of educating the new hire about the company and area of work.

OSHA See *Occupational safety and Health Administration*.

Otic Agents used to treat conditions of the ear.

Over-the-counter (OTC) Agent or product available without a prescription; nonprescription.

P&T Committee *See* Pharmacy and Therapeutics Committee.

parenteral A drug administered that bypasses the digestive system

parenteral administration Medications delivered outside of the gastrointestinal system.

parenteral nutrition Combination of amino acids, dextrose, fats, vitamins, minerals, electrolytes, and water administered intravenously.

passive transport Most common method for a drug to cross a membrane.

pastille Molded lozenges

patent Official document conferring a right or privilege to license.

pathogen Microbial agent causing disease.

percent Parts per 100.

personal digital assistant (PDA) Handheld device that runs on its own battery power so that it may be used anywhere.

pharmaceutical care plan Plan developed by the pharmacist at the beginning of therapy for a home infusion patient. The care plan is developed to accomplish the goals of the drug therapy and minimize drug-related problems. It is also known as a care plan.

pharmacokinetics Study of the absorption, distribution, metabolism, and elimination of drugs.

Pharmacy and Therapeutics (P&T) Committee Hospital committee chaired by a physician and composed of physicians, nursing staff, and pharmacists, who establish and maintain a listing of approved drugs for use in a hospital.

policy and procedures Manual containing regulations of the facility including how the regulations are performed.

potency Measure of the strength or concentration of a drug to produce a specific effect.

potentiation Process where one drug increases the potency or strength of another medication and the effect is greater than the effect of each drug prescribed alone.

preceptor Pharmacist or pharmacy technician that supervises students on a daily basis during the externship.

preferred provider organization (PPO) Managed-care organization that provides health care services to enrolled members for a discounted fee.

prescription A written directive for the preparation and administration of a remedy.

probation Trial period that often must be completed prior to permanent hiring.

product rotation Placing the merchandise with the shortest amount of time remaining before the manufacturer's expiration in a location to be purchased and used before the product expires.

professionalism Quality of being a professional (positive, proactive, competent).

program director Individual responsible for the administration of the pharmacy technician program.

prophylactic dose Dose given to prevent a situation from developing.

prophylaxis postexposure prophylaxis Using preventative measures, such as medications, to prevent a disease or infection after a person has had an accidental exposure to the disease or infection.

proportion Expression demonstrating that two ratios are equivalent.

proprietary blend Mixture of various herbal, vitamin, and mineral agents to form a component of a specific product.

proprietary drug Denoting a medicine protected against free competition as to name, composition, or manufacturing process by patent, trademark, copyright, or secrecy. Also known as a brand name or trade drug.

Protected Health Information (PHI) Individually identifiable health information transmitted or maintained in any form or medium.

protocol Written guidelines for patient care to meet specific criteria.

proxemics Study of the nature, degree, and effect of the spatial separation individuals naturally maintain (as in various social and interpersonal situations).

pulmonary Inhaled into the lungs.

pyrogens Fever-producing substance by microorganisms.

ratio Comparison of two quantities having the same type of units.

receiver Individual who responds to the sender's communication.

receptor Specific site of drug or chemical action.

receptor site Identifies the exact cell site on a specific cell where a drug produces its effect.

reconstitution Addition of a diluent (usually sterile water) to dissolve or suspend a powder in a liquid.

rectal Inserted into the rectum of the body by way of the anus.

registering Process of making a list or being included on an existing list. In many states, a pharmacy technician may be required to register with the state board of pharmacy. The technician must submit an application, which indicates the PTCB certification number and its expiration date, if the individual took a state pharmacy technician examination, or if he or she completed a pharmacy board approved training program. The registration process may vary among states.

regulatory agency Agency established by an executive branch of government. Regulatory agencies affecting the practice of pharmacy include the FDA, DEA, and OSHA.

regulatory statute Licensing statute enacted to protect the public.

respondeat superior Latin term meaning "let the master answer;" a key doctrine in the law of agency, states that a principal (employer) is responsible for the actions of his or her agent (employee) in the course of employment.

resume Professional document consisting of a listing of an individual's educational, work, and personal experiences qualifying him or her for a job.

reverse distributor Pharmacy wholesaler capable of accepting expired controlled substances for destruction.

Roman numerals System that uses the letters I, V, X, L, C, D, and M to represent numbers.

sender Individual who initiates the communication.

sepsis Bacterial infection disseminated in the bloodstream.

side effect Drug effect other than the therapeutic effect that is undesirable but not harmful.

site of action Place in the body where the drug produces its effect.

solution A solution is a homogenous mixture that is prepared by dissolving a solid, liquid, or gas in another liquid.

Standard of Care Watchfulness, attention, caution, and prudence that a reasonable person in the circumstances would exercise.

standardization Consistency of components of the active ingredient from batch to batch and from manufacturer to manufacturer.

stat order Medication order for immediate administration.

statute Written law enacted by the legislative branch of the federal or state governments that establishes certain courses of conduct that must be adhered to by covered parties.

sterile Absence of pathogens and contaminants.

subcutaneous Injection administered into the fatty tissue layer under the skin.

sublingual Placed under the tongue.

suppository A solid medication dosage formulated to be inserted intothe rectum, vagina, or urethra.

subcutaneous Injection administered into the fatty tissue layer under the skin.

sublingual Placed under the tongue.

suppository A solid medication dosage formulated to be inserted into the rectum, vagina, or urethra.

surfactant An emulsifying agent that stabilizes an emulsion from preventing small droplets from becoming large droplets.

suspensions Suspensions are liquid preparations consisting of solid particles dispersed throughout a liquid phase in which the particles are not soluble.

syrup A concentrated solution of sugar in water or other aqueous solutions with or without flavoring agents and medicinal substances.

tablet A solid pharmaceutical dosage form prepared by compression or molding.

therapeutic index (TI) Ratio of lethal dose 50 (LD50) compared to the effective dose 50 (ED50).

tincture Alcoholic or hydro-alcoholic solutions prepared from vegetable or chemical substances. tincture Alcoholic or hydro-alcoholic solutions prepared from vegetable or chemical substances.

total parenteral nutrition (TPN) Nutritional support (calories, proteins, multivitamins) administered intravenously; also known as hyperalimentation.

toxic effects More serious than either a side or adverse effect. it may be extremely dangerous and may become fatal if it continue in an individual.

TPN See *total parenteral nutrition.*

transdermal The passage of therapeutic quantities of medications through the skin and into systemic circulation.

triturate To crush or grind solid particles using a mortar and pestle to decrease particle size for ease of incorporation into a compounded preparation.

troche Compressed lozenges.

unit-dose Medication packaged in a single dose.

urethral Inserted into the male or female urethra.

U.S. Pharmacopeia (USP) United States Pharmacopeia (USP) is an official public standards–setting authority for all prescription and over-the-counter medicines and other health care products manufactured or sold in the United States.

USP/NF 797 Set of enforceable standards and guidelines for sterile compounding.

USP <797> First set of official and enforceable regulations involving sterile compounding.

Vaccine Adverse Event Reporting System (VAERS) Cooperative program for vaccine safety of the Centers for Disease Control and Prevention (CDC) and the Food and Drug Administration (FDA). VAERS is a postmarketing safety surveillance program, collecting information about adverse events (possible side effects) that occur after the administration of U.S. licensed vaccines.

vaginal Inserted into the vagina.

VAERS See *Vaccine Adverse Event Reporting System*.

vasoconstriction Constriction of blood vessels.

velocity report Also known as an 80/20 report, which is a detailed summary of purchasing history, where 80% of purchasing dollars are spent on 20% of the products.

Verified Internet Pharmacy Practice Site (VIPPS) Program developed by the National Association of Boards of Pharmacy (NABP) to direct the safety of the practice of pharmacy.

xerostomia Dry mouth.

Young's Rule Method for calculating a child's dose based upon the child's age and the recommended adult dose of a particular drug.

Credits

Photo Credits

Chapter 1

Opener: ©Royalty-Free/Corbis; p. 6 (a): ©Burke/Triolo/Brand X Pictures/JupiterImages RF; p. 6 (b): ©Ryan McVay/Getty Images RF; p. 6 (c): ©Fototeca Storica Nazionale/Getty Images RF; p. 6 (d): ©Kent Knudson/PhotoLink/Getty Images RF; p. 8 (*top*): ©Comstock Images/PictureQuest RF; 1.1: ©Keith Brofsky/Getty Images RF; 1.2-1.3: ©Total Care Programming, Inc.; 1.4: ©Comstock Images/PictureQuest RF; 1.5 (*left*): ©PhotoDisc/Getty Images RF; 1.5 (*right*): ©Royalty-Free/Corbis; 1.6a: ©Total Care Programming, Inc.; 1.6b: ©Royalty-Free/Corbis; 1.6c-d: ©Comstock Images/PictureQuest RF; 1.7: ©The McGraw-Hill Companies, Inc./Andrew Resek, photographer; 1.8: ©Stockbyte/PunchStock RF; 1.9: ©Comstock/PunchStock RF; 1.10-1.11: ©Royalty-Free/Corbis.

Chapter 2

Page 29: ©Total Care Programming, Inc.; p. 30: ©Dynamic Graphics/JupiterImages RF; 2.1: ©Geostock/Getty Images RF; p. 33: ©Sean Justice/Corbis RF; 2.3-2.4: CDC/Janice Haney Carr; 2.5a-b: ©The McGraw-Hill Companies, Inc./Jill Braaten, photographer; 2.6 (*left*): ©davidkellycrow.com; 2.6 (*right*): ©Total Care Programming, Inc.; p. 41: ©The McGraw-Hill Companies, Inc./Christopher Kerrigan, photographer; 2.9: ©The McGraw-Hill Companies, Inc./Chris Hammond, photographer; 2.10: CDC/James H. Steele; 2.11: Dr. Fred Murphy, 1975, Centers for Disease Control and Prevention; 2.12: ©Total Care Programming, Inc.; 2.13: ©Chase Jarvis/Getty Images RF; 2.14 (*left, right*): ©Total Care Programming, Inc.; 2.16: ©Comstock Images/PictureQuest RF.

Chapter 3

Page 56 (*top*): ©Total Care Programming, Inc.; p. 56 (*bottom*): ©Stockbyte/PunchStock RF; 3.2: ©Royalty-Free/Corbis; 3.3: ©Corbis RF; p. 60 (a): ©Digital Vision RF; p. 60 (b): ©Brand X Pictures/PunchStock RF; p. 60 (c): ©Getty Images RF; p. 60 (d): ©Stockbyte/PunchStock RF; p. 61 (e): ©Brand X Pictures/PunchStock RF; p. 61 (f): ©Royalty-Free/Corbis; 3.4: ©Comstock Images/PictureQuest RF; 3.5-3.9: ©Total Care Programming, Inc.; 3.10-3.11: ©Royalty-Free/Corbis; 3.12-3.13: ©Comstock Images/JupiterImages RF; 3.14: ©Total Care Programming, Inc.; 3.15 (a): ©Comstock/Corbis RF; 3.15 (b): ©PhotoDisc/Getty Images RF; 3.16: ©Total Care Programming, Inc.; 3.17: ©BananaStock/PunchStock RF; 3.18: ©Comstock Images/PictureQuest RF.

Chapter 4

Figure 4.1: ©Royalty-Free/Corbis; p. 82: ©Total Care Programming, Inc.; 4.2: ©Total Care Programming, Inc.; 4.3: Library of Congress; 4.4: Library of Congress Prints & Photographs Division (LC-USZ62-102090); 4-5: ©Comstock Images/PictureQuest RF; 4.6-4.8: ©Total Care Programming, Inc.; 4.9: ©The McGraw-Hill Companies, Inc./Elite Images; 4.10: ©Total Care Programming, Inc.; 4.16: ©Creatas/PunchStock RF; 4.17 (*top*): ©PhotoDisc/Getty Images RF; 4.17 (*bottom*): ©Don Farrall/Getty Images RF; 4.18: ©Royalty-Free/Corbis; 4.19: ©Total Care Programming, Inc.

Chapter 5

Opener: ©PhotoLink/Getty Images RF; p. 128: ©Comstock Images/PictureQuest RF.

Chapter 6

Page 171: ©Keith Brofsky/Getty Images RF; p. 172: ©Don Farrall/Getty Images RF; p. 173: ©Royalty-Free/Corbis; p. 176: ©Brand X Pictures/PunchStock RF; p. 178: ©Steve Allen/Getty Images RF; p. 180: ©Stockdisc/PunchStock RF; p. 184: ©Brand X Pictures RF; p. 187, 188: ©Royalty-Free/Corbis; p. 189 (*top*): ©PhotoDisc/Getty Images RF; p. 189 (*bottom*): ©Brand X Pictures/PunchStock RF.

Chapter 7

Page 197: ©Stockdisc/PunchStock RF; 7.7: CDC/Janice Haney Carr; 7.8: ©Royalty-Free/Corbis; 7.10: ©Nick Koudis/Getty Images RF.

Chapter 8

Figure 8.1: ©The McGraw-Hill Companies, Inc./Elite Images; 8.2: ©The McGraw-Hill Companies, Inc./Christopher Kerrigan, photographer; p. 228: ©Corbis RF; 8.3-8.4: ©Creatas/PunchStock RF; 8.5-8.6: ©The McGraw-Hill Companies, Inc./Jill Braaten, photographer; 8.7: ©Royalty-Free/Corbis; 8.8: ©McGraw-Hill Companies, Inc.; 8.9: ©The McGraw-Hill Companies, Inc./Jill Braaten, photographer; 8.10: ©David Tietz/Editorial Image, LLC RF; 8.11: Centers for Disease Control; 8.12: ©Robert Manella for MMH; 8.13 ©The McGraw-Hill Companies, Inc./Ken Karp, photographer; 8.14: Centers for Disease Control/Dr. Lucille K Georg; 8.15: Image courtesy of the Centers for Disease Control and Prevention, Frank Collins, PhD.; 8.16: ©Comstock Images/PictureQuest RF; 8.17-8.18: ©PhotoDisc/Getty Images RF; 8.19: ©The McGraw-Hill Companies, Inc.; 8.20: ©The McGraw-Hill Companies, Inc./Photo by Eric Misko, Elite Images Photography; 8.21: ©The McGraw-Hill Companies, Inc./Jill Braaten, photographer; 8.22: ©Chris Kerrigan RF; 8.23: ©Stockbyte/PictureQuest RF; 8.24: ©The McGraw-Hill Companies, Inc./Jill Braaten, photographer.

Chapter 9

Page 251 (*top*, a): ©Royalty-Free/Corbis; p. 251 (b): ©Thinkstock/PunchStock RF; p. 252 (c): ©Nancy R. Cohen/Getty Images RF; p. 252 (d): ©PhotoAlto/PunchStock RF; p. 252 (e): ©Royalty-Free/Corbis; p. 252 (f): ©Jack Star/PhotoLink/Getty Images RF; p. 252 (g): ©LifeART/Fotosearch RF; p. 252 (h): ©Digital Vision RF; p. 252 (i): ©The McGraw-Hill Companies, Inc./Jill Braaten, photographer; p. 252 (j): ©Royalty-Free/Corbis; p. 252 (k): ©Dynamic Graphics/JupiterImages RF; p. 252 (l): ©Keith Brofsky/Getty Images RF; p. 252 (m): ©Stockbyte/PunchStock RF; p. 252 (n): ©Duncan Smith/Getty Images RF; p. 253: ©Royalty-Free/Corbis; 9.1-9.2: ©The McGraw-Hill Companies, Inc./Jill Braaten, photographer; p. 257 (a): ©D. Hurst/Alamy RF; p. 257 (b): ©Valerie Giles/Photo Researchers, Inc.; p. 257 (c): ©Valentyn Volkov/

Alamy RF; p. 257 (d): ©DAJ/Getty Images; p. 258 (e): ©Envision/Corbis; p. 258 (f): ©Brand X Pictures/PunchStock RF; p. 258 (g): ©Robert George Young/Getty Images RF; p. 258 (h): ©Royalty-Free/Corbis; p. 258 (i): ©Robert Medvedenko/Getty Images; p. 258 (j): ©Maximilian Stock Ltd./Photo Researchers, Inc.; p. 258 (k): ©Medicimage/Visuals Unlimited; p. 258 (l): ©2009 Steven Foster; p. 258 (m): ©Gilbert S. Grant/Photo Researchers, Inc.; p. 258 (n): ©Per Arvid Aasen/Getty Images; p. 259 (o): ©Dr. John D. Cunningham/Visuals Unlimited; p. 259 (p): ©Victoria Firmston/Getty Images; p. 259 (q): ©Dr. Peter J. Llewellyn; p. 259 (r): ©Linda Lewis/Getty Images; 9.3: ©David Tietz/Editorial Image, LLC RF; 9.4: ©The McGraw-Hill Companies Inc./John Flournoy, photographer.

Chapter 10

Opener: ©Brand X Pictures/PunchStock RF; p. 269: Ken Karp for MMH; 10.1: ©PhotoDisc/Getty Images RF; 10.6: ©Corbis RF; 10.8: ©Ken Lax; 10.9: Ken Karp for MMH; 10.10: ©Brand X Pictures/PunchStock RF; 10.11: ©Total Care Programming, Inc.; 10.12: Copyright ©1978–2009 Lexi-Comp, Inc.; 10.13: ©Brand X Pictures/PunchStock RF; 10.14: Copyright ©1978–2009 Lexi-Comp, Inc.; 10.15: ©Total Care Programming, Inc.; 10.16: ©Digital Vision/Superstock RF; 10.17: ©PhotoDisc/Getty Images RF; 10.18: Copyright ©1978–2009 Lexi-Comp, Inc.; 10.19: ©Total Care Programming, Inc.; 10.20: ©The McGraw-Hill Companies, Inc./Jill Braaten, photographer; 10.21: ©Stockdisc/PunchStock RF; 10.22: ©The McGraw-Hill Companies, Inc./Christopher Kerrigan, photographer; 10.23: ©Royalty-Free/Corbis; 10.24: ©The McGraw-Hill Companies, Inc./Christopher Kerrigan, photographer; 10.25: ©Stockdisc/PunchStock RF; 10.26: ©The McGraw-Hill Companies, Inc./Jill Braaten, photographer; 10.27: ©Dynamic Graphics/JupiterImages RF; 10.28: ©Royalty-Free/Corbis.

Chapter 11

Page 297 (*top*)-11.12: ©Total Care Programming, Inc.; 11.13a: ©Randy Allbritton/Getty Images RF; 11.13b: ©Thermal Angel Blood Warmer; 11.14: ©Total Care Programming, Inc.

Chapter 12

Figure 12.1: ©Brand X Pictures RF; p. 315: ©Suza Scalora/Getty Images RF; 12.2: ©Royalty-Free/Corbis; 12.4-12.5: ©Royalty-Free/Corbis; 12.6: ©Brand X Pictures RF; 12.7: ©amana images inc./Alamy RF; 12.8: ©Blend Images RF; 12.9: ©Don Farrall/Getty Images RF; 12.10: ©Total Care Programming, Inc.; 12.11: ©Comstock Images/PictureQuest RF.

Chapter 13

Page 347-348: ©Total Care Programming, Inc.; 13.2: http://www.ncbi.nlm.nih.gov/pubmed/ Database resources of the National Center for Biotechnology Information; 13.3: ©Quantros, Inc.; 13.4: Courtesy of USP; 13.5: U.S. Food and Drug Administration; 13.6: Courtesy of USP; 13.7: ©GO INfusion LLC; 13.8-13.10: ©2009 Pysicians' Desk Reference Inc. All Rights Reserved; 13.11: Used with permission of the American Academy of Pediatrics, Red Book® 2009 Report of the Committee on Infectious Diseases, 28th Edition, American Academy of Pediatrics, 2009; 13.12: ©Comstock/PunchStock RF.

Chapter 14

Opener: ©Comstock/JupiterImages RF; p. 374: ©Total Care Programming, Inc.; 14.1-14.2: ©Royalty-Free/Corbis; 14.3: ©The McGraw-Hill Companies, Inc./Andrew Resek, photographer; 14.4: ©Stockdisc/PunchStock RF; 14.7: ©Total Care Programming, Inc.; 14.8: ©PhotoDisc/Getty Images RF; 14.9-14.13: ©Total Care Programming, Inc.

Chapter 15

Page 398: ©Ryan McVay/Getty Images RF; p. 399 (*top*): ©Stockbyte/PunchStock RF; p. 399 (*bottom*)-400: U.S. Drug Enforcement Administration; 404: ©liquidlibrary/PictureQuest RF; p. 406: ©PhotoDisc/Getty Images RF; 15.3: Pyxis® DuoStation system from CareFusion, Corp.; 15.4: Accuflex® OnDemand® by MTS Medication Technologies®; 15.5: ©Total Care Programming, Inc.

Chapter 16

Page 413: ©Stockdisc/PunchStock RF; 16.1: ©Keith Brofsky/Getty Images RF; 16.2: ©The McGraw-Hill Companies, Inc./Rick Brady, photographer; 16.3: ©Total Care Programming, Inc.; 16.4: ©Comstock/PictureQuest RF; 16.5: ©Stockdisc/PunchStock RF; 16.6: ©Comstock/Alamy RF; 16.7: ©Royalty-Free/Corbis; 16.8: ©Comstock/PictureQuest RF; 16.9: ©Digital Vision/PunchStock RF; 16.10: ©Royalty-Free/Corbis; 16.11: ©Brand X Pictures/PunchStock RF; 16.12: ©Brand X Pictures/PunchStock RF; 16.13: ©Royalty-Free/Corbis.

Chapter 17

Page 440: ©Royalty-Free/Corbis; 17.1-17.3: ©Total Care Programming, Inc.; 17.4: ©The McGraw-Hill Companies, Inc./Andrew Resek, photographer; 17.5: ©Ryan McVay/Getty Images RF; 17.6: ©Royalty-Free/Corbis; 17.7: ©Total Care Programming, Inc.; 17.10: ©Royalty-Free/Corbis; 17.11: ©Image Source/Getty Images RF.

Chapter 18

Opener: ©BananaStock/JupiterImages RF; 18.1: ©Total Care Programming, Inc.; p. 470: ©BananaStock/JupiterImages RF; 18.2 – 18.3: ©Total Care Programming, Inc.; 18.4: ©C Squared Studios/Getty Images RF; 18.5: ©Thinkstock/agefotostock RF; 18.6: ©Getty Images/Image Source RF; 18.9: ©C. Sherburne/PhotoLink/Getty Images RF; 18.10: ©Getty Images/PhotoDisc RF; 18.11: ©Flying Colours Ltd/Digital Vision/Getty Images RF; 8.12: ©Digital Vision RF.

Chapter 19

Page 487: ©Stockdisc/PunchStock RF; 19.1: ©Thinkstock/Getty Images/Ron Chapple RF; 19.2: ©BananaStock/PictureQuest RF; 19.3: ©Steve Cole/Getty Images RF; 19.5: ©Comstock/JupiterImages RF; 19.6: ©Digital Vision/Getty Images RF.

Line Art and Text Credits

Chapter 1

Page 4: PTCB Knowledge Statements, Table 1-3, Table 1-4, The Pharmacy Technician Certification Board.

Chapter 2

Figure 2.8: Courtesy of the Office of Infectious Disease Services of Arizona; 2.15: Booth, Medical Assisting 3e; p. 39, Pharmacy Infection Control Policies and Procedures, The Joint Commission, Source CP Coe, JP Uselton: *Preparing the Pharmacy for a Joint Commission Survey,* 5th ed. Bethesda, MD: ASHP, 2003, pg. 106.

Chapter 3

Figure 3.1: Booth, Medical Assisting, 3e; Table 3-2: *Source:* Adapted with permission from Michael A. Aun, *Thirteen Customer Service Facts*, © 2006.

Chapter 4

Figure 4.8: Booth, Math and Dosage, 3e; Table 4-2: Copyright © The Joint Commission, 2009. Reprinted with permission; p. 81, Code of Ethics for Pharmacists: *Journal of the American Pharmacists Association* by American Pharmacists Association, Copyright 2009 by AMERICAN PHARMACISTS ASSOCIATION (J). Reproduced with permission of AMERICAN PHARMACISTS

ASSOCATION (J) in the format Textbook via Copyright Clearance Center.; p. 82, Code of Ethics for Pharmacy Technicians: Institute for the Certification of Pharmacy Technicians.

Chapter 5

Figure 5.1, 5.4, 5.5, 5.6, 5.7: Booth, Math and Dosage, 3e; 5.2: Courtesy TEVA Pharmaceuticals; 5.3: Courtesy JHP Pharmaceuticals; 5.8: Courtesy Bayer Corporation; 5.9: Courtesy Ortho-McNeil-Janssen Pharmaceuticals; p. 165: Courtesy Forest Pharmaceuticals, Inc.

Chapter 6

Figure 6.1, 6.2, 6.3, 6.4: Hinter / Nagle, Pharmacology: An Introduction, 5e.

Chapter 7

Figure 7.1, 7.2, 7.3, 7.4, 7.5, 7.6, 7.9: Booth, Medical Assisting, 3e.

Chapter 10

Figure 10.2a: © Pfizer, Inc. Reproduced with permission; 10.2b, 10.3, 10.4, 10.7: Booth, Medical Assisting, 3e; 10-5: Reprinted with the permission of Roche Laboratories Inc. All rights reserved.

Chapter 12

Table 12-6: Institute for Safe Medication Practices, used with permission.

Chapter 15

Figure 15.1: Booth, Math and Dosage, 3e. Table 15-2: Copyright © The Joint Commission, 2009, Reprinted with permission.

Chapter 18

Figure 18.8: Booth, Medical Assisting, 3e.

Appendix B

Page 493: Adapted from The Joint Commission, National Safety Goal: Identify and, at a minimum, annually review a list of look-alike/sound-alike drugs used in the organization, and take action to prevent errors involving the interchange of these drugs. 2006–2008 and ISP Quality Review, No. 79, April 2004.

Index

A

AAP Red Book: Report of the Committee on Infectious Diseases, 358
Abbreviated New Drug Application (ANDA), 105–106
Abbreviations
  common prescription, 379
  dosage forms, 290
  Institute for Safe Medication Practices (ISMP) list of error-prone, 325–327
  pharmacy, 149–152
  TJC's Official Do Not Use List of, 405
Absorbing surface area, 179
Absorption, 176, 178–181
  bioavailability and, 181
  blood flow to site of, 179
  defined, 178
  route of administration and, 179–181
Abstinence syndrome, 190
Academy of Managed Care Pharmacy on defining managed care, 423
Acceptance as stage of dying, 69
Access the Pharmacy Technician Certification Board, 491
Accreditation, 7, 18
Accreditation Council of Pharmacy Education (ACPE), 361
Accrediting Bureau of Health Education Schools (ABHES), 18
Acetaminophen, 170, 200, 231
Acetic acid, 279
Achromycin, 276
Acidic medications, 177
Acids, 177
Acquired immunodeficiency syndrome (AIDS), 68
Active listening, 59
Active transport, 178
Active tubular secretion, 185
Acupressure, 251
Acupuncture, 251
Adaptation, neuronal, 187
Addition, 188
ADIS LMS Drug Alerts, 350
Adjudication
  defined, 384
  in mail-order pharmacy, 430
  online, 390–391
ADME (absorption, distribution, metabolism, and elimination) process, 176, 204
Administration errors, 319
Administration sets and drop factor, 161–162
Adrenal steroids, 210, 212
Adulteration, 86–87, 255
Adverse drug reactions
  associated with aspirin and nonsteroidal anti-inflammatory agents, 230–231
  common, of antiretroviral agents for HIV PEP, 41
Adverse effects, 172, 196
Adverse Event Reporting System (AERS), 360
Aerosols, 289
Affinity, 173
Age, dosing and, 186–187
Agency for Health Care Policy and Research (AHCPR), 432
Agonists, 173
AHFS Drug Information, 358
Airborne diseases, 33
  precautions in spread of, 33
Air Force, pharmacists in, 432
Alcohol, 198
Alcohol, Tobacco, Firearms and Explosives, Bureau of, 117
Alka-Seltzer, 276
Alkylating agents, 219
Allergic responses, 189
Alligation, 157, 302
Alligation medial, 157–158
Allopurinol, 200
Aloe, 257
Alopecia agents, 237
Alpha-1 adrenergic blockers, 206
Alpha-glucosidase inhibitors, 212
Alternative medicine, 253
Aluminum hydroxide, 233
Ambulatory pharmacies, 376
American Association of Colleges of Pharmacy (AACP), 7, 16
American Association of Pharmacy Technicians (AAPT), 493
American Council of Pharmacy Education (ACPE), 67
American Drug Index, 359
American Heart Association (AHA), CPR training offered by, 42
American Journal of Health-System Pharmacy, 347
American Pharmaceutical Association (APhA), 6, 7, 66
  on pharmacy mission, 5
  on training, 16
American Pharmacists Association (APhA), 6, 340, 360, 493
American Red Cross, CPR training offered by, 42
American Society of Consultant Pharmacists (ASCP), 22, 417
American Society of Health-System Pharmacists (ASHP), 7, 45, 301, 432, 493
  on externship, 470
  on hazardous drugs, 45, 408
  as source of continuing education, 490
  Task Force on Technical Personnel in Pharmacy, 18
  on training programs, 16, 469–471
Amino acids, 261
  in total parenteral nutrition (TPN), 308
Aminoglycosides, 213, 214, 215
Amoxil, 276
Anabolic Steroid Control Act (2004), 112
Analgesics, 198, 200, 221, 230–232, 243
  in home infusion, 419
Anaphylactic reaction, 189
Anesthetics, 198, 200, 221
Anger as stage of dying, 69
Angiotensin-converting enzyme (ACE) inhibitors, 198, 203, 206
Angiotensin receptor blockers, 206
Antacids, 208, 209, 233
Antagonism, 188
Antagonist, 173
  competitive, 173
Antazoline, 240
Anthrax, 43
Anti-acne agents, 221, 237
Anti-allergy agents, 221
Antianginal medications, 203–204
Antianxiety agents, 198
Antiarrhythmic medications, 203
Antibacterials, 221, 237–238
Antibiotics, 180, 197, 219, 221
  bactericidal, 213
  beta-lactam, 214
  in home infusion, 419
Anticholinergic effects, 242
Anticoagulant agents, 205, 206
Anticonvulsants, 198, 200, 201, 202
Anti-dandruff agents, 238–239
Antidepressants, 198, 201
Antidiabetic agents, 210, 212
Antidiarrheals, 208, 209, 234

Antiemetics, 208, 209, 234–235
Antiepileptics, 200
Antiflatulents, 235
Antifungals, 213, 214, 221, 236, 239
Antigout medications, 198, 202
Antihelmintic agents, 215
Antihemorrhoidals, 235
Antihistamines, 197, 198, 201, 207, 239, 244
Antihistaminets, 232
Antihyperlipidemic agents, 205, 206
Antihypertensives, 203, 205, 206
Anti-infective medications, 213–218
Anti-inflammatory agents, 200, 221
Antimetabolites, 219
Antimicrobial agents, 213–214, 216
Antimicrobial preservatives, 284
Antineoplastic medications, 218–219
  in home infusion, 419
Antiparasitics, 220, 221
Anti-Parkinson's agents, 198, 200, 201, 202
Antiplatelet agents, 205, 206
Antiprotozoal agents, 215
Antipruritics, 221
Antipsoriatics, 220, 221
Antipsychotics, 198, 201
Antipyretics, 230
Antiretroviral agents, 215
  common adverse drug reactions of, for HIV PEP, 41
  defined, 40
Antiseptics, 36–37, 215, 218
  hand hygiene and, 36
Antithrombotic agents, 205
Antithyroid agents, 210, 212
Antitussives, 244
Antivirals, 214, 221
Anusol HC ointment, 272
Anxiolytics, 198
Aplisol, 272
Apothecary system of measurement, 136
  conversions in, 137
Appearance in professionalism, 472
Application process, 476
  completing forms, 479
Approved Drug Products with Therapeutic Equivalence Evaluations (Orange Book), 351
Aqueous drugs, 180
Arabic numbers, 129
Arginine, 262
Armed Forces, 16
Army, pharmacists in, 432
Aromatherapy, 252
Artificial tears, 240
Aseptic technique, 304–306, 307
  defined, 34, 296, 406
ASHP Statement on Supportive Personnel in Hospital Pharmacy, release of, 7
Assisted-living facilities, 413
Associate degree programs, 17
Atrovent, 289
Attitude, 67
  in externship, 472
  positive, 67
Automatic pill counting machines in mail-order pharmacy, 430
Automation, 406
Avian flu, 43
Avoirdupois system of measurement, 136–137
  conversions in, 137
Ayurvedic medicine, 251, 252
Azithromycin, 171

B

Bactericidal antibiotics, 213
Balances, 139
  Class A, 139
  electronic, 139
Barbiturates, 201
Bar coding, 332, 406
  in mail-order pharmacy, 430
Bargaining as stage of dying, 69
Bases, 177
Basic medications, 177
Benadryl, 189
Benzalkonium chloride, 283
Benzocaine, 242
Benzodiazepines, 197, 201
Benzoyl peroxide, 237, 279
Beta adrenergic blockers, 203, 206
Beta carotene, 262
Beta-lactam antibiotics, 213, 214
Betoptics, 290
Bicillin LA, 272
Bid price, 450
Biennial inventory, 443
Bilberry, 257
Bile acid binding resins, 206
Binders, 275
Bingo cards, 415
Bioavailability, 181
Biological, 352
Biological Abstracts, 349
Biologically equivalent, 181
Biological response modifiers in home infusion, 419
Biological safety cabinets, 46
Biomedical Service Corps, 432
Bioresearch, 349
BIOSIS Previews, 349
Biotechnology, 351
Bioterrorism, biological agents associated with, 43–44
Biotransformation, 184
Bipolar affective disorder, 199
Birth defects, drugs associated with, 184
Bisphosphonates, 210
Black cohosh, 257
Blanket authorization
  for destruction of controlled substances, 97
  issuance by Drug Enforcement Administration, 456–457
Blended unit-dose system, 415
Blister cards, 415
Bloodborne diseases, 31
  standard precautions for, 31
Bloodborne pathogens, 31, 44
Blood-brain barrier, 186–187
Blood flow to site of absorption, 179
Bloodstream infections, 34
Board and care homes, 414
Body fluids, contact with, 35
Body language, 60–61
Body size, dosing and, 187
Body surface area (BSA), 148
Bonine, 233
Brand name of drug, 171
  generic versus, 383–384
Breast milk, drugs found in, 186
Breathing, 207
Broad-spectrum antibacterial coverage, 238
Brompheniramine, 244
Bronchodilators, 207
Buccal administration, 271
Buffering agents, 289–290
Butoconazole, 236

C

Calcium channel blockers, 203, 206
Calcium gluconate, 142
Callus removal agents, 238
Candida species, 34
Canker sore agents, 241–242
Capitation-based reimbursement system, 425
Capsicum peppers (Capsaicin), 257
Capsules, 276
Carbacephems, 214, 216
Carbamide peroxide, 242
Carbapenems, 214, 215
Carboxymethylcellulose, 240, 242
Carcinogenesis, 354
Cardiac care units (CCUs), 398
Cardiac glycosides, 203
Cardiopulmonary resuscitation (CPR), 42
Cardiovascular system medications, 203–204
Cassettes, 406
Castor oil, 286
Catapres-TTS, 280
Catechol-0-methyltransferase (COMT) inhibitors, 200
Cathartics, 209
Caventou, 6
Ceiling effect of a drug, 174–175
Cells, target, 172
Cellulitis, 238
Center for Biologics Evaluation and Research (CBER), 360
Centers for Disease Control and Prevention (CDC), 29–30, 42, 432
  administration of Vaccine Adverse Event Reporting System (VAERS), 335
Centers for Medicare and Medicaid Services (CMS), 400
Central fill pharmacy, 431
Centralized pharmacy, 399
Centrally acting agents, 206
Central nervous system (CNS), 198
Central nervous system (CNS) agents, 198–203, 232–233
Central nervous system (CNS) stimulants, 189
Cephalosporins, 197, 214, 216
Cerumenex, 274
Certification, 491
  defined, 7, 486

Cetirizine, 207
Chain pharmacies, 85, 375–376
defined, 19
inventory management in, 444
Chamomile, 257
Chaste tree, 258
Chemically equivalent, 181
Chemical name of drug, 170–171
Chemotherapeutic agents, 309
Chemotherapy, 308–309
Chewable tablets, 276
Child-resistant packaging, 102, 229
Chinese medicine, 251, 252, 253
Chlorpheniramine, 207, 244
Chondroitin sulfate, 262
Claritin, 232
Claritin RediTab, 276
Clark's Rule, 148
Class A balances, 139, 298
Class I recall, 460
Class II recall, 460
Class III recall, 460
Classifieds, 473
Clemastine, 244
Clindamycin, 279
Clinical coordinator, 470
Clinical trials, 114–115, 457
types of, 114
Clobetasol, 279
Clotrimazole, 236, 239
Cocaine, 199
Codeine, 170
Code of ethics
for pharmacists, 81–82
for pharmacy technicians, 82–83
Code of Federal Regulations, 229
Co-insurance, 390
Colchicine, 200
Cold sore agents, 241–242
Colonic therapy, 252
Coloring agents, 275
Coly-Mycin M Parenteral, 272
Combat Methamphetamine Epidemic Act (2003), 227
Common prescription abbreviations, 379
Communication, 56–58
barriers in, 58
customer service and, 71–72
defined, 56
downward, 57
lateral, 57–58
nonverbal, 56
obstacles, 62–63
one-on-one, 57
types of, 58–63
upward, 57
verbal, 58–59
written, 62
Community hospitals, 398
Community pharmacies, duties of pharmacy technicians in, 10–12
Community (retail) setting, 19–20
Compassion, 69
Compassionate health care, 68–70
Competitive antagonists, 173
Complementary and alternative modalities, 251–262
defined, 253
dietary supplements, 254–257, 258–259
critical issues of use, 255–256
herbal preparations, 256–257, 257–259
minerals, 260–261
nonherbal dietary supplements, 261, 262
vitamins, 260, 261
examples of, 251–252
significance of, 253–254
Compliance (bid) report, 451
Compounding, 8, 296–309
alligation medial, 157–158
dilution, 156–157
extemporaneous, 296, 297–300
records on, 418
reducing and enlarging formula, 155–156
specific gravity, 158, 159
sterile, 296–297, 301–304, 407
Comprehensive Drug Abuse Prevention and Control Act (Controlled Substance Act, 1970), 89–102, 376
controlled substance inventories, 97
controlled substance prescription refills, 94
controlled substance record retention, 99–100
destruction of controlled substances, 97
drug schedules, 89–90
emergency dispensing of Schedule II medications, 94
exempt narcotics, 95
mailing of controlled substances, 102
methods of receiving controlled substance prescription, 93
ordering of controlled substances, 95
partial dispensing of controlled substances, 93–94
prescription label for controlled substances, 94–95
prescription requirements for controlled substances, 90
transferring prescription for controlled substances, 94
Comprehensive Methamphetamine Control Act (1996), 109
Computerized physician order entry (CPOE), 389, 403
Computer systems, 383
in retail pharmacy, 389–391
Concentration, 178
Conflict, 70–71
Conjugation, 184
Consultant pharmacists, 22
Consumerism, 226
Containers, 387–388
Contamination, 255
Continual stress, 74
Continuing education, 9, 490–492
Continuous quality improvement (CQI), 333–334
Contraceptives, 236
Contracts in hospital inventory management, 450–451
Contraindication
defined, 196
drug, 172
drug-disease, 172
Controlled-release (CR) tablets, 275
Controlled Substance Act, 117
maintenance of current copy by pharmacy, 347
Controlled substances, 452–457
defined, 89, 199
destruction of, 97
blanket authorization for, 97
examples of, 91–92
in hospitals, 456
inventories of, 97
mailing of, 102
methods of receiving prescription, 93
ordering of, 95
partial dispensing of, 93–94
prescription label for, 94–95
prescription refills, 94
prescription requirements for, 90
record retention, 99–100
theft of, 100
transferring prescription for, 94
Conversion factors, 134, 139–140
using, 140–141
Co-pay, 390
Corn removal agents, 238
Correctional facilities, 413
Cort-Dome enema, 283
Cort enemas, 272
Corticosteroids, 207, 221, 239
Cortisporin otic suspension, 274
Cosmeceuticals, 352
Cosmetic mouthwashes, 282
Cosolvents, 282
Costco, 376
Cost-containment strategies of managed-care organizations, 426–427
Coumadin, 178, 275
Covera HS, 275
Cover letter, 476, 477
Cover sheet, fax, 478
CPR requirements, 42–45
"Crack" cocaine, 189
Craigie, Andrew, 6
Creams, 278
Creatine, 262
Credentialing, 18–19
Cross tolerance, 187
Crystal therapy, 252
Cultural differences, 58
Customers
barriers of communication for, 63
external, 65
internal, 65–66
types of, 65–66
Customer service, 63–73, 391–392
defined, 56, 64
facts on, 64
at pharmacy, 64–65
quality, 66–68
solutions for, 71–73
CVS, 19, 375–376
Cycle-fill system, 415
Cylindrical graduates, 138

Cytochrome P-450, 188
Cytomegalovirus, 35

D

Dalmane, 276
Databases, 349
 specialized, 350
DAW (dispense as written) codes, reimbursement and, 384
Days supply, 153–154
Decadron Ophthalmic Solution, 290
Decentralized pharmacy, 399
Decimals
 converting fractions to, 131–132
 equivalencies of, 133
Decongestants, 244
Defense, U.S. Department of, 24
 pharmacy in, 432
Dehydroepiandrosterone (DHEA), 262
Delayed-release tablets, 276
Denial as stage of dying, 69
Denominator, 130
Depression as stage of dying, 69
Dermatitis, 239
Dermatitis agents, 239
Dermatologic agents, 220, 221
Derwent Drug File, 350
Desired dose, 144
Desloratadine, 207
Desoximethasone, 279
Dextromethorphan (DMX), 244
Diabetes mellitus, 210
Diazepam, 197
Dietary Supplement Health and Education Act (DSHEA) (1994), 86, 108, 254
Dietary supplements, 205, 206, 246, 251, 254–259
 critical issues of use, 255–256
 defined, 253
 herbal preparations, 256–257, 257–259
 minerals, 260–261
 nonherbal, 261, 262
 vitamins, 260, 261
Dietitian as member of infusion team, 420
Diffusion, 177
Digoxin, 170
Dilantin, 178
Diluents, 156, 275, 302, 308
Dilution, 156–157
 defined, 156
 solving problems involving, 157–158
Dimensional analysis, 134
Diogenes FDA Regulatory Updates, 350
Dioscorides, 6
Diphenhydramine, 207, 244
Diploma and certificate programs, 16–17
Disease management, 424
Disinfectants, 215, 218
Disintegrants, 275
Disintegration, 178
Dispensing, 331–332
 errors in, 319
 in mail-order pharmacy, 430
Disperse systems, 285–286
Disposable protective wear, 37
Distribution, 181–184
 passage of drugs into and across cells, 182–184
Diuretics, 198, 203, 204–205, 206
Divisibility tests of number, 131
Doctor's information, entering, in processing prescriptions, 383–384
Documentation and reporting outside organization, 42
Dopamine, 199
Dosage calculations, 144–149
 body surface area, 148
 determining desired dose, 145–147
 pediatric dosing, 148
Dosage forms
 abbreviations for, 290
 aerosols, 289
 available for administration by various routes of administration, 291
 capsules, 276–277
 creams, 278
 defined, 199
 douche, 283
 elixirs, 284–285
 enemas, 283
 gel (jellies), 279
 inhalants, 288–289
 injectable parenteral preparations, 286–287, 288
 nasal solutions, 282
 ointments, 278
 ophthalmic preparations, 289–290
 optic solutions, 283
 pastilles, 277
 pellets (implants), 280
 solutions, 281–282
 storage of, 276
 suppositories, 280
 suspensions, 286
 syrups, 284
 tablets, 275–276
 tinctures, 285
 topical solutions, 282
 transdermal drug delivery systems, 279–280
 troches, 277
 vaginal inserts, 281
Dosage ordered, 144
Dose
 desired, 144
  determining, 145–147
 loading, 175
 maintenance, 175
 prophylactic, 175
Dose-response, 174–175
Dosing, 186–190
 age in, 186–187
 body size in, 187
 drug interactions in, 188
 factors affecting drug, 187–188
 pediatric, 148
 sex in, 187
 timing of administration in, 187
 tolerance in, 187
Double gloving, 46
Douches, 283
 defined, 283
 eye, 283
 pharyngeal, 283
 vaginal, 283
Downsizing, 486
Downward communication, 57
Dramamine (dimenhydrinate), 233
Drop factor, 161–162
 calculating, 162
Droplets, precautions with, 33
Drug addiction, 189–190
Drug allergies, 189
Drug classifications, 196–221
 anti-infective medications, 213–218
 antineoplastic medications, 218–219
 cardiovascular system medications, 203–204
 central nervous system medications, 198–203
 dermatologic agents, 220, 221
 endocrine system medications, 210–213
 gastrointestinal system medications, 208–209
 immune system medications, 219, 220
 ophthalmic agents, 220, 221
 renal/vascular system medications, 204–205, 206
 respiratory system medications, 207
Drug contraindication, 172
Drug delivery system of long-term care facility, 414
Drug dependence, 189–190
Drug-disease contraindication, 172
Drug Enforcement Administration (DEA), 117–118, 331, 399, 452, 454–455
 Form 41, 97, 455, 456
 Form 222, 95, 96, 452–453, 456
 Form 224, 452
 issuance of blanket authorization by, 456–457
 numbers of, 90
 transmission of Schedule II medications and, 416
Drug Facts and Comparisons (F & C), 353
Drug interactions, 188
Drug labels, 154–155
Drug Listing Act (1972), 103–104
Drug manufacturer, 65
Drug orders, 401–404
Drug Price Competition and Patent Term Restoration Act (1984), 105–106
Drug recalls, 460–461
 Food and Drug Administration and, 434
Drug-receptor interaction, 197
Drug Reimbursement Information, 356
Drugs, 170–171
 bioavailability testing on all, 181
 birth defects associated with, 184
 brand name of, 171
 ceiling effect of, 174–175
 chemical name of, 170–171
 defined, 170
 generic name of, 171
 intended effect of, 172
 investigational, 457–459
 legend, 87–88
 oral administration of, 185
 passage of, into and across, 182–184
 placental transfer of, 183–184

Drugs *(cont)*
potency of, 173–175
prescription or legend, 88–89
pulmonary absorption of a, 180
renal elimination of, 185
therapeutic effect of a, 172
Drug schedules, 89–90
Drug screening, 479
Drug Topics, 360
Drug utilization evaluation (DUE), 22, 384–385
defined, 384–385
Drug utilization review (DUR) programs, 107
Dual co-insurance, 390
Durham-Humphrey Amendment (1952), 87–89, 376
Dyclonine, 242
Dying, stages of, 69

E

Eardrops, 283
Ebers Papyrus, 6
Echinacea, 258
Ecotrin, 276
ED50 (effective dose 50), 172
Effervescent tablets, 276
Efficacy, 173
E-Health Initiative, 330
80/20 report, 451
Electrolytes, 142
Electronic balances, 139
Electronic orders, 403
Electronic prescribing, 330–331
Elimination, 176, 185–186
rate of, 176
Elixirs, 284–285
EMBASE, 349
Emergency Action Plan (EAP), 44
Emergency medications, examples of, 415–416
Emergency Use Investigational New Drug, 458
Emesis, 234
Emollient agents, 221
Empathy
defined, 59
displaying, 59–60
Employee evaluation, 489
Employee's work record, employee's evaluation in, 489
Employment agencies, 473
Emulsification, 286
Emulsions, 285–286
E-mycin, 276
Encoding, 57
Endocrine system medications, 210–213
Enemas
defined, 283
evacuant, 283
retention, 283
Enteral administrations, 179
Enteric-coated tablets, 276
Enterohepatic (intestinal) pathway, 185
Environment, 62
as barrier in communication, 62
Enzyme induction, 185
Enzyme inhibition, 185
Epocrates, 361
Epstein-Barr virus (EBV), 35
Errors
defined, 314
in dispensing medications, 314
external, 321
judgment, 319
knowledge-based, 321
medication, 314–340
Erythropoietin, 170
Escherichia coli, 34
Eskalith, 199
Estraderm, 280
Estradiol, 274
Ethics, 81–83
Ethnic medicine, 252
Etiology, 358
Evacuant enemas, 283
Exam for the Certification of Pharmacy Technicians (ExCPT), 491
Excipients, 226, 227, 281
Exempt narcotics, 95
Expiration dates, checking, 447
Extemporaneous compounding, 297–300
defined, 296
equipment and tools, 298, 299
sterile, 301–304
techniques, 298–300
Extended-care facilities (ECFs), 21, 413
Extended-release (ER) tablets, 275
External customers, 65
External errors, 321
Externships, 470
defined, 9, 470
expectation of candidates, 471–472
for pharmacy technician programs, 470–471
professionalism on, 471–472
Eye douche, 283

F

Failure mode and effects analysis (FMEA), 323
Fax cover sheet, 478
Fax transmission of resume, 476
FDA Modernization Act (1997), 109
F-D-C Reports, 350
Fecal-oral transmission, 35
Federal Bureau of Investigation (FBI), 42
Federal Food, Drug and Cosmetic Act (1938) (FDC), 86–87, 104, 111, 113, 115, 351, 376
Federal law, 84
Federal pharmacy, 432–434
Defense, U.S, Department of, 432
laws covering, 85–113
marketing in, 434
pharmaceutical sales in, 434
Public Health Service, 432–433
Veterans Administration (VA), 433
Federal Register, 229
Federal Trade Commission (FTC), 116–117
Feedback, 57
absence or lack of, 58
Fexofenadine, 207
Fibric acid derivatives, 206
Fire Prevention Plan (FPP), 44–45
First aid requirements, 42–45
First-pass metabolism, 185
Flavoring agents, 275
Fleet's enema, 283
Flonase, 289
Flow of service, 377–389
Flow rates, 160–161
FluMist, 274
Fluorides, 242
Fluoroquinolones, 213, 214, 215
Folic acid, 261
Folk medicine, 252
Folliculitis, 238
Food additives, 433
Food and Drug Administration (FDA), 113–117, 309, 433
administration of Vaccine Adverse Event Reporting System (VAERS), 335
approval of over-the-counter drugs, 226
authority to establish good manufacturing processes for dietary supplements, 254, 255
on bioavailability testing of drugs, 181
categorization of antiseptic drug products, 36–37
creation of, 86
defined, 86
Form 3500A for mandatory reporting, 337
Form 3500 for voluntary reporting, 336
Internet references of, 360
investigational drugs and, 457
pharmaceutical industry and, 434
pregnancy categories established by, 190
role in classification of drugs, 197
Safety Information and Adverse Event Reporting Program of, 335
Foodborne pathogens, 44
Formula, reducing and enlarging, 155–156
Formularies, 401, 426–427, 449–450
defined, 350, 401
utilization of, by prescription benefits manager, 389–390
Fractions
converting to decimals, 131–132
equivalencies of, 133
improper, 131
in mathematical concepts, 130–131
proper, 130–131
Franchise pharmacies, 376
defined, 19
inventory management in, 444
Frederick II of Hohenstaufen, 6
Free Online Education for Healthcare Profession as source of continuing education, 490

G

Galen, 6
Gamma amino butyric acid (GABA), 197
Gargles, 281
Garlic, 257, 258

Gastrointestinal system agents, 208–209, 233–235, 234
Gelatin capsules, 298
Gelatin-coated tablets, 276
Gels (jellies), 279
General anesthetics, 198, 200, 202, 273
Generic name of drug, 171
 brand versus, 383–384
Genital itching, agents for, 236
Genitourinary system agents, 235–236, 237
Giardia, 35
Ginger, 257, 258
Gingko, 257, 258
Ginseng, 257, 258
Glaucoma, agents for, 221
Glomerulonephritis, 189
Glomerulopathy, 189
Glucocorticoids, 210, 239
Glucosamine, 262
Glycerin, 240
Glycylcycline, 216
Goldenseal, 258
Gonadal hormones and oral contraceptives, 210, 212
Goodman and Gilman's The Pharmacologic Basis of Therapeutics, 348, 358
Good Manufacturing Practices (GMPs), 115–117, 116
 FDA enforcement of, 254, 255
Gout, 200
Gravity, specific, 158, 159
Green tea, 258
Group model health maintenance organizations (HMOs), 425
Group purchasing organization (GPO), 450

H

H2 blockers, 208, 209
Habit, 68
Half-life (t1/2), 176
Handbook on Injectable Drugs, 358
Hand hygiene, 34
Hand hygiene antiseptic agents, 36
 characteristics and antimicrobial spectrum of, 37
Hand washing
 disease containment and, 35
 technique in, 35–37
Harrison Narcotic Act (1914), 86
Hazardous drugs, 45, 48
 disposal of, 50
Hazardous material
 drugs as, 45
 handling of, 46–48
 storage of, 45
Health care, compassionate, 68–70
Health care workers, National Institute for Occupational Safety and Health (NIOSH) recommendations for, 49–50
Health Insurance Portability and Accountability Act (2003) (HIPAA), 15, 70, 108–109, 376
Health maintenance organizations (HMOs), 389, 425
 defined, 385
 group model of, 425
 network model of, 425
 staff model of, 425
HealthSTAR, 361
Hematologic agents, 205, 206
Hematopoietic stimulants, 206
Hepatic, 184
Hepatitis A, 35
Hepatitis B virus (HBV), 31
Hepatitis C virus (HCV), 31
Hepatoxicity, 189
 nephrotoxicity and, 189
Herbal preparations, 256–257, 257–259
Hermetic container, 448
Heroin, 189, 199
High-alert medications, 328–329
Highest Ranking Criticality Indexes, 323
Histamine, 172
Histamine 2 receptor blockers, 209, 233
HMG-CoA reductase inhibitors, 206
Home diagnostic, 246
Home health care environment, pharmacists working in, 9
Home infusion, 418
 commonly used medications in, 419
Home infusion pharmacy, 23, 418–423
 managed-care, 423–428
 pharmacist in, 427–428
 pharmacist responsibilities in, 420–422
 pharmacy technicians in, 422–423, 427–428
 team in, 418–420
Homeopathy, 252
Home remedies, 252
Horizontal laminar flow, 302
Hormonal agents, 219
Hormonal supplementation agents, 211
Hospital/institutional setting, 20–21
Hospital inventory management, 449–462
Hospital pharmacy technicians, responsibilities of, 20–21
Hospitals, 397–409, 398
 community, 398
 controlled substances in, 456
 electronic orders in, 403
 formulary in, 401
 investigational drugs in, 459
 medication orders in, 401–404
 pharmacy and therapeutics committee in, 401
 policy and procedure manual in, 400
 safety committee in, 39
 teaching, 398
Household system of measurement, 137–139
 conversions in, 137
Human immunodeficiency virus (HIV), 31
 monitoring patient, 41
 postexposure prophylaxis (PEP), 41
 procedures for prophylaxis, 41–42
Hydrogen peroxide, 242
Hydroxyethyl cellulose, 240, 242
Hydroxyzine, 207
Hyperreactivity, 173
Hypersensitivity, 189
Hyperthyroidism, 210
Hypnotic agents, 198–199
Hyporeactivity, 173
Hypothyroidism, 210

I

Ident-A-Drug, 358
Idiosyncrasy, 173
Illinois Council of Health System Pharmacists (ICHP), 7
Imaging systems in mail-order pharmacy, 430
Immune system medications, 219, 220
Immunomodulators, 219
Immunosuppressive agents, 219
Improper fraction, 131
Improper preparation, 255
Incident report, 31, 39–40
 sample, 32
Independent pharmacies, 376
 defined, 19
 inventory management in, 444
Independent practice association (IPAs), 425
 defined, 389
Indian Health Service (IHS), 433
Indication, 197
Indigestion, agents for, 233
Indocin, 276
Infection control, 306–308
Infections, nosocomial, 34
Infectious diseases
 common, 30–31
 prevention of spreading, 34–38
Infusions containing medications, 162–163
Infusion therapy, 23
Inhalants, 288–289
Inhalation products, 273
Inhalers, 180
Initial inventory, 443
Injectable administration, 272–273
Injectable parenteral preparations, 286–287, 288
Inpatient setting. *See* Hospitals
Insomnia, agents for, 232
Instant disintegrating/dissolving tablets, 276
Institute for Safe Medication Practices (ISMP)
 defined, 323
 list of error-prone abbreviations, symbols, and dose designations, 325–327
 list of high-alert medications, 328–329
Institute for the Certification of Pharmacy Technicians (ICPT), 491
Institute of Medicine (IOM), 323
 release of *To Err Is Human,* 314
Institute for Safe Medication Practices, establishment of Patient's Five Rights of Medication, 128
Insulins, 210, 212, 272–273
Intal inhaler, 289
Integrase inhibitors, 41
Integrative medicine, 251, 253
Integumentary system agents, 236–239, 238
Intended effect of a drug, 172
Intensive care units (ICUs), 398

Interactions, 196
Intermediate-care facilities (ICFs), 21–22, 413
Internal customers, 65–66
International time, 143
International units, 142
Internet, 431
Internet Grateful Med, 349
Internet pharmacy, 431
Internship, 9
Interviewing, 479–482
Intra-arterial administration, 180
Intradermal injections, 272
Intramuscular administration, 180, 272
Intraperitoneal administration, 180
Intrathecal administration, 180
Intravenous additive solutions, 305–306
Intravenous administration, 179
  defined, 272
Intravenous applications
  administration sets and drop factor, 161–162
  calculating drop factor, 162
  flow rates, 160–161
  infusions containing medications, 162–163
Intravenous infusions, 301
Intravenous injections, 272
  defined, 272
Intravenous medications, 180
Intravenous piggyback, 301
Inventory
  biennial, 443
  defined, 439
  initial, 443
  in long-term care pharmacy, 414
  perpetual, 443
  pharmacy, 439
  physical, 442–443
Inventory management, 438–461
  drug recalls, 460–461
  importance of, 440
  periodic automatic replenishment in, 441–442
  physical inventory in, 442–443
  retail, 444–449
Inventory turnover rates, 442
Investigation, phrases of, 458–459
Investigational drugs, 457–459
  in hospital setting, 459
Investigational New Drug (IND), 457, 458
  types of, 458
Investigator, 457
Investigator Investigational New Drug (IND), 458
In-windows, 376
Ionized, 176
Iowa Drug Information Service, 350
Iridology, 252
Isotonicity, 289
Isotretinoin Safety and Risk Management Act (2004), 111–112

J

JAMA: Journal of the American Medical Association, 347
JAPhA, 360
Jaundice, 189
Job security, professionalism and, 486
Joint Commission (TJC), 18, 111, 118–119, 309, 317, 383, 399–400
  accreditation of infusion pharmacies and, 419
  Official Do Not Use List of Abbreviations, 405
  Patient Safety Goals, 323
  standards of, 29
    for infection control, 38
Joint Commission Journal on Quality and Safety, 317
Joint Commission on Accreditation of Healthcare Organizations (JCAHO), 18, 111, 309, 317, 383, 399–400
JPharmSci, 360
Judgment error, 319

K

Kaolin-pectin, 208
Kava, 257, 258
Kefauver-Harris Amendment (1962), 89, 376
Ketolides, 214, 216
Kinesics, 61
Klebsiella species, 34
Knowledge-base and understanding, 66–67
Knowledge-based error, 321
Kübler-Ross, Elizabeth, 69

L

Labeling, 87
  packaging and, 332
Labor induction, 211
Lacrimal fluid, 289
Lactobacillus, 262
Laminar flow hood, 302, 407
Language problems, 58
Lanoxin, 275
Large-volume parenterals (LVPs), 287
Lateral communication, 57–58
Latex gloves, 46
Laws, 83–85
  defined, 83
  federal, 84
  federal pharmacy, 85–113
  state, 84
  tort, 84–85
Laxatives, 209, 235
LD50 (lethal dose 50), 172
Leapfrog Group, 330
Legend drugs, 87–89, 199
Levigation, 299
Levodopa, 200
Licensure
  defined, 18
  of mail-order pharmacy, 430–431
  proof of state, 478–479
Lidocaine, 180, 242
Light-resistant packaging, 448
Limitations as cost-containment strategy in managed-care pharmacy, 427
Lipid-soluble drug, 184
Listening, active, 59
Lithane, 199
Lithium, 178, 199
Lithobid, 199
Lithonate, 199
Loading dose, 175
Local anesthetics, 198, 200, 202, 239, 242
Local effect, 270
Long-term care facilities (LTCFs), 21, 399
  drug delivery system of, 414
  examples of, 413
Long-term care pharmacy, 21–23, 413–418
  legal requirements of, 415–416
  pharmacy technicians in, 417–418
Loop, 206
Loperamide, 208, 234
Loratadine, 207, 244
Lubricants, 275
Lysergic acid diethylamide (LSD), 199

M

Maalox, 233
Macrolides, 214, 216
Magnesium hydroxide, 233
Magnesium sulfate, 142
Mail-order pharmacy, 22–23, 428–431
  advantages of, 429
  disadvantages of, 429
  licensure of, 430–431
  pharmacy technicians in, 431
  technology in, 430
  workflow in, 429–430
Maintenance dose, 175
Major tranquilizers, 199
Malpractice, 85
Managed care, 423
Managed-care organizations, 424–426
  cost-containment strategies of, 426–427
Managed-care pharmacy, 23, 423–428
Manual for Hospital Pharmacy Technicians: A Programmed Course in Basic Skills, 7
Manufacturer/Wholesaler Information, 356
Marijuana, 189
Marketing in pharmaceutical industry, 434
Market withdrawal, 460
Marshall Apothecary shop, 6
Massachusetts Coalition for the Prevention of Medical Errors, 319
Massage therapy, 252
Masters, Wardens, and Society of the Art and Mystery of the Apothecaries of the City of London, 6
Material Safety Data Sheets (MSDS), 47, 103
Mathematical concepts
  converting fractions to decimals, 131–132
  converting number to a percent, 132
  dimensional analysis in, 134
  fractions in, 130–131
  percent in, 132–133
  proportion, 133–134
  ratio in, 132
McNeil Laboratories, 460
MDMA (3,4-Methylenedioxymethamphetamine) ("Ecstasy"), 199

Measurement systems
apothecary, 136
avoirdupois, 136–137
household, 137–139
metric, 135–136
temperature, 142–143
units of, 135–141
Mechanism of action, 173
Medicaid, 426
Medicaid Tamper Resistant Prescription Pad Law, 112–113
Medical Device Amendments (1976), 104
Medical devices, 104
safety alerts for, 460
Medical Service Corps., 432
Medicare
Part A, 425
Part B, 425
Part C, 425
Medicare Modernization Act (MMA) (2003), 110, 376
Medication(s)
acidic, 177
anti-infective, 213–218
antineoplastic, 218–219
basic, 177
cardiovascular system, 203–204
central nervous system (CNS), 198–203
endocrine system, 210–213
gastrointestinal system, 208–209
high-alert, 328–329
immune system, 219, 220
infusions containing, 162–163
over-the-counter (OTC), 88
packaging and storage of, in retail inventory management, 447–449
parenteral, 406–407
reconciliation of, 407–408
renal/vascular system, 204–205, 206
respiratory system, 207
storage of, 142
Medication administration records (MARs), 398
Medication dosing, 173–175
Medication errors, 314–340
administration, 319
assessment of, 324
categories of, 316
consequences of, 321–322
defined, 314–315
dispensing, 319
electronic orders and, 403
facts on, 317
identifying, 323
organizational, 320–321
prescribing, 317–318
preventing, 325–334
bar coding, 332
continuous quality improvement, 333–334
dispensing, 331–332
electronic, 330–331
labeling and packaging, 332
pharmaceutical industry assistance, 333
prescription scanning, 333
prescription writing, 329
verbal prescriptions, 329–330
reducing, 323–329, 325–327
regulatory oversight, 334–340
MEDMARX, 339
MedWatch, 335
patient role in reduction of, 340
USP-ISMP Medication Errors Reporting Program (MERP), 339–340
Vaccine Adverse Event Reporting System (VAERS), 335
from verbal orders, 402
from written orders, 402
Medication Management Standards, 323
Medication (drug) orders, 152–153
processing, 405–408
Medicine Shoppe, 19, 376
MEDLINE, 349
Medline Plus, 361
MEDMARX, 320, 323, 339, 349
defined, 319
features of, 339
MedWatch, 335, 360
Melatonin, 262
Merck Index, 352–353
Metabolism, 184–185
first-pass, 185
hepatic microsomal drug-metabolizing system, 184–185
Metered-dose inhalant (MDI), 289
Methamphetamine, 199
Methicillin-resistant *Staphylococcus aureus* (MRSA), 34
Metoclopramide, 208
Metric system of measurement, 135–136
prefixes in, 136
Michigan Pharmacists Association (MPA), 7
Miconazole, 236, 239
Military time, 143
Milk thistle, 258
Millis Report, 347
Minerals, 260–261
Minimum Competencies for Institutional Pharmacy Technicians with Training Guidelines, 7
Min/Max, 445
Misbranding, 87
Misidentification, 255
Mithridates, 6
Mitotic inhibitors, 219
Mixed messages, 58
Model Curriculum for Pharmacy Technician Training, 16
Modified unit-dose system, 415
Moisturizers, 220
Monoamine oxidase inhibitors (MAOIs), 199, 200
Monobactams, 214
Monoclonal antibody, 352
Monographs, 115, 351
Monophasic and multiphasic products, 210
Morphine, 188
Motion sickness, agents for, 233, 234
Motrin, 275
Mouthwashes, 281–282
Movement disorders, agents for, 198, 200
Multi-drug-resistant pathogens, defined, 34
Multiple-dose containers, 287, 290, 448
Multiple tiered co-payments, 390
Multiple-unit containers, 448
Muscle relaxants, 198, 200
Muse, 280
Mutagenesis, 354
Mycelex Troche, 271, 277
Mydriasis, 241
Myelosuppression, 218
Mylicon drops, 286

N

Naloxone, 173
Naphazoline, 245
Narcan (naloxone), 188
Narcotic analgesics, 198, 200, 202, 203
Narcotics, 89
Nasal administration, 274
NasalCrom, 289
Nasal decongestants, 244–245
Nasal solutions, 282
National Association of Boards of Pharmacy (NABP), 6, 18, 120, 431, 492
National Association of Chain Drug Stores (NACDS), 16, 320, 491
National Association of Retail Druggists (NARD), 7
National Center for Competency Testing (NCCT), 479, 491
National Center for Complementary and Alternative Medicine, 260
National Childhood Vaccine Injury Act (NCVIA) (1986), 335
National Community Pharmacists Association (NCPA), 491
National Coordinating Council for Medication Error Reporting and Prevention (NCC MERP), 314–315, 329
National Council on Prescription Drug Programs (NCPDP), 330
National Drug Code (NDC), 104
National Drug Code (NDC) number, 386
National Formulary (NF), 135, 351
National Institute for Occupational Safety and Health (NIOSH), recommendations for health care workers, 49–50
National Institutes of Health (NIH), 433
National Pharmacy Technician Association (NPTA), 493
as source of continuing education, 490
National Provider's Identifier, 385–388
National Quality Forum, 323
Navy, pharmacists in, 432
NDA Pipeline: New Drugs, 350
Nebulizers, 180, 288
Negative stress, 73
Negligence, 321–322
defined, 84–85, 321
Neofax, 359
Neomycin oral solution or tablets, 214
Nephrotoxicity, 189
hepatoxicity and, 189
Networking, 473
Network model health maintenance organizations (HMOs), 425
Neuroleptic agents, 199
Neuronal adaptation, 187
New Drug Application (NDA), 86

New England Journal of Medicine, 347
Niacin, 261
NicoDerm, 280
Nitroglycerin, 204, 274
Nitrostat, 271
Nomogram, 148, 149
Nonherbal dietary supplements, 261, 262
Non-legend medications, 88
Nonnarcotic analgesics, 198, 202
Nonnucleoside reverse transcriptase inhibitors (NNRTIs), 41
Nonprescription antihistamines, 232
Nonresident pharmacy, 430
Nonsteroidal anti-inflammatory drugs (NSAIDS), 198, 200, 202, 203, 230
Nonsynthetic reaction, 184
Nonverbal communication, 56, 60–62
Norplant, 280
Nosocomial infections, 34
  defined, 30
Nucleoside reverse transcriptase inhibitors (NRTIs), 41
Number
  converting to percent, 132
  divisibility tests of, 131
Numbering systems, 129
Numerator, 130
Nurse, 65
  as member of infusion team, 420
Nursing care in long-term care facilities, 414
Nursing facilities, 413
Nursing home, 21
Nursing staff, communication with, 408–409
Nutraceutical, 352

O

Occupational Safety and Health Act (1970), 103
Occupational Safety and Health Administration (OSHA), 118
  compliance with, 408
  defined, 30
  on disposal of hazardous drugs, 50
  requirements for hazardous drugs, 46–47
Oculesics, 62
Official Do Not Use List of Abbreviations, 405
Oil-in-water emulsions, 278
Ointments
  defined, 278
  preparation of, 299–300
Omega-3 fatty acids, 262
Omeprazole (Prilosec), 233
Omnibus Budget Reconciliation Act (1987) (OBRA-87), 106–107
  requirements for pharmacy, 416
Omnibus Budget Reconciliation Act (1990) (OBRA-90), 10, 107–108, 332, 348, 376
Omnicell, 406
On Death and Dying (Kübler-Ross), 69
One-on-one communication, 57
  barriers to, 62
Online adjudication, 390–391, 427
On-the-job training, 16, 17–18, 486–489
Ophthalmic administration, 274, 289
Ophthalmic agents, 220, 221, 289–290
Ophthalmic antihistamines, 240
Ophthalmic decongestants, 240–241
Ophthalmic lubricants, 240
Oral administration of drug, 179, 185, 270–271
Oral antidiabetic agents, 212
Oral contraceptive agents, 211, 212
Oral/dental care agents, 241–242, 243
Oral medications, 271, 281
Oral pain, 242
Oral solutions, 281
Oral suspensions, 286
Order entry
  in mail-order pharmacy, 430
  in retail inventory management, 445
Order/rotating stock, receiving in retail inventory management, 446
Organizational causes of errors, 320–321
Orientation, 486
Orphan Drug Act (ODA) (1983), 105
Orphan drugs, 105
OSHA Technical Manual, 45, 47
Osteoporosis agents, 210
Otic agents, 221, 242, 243, 274, 283
Outdated and damaged stock in retail inventory management, 447
Outpatient pharmacies (ambulatory pharmacies), 376
Out-windows, 376
Over-the-counter (OTC) medications, 9, 88, 226–246, 392
  defined, 226
  legal requirements for, 227–229
  packaging of, 228–229
  types of, 230–246
Oxymetazoline, 245
Oxytocic agents, 211, 213

P

Package inserts, 47
Packaging, 332, 430
  types of, 448
Pain relievers, 231
Parenteral hormonal contraceptives, 211
Parenteral medications, 179–181, 271, 406–407
  defined, 271
  in home infusion, 419
Parkinson's disease, 200
Passion flower, 259
Passive reabsorption, 185
Passive transport, 177
Passive tubular reabsorption, 185
Pastille, 277
Patent, 105
Pathogen, 30
Patient consultation area, 376
Patient Product Insert (PPI), 115, 354, 388
Patients, 55, 65
  confidentiality and privacy of, 70
  entering information in processing prescription, 383
  Five Rights of Medication for, 128
  Joint Commission goals to improve safety of, 323
  in medication error reduction, 340
  mental or physical disabilities of, 58
  monitoring of IV therapy, by infusion pharmacist, 421
  preoperative skin preparation of, 36
Patient service representative as member of infusion team, 420
Patriot Act (2006), 227
PDR Drug Guide for Mental Health Professionals, 355
PDR for Herbal Medications, 355
PDR for Nonprescription Drugs, Dietary Supplements, and Herbs, 355
PDR for Nutritional Supplements, 355
PDR for Ophthalmic Medicines, 355
PDR Pharmacopoeia Pocket Guide, 355
Pediatric dosing, 148
Pediculosis, 239
Pelletier, 6
Pellets (implants), 280
Penicillins, 214, 215
Pen T-Sao (Shen Nung), 6
Percent(s), 132
  equivalencies of, 133
  in mathematical concepts, 132
  number converting to, 132
Percent volume-in-volume, 132
Percent weight-in-volume, 132
Percent weight-in-weight, 132
Periodic automatic replenishment, in inventory management, 441–442
Permethrin, 239
Perpetual inventory, 443
Personal barriers in communication, 63
Personal care, 414
  in long-term care facilities, 414
Personal digital assistant (PDA), 361
Personal portfolio, 478
Personal protective equipment (PPE), 46
  OSHA requirements for use of, 408
Pesticides, 433
PharmaCE as source of continuing education, 490
Pharmaceutical care plan, 421
Pharmaceutical industry, 24, 433–434
  assistance of, 333
Pharmaceutical News Index, 350
Pharmaceutical sales in pharmaceutical industry, 434
Pharmacies
  central fill, 431
  centralized, 399
  chain, 19, 85
  customer service at, 64–65
  decentralized, 399
  defined, 5
  federal, 432–434
  franchise, 19
  home infusion, 23, 418–423
  independent, 19
  Internet, 431
  long-term care, 21–23, 413–418
  mail-order, 22–23, 428–431
  managed-care, 23, 423–428
  medication errors committed by, 319

mission of, 5
nonresident, 430
physical appearance of, 62
practice of, 8–15
retail, 9
stress in, 73–75
Pharmacists, 8–9
code of ethics for, 81–82
consultant, 22
home infusion responsibilities of, 420–422
as member of home infusion team, 419
pharmacy calculations and, 127
role of, in managed care, 427–428
Pharmacodynamic tolerance, 187
Pharmacokinetics, 176–178
Pharmacokinetic tolerance, 187
Pharmacology, 172
terms associated with, 171–175
Pharmacy abbreviations, 149–150, 151–152
Pharmacy and Therapeutics (P&T) Committee, 426, 449–450
defined, 401, 449
of managed-care organization, 427
Pharmacy benefit manager (PBM), 424–425
Pharmacy Choice as source of continuing education, 490
Pharmacy incident report form, 40
Pharmacy Internet Web Sites, 362–363
Pharmacy inventory, 439
Pharmacy layout, 61–62
Pharmacy Now as source of continuing education, 490
Pharmacy practice, development of modern-day, 5, 6, 7
Pharmacy practice settings, pharmacy technician responsibilities and, 19–24
Pharmacy school, curriculum at, 8
Pharmacy Technician Certification Board (PTCB), 7, 493
Pharmacy Technician Certification Examination (PTCE), 18
successful completion of, 478–479
Pharmacy Technician Certification Examination (PTCE), 18, 491
Pharmacy technicians, 10–14
in care and cleaning of laminar flow hood, 304
characteristics of, 14–15
code of ethics for, 82–83
communication skills of, 55
in community pharmacies, 10–12
drug classification and, 197–198
duties of, 10
in extemporaneous compounding, 298
finding a position, 473
in home infusion pharmacy, 422–423
in hospital/institutional setting, 12–14
infection control and, 308
in long-term care pharmacy, 417–418
in mail-order pharmacy, 431
in managed care, 427
milestones for, 7
occupational outlook for, 14
pharmacy calculations and, 127
pharmacy practice settings and responsibilities of, 19–24
primary role of, 8
responsibilities of, 487
safety role of, 29–30
in sterile compounding, 302, 309
training programs for, 16–19, 469–472
Pharmacy Technicians Educators Council (PTEC), 16, 494
Pharmacy technicians–inpatient setting, 404–409
communication with nursing staff, 408–409
compliance with OSHA guidelines, 408
processing medication orders, 405–408
responsibilities of, 404
Pharmacy technicians programs
expectations of student externship candidates, 471–472
externships for, 470–471
Pharmacy Times, 361
Pharmacy Today, 360
Pharmacy units of measurement, 135–141
apothecary system of measurement, 136
avoirdupois system of measurement, 136–137
conversion factors, 139–140
household system of measurement, 137–139
metric system of measurement, 135–136
Pharmaprojects, 350
PharmD degree, 9
Pharyngeal douches, 283
Phenazopyridine, 236
Phenergan suppositories, 272
Pheniramine, 240
Phenylephrine (PE), 244, 245
Physical dependence, 189–190
Physical distractions, 58
Physical exam, 479
Physical inventory in inventory management, 442–443
Physician, 65
as member of home infusion team, 419
Physicians' Desk Reference (PDR), 353–354
Physician's orders and prescriptions
days supply, 153–154
drug labels, 154–155
medication order, 152–153
pharmacy abbreviations, 149–150, 151–152
prescription order, 152
Pill counting, 386–387
Placental transfer of drugs, 183–184
Pneumonia, 33
Podofilox, 279
Poison Control Act, 376
Poison Prevention Packaging Act (1970), 102–103
Poisons, 433
Position, finding, 473
Positive attitude, 67
Positive stress, 73
Postexposure prophylaxis (PEP), 31, 41
Potassium channel blockade, 203
Potassium chloride, 142
for oral solution, 281
Potassium nitrate, 242
Potassium-sparing, 206
Potency, 173
Potency of drug, 173–175
Potentiation, 188
Preceptor, 470
Pre-employment requirements
completing application form, 479
drug screening, 479
interviewing, 479–482
physical exam, 479
proof of state registration or licensure, 478–479
Preferred provider organizations (PPOs), 389, 425
Pregnancy, 190
Pregnancy test, 246
Premarin, 170
Prescribing errors, 317–318
Prescription benefits managers (PBMs), utilization of formulatory system, 389–390
Prescription claims, 427
Prescription Drug Marketing Act (1987), 106
Prescription drugs, 9, 88–89
Prescription errors, 69–70. *See also* Medication errors
Prescription filling, 386–388
Prescription item in mail-order pharmacy, 430
Prescription order, 152
Prescription pickup, 388–389
Prescription processing, 377–378
Prescription requirements for controlled substances, 90
Prescriptions
components of, 152
defined, 88
interpreting, 380
processing, 383–385
receiving, 378
verbal, 329–330
Prescription scanning, 333
Prescription writing, 329
Primary literature for pharmacies, 347
Primary reference source, 349
PRN orders, 406
Probation, 489
Probenecid, 200
Prochlorperazine, 208
Product Identification Guide, 356
Product rotation, 446
Professionalism, 66, 471–472
job security and, 486
responsibility as aspect of, 486–487
Professional organizations, 492–493
Professional relationship in externship, 472
Professional's Handbook of Complementary and Alternative Medicines, 358–359
Program director, 470
Proof of state registration or licensure, 478–479
Proper fraction, 130–131
Prophylactic dose, 175
Proportion in mathematical concepts, 133–134
Proprietary blend, 257

Proprietary drug, 88
Prostaglandin, 172
Protease inhibitors, 41
Protected Health Information (PHI), 108
Protective wear, 37
Protocol, 114, 401
Proton pump inhibitors, 208, 209, 233
Proventil inhalation aerosol, 289
Proxemics, 61–62
Pseudoephedrine (PSE), 244
Pseudomonas aeruginosa, 34
Psychiatric hospitals, 414
Psychiatric medications, 198, 199
Psychomimetic drugs, 199
Psychomotor stimulants, 198, 199, 201
PubMed, 349
Pulmonary absorption of a drug, 180
Pulmonary inhalation, 273
Punch cards, 415
Punch method, 276
Pure Food and Drug Act (1906), 86
Pyrethrum extract, 239
Pyrithione zinc, 238
Pyrogens, 273
Pyxis, 331, 406

Q

QTC/Non-Drug Product Listings, 356
Quality assurance check in mail-order pharmacy, 430
Quality customer service, 66–68
Quinine, 170

R

Rare disease, 105
Ratios
  defined, 132
  equivalencies of, 133
  in mathematical concepts, 132
Rebound nasal congestion, 245
Receiver, 57
Receptor, 197
Receptor site, 173
Recommended Dietary Allowances (RDAs), 260
Reconstitution, 308
Rectal medications, 179, 272
Rectal suppositories, 280
Red Book, 356
Redistribution, 183
Referencing, 346–364
  commonly used pharmacy reference books, 350–359
  Internet references, 360–363
  personal digital assistants (PDAs), 361
  pharmacy software, 361
  types of sources, 347–349
Registration, 18–19, 491–492
  proof of state, 478–479
Regulatory agencies
  clinical drug studies and, 114–115
  Drug Enforcement Administration, 117–118
  Food and Drug Administration, 113–117
  Good Manufacturing Practices, 115–117
  Joint Commission, 118–119
  monographs and, 115
  National Association of Boards of Pharmacy, 120
  Occupational Safety and Health Administration, 118
  Patient Package Inserts, 115
  state boards of pharmacy, 119
Regulatory oversight, 334–340
Reimbursement, DAW codes and, 384
Reimbursement specialist as member of infusion team, 420
Rejection, common causes of, 390
Remington's Pharmaceutical Sciences: The Science and Practice of Pharmacy, 348, 357
Renal elimination of drugs, 185
Renal/vascular system medications, 204–205, 206
Reservoir, 183
Residential care, 414
Residents, 398
Respiration, 207
Respiratory inhalants, 207
Respiratory secretions, indirect contact with, 35
Respiratory syncytial virus (RSV), 35
Respiratory system agents, 207, 242–245
Respondeat superior, 85
Responsibility as aspect of professionalism, 486–487
Resumes, 473–475
  components of, 474
  defined, 473
  distributing, 476, 478
  fax transmission of, 476
  sample, 475
  tips to writing, 475
Retail inventory management, 444–449
Retail pharmacy, 9, 372–392
  computer usage in, 389–391
  customer service in, 391–392
  flow of service, 377–389
  over-the-counter medications in, 392
  types of, 375–376
Retention enemas, 283
Reverse distributor, 454
Rite Aid, 19
Rogaine (minoxidil), 237
Roman numerals, 149
  converting, 129
  defined, 129
  interpreting, 130
Routes of administration, 179–181, 270
  buccal, 271
  dosage forms available for administration by various, 291
  injectable, 272–273
  nasal, 274
  ophthalmic, 274
  optic, 274
  oral, 270–271
  pulmonary inhalation, 273
  rectal, 272
  sublingual, 271
  topical, 274
Rowasa enema, 283
Rule-based errors, 321
RxProduct Listings, 356
Rx Times, 361

S

Safe Medical Devices Act (1990), 423
Safety caps, 229
St. John's wort, 257, 259
St. Joseph's Chewable Aspirin, 276
Salicylic acid, 238
Salmonella, 35
Saw palmetto, 259
Schedule I drugs, 89–90
Schedule II drugs, 90, 93, 97, 331, 416
  emergency dispensing of, 94
  need for perpetual inventory on, 443
  prescriptions for, 381
Schedule III drugs, 90, 97, 112
  need for perpetual inventory on, 443
  prescriptions for, 381
Schedule IV drugs, 90, 97
  need for perpetual inventory on, 443
Schedule V drugs, 90, 95, 97
  need for perpetual inventory on, 443
  prescriptions for, 381
Scopolamine, 274
Screening in mail-order pharmacy, 430
Secondary sources of reference material, 347
Sedative, 198
Sedative-hypnotic drugs, 198–199
SEDBASE, 350
Seizure medication, 200
Selective serotonin reuptake inhibitors (SSRIs), 173, 199, 201
Selenium sulfide, 238
Semicid, 281
Semmelweis, Ignaz, 34
Sender, 57
Senna, 259
Sensitive teeth, 242
Sepsis, 306
Serotonin, 199, 208
Serotonin-norepinephrine reuptake inhibitors (SNRIs), 199
Serturner, Friedrich Wilhelm Adam, 6
Sex, dosing and, 187
Shark cartilage, 262
Shelter care, 414
Shen Nung, 6
Sherley Amendment (1912), 86
Shigella, 35
Side effects, 189–190
  allergic responses, 189
  defined, 172
  drug dependence, 189–190
  hepatoxicity and nephrotoxicity, 189
Silver nitrate, 170
Single-dose container, 287, 448
Single-unit container, 448
Site of action, 173
Skilled nursing facilities (SNFs), 21, 414
Smoking cessation agents, 246
Social distance, 61
Sodium bicarbonate, 283
Sodium borate solution, 283

Sodium channel blockade, 203
Sodium chloride, 142
Solubility, 178
Solutions, 281–282
  defined, 281
  nasal, 282
  otic, 283
  topical, 282
Soy, 261, 262
Special facilities for elderly people, 414
Specialization, 409
Specialized databases, 350
Specific gravity, 158, 159
Speech, clear, 59
Spermicide, 236
Spirulina, 262
Sponsor, 457
Sponsor-investigator, 457
Stadol NS, 274
Staff model health maintenance organizations (HMOs), 425
Standardization, 255
Standard precautions, 31
Standard treatment, 115
Stannous fluoride, 279
Staphylococcal species, 35
State boards of pharmacy, 119, 399
State law, 84
Stat orders, 406
Sterile compounding, 301–304, 407
  agencies/regulations governing, 309
  defined, 296–297
  equipment used in, 302–304, 303
  techniques used in, 304–309
Stress
  continual, 74
  management of, 487–488
  negative, 73
  in pharmacy, 73–75
  positive, 73
  potential causes of, 74
  reducing, 74–75
Strontium chloride, 242
Subacute care units, 414
Subcutaneous (sub-Q) administration, 179, 180, 272
Sublingual administration, 179, 271
Substance Abuse and Mental Health Services Administration (SAMSHA), 433
Sucralfate (Carafate), 209
Sucrets, 277
Sulfinpyrazone, 200
Sulfonamides, 214, 216
Sulfonylureas, 213
Sulfur, 238
Summer's Eve, 283
Sunscreens, 239
Supersensitivity, 173
Suppositories
  defined, 280
  preparation of, 300
  rectal, 280
  urethral, 280
  vaginal, 280
Suremed, 406
Surfactants, 282
Surgical hand scrub, 37
Suspensions, 286
Synergism, 188
Synthetic reactions, 184
Synthroid, 275
Syrup of ipecac, 235
Syrups, 284
Systemic effect, 270

T

Tablets
  defined, 275
  storage of, 276
  sublingual, 271
  types of, 275–276
Tachyphylaxis, 173
Tamper-evident packaging, 228, 448
Tar derivatives, 238
Target, 376
Target cells, 172
Teaching hospitals, 398
Tea tree oil, 259
Technical error, 321
Tegretol, 276
Telazon, 445, 453
Telephone etiquette, 72–73
Temperature
  measurement of, 142–143
  in retail inventory management, 449
Tenormin, 272
Teratogens, 190
Terminally ill, 68–69
Tertiary sources of reference materials, 348
Tetracaine, 242
Tetracyclines, 214, 216
Theophrastus, 6
Therapeutic effect of a drug, 172
Therapeutic-equivalent drugs, 181, 450
Therapeutic index (TI), 172
Therapeutic mouthwash, 281–282
Therapeutic response, 179
Thiazide, 206
Third-party providers, 389–390
Thrombolytic agents, 206
Thyroid medications, 210, 212
Tight containers, 448
Time conversions, 143–144
Time management, 488–489
Timing of administration, dosing and, 187
Timolol maleate, 279
Timoptic, 274, 290
Tinctures, 285
Tioconazole, 236
Tobrex, 290
Tocolytic agents, 211, 213
To Err Is Human, release of, by Institute of Medicine (IOM), 314
Tolerance, 173
  cross, 187
  dosing and, 187
  pharmacodynamic, 187
  pharmacokinetic, 187
Tolnaftate, 239, 279
Toothache, 242
Topical medications, 180–181, 274, 282
Topics in Health Information Management, 330
Tort law, 84–85
Total parenteral nutrition (TPN), 272, 308, 422
  defined, 308
Toxic effect, 172
TOXLIT, 350
Training, on-the-job, 16, 17–18, 486–489
Training Guidelines for Hospital Pharmacy Supportive Personnel, release of, 7
Transdermal drug delivery system (TDDS), 279–280
Transderm-Nitro, 280
Transderm Scop, 280
Transitioning of over-the-counter (OTC) agents, 229
Trichogenics, 220
Tricyclic antidepressants, 199, 201
Triprolidine, 244
Trissel's Stability of Compounded Formulations, 359
Triturate, 299
Troche, 277
Tuberculosis, 33
Tubular necrosis, 189
Tubular secretion, 185
Turn-around system, 415
Tylenol, 275
  market withdrawal for products, 460

U

Ubiquinone coenzyme Q10, 262
Undecylenic acid, 239
Unionized, 176
Unit-dose container, 448
Unit-dose systems, 406
  types of, 415
United States Adopted Name (USAN), 171
U.S. Pharmacist, 361–362
United States Pharmacopeia (USP)
  conversions for weights and measures, 138
  defined, 320
  Dictionary of USAN and International Drug Names, 352
  dietary supplements and ingredients section of, 351
  emulsions definition of, 285
  metric system of measurement in, 135
  on packaging and containers of medications, 447
  percentage of active ingredients and, 132
  publishing of USP <797>, 309
  as standards setting authority, 320
  therapeutic equivalent codes of, 182
  USP Chapter <797> Guidebook to Proposed Revision Guidelines, 110–111, 309, 357
United States Pharmacopeia (USP)-Institute for Safe Medication Practices (ISMP), Medication Errors Reporting Program (MERP), 339–340

United States Pharmacopeia–National Formulary (USP–NF), 111, 350–351
  maintenance of current copy by pharmacy, 347
U.S. Public Health Service, pharmacy in, 432–433
Unit-of-use container, 448
Units of measurement, 142
  electrolytes, 142
  international units, 142
  temperature, 142–143
  time conversions, 143–144
Universal precautions, 306
Unlisted Drugs, 350
Upward communication, 57
Urethral suppositories, 280

V

Vaccine Adverse Event Reporting System (VAERS), 335, 360
  defined, 335
  reporting form of, 338
Vaginal, 280
Vaginal douches, 283
Vaginal inserts, 281
Vaginal suppositories, 280
Valerian, 257, 259
Valium, 272
Vasoconstriction, 244
Vasodilators, 203, 206
Velocity report (80/20 report), 451
Ventilation, 207
Verbal communication, 58–59
  tools for, 59
Verbal prescriptions, 329–330
Verified Internet Pharmacy Provider Site (VIPPS), 431
Vertical flow hoods, 302–303
Veterans Administration (VA) hospital, 20
Veterans Affairs, U.S. Department of, pharmacy in, 433
Vitamin A, 261
Vitamin B_1, 261
Vitamin B_6, 261
Vitamin B_{12}, 261
Vitamin C, 261
Vitamin D, 261
Vitamin E, 261
Vitamin K, 261
Vitamins, 260, 261
Volumes, measurement of, 138

W

Walgreen's, 19, 375–376
Walmart, 376
Warehouse and delivery staff as member of infusion team, 420
Wart removal agents, 221, 238
Water-in-oil (W/O) emulsions, 278
Water-soluble form of drug, 184
Web Sites, pharmacy Internet, 362–363
Weight-loss agents, 246
Well-closed container, 448
The White Paper on Pharmacy Student Professionalism, 66
The White Paper on Pharmacy Technicians 2002: Needed Changes Can No Longer Wait, 7
Wholesalers in retail inventory management, 444–445
Wild yam, 259
Witch hazel, 259
Withdrawal syndrome, 190
Word of mouth, 473
Work ethic, 68
Written communication, 62
Written orders, 402–403

X

Xalatan, 274
Xerostomia, 241, 242
Xylometazoline, 245

Y

Yeast infection, 236
Young's Rule, 148

Z

Zithromax, 170–171
Z-Pak (azithromycin), 175